S0-CAB-319

SIGNS AND SYMPTOMS
HANDBOOK

SIGNS AND SYMPTOMS

HANDBOOK

Springhouse Corporation
Springhouse, Pennsylvania

STAFF FOR THIS VOLUME

CLINICAL STAFF

Clinical Director
Barbara McVan, RN

Clinical Editors
Helen Hahler D'Angelo, RN, MSN
Nina Poorman Welsh, RN

PUBLICATION STAFF

Executive Director, Editorial
Stanley Loeb

Executive Director, Creative Services
Jean Robinson

Design
John Hubbard (art director), Stephanie
Peters (associate art director),
Julie Carleton Barlow

Editing
Regina Ford (project manager),
Kathy Goldberg

Copy Editing
David Moreau (manager), Edith
McMahon (supervisor), Nick Anastasio,
Keith de Pinho, Diane Labus,
Doris Weinstock, Debra Young

Art Production
Robert Perry (manager), Anna Brindisi,
Loretta Caruso, Donald Knauss,
Christina McKinley, Robert Wieder

Typography
David Kosten (manager), Diane Paluba
(assistant manager), Brenda Mayer,
Robin Rantz, Brent Rinedoller, Joyce
Rossi-Biletz, Nancy Wirs

Manufacturing
Deborah Meiris (manager), T.A. Landis

Project Coordination
Aline Miller (supervisor), Maureen
Carmichael, Elizabeth B. Kiselev

The clinical procedures described and recommended in this publication are based on research and consultation with nursing, medical, and legal authorities. To the best of our knowledge, these procedures reflect currently accepted practice; nevertheless, they can't be considered absolute and universal recommendations. For individual application, all recommendations must be considered in light of the patient's clinical condition and, before administration of new or infrequently used drugs, in light of latest package-insert information. The authors and the publisher disclaim responsibility for any adverse effects resulting directly or indirectly from the suggested procedures, from any undetected errors, or from the reader's misunderstanding of the text.

Some material in this book was adapted from *Signs & Symptoms* (Nurse's Reference Library®), © 1986 by Springhouse Corporation.
Authorization to photocopy items for internal or personal use, or the internal or personal use of specific clients, is granted by Springhouse Corporation for users registered with the Copyright Clearance Center (CCC) Transactional Reporting Service, provided that the base fee of $00.00 per copy, plus $.75 per page, is paid directly to CCC, 27 Congress St., Salem, Mass. 01970. For those organizations that have been granted a photocopy license by CCC, a separate system of payment has been arranged. The fee code for users of the Transactional Reporting Service is 0874341434/88 $00.00 + $.75.

© 1988 by Springhouse Corporation. All rights reserved. No part of this book may be used or reproduced in any manner whatsoever without written permission except for brief quotations embodied in critical articles and reviews. Printed in the United States of America. For information write Springhouse Corporation, 1111 Bethlehem Pike, Springhouse, Pa. 19477.

SSSC-021091

Library of Congress Cataloging-in-Publication Data
Signs and symptoms handbook.
    Includes bibliographies and index.
    1. Diagnosis—Handbooks, manuals, etc. 2. Nursing—Handbooks, manuals, etc. 3. Symptomatology—Handbooks, manuals, etc. I. Springhouse Corporation. [DNLM: 1. Diagnosis—handbooks. 2. Diagnosis—nurses' instruction. 3. Nursing Assessment—handbooks. WY 39 S578]
RT48.5.S54 1988   616.07′5   87-32107
ISBN 0-87434-143-4 (Soft)   ISBN 0-87434-190-6 (Flex)

CONTENTS

ADVISORY BOARD, CONTRIBUTORS, AND CONSULTANTS

ADVISORY BOARD

Lillian S. Brunner, RN, MSN, ScD, FAAN, Nurse/Author, Brunner Associates, Inc., Berwyn, Pa.

Donald C. Cannon, MD, PhD, Resident in Internal Medicine, University of Kansas, School of Medicine, Wichita

Luther Christman, RN, PhD, Dean, Rush College of Nursing; Vice-President, Nursing Affairs, Rush–Presbyterian–St. Luke's Medical Center, Chicago

Kathleen A. Dracup, RN, DNSc, FAAN, Associate Professor, School of Nursing, University of California at Los Angeles

Stanley J. Dudrick, MD, FACS, Professor, Department of Surgery, and Director, Nutritional Support Services, University of Texas Medical School at Houston; St. Luke's Episcopal Hospital, Houston

Halbert E. Fillinger, MD, Assistant Medical Examiner, Philadelphia County

M. Josephine Flaherty, RN, PhD, Principal Nursing Officer, Department of National Health and Welfare, Ottawa

Joyce LeFever Kee, RN, MSN, Associate Professor, College of Nursing, University of Delaware, Newark

Dennis E. Leavelle, MD, Associate Professor, Mayo Medical Laboratories, Mayo Clinic, Rochester, Minn.

Roger M. Morrell, MD, PhD, FACP, Professor, Neurology and Immunology/Microbiology, Wayne State University, School of Medicine, Detroit; Chief, Neurology Service, Veterans Administration Medical Center, Allen Park, Mich.; Diplomate, American Board of Psychiatry and Neurology

Ara G. Paul, PhD, Dean, College of Pharmacy, University of Michigan, Ann Arbor

Rose Pinneo, RN, MS, Associate Professor of Nursing and Clinician II, University of Rochester, N.Y.

Thomas E. Rubbert, BSL, LLB, JD, Attorney-at-Law, Pasadena, Calif.

Maryanne Schreiber, RN, BA, Product Manager, Patient Monitoring, Hewlett-Packard Co., Waltham (Mass.) Division

Frances J. Storlie, RN, PhD, ANP, Director, Personal Health Services, Southwest Washington Health District, Vancouver

Claire L. Watson, RN, Clinical Documentation Associate, IVAC Corp., San Diego

CONTRIBUTORS

Deborah G. Althoff, RN, BSN, CNOR, Operating Room Staff Nurse, Rutland (Vt.) Regional Medical Center

Sherry L. Altschuler, PhD, Chief, Audiology/Speech Pathology, Veterans Administration Hospital, Philadelphia

Linda M. Appenheimer, RN, MS, Unit Leader/Assistant Professor, College of Nursing, Rush–Presbyterian–St. Luke's Medical Center, Chicago

Charold L. Baer, RN, PhD, Professor, Oregon Health Sciences University, Portland

Roxanne Aubol Batterden, RN, CCRN, Primary Nurse II, Surgical ICU, University of Maryland Medical Systems, Baltimore

Barbara Gross Braverman, RN, MSN, CS, Psychiatric Clinical Nurse Specialist, Medical College of Pennsylvania, Philadelphia

Sally A. Brozenec, RN, MS, Practitioner–Teacher, Rush University of Chicago

June M. Buckle, RN, MSN, Assistant Director of Nursing, Department of Medicine, The Johns Hopkins Hospital, Baltimore

Laura J. Burke, RN, MSN, Cardiovascular Clinical Nurse Specialist, St. Luke's Hospital, Milwaukee

Dorothea Caldwell, MPH, NP, Nurse Practitioner, Rockefeller University, New York

Mimi Callanan, RN, MSN, Epilepsy Clinical Specialist, Mid-Atlantic Regional Epilepsy Center, Medical College of Pennsylvania, Philadelphia

Jeanette K. Chambers, RN, MS, CS, Renal Clinical Nurse Specialist, Riverside Methodist Hospital, Columbus, Ohio

Mary Katherine Crathern, RN, BSN, Assistant Professor, New Hampshire Vocational Technical Institute, Berlin

Betty Dale, RN, BSN, Head Nurse, Urology, University of Minnesota Hospitals and Clinics, Minneapolis

Nancy B. Davis, RN, BSN, FNP, Nurse Practitioner and RN First Assistant, Cardiovascular and Chest Surgical Associates, Boise, Idaho

Linda J. Dec, RN, ADN, Staff Nurse, Medical City Dallas Hospital

Gloria Ferraro Donnelly, RN, PhD, FAAN, Chairman, Department of Nursing, La Salle University, Philadelphia

Linda M. Duffy, RN, MS, CURN, CANP, Clinical Specialist for Urology, Veterans Administration Medical Center, Minneapolis

Elizabeth A. Ely, RN, MS, Assistant Professor of Nursing, University of New Hampshire, Durham

Susan Hann Eshleman, RN, MS, MSN, Neurosensory Nursing Instructor, Chester County Hospital School of Nursing, West Chester, Pa.

Roslyn M. Gleeson, RNC, MSN, Clinical Specialist/Nursing of Children, Alfred I. duPont Institute, Wilmington, Del.

Susan Gauthier, RN, MSN, Assistant Professor, Department of Nursing, College of Allied Health Professions, Temple University, Philadelphia

Sandra K. Crabtree Goodnough, RN, MSN, Pulmonary Clinical Nurse Specialist, Hermann Hospital, Houston; Assistant Professor, School of Nursing, University of Texas Health Science Center at Houston

Diana W. Guthrie, RN, C, PhD, FAAN, Associate Professor/Diabetes Nurse Specialist, University of Kansas School of Medicine, Wichita

Mary Chapman Gyetvan, RN, BSEd, Clinical Consultant, Springhouse Corporation, Springhouse, Pa.

Marcia J. Hill, RN, MS, Clinical Practitioner/Teacher, Methodist Hospital, Houston; Clinical Assistant Professor, Baylor College of Medicine, Houston

Esther Holzbauer, OSB, MSN, Assistant Professor, Nursing, Mount Marty College, Yankton, S.D.

Kathryn M. Kater, RN, MSN, Neuro-Cardiothoracic Clinical Specialist, Barnes Hospital, St. Louis

Lee Ann Kelly, RN, MS, PNP, Head Nurse, Antepartum/Postpartum, Hermann Hospital, Houston

Mary Ann Myrick King, RN, BSN, Staff Nurse, Outpatient Dermatology Clinic, Veterans Administration Medical Center, Washington, D.C.

JoAnne Konick-McMahan, RNC, BSN, Level 4 Staff Nurse, Hospital of the University of Pennsylvania, Philadelphia

Susan L.W. Krupnick, RN, MSN, CCRN, CEN, CS, Administrator, Education Division, and Independent Clinical Nurse Specialist (Psychiatry), Skilled Nursing, Inc., Springhouse, Pa.

Karen A. Landis, RN, MS, CCRN, Pulmonary Clinical Nurse Specialist, Lehigh Valley Hospital Center, Allentown, Pa.

Melvina J. Lohmann, RNC, MEd, ANP, Assistant Professor of Nursing, Cedar Crest College, Allentown, Pa.

Chris Platt Moldovanyi, RN, MSN, Clinical Nurse Specialist, Endocrinology, Cleveland Clinic Foundation

Mary Lou Moore, RNC, PhD, ACCE, FAAN, Nurse Researcher/Educator, Bowman Gray School of Medicine, Winston-Salem, N.C.

Janice Overdorff, RN, BSN, Administrative Nurse III, University of Illinois, Chicago

Amy Perrin-Ross, RN, MSN, CNRN, Clinical Nurse Specialist, Neuroscience, Loyola University Medical Center, Maywood, Ill.

Frances W. Quinless, RN, PhD, Assistant Professor, Rutgers University College of Nursing, Newark, N.J.

Patricia L. Radzewicz, RN, BSN, Head Nurse, University of Illinois Eye and Ear Infirmary, Chicago

Dennis G. Ross, RN, MSN, MAE, CNOR, Associate Professor of Nursing, Castleton (Vt.) State College

Linda C. Rothfield, RN, MSN, CANP, Specialty Instructor II, The Johns Hopkins Hospital, Baltimore

Susan Rumsey, RN, BSN, MPH, Perinatal Outreach Education Coordinator, Wake Area Health Education Center, Raleigh, N.C.

Mary Jo Sagaties, RN, MSN, FNP-C, Nurse Practitioner/Ophthalmic Photographer, Leahey Eye Clinic, Lowell, Mass.; PhD Candidate, Boston University School of Medicine

Sheron L. Salyer, RNC, BSN, Perinatal Research Nurse, Vanderbilt Medical Center, Vanderbilt University School of Medicine, Nashville, Tenn.

Kay Freeman Sauers, RN, BSN, MS, Clinical Nurse Specialist in Orthopedics, Trauma Rehabilitation Center/Montebello Hospital Center, Baltimore

Kristine Ann Scordo, RN, BSN, MS, Clinical Nurse Specialist, Cardiology, Bethesda Hospital, Cincinnati

Karen N. Shine, RN, BSN, Quality Assurance–Risk Management Coordinator, Dana-Farber Cancer Institute, Boston

Katherine Small, RN, MS, Nurse Supervisor, University of Maryland Hospital, Baltimore

Carol E. Smith, RN, PhD, Associate Professor, University of Kansas School of Nursing, Kansas City

June L. Stark, RN, BSN, CCRN, Critical Care Instructor/Renal Nurse Consultant, New England Medical Center, Boston

Clare M. Stearns, RN, MS, CNOR, ARNP, Orthopedic Nurse Practitioner, St. Luke Medical Center, Berlin, N.H.; Adjunct Faculty, Department of Nursing, University of New Hampshire, Durham

Christina M. Stewart, RN, MSN, CNRN, CCRN, Clinical Nurse Specialist, Loyola University of Chicago, Maywood, Ill.

Frances J. Storlie, RN, PhD, CANP, Director, Personal Health Services, Southwest Washington Health District, Vancouver

Arlene B. Strong, RN, MN, ANP, Cardiac Clinical Specialist, Adult Nurse Practitioner, Anticoagulation Clinic, Veterans Administration Medical Center, Portland, Ore.

Alicia Alphin Tollison, RNCS, BSN, MN, Educational Coordinator, Alexandria (Va.) Hospital

Naomi Walpert, RN, MS, Clinical Nurse Specialist for Endocrinology and Metabolism, Sinai Hospital, Baltimore

Maryann Banko Wee, RN, BSN, Risk Management Consultant, Virginia Professional Underwriters, Inc., Jackson, Miss.

Bunny Weiss, RN, BSN, Urology Nurse Specialist, Albert Einstein Medical Center–Northern Division, Philadelphia

Janette R. Yanko, RN, MN, CNRN, Neurological/Neurosurgical Clinical Specialist, Youngstown (Ohio) Hospital Association

CLINICAL CONSULTANTS

Roslyn M. Gleeson, RNC, BS, MSN
Spinal Dysfunction Clinical Specialist
Alfred I. duPont Institute
Wilmington, Del.

Carol E. Smith, RN, PhD
Associate Professor
University of Kansas School of Nursing
Kansas City

Anne L. Wagner, RN, BS
Staff Nurse—Post Anesthesia Room
Strong Memorial Hospital
Rochester, N.Y.

FOREWORD

You probably know nurses who can recognize a new sign or symptom in virtually any patient and can quickly pinpoint its probable cause. These nurses always seem to know just what to assess and just what their findings may mean. This skill, once uncommon as a prerequisite of nursing practice, is becoming increasingly important to health care professionals. Why? One important reason is the impact of sweeping changes in our health care system. Cost-containment policies and their ever-increasing demands on your time are making it harder than ever to properly care for the growing number of gravely ill patients. You're constantly pressed to expand the scope of your duties, pressuring you to improve your present skills and acquire new ones.

To meet these challenges confidently, you obviously need more than a passing familiarity with the most common disease signs and symptoms. You need comprehensive information on how to recognize and interpret even the most subtle indicators of disease. You also need to know what to assess after you've identified them—and, if necessary, how to intervene to prevent or contain complications. And, of course, you need to know what a sign or symptom forecasts about your patient's condition.

SIGNS AND SYMPTOMS HANDBOOK puts this body of knowledge at your fingertips. This handy reference covers 550 signs and symptoms, ranging from common indicators of disease, such as fever and vomiting, to less common indicators, such as nystagmus and tracheal deviation. What's more, the volume's alphabetical arrangement helps you quickly locate any sign or symptom.

Each sign or symptom is covered in a standard format, beginning with a *Description* that defines and describes the sign or symptom, discusses its significance and incidence, and summarizes its possible causes. When appropriate, it also alerts you to key differences between adult and pediatric patients in a sign's significance or severity. For an elicited sign, such as Kernig's sign, this section also describes the technique for evoking a response.

When appropriate, a section called *Mechanism* follows. This brief section explains the pathophysiology of the sign or symptom. The next section, *Possible causes,* covers medical disorders, environmental factors, drugs, treatments, and tests that can produce the sign or symptom.

The following section, *Clinical considerations,* discusses pertinent nursing care measures: monitoring the patient for signs of complications, promoting comfort, administering drugs, and carrying out patient teaching. This section also reviews diagnostic tests the patient may undergo.

A special feature in SIGNS AND SYMPTOMS HANDBOOK is the "Diseases and Disorders Profile." This handy chart highlights the typical signs and symptoms of 100 major diseases and disorders.

SIGNS AND SYMPTOMS HANDBOOK is a well-organized, comprehensive reference. I heartily recommend it to nurses, students, and other health care professionals who wish to confirm, update, and expand their knowledge of this clinically significant subject.

The times demand this knowledge—and SIGNS AND SYMPTOMS HANDBOOK delivers it.

**Gloria Ferraro Donnelly,
RN, PhD, FAAN**

EVALUATING A SIGN OR SYMPTOM

The step-by-step procedure illustrated below may be used as a guide to interpreting and evaluating a sign or symptom. It begins with identification of the sign or symptom and ends with helping to establish a differential diagnosis.

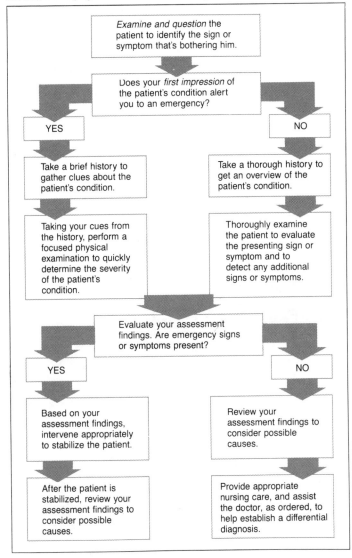

Examine and question the patient to identify the sign or symptom that's bothering him.

Does your *first impression* of the patient's condition alert you to an emergency?

YES

NO

Take a brief history to gather clues about the patient's condition.

Take a thorough history to get an overview of the patient's condition.

Taking your cues from the history, perform a focused physical examination to quickly determine the severity of the patient's condition.

Thoroughly examine the patient to evaluate the presenting sign or symptom and to detect any additional signs or symptoms.

Evaluate your assessment findings. Are emergency signs or symptoms present?

YES

NO

Based on your assessment findings, intervene appropriately to stabilize the patient.

Review your assessment findings to consider possible causes.

After the patient is stabilized, review your assessment findings to consider possible causes.

Provide appropriate nursing care, and assist the doctor, as ordered, to help establish a differential diagnosis.

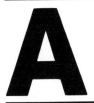

A

Aaron's sign

Description
Aaron's sign is pain in the chest or abdominal area that is elicited by applying gentle but steadily increasing pressure over McBurney's point. A positive sign indicates appendicitis.

Abadie's sign

Description
Abadie's sign is spasm of the levator muscle of the upper eyelid. This sign may be slight or pronounced and may affect one eye or both. It reflects an exophthalmic goiter in Graves' disease.

Abdominal mass

Description
An abdominal mass is a localized swelling in one of the abdominal quadrants. Often detected on routine physical examination, this sign typically develops insidiously and may represent an enlarged organ, a neoplasm, an abscess, a vascular defect, or a fecal mass.

Distinguishing an abdominal mass from normal structures requires skillful palpation. At times, palpation must be repeated with the patient in a different position or performed by a sec-

ond examiner to verify initial findings. A palpable abdominal mass is an important clinical sign and usually represents a serious—and perhaps life-threatening—disorder.

Possible causes
Cardiovascular
Abdominal aortic aneurysm. This disorder may persist for years, producing only a pulsating periumbilical mass with a systolic bruit over the aorta. However, it may become life-threatening if the aneurysm expands, its walls weaken, and it ruptures; then, it produces severe abdominal and back pain. After rupture, the aneurysm no longer pulsates.

Gastrointestinal
Cholecystitis. Deep palpation below the liver border may detect a smooth, firm, sausage-shaped mass. However, in acute inflammation, the gallbladder is usually too tender to palpate, so other associated signs and symptoms are more reliable indicators of this disorder.

Cholelithiasis. Usually, a stone-filled gallbladder produces a painless right upper quadrant mass that is smooth and sausage-shaped.

Colonic cancer. A right lower quadrant mass may occur in cancer of the right colon. Occasionally, cancer of the left colon causes a palpable left lower quadrant mass.

Crohn's disease. In this disorder, tender, sausage-shaped masses are usually palpable in the right lower quadrant and, at times, in the left lower quadrant.

Abdominal Mass: Locations and Causes

The location of an abdominal mass provides an important clue to the causative disorder. Here are the disorders responsible for abdominal masses and the quadrants where the masses occur.

Right upper quadrant
- Aortic aneurysm (epigastric area)
- Cholecystitis/cholelithiasis
- Gallbladder, gastric, hepatic carcinoma
- Hepatomegaly
- Hydronephrosis
- Pancreatic abscess/pseudocysts
- Renal cell carcinoma

Left upper quadrant
- Aortic aneurysm (epigastric area)
- Gastric carcinoma (epigastric area)
- Hydronephrosis
- Pancreatic abscess (epigastric area)
- Pancreatic pseudocysts (epigastric area)
- Renal cell carcinoma
- Splenomegaly

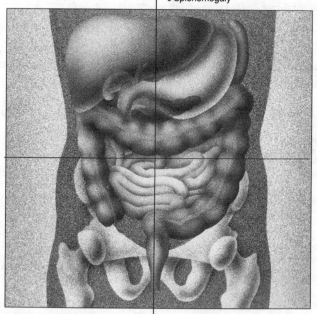

Right lower quadrant
- Bladder distention (suprapubic area)
- Colonic cancer
- Crohn's disease
- Ovarian cyst (suprapubic area)
- Uterine leiomyomas (suprapubic area)

Left lower quadrant
- Bladder distention (suprapubic area)
- Colonic cancer
- Diverticulitis
- Ovarian cyst (suprapubic area)
- Uterine leiomyomas (suprapubic area)
- Volvulus

Diverticulitis. Most common in the sigmoid colon, this disorder may produce a left lower quadrant mass.

Gallbladder carcinoma. This disorder may produce a moderately tender, irregular mass in the right upper quadrant. Accompanying it is chronic, progressively severe epigastric or right upper quadrant pain that may radiate to the right shoulder.

Gastric carcinoma. Advanced gastric carcinoma may produce an epigastric mass.

Hepatic carcinoma. This disorder produces a tender, nodular mass in the right upper quadrant or right epigastric area accompanied by severe pain.

Hepatomegaly. This produces a firm, blunt, irregular mass in the epigastric region or below the right costal margin.

Pancreatic abscess. Occasionally, this disorder may produce a palpable epigastric mass accompanied by epigastric pain and tenderness.

Pancreatic pseudocysts. After pancreatitis, pseudocysts may form on the pancreas, causing a palpable nodular mass in the epigastric area.

Splenomegaly. The lymphomas, leukemias, hemolytic anemias, and inflammatory diseases are among the many disorders that may cause splenomegaly. Typically, the smooth edge of the enlarged spleen is palpable in the left upper quadrant.

Genitourinary

Bladder distention. A smooth, rounded, fluctuant suprapubic mass is characteristic. In extreme distention, the mass may extend to the umbilicus.

Hydronephrosis. Enlarging one or both kidneys, this disorder produces a smooth, boggy mass in one or both flanks.

Renal cell carcinoma. Usually occurring in only one kidney, this disorder produces a smooth, firm, nontender mass near the affected kidney. Accompanying it are dull, constant abdominal or flank pain and hematuria.

Obstetrics-Gynecology

Ovarian cyst. A large ovarian cyst may produce a smooth, rounded, fluctuant mass resembling a distended bladder in the suprapubic region.

Uterine leiomyomas (fibroids). If large enough, these common, benign uterine tumors produce a round, multinodular mass in the suprapubic region. Most often, the patient's chief complaint is menorrhagia.

Clinical considerations

If the patient has a pulsating midabdominal mass and severe abdominal pain:

• An aortic aneurysm should be suspected and the physician notified immediately.

• Vital signs and urinary output should be monitored frequently.

• The patient should be observed for signs of shock, such as tachycardia, hypotension, and cool, clammy skin.

• Fluid replacement should be anticipated.

• Emergency equipment should be kept on hand.

• Because the patient may require emergency surgery, food and fluids should be withheld, as ordered, until the physician can fully examine the patient.

• If surgery is necessary, the patient should be prepared accordingly.

If the patient's abdominal mass does not suggest an aortic aneurysm:

• A complete history should be obtained and an abdominal examination performed.

• The patient's position should be noted when the mass is located; some masses can be detected only with the patient supine; others require a side-lying position.

• A pelvic or rectal examination may be performed.

• Diagnostic tests may include blood and urine studies, abdominal X-rays, barium enema, computed tomography, ultrasonography, angiography, radioisotope scans, and gastroscopy or sigmoidoscopy.

• Because discovery of an abdominal mass often causes anxiety, emotional support should be provided to the patient and his family as they await the diagnosis.

• The patient should be positioned comfortably, and drugs for pain or anxiety administered, as ordered.

Abdominal rigidity
(Abdominal muscle spasm, involuntary guarding)

Description

Abdominal rigidity refers to abnormal muscle tension or inflexibility of the abdomen. Detected by palpation, rigidity may be voluntary or involuntary. Voluntary rigidity reflects the patient's fear or nervousness upon palpation, while involuntary rigidity reflects potentially life-threatening peritoneal irritation or inflammation. Voluntary rigidity may be difficult to distinguish from involuntary rigidity in a child if associated pain makes the child restless, tense, or apprehensive.

Involuntary rigidity most commonly results from GI disorders, but may also result from pulmonary and vascular disorders and from the effects of insect toxins. Usually, it occurs with nausea, vomiting, and abdominal tenderness, distention, and pain.

Possible causes

Respiratory
Pneumonia. In lower lobe pneumonia, severe upper abdominal pain and tenderness accompany rigidity that diminishes with inspiration.

Cardiovascular
Dissecting abdominal aortic aneurysm. Mild-to-moderate abdominal rigidity occurs in this life-threatening disorder. Typically it is accompanied by constant upper abdominal pain that may radiate to the lower back.

Gastrointestinal
Mesenteric artery ischemia. Two to three days of persistent, low-grade abdominal pain and diarrhea precede abdominal rigidity in this life-threatening disorder. Rigidity occurs in the central or periumbilical region and is accompanied by severe abdominal tenderness, fever, and signs of shock such as tachycardia and hypotension.

Peritonitis. Depending on the cause of peritonitis, abdominal rigidity may be localized or generalized. For example, if an inflamed appendix causes local peritonitis, rigidity may be localized in the right lower quadrant. If a perforated ulcer causes widespread peritonitis, rigidity may be generalized and, in severe cases, boardlike.

Environmental
Insect toxins. Insect stings and bites, especially black widow spider bites,

---

Recognizing Voluntary Rigidity

Distinguishing voluntary and involuntary abdominal rigidity is a must for accurate nursing assessment. This comparison can be used to quickly tell the two apart.

Voluntary rigidity is:
• usually symmetric
• more rigid on inspiration (expiration causes muscle relaxation)
• eased by relaxation techniques, such as positioning the patient comfortably and talking to him in a calm, soothing manner
• painless when the patient sits up using his abdominal muscles alone

Involuntary rigidity is:
• usually asymmetric
• equally rigid on inspiration and expiration
• unaffected by relaxation techniques
• painful when the patient sits up using his abdominal muscles alone.

release toxins that can produce generalized, cramping abdominal pain usually accompanied by rigidity.

Clinical considerations

- The patient's vital signs should be taken quickly and the physician notified immediately.
- Emergency intervention should be anticipated even though the patient may not appear gravely ill or have markedly abnormal vital signs.
- Because emergency surgery may be necessary, the patient should be prepared for laboratory tests and X-rays, and food and fluids withheld, as ordered.

If the patient's condition allows further assessment:

- A history should be taken and an abdominal examination performed.
- A pelvic or rectal examination may also be done.
- Diagnostic tests may include blood, urine, and stool studies; chest and abdominal X-rays; peritoneal lavage; and gastroscopy or colonoscopy.
- The patient should be positioned as comfortably as possible and monitored closely for signs and symptoms of shock.
- Analgesics should be withheld, as ordered, until a tentative diagnosis is made because they may mask symptoms.

Accessory muscle use

Description

The accessory muscles—the sternocleidomastoid, scalene, pectoralis major, trapezius, internal intercostals, and abdominal muscles—help the diaphragm maintain respiration when breathing requires *extra* effort. Some accessory muscle use normally takes place during singing, talking, coughing, defecating, and exercising. However, more pronounced use of these muscles may signal acute respiratory distress. It may also result from chronic respiratory disease or the effects of

tests and treatments. Typically, the extent of accessory muscle use reflects the severity of the underlying cause.

Possible causes

Central nervous system

Amyotrophic lateral sclerosis. Typically, this progressive motor neuron disorder affects the diaphragm, but not the accessory muscles. As a result, increased accessory muscle use is characteristic. It is accompanied by fasciculations, muscle atrophy and weakness, spasticity, bilateral Babinski's reflex, and hyperactive deep tendon reflexes.

Spinal cord injury. Increased accessory muscle use may occur, depending on the location and severity of injury. Injury below L1 typically does not affect the diaphragm or accessory muscles, whereas injury between C3 and C5 affects only the upper respiratory muscles and diaphragm, causing increased accessory muscle use.

Respiratory

Adult respiratory distress syndrome. In this life-threatening disorder, accessory muscle use increases in response to hypoxia. It is accompanied by intercostal, supracostal, and sternal retractions on inspiration and by grunting on expiration.

Airway obstruction. Acute upper airway obstruction can be life-threatening—fortunately, most obstructions are subacute or chronic. Typically, this disorder increases accessory muscle use. Its most telling sign, however, is inspiratory stridor.

Asthma. During acute asthmatic attacks, the patient usually displays increased accessory muscle use. Accompanying it are severe dyspnea, tachypnea, wheezing, productive cough, nasal flaring, and cyanosis.

Chronic bronchitis. In this form of chronic obstructive pulmonary disease (COPD), increased accessory muscle use is preceded by productive cough and exertional dyspnea. It is accompanied by wheezing, basal crackles, tachypnea, neck vein distention, prolonged expiration, barrel chest, and clubbing.

Diffuse infiltrative (or fibrotic) lung disease. In this disorder, progressive pulmonary degeneration eventually increases accessory muscle use. Typically, though, progressive dyspnea on exertion is the chief complaint.

Emphysema. Increased accessory muscle use occurs with progressive dyspnea on exertion and minimally productive cough in this form of COPD.

Pneumonia. Bacterial pneumonia most commonly produces increased accessory muscle use. Initially, however, this infection produces sudden high fever with chills.

Pulmonary edema. In acute pulmonary edema, increased accessory muscle use is accompanied by dyspnea, tachypnea, orthopnea, crepitant crackles, wheezing, and a cough productive of pink, frothy sputum.

Pulmonary embolism. Although signs and symptoms vary with the size, number, and location of the emboli, this life-threatening disorder may cause increased accessory muscle use. More commonly, however, it produces dyspnea and tachypnea, which may be accompanied by pleuritic or substernal chest pain.

Thoracic injury. Increased accessory muscle use may occur, depending on the type and extent of injury.

Diagnostic tests
Pulmonary function tests can increase accessory muscle use.

Treatments
With incentive spirometry and intermittent positive pressure breathing, accessory muscle use typically increases.

Clinical considerations

If the patient has signs or symptoms of acute respiratory distress, such as decreased level of consciousness, shortness of breath when speaking, tachypnea, intercostal and sternal retractions, cyanosis, external breath sounds like wheezing or stridor, diaphoresis, nasal flaring, and extreme apprehension or agitation:

• A quick respiratory assessment should be performed and the physician notified immediately.

• Emergency intervention may be necessary to restore airway patency and adequate respiratory function.

If the patient is not in distress:

• A complete history should be obtained and a detailed chest examination performed.

• Diagnostic tests may include pulmonary function studies, chest X-rays, lung scans, arterial blood gas analysis, complete blood count, and sputum culture.

• Because labored breathing can make the patient apprehensive, emotional support should be provided.

• If the patient is alert, the head of the bed should be elevated to make breathing as easy as possible.

• The patient should be allowed to get plenty of rest and encouraged to increase fluid intake to liquefy secretions.

• Oxygen should be administered, as ordered.

Adipsia

Description

Adipsia is the abnormal absence of thirst. This sign commonly occurs in hypothalamic injury or tumor, head injury, bronchial tumor, and cirrhosis.

Agitation

Description

Agitation refers to a state of hyperarousal, increased tension, and irritability that can lead to confusion, hyperactivity, and overt hostility. This common sign can result from various disorders, pain, fever, anxiety, drug use and withdrawal, and hypersensitivity reactions. It can arise gradually or suddenly and last for minutes or months. Whether it is mild or severe, agitation worsens with increased fever, pain, stress, or external stimuli.

By itself, agitation merely signals a change in the patient's condition. But when considered in light of the history, current status, and other signs and symptoms, it becomes a more useful indicator of a developing disorder.

Possible causes

Central nervous system

Dementia. Mild-to-severe agitation can result from many common syndromes, such as Alzheimer's disease and Huntington's chorea. Agitation may present as a decrease in memory, attention span, problem-solving ability, and alertness.

Hepatic encephalopathy. Agitation occurs only with fulminating encephalopathy.

Increased intracranial pressure (ICP). No matter what causes increased ICP, agitation usually precedes other symptoms.

Organic brain syndrome. In this syndrome, agitation is manifested as hyperactivity, emotional lability, confusion, and memory loss.

Post–head trauma syndrome. Shortly after or even years after injury, mild-to-severe agitation develops, characterized by disorientation, loss of concentration, angry outbursts, and emotional lability.

Genitourinary

Chronic renal failure. Moderate-to-severe agitation occurs with this disorder, marked especially by confusion and memory loss.

Hematologic

Hypoxemia. Beginning as restlessness, agitation rapidly worsens.

Metabolic

Vitamin B₆ deficiency. Agitation can range from mild to severe in this deficiency.

Immunologic

Hypersensitivity reaction. Moderate-to-severe agitation appears, possibly as the first sign of a reaction. Depending on the reaction's severity, agitation may be accompanied by urticaria, pruritus, and facial and dependent edema.

In *anaphylactic shock,* a potentially life-threatening hypersensitivity reaction, agitation occurs rapidly along with apprehension or uneasiness, urticaria or diffuse erythema, warm moist skin, paresthesias, pruritus, edema, dyspnea, wheezing, stridor, hypotension, and tachycardia.

Drugs

Mild-to-moderate agitation, frequently dose-related, develops as a side effect of central nervous system stimulants—especially appetite suppressants, such as amphetamines and amphetamine-like drugs; sympathomimetic drugs such as ephedrine, caffeine, and theophylline.

In *alcohol withdrawal syndrome,* mild-to-severe agitation occurs. In *delirium tremens,* the potentially life-threatening stage of alcohol withdrawal, severe agitation occurs with visual hallucinations, insomnia, diaphoresis, and depression.

In *drug withdrawal syndrome,* mild-to-severe agitation occurs along with related findings that vary with the specific drug.

Diagnostic tests

Reaction to the contrast medium injected during various diagnostic tests produces moderate-to-severe agitation along with other signs of hypersensitivity.

Clinical considerations

• The severity of the patient's agitation should be determined by assessing the number and quality of agitation-induced behaviors, such as emotional lability, confusion, memory loss, hyperactivity, and hostility.

• A history should be obtained from the patient, if possible, or from a family member.

• Vital signs should be recorded and a neurologic assessment performed as a baseline for future comparison.

• Diagnostic tests, such as computed tomography scanning, skull X-rays, magnetic resonance imaging, and blood studies, may be performed.

• Because agitation can be an early sign of diverse disorders, the patient's vital signs and neurologic status should be monitored while the cause is being determined.

• Stressors, which can increase agitation, should be minimized or eliminated by providing adequate lighting, a calm environment, and ample time to sleep.

• The patient should be encouraged to discuss his feelings.

• Restraints should be used sparingly, since they tend to increase agitation.

Agnosia

Description
Agnosia is the inability to recognize and interpret sensory stimuli. *Auditory agnosia* refers to the inability to recognize familiar sounds. *Astereognosis,* or *tactile agnosia,* is the inability to recognize objects by touch or feel. *Anosmia* is the inability to recognize familiar smells; *gustatory agnosia,* the inability to recognize familiar tastes. *Visual agnosia* refers to the inability to recognize familiar objects by sight. *Autotopagnosia* is the inability to recognize body parts. *Anosognosia* refers to the denial or lack of awareness of a disease or defect (especially paralysis).

Agnosias stem from lesions that affect the association areas of the parietal sensory cortex. They are common sequelae of cerebrovascular accidents.

Agraphia

Description
Agraphia is the inability to express thoughts in writing. *Aphasic agraphia*

is associated with spelling and grammatical errors, whereas *constructional agraphia* refers to the reversal or incorrect ordering of correctly spelled words. *Apraxic agraphia* refers to the inability to form letters in the absence of significant motor impairment.

Agraphia commonly results from cerebrovascular accidents.

Allis' sign

Description
In an adult, Allis' sign is relaxation of the fascia lata between the iliac crest and greater trochanter due to fracture of the neck of the femur. To detect this sign, the examiner places a finger over the area between the iliac crest and greater trochanter and presses firmly. If the finger sinks deeply into this area, Allis' sign is present.

In an infant, Allis' sign refers to unequal leg lengths due to hip dislocation. To detect this sign, the examiner places the infant on his back with his pelvis flat, both legs flexed at the knee, and the hips even with the feet. If the height of the knees differs, hip dislocation in the leg with the shorter knee height should be suspected.

Alopecia
(Hair loss)

Description
Alopecia is partial or complete loss of hair. Occurring most often on the scalp, alopecia usually develops gradually and may be diffuse or patchy.

Alopecia normally occurs in the first six months of life. It may involve sudden, diffuse hair loss or gradual thinning that is hardly noticeable. Normally, everyone loses about 50 hairs a day, and these hairs are replaced by new ones. However, aging, genetic predisposition, and hormonal changes may contribute to gradual recession of the hairline and hair thinning. This nonpathologic alopecia occurs in about 40% of adult men and may also occur in postmenopausal women. In men, hair loss commonly affects the temporal areas, producing an M-shaped hairline. In women, diffuse thinning marks the centrofrontal area. In both sexes, hair loss also occurs on the trunk, pubic area, axillae, arms, and legs. Another normal pattern of alopecia occurs 2 to 4 months postpartum. This temporary diffuse hair loss on the scalp may be scant or dramatic and possibly accentuated at the frontal areas. Acute anxiety, high fever, and even certain hair styles or grooming methods may also cause alopecia.

Abnormal patterns of alopecia can be classified as scarring or nonscarring. Probably the most common cause of alopecia is use of antineoplastic drugs. However, alopecia may also result from use of other drugs; radiotherapy; skin, connective tissue, endocrine, nutritional, and psychological disorders; neoplasms; infection; burns; and the effects of toxins.

Mechanism

Scarring alopecia, or permanent hair loss, results from hair follicle destruction, which smooths the skin surface, erasing follicular openings. Nonscarring alopecia, or temporary hair loss, results from hair follicle damage that spares follicular openings, allowing future hair growth.

Possible causes

Cardiovascular

Arterial insufficiency. Patchy alopecia occurs in this disorder, typically on the legs, feet, and toes. It is accompanied by thin, shiny, atrophic skin and thickened nails.

Progressive systemic sclerosis. A late sign in this disease, permanent alopecia is accompanied by thickening of the skin, especially on the arms and hands. The skin appears taut and shiny and loses its pigment.

Endocrine

Hypopituitarism. Gonadotropin deficiency in the female causes sparse or absent pubic and axillary hair accompanied by infertility, amenorrhea, and breast atrophy. A similar deficiency in the male decreases facial and body hair and causes infertility, decreased libido, poor muscle development, and undersized testes, penis, and prostate gland.

Hypothyroidism. In this disorder, the hair on the face, scalp, and genitals thins and becomes dull, coarse, and brittle. Most characteristic, though, is loss of the outer third of the eyebrows. Typically, alopecia is preceded by fatigue, constipation, cold intolerance, and weight gain.

Thyrotoxicosis. Diffuse hair loss, possibly accentuated at the temples, occurs with this disorder. Hair becomes fine, soft, and friable.

Musculoskeletal

Lupus erythematosus. In both discoid and systemic lupus, hair tends to become brittle and may fall out in patches. Short, broken hairs ("lupus hairs") commonly appear above the forehead.

Myotonic dystrophy. Premature baldness characterizes the adult form of this muscular dystrophy. However, myotonia—the inability to normally relax a muscle after its contraction—is its primary sign.

Respiratory

Sarcoidosis. This disorder may produce scarring alopecia if it infiltrates the scalp.

Skin

Alopecia areata. Well-circumscribed patches of nonscarring scalp alopecia usually occur in this disorder, without skin changes. Occasionally, however, the patches also appear on the beard, axillae, pubic area, arms, legs, or the entire body (alopecia universalis). "Exclamation point" hairs—loose hairs with rough, brushlike tips on narrow, less-pigmented shafts—typically border expanding patches of alopecia. Although this disorder is recurrent, hair growth usually returns after several months.

Alopecia mucinosa. This uncommon disorder causes hair loss with follicular papules or plaques primarily on the head and neck; keratin and oil commonly plug these follicles.

Cutaneous T-cell lymphoma. Common in older patients, this disorder may be associated with alopecia mucinosa in its first, or premycotic, stage. Scattered papules or plaques may occur on clothed areas, such as breasts and buttocks, or a zebra-like pattern of scaly erythema may form on the trunk. Alopecia may persist through the plaque and tumor stages.

Dissecting cellulitis of the scalp. Resulting from infection, this disorder is characterized by small nodules that eventually rupture and drain. Keloid formation during healing causes permanent alopecia.

Exfoliative dermatitis. In this transient disorder, loss of scalp and body hair is preceded by several weeks of generalized scaling and erythema.

Folliculitis decalvans. This rare disorder eventually causes scarring alopecia, especially on the scalp, axillae, groin, and beard. It is characterized by inflamed hair follicles with small pustules, erythema, and scaling that leave smooth, shiny, depressed scars.

Fungal infections. Tinea capitis (ringworm), the most common fungal infection, produces irregular balding areas, scaling, and erythematous lesions.

Lichen planus. Occasionally, this skin disorder produces patchy hair loss on the scalp with skin inflammation.

Seborrheic dermatitis. Erupting in areas with many sebaceous glands and skin folds, this disorder most commonly produces hair loss on the scalp. Alopecia begins at the vertex and frontal areas and may spread to other scalp areas.

Metabolic

Protein deficiency. This disorder produces brittle, fine, dry, and thinning hair and, occasionally, changes in its pigment.

Infectious diseases

Secondary syphilis. This infection produces temporary, patchy hair loss that gives the scalp and beard a "moth-eaten" appearance. It also produces loss of eyelashes and eyebrows. Accompanying alopecia is a pruritic rash that may be macular, papular, pustular, or nodular.

Neoplastic

Hodgkin's lymphoma. Permanent alopecia may occur if the lymphoma infiltrates the scalp. It is accompanied by edema, pruritus, and hyperpigmentation.

Skin metastases. Occasionally, cancer from an internal site, such as the lung, metastasizes to the skin, causing scarring alopecia that may develop slowly along with scalp induration and atrophy.

Environmental

Arsenic poisoning. Most common in chronic poisoning, alopecia is diffuse and mainly affects the scalp.

Burns. Full-thickness or third-degree burns completely destroy the dermis and epidermis, leaving translucent, charred, or ulcerated skin. Scarring or keloid formation associated with these burns causes permanent alopecia.

Thallium poisoning. This type of poisoning produces diffuse, but temporary, hair loss on the scalp.

Drugs

Chemotherapy especially can cause alopecia. For example, bleomycin, cyclophosphamide, dactinomycin, daunorubicin, doxorubicin, fluorouracil, and methotrexate may cause patchy, reversible alopecia a few weeks after administration. Usually, hair loss is limited to the scalp, but with long-term chemotherapy, the axillae, arms, legs, face, and pubic area may also shed hair. New hair, which may differ in thickness, texture, and color from the patient's normal hair, may begin to grow after discontinuing the drug or between successive treatments.

Other common drugs may cause diffuse hair loss on the scalp a few weeks after administration. These include oral contraceptives, colchicine, heparin, warfarin, excessive doses of vitamin A, trimethadione, indomethacin, methysergide, valproic acid, carbamazepine, gentamicin, allopurinol, lithium, beta-adrenergic blockers, and antithyroid drugs. Hair growth usually returns when these drugs are discontinued.

Treatments
Like certain drugs, radiotherapy produces temporary, reversible hair loss a few weeks after exposure. Because X-rays damage hair follicles at the site of therapy, head or scalp X-rays cause the most obvious hair loss.

Clinical considerations
• A history should be obtained and a physical examination of the skin, including the extent and pattern of hair loss, should be performed.
• The physician may order a skin biopsy to determine the cause of the alopecia, especially if skin changes are evident. Microscopic examination of a plucked hair may also aid diagnosis.
• Alopecia can have a devastating impact on the patient's self-image, especially if it is extensive and sudden, as with antineoplastic drugs. To reduce anxiety, the patient should be told what to expect and, if appropriate, reassured that the hair will grow back.
• Occasionally, scalp hypothermia methods, such as a cryogen- or ice-filled cap or a scalp tourniquet, may be used before, during, and after drug administration to cause scalp vasoconstriction and to decrease drug delivery to the hair follicles. However, these methods are contraindicated in cancers with circulating malignant cells, such as lymphoma, or with scalp metastases.
• In patients with partial baldness or alopecia areata, topical application of minoxidil (a common antihypertensive drug) for several months may stimulate localized hair growth. However, hair loss may recur if the drug is discontinued.
• Gentle hair care should be encouraged to avoid further hair loss.
• A wig, cap, or scarf should be suggested, if appropriate.
• The patient should be advised to cover his head in cold weather to prevent loss of body heat.

Ambivalence

Description
Ambivalence is simultaneous existence of conflicting feelings about a person, idea, or object. It causes uncertainty or indecisiveness about which course to follow. Severe, debilitating ambivalence can occur in schizophrenia.

Amenorrhea

Description
Amenorrhea—the absence of menstrual flow—can be classified as primary or secondary. In *primary amenorrhea*, menstruation fails to begin before age 18. In *secondary amenorrhea*, it begins at an appropriate age but later ceases for 3 or more months in the absence of normal physiologic causes, such as pregnancy, lactation, and menopause.

Pathologic amenorrhea results from anovulation or physical obstruction to menstrual outflow, such as from an imperforate hymen, cervical stenosis, or intrauterine adhesions. Anovulation itself may result from hormonal imbalance, debilitating disease, stress or emotional disturbances, demanding and continuous exercise, malnutrition, obesity, and anatomic abnormalities, such as genetic absence of the ovaries or uterus. Amenorrhea may also result from certain treatments.

How Amenorrhea Develops

A disruption at any point in the menstrual cycle can produce amenorrhea, as illustrated in the flowchart below.

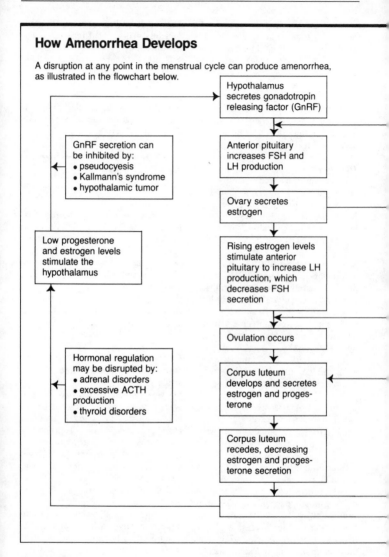

Mechanism
See *How Amenorrhea Develops*.

Possible causes
Endocrine
Adrenal tumor. Amenorrhea may be accompanied by acne, thinning scalp hair, hirsutism, increased blood pressure, and truncal obesity.

Adrenocortical hyperplasia. Amenorrhea precedes characteristic cushingoid signs, such as truncal obesity, moon face, buffalo hump, bruises, purple striae, and widened pulse pressure.

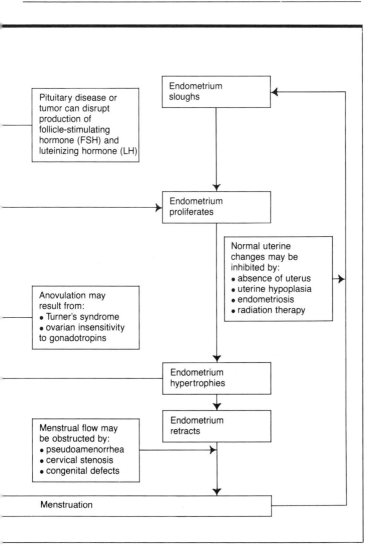

Adrenocortical hypofunction. Besides amenorrhea, this disorder may cause fatigue, irritability, weight loss, nausea, vomiting, and orthostatic hypotension.

Amenorrhea-lactation disorders. These disorders, such as Forbes-Albright and Chiari-Frommel syndromes, produce secondary amenorrhea accompanied by lactation in the absence of breast-feeding.

Hypothalamic tumor. Besides amenorrhea, a hypothalamic tumor can cause endocrine and visual field defects, gonadal underdevelopment or dysfunction, and short stature.

Hypothyroidism. Deficient thyroid hormone levels can cause primary or secondary amenorrhea.

Kallmann's syndrome. This rare familial form of hypothalamic dysfunction causes primary amenorrhea and infantile sexual development.

Ovarian insensitivity to gonadotropins. This hormonal disturbance leads to amenorrhea and an absence of secondary sex characteristics.

Pituitary infarction. This disorder usually causes postpartum failure to lactate and to resume menses.

Pituitary tumor. Amenorrhea may be the first sign of several types of pituitary tumor.

Thyrotoxicosis. Thyroid hormone overproduction may result in amenorrhea.

Genetic

Mosaicism. This genetic disorder results in primary amenorrhea and absence of secondary sex characteristics.

Testicular feminization. Primary amenorrhea may signal this form of male pseudohermaphroditism. The patient, outwardly female but genetically male, shows breast and external genital development, but scant or absent pubic hair.

Turner's syndrome. Primary amenorrhea and failure to develop secondary sex characteristics may signal this syndrome of genetic ovarian dysgenesis.

Psychiatric

Anorexia nervosa. This psychological disorder can cause either primary or secondary amenorrhea.

Obstetrics-Gynecology

Asherman's syndrome. This relatively rare sequela of vigorous curettage produces secondary amenorrhea.

Cervical stenosis. An uncommon disorder, cervical stenosis obstructs menstrual flow, producing amenorrhea.

Congenital absence of the ovaries. This anomaly results in primary amenorrhea and absence of secondary sex characteristics.

Congenital absence of the uterus. Primary amenorrhea occurs with this disorder.

Corpus luteum cysts. Often causing sudden amenorrhea, these cysts may also produce acute abdominal pain and breast swelling.

Pelvic inflammatory disease (PID). Rarely, PID destroys the ovaries and produces secondary amenorrhea.

Polycystic ovary syndrome. Typically menarche occurs at a normal age, followed by irregular menstrual cycles, oligomenorrhea, and secondary amenorrhea. Or periods of profuse bleeding may alternate with periods of amenorrhea.

Pseudoamenorrhea. An anatomic anomaly, such as imperforate hymen, obstructs menstrual flow, causing primary amenorrhea and possibly abdominal cramps.

Sertoli-Leydig cell tumor. This ovarian tumor may produce amenorrhea.

Uterine hypoplasia. Primary amenorrhea results from underdevelopment of the uterus.

Vaginal agenesis. A rare cause of primary amenorrhea, this anomaly may also produce cyclic moliminal symptoms but without abdominal pain.

Drugs

Cyclophosphamide, busulfan, chlorambucil, and phenothiazines may cause amenorrhea. Oral contraceptives may cause anovulation and amenorrhea after discontinuation.

Treatments

Irradiation of the abdomen may destroy the endometrium or ovaries, causing amenorrhea. Surgical removal of both ovaries or the uterus produces amenorrhea.

Clinical considerations

• A complete health history including a menstrual history should be obtained.

• A physical examination, including a pelvic examination, will be performed.

• In patients with secondary amenorrhea, physical and pelvic examinations must rule out pregnancy before diagnostic testing begins. Typical tests include progestin withdrawal, serum hormone and thyroid function studies, and endometrial biopsy.

• After diagnosis, the patient's questions about the type of treatment that will be provided and its expected outcome should be answered.

• Because amenorrhea can cause severe emotional distress, emotional support should be provided. The patient should be encouraged to discuss her fears, and, if necessary, referred for psychological counseling.

Amnesia

Description

Amnesia—a disturbance in or loss of memory—may be partial or complete, and anterograde or retrograde. Anterograde amnesia denotes memory loss for events that occurred *after* onset of the causative trauma or disease; retrograde amnesia denotes memory loss for events that occurred *before* onset. Depending on the cause, amnesia may arise suddenly or slowly and may be temporary or permanent.

Organic, or *true, amnesia* results from temporal lobe dysfunction and characteristically spares patches of memory. A common symptom in patients with seizures and head trauma, organic amnesia can also be an early indicator of Alzheimer's disease. *Hysterical amnesia* has a psychogenic origin and characteristically causes complete memory loss. *Treatment-induced amnesia* is usually transient.

Possible causes

Central nervous system

Alzheimer's disease. This disease usually begins with organic retrograde amnesia, which progresses slowly over many months or years to include anterograde amnesia, producing severe and permanent memory loss.

Cerebral hypoxia. After recovery from hypoxia (brought on by such conditions as carbon monoxide poisoning or acute respiratory failure), the patient may experience total amnesia for the event, along with sensory disturbances, such as numbness and tingling.

Head trauma. Depending on the trauma's severity, amnesia may last for minutes, hours, or longer. Usually, amnesia for the event persists, as well as brief retrograde and longer anterograde amnesia. Severe head trauma can cause permanent amnesia or difficulty in retaining recent memories.

Herpes simplex encephalitis. Recovery from this disease often leaves the patient with severe and possibly permanent amnesia.

Seizure. In temporal lobe seizures, amnesia occurs suddenly and lasts for several seconds to minutes. The patient may recall an aura or nothing at all.

An irritable focus on the left side of the brain primarily causes amnesia for verbal memories; an irritable focus on the right side of the brain, graphic *and* verbal amnesia.

Vertebrobasilar circulatory disorders. Vertebrobasilar ischemia, infarction, embolus, or hemorrhage typically causes complete amnesia that begins abruptly, lasts for several hours, and ends abruptly.

Wernicke-Korsakoff syndrome. Retrograde and anterograde amnesia can become permanent without treatment in this syndrome.

Psychiatric

Hysteria. Hysterical amnesia, a complete and long-lasting memory loss, begins and ends abruptly. It is typically accompanied by confusion.

Drugs

Anterograde amnesia can be precipitated by general anesthetics, especially fentanyl, halothane, and isoflurane; barbiturates, most commonly thiopental and pentobarbital; and certain benzodiazepines, especially triazolam.

Treatments

Sudden onset of retrograde or anterograde amnesia occurs with electroconvulsive therapy. Typically, the amnesia lasts for several minutes to several hours, but severe, prolonged amnesia occurs with treatments given frequently over a prolonged period.

Usually performed on only one lobe, temporal lobe surgery causes brief, slight amnesia. However, removal of both lobes leaves permanent amnesia.

Clinical considerations

• A history should be obtained with the help of family and friends and a neurologic assessment performed.

• The patient's recent, intermediate, and remote memory should be tested, as ordered, by asking appropriately selected questions.

• Diagnostic tests, such as computed tomography scan, electroencephalography, or cerebral angiography may be performed.

• Reality orientation should be provided for the patient with retrograde amnesia, and family members should be encouraged to help by supplying familiar photos, objects, or music.

• Patient-teaching techniques must be adjusted for the patient with anterograde amnesia since he cannot acquire new information. His family should be included in teaching sessions. In addition, all instructions—particularly medication dosages and schedules—should be written down so the patient will not have to rely on his memory.

• Basic needs, such as safety, elimination, and nutrition, must be considered for the patient with severe amnesia. If necessary, placement in an extended-care facility can be arranged.

Amoss' sign

Description

Amoss' sign is a sparing maneuver to avoid pain upon flexion of the spine. To detect this sign, the examiner asks the patient to rise from a supine to a sitting position. If the patient supports himself by placing his hands far behind him on the examining table, this sign is present.

Analgesia

Description

Analgesia is the absence of sensitivity to pain. It is an important sign of central nervous system disease, often indicating a specific type and location of spinal cord lesion. It always occurs with loss of temperature sensation (thermanesthesia), since these sensory nerve impulses travel together in the spinal cord. It can also occur with other sensory deficits, such as paresthesia, loss of proprioception and vibratory sense, and tactile anesthesia in various disorders involving the peripheral nerves, spinal cord, and brain. However, when accompanied only by thermanesthesia, analgesia points to an incomplete lesion of the spinal cord.

Analgesia can be partial or total below the level of the lesion, and unilateral or bilateral, depending on the cause and level of the lesion. Its onset may be slow and progressive with a tumor, or abrupt with trauma. Often transient, analgesia may resolve spontaneously.

Possible causes

Central nervous system

Anterior cord syndrome. In this syndrome, analgesia and thermanesthesia occur bilaterally below the level of the lesion, along with flaccid paralysis and hypoactive deep tendon reflexes.

Central cord syndrome. Typically, analgesia and thermanesthesia occur bilaterally in several dermatomes, frequently extending in a capelike fashion over the arms, back, and shoulders.

With brain stem involvement, additional findings may include facial analgesia and thermanesthesia, vertigo, nystagmus, atrophy of the tongue, and dysarthria.

Spinal cord hemisection. Contralateral analgesia and thermanesthesia occur below the level of the lesion.

Testing for Analgesia

By carefully and systematically testing a patient's sensitivity to pain, the examiner can determine whether his nerve damage has a segmental or peripheral distribution and help locate the causative lesion.

The examiner tells the patient to relax, and explains that she is going to lightly touch areas of his skin with a small pin. She has him close his eyes, then applies the pin firmly enough to produce pain without breaking the skin. (She can practice on herself first to learn how to apply the correct pressure.)

Starting with the patient's head and face, she moves down his body, pricking his skin on alternating sides. The patient should report when he feels pain. Occasionally the examiner should use the blunt end of the pin and vary her test pattern to gauge the accuracy of his response.

The examiner documents the findings thoroughly, clearly demarcating any areas of lost pain sensation on either a dermatome chart (page 18) or on appropriate peripheral nerve diagrams (below).

Peripheral nerves

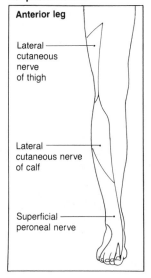

Anterior leg

Lateral cutaneous nerve of thigh

Lateral cutaneous nerve of calf

Superficial peroneal nerve

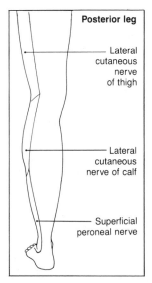

Posterior leg

Lateral cutaneous nerve of thigh

Lateral cutaneous nerve of calf

Superficial peroneal nerve

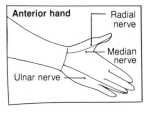

Anterior hand

Radial nerve

Median nerve

Ulnar nerve

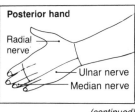

Posterior hand

Radial nerve

Ulnar nerve

Median nerve

(continued)

Testing for Analgesia (continued)
Dermatomes

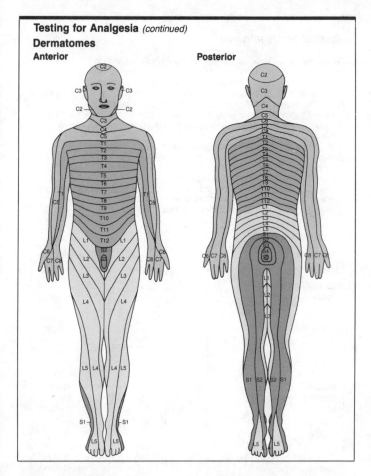

Anterior

Posterior

Drugs

Analgesia may occur with use of topical and local anesthetics, although numbness and tingling are more common.

Clinical considerations

If the patient complains of unilateral or bilateral analgesia over a large body area, accompanied by paralysis:

• A spinal cord injury should be suspected and the physician notified immediately.

• The patient's spine must be immobilized in proper alignment, using a cervical collar and a long backboard if possible. If a collar or backboard is not available, the patient should be positioned supine on a flat surface, and sandbags placed around his head, neck, and torso.

• Extreme caution must be used when moving the patient to prevent exacerbating spinal injury.

• Respiratory status must be monitored continuously, since a complete lesion above the T6 level may cause diaphragmatic and intercostal muscle paralysis.

• Emergency equipment should be kept close by for use in case respiratory failure occurs.

Once the patient's spine and respiratory status are stabilized—or if the analgesia is less severe and is not accompanied by signs of spinal cord injury:

• A history should be obtained and a complete neurologic assessment performed.

• A more thorough assessment of pain sensitivity may be necessary (see *Testing for Analgesia,* pp. 17 and 18).

• Spine X-rays will be taken.

• Further injury to the patient must be prevented because analgesia can mask injury or developing complications.

• Formation of decubiti may be prevented through meticulous skin care, massage, use of lamb's wool pads, and frequent repositioning, especially when significant motor deficits hamper the patient's movement.

• Scalding should be avoided by testing the patient's bathwater temperature before he bathes; he should be advised to test it at home using a thermometer or a body part with intact sensation.

Anesthesia

Description

Anesthesia is the absence of cutaneous sensation of touch, temperature, and pain. This sensory loss may be partial or total, unilateral or bilateral. To detect anesthesia, the examiner asks the patient to close his eyes. Then she touches him and asks him to specify the location. If the patient's verbal skills are immature or poor, she should watch for movement or changes in facial expression in response to touch.

Anhidrosis

Description

Anhidrosis is an abnormal deficiency of sweat in response to heat. It can be generalized (complete) or localized (partial). Generalized anhidrosis can lead to life-threatening impairment of thermoregulation. Localized anhidrosis rarely interferes with thermoregulation, since it affects only a small percentage of the body's eccrine (sweat) glands.

Anhidrosis results from neurologic and skin disorders; congenital, atrophic, or traumatic changes to sweat glands; and use of certain drugs.

Anhidrosis may go unrecognized until significant heat or exertion fails to raise sweat. However, localized anhidrosis often provokes compensatory hyperhidrosis in the remaining functional sweat glands. Often the patient's chief complaint, this hyperhidrosis can flood the skin surface, masking areas of sweat gland deficiency.

Mechanism

Neurologic disorders disturb central or peripheral nervous pathways that normally activate sweating, causing retention of excess body heat and perspiration. The absence, obstruction, atrophy, or degeneration of sweat glands can produce anhidrosis at the skin surface, even if neurologic stimulation is normal.

Possible causes
Central nervous system
Cerebral lesions. Cerebral cortex and brain stem lesions may cause anhidrotic palms and soles, along with various motor and sensory disturbances specific to the site of the lesions.

Horner's syndrome. A supraclavicular spinal cord lesion produces unilateral facial anhidrosis with compensatory contralateral hyperhidrosis.

Peripheral neuritis. Anhidrosis over the legs often appears with compensatory hyperhidrosis over the head and neck.

Shy-Drager syndrome. This degenerative neurologic syndrome causes ascending anhidrosis in the legs.

Spinal cord lesions. Anhidrosis may occur symmetrically below the level of the lesion, with compensatory hyperhidrosis in adjacent areas.

Skin

Miliaria crystallina. This usually innocuous form of miliaria causes anhidrosis and tiny, clear, fragile blisters, usually under the arms and breasts.

Miliaria profunda. If severe and extensive, this form of miliaria can progress to life-threatening anhidrotic asthenia. Typically, though, it produces localized anhidrosis with compensatory facial hyperhydrosis.

Miliaria rubra (prickly heat). Like miliaria profunda, this common form of miliaria can progress to life-threatening anhidrotic asthenia if it is severe and extensive. Typically, though, it produces localized anhidrosis.

Environmental

Anhidrotic asthenia (heatstroke). This life-threatening disorder causes acute, generalized anhidrosis. In early stages, sweating may still occur and the patient may be rational, but his rectal temperature may already exceed 102.2° F. Associated signs and symptoms include severe headache and muscle cramps, which later disappear; fatigue; nausea and vomiting; dizziness; palpitations; substernal tightness; and elevated blood pressure followed by hypotension. Within minutes, anhidrosis and hot, flushed skin develop, accompanied by tachycardia, tachypnea, and confusion progressing to loss of consciousness.

Burns. Depending on their severity, burns may cause permanent anhidrosis in affected areas.

Clinical considerations

If the patient has generalized anhidrosis; hot, flushed skin; a rectal temperature above 102.2° F. (39° C.); tachycardia; tachypnea; and decreased level of consciousness:

• Anhidrotic asthenia should be suspected and the physician notified immediately.

• Rapid cooling measures and fluid replacement should be initiated, as ordered.

• The patient should be placed in an air-conditioned room.

• Vital signs and neurologic status should be monitored frequently until the patient's temperature drops below 102° F.

If anhidrosis is localized or the patient reports local hyperhidrosis or unexplained fever:

• A history should be obtained and a physical examination performed.

• Because even a careful assessment can be inconclusive, specific tests may be needed to evaluate anhidrosis. These include wrapping the patient in an electric blanket or placing him in a heated box to observe the skin for sweat patterns, applying topical agents that detect sweat on the skin, or administering systemic cholinergic drugs, which stimulate sweating.

• The patient with anhidrosis should be advised to remain in cool environments, to move slowly during warm weather, and to avoid strenuous exercise and hot foods.

Anisocoria

Description

Anisocoria is a difference of 0.5 to 2 mm in pupil size. Anisocoria occurs normally in about 2% of people, in whom the pupillary inequality remains constant over time and despite changes in light. However, if anisocoria results from fixed dilation or constriction of one pupil or slowed or impaired constriction of one pupil in response to light, it may indicate neurologic disease.

Anorexia

Description

Anorexia is a lack of appetite in the presence of a physiologic need for food. A common symptom of GI and endocrine disorders, it is also characteristic of certain severe psychological disturbances. This symptom can also result from such factors as anxiety, chronic pain, poor oral hygiene, increased blood temperature due to hot weather or fever, and alterations in taste or smell that normally accompany aging. Anorexia can result from drug therapy or abuse, too. Short-term anorexia rarely jeopardizes the patient's health. However, chronic anorexia can lead to life-threatening malnutrition.

Possible causes

Endocrine

Adrenocortical hypofunction. In this disorder, anorexia may begin slowly and subtly, causing gradual weight loss.

Hypopituitarism. Anorexia usually develops slowly in this disorder. Its accompanying signs vary with the disorder's severity and the number and type of deficient hormones.

Hypothyroidism. Anorexia is common and usually insidious in thyroid hormone deficiency.

Ketoacidosis. Anorexia usually arises gradually and is accompanied by dry, flushed skin; fruity breath odor; polydipsia; hypotension; weak, rapid pulse; dry mouth; abdominal pain; and vomiting.

Gastrointestinal

Appendicitis. Anorexia closely follows the abrupt onset of generalized or localized epigastric pain, nausea, and vomiting. It can continue as pain localizes in the right lower quadrant (McBurney's point) and other signs appear.

Cirrhosis. Anorexia occurs early and may be accompanied by weakness, nausea, vomiting, constipation or diarrhea, and dull abdominal pain. It continues after these early signs subside and is accompanied by lethargy, slurred speech, bleeding tendencies, ascites, severe pruritus, dry skin, poor skin turgor, hepatomegaly, fetor hepaticus, jaundice, edema of the legs, and right upper quadrant pain.

Crohn's disease. Chronic anorexia causes marked weight loss.

Gastritis. In *acute gastritis,* the onset of anorexia may be sudden; in *chronic gastritis,* it is insidious.

Hepatitis. In *viral hepatitis,* anorexia begins in the preicteric phase, accompanied by fatigue, malaise, headache, arthralgia, myalgia, photophobia, cough, sore throat, rhinitis, nausea and vomiting, mild fever, hepatomegaly, and lymphadenopathy. It may continue throughout the icteric phase, along with mild weight loss, dark urine, clay-colored stools, jaundice, right upper quadrant pain, and, possibly, irritability and severe pruritus.

In *nonviral hepatitis,* anorexia and its accompanying signs usually resemble those of viral hepatitis but may vary depending on the causative agent and the extent of liver damage.

Genitourinary

Chronic renal failure. Chronic anorexia is common and insidious. It is accompanied by changes in all body systems.

Metabolic

Pernicious anemia. In this disorder, insidious anorexia may cause considerable weight loss.

Psychiatric

Alcoholism. Chronic anorexia commonly accompanies alcoholism, eventually leading to malnutrition.

Anorexia nervosa. Chronic anorexia begins insidiously and eventually leads to life-threatening malnutrition, evidenced by skeletal muscle atrophy, loss of fatty tissue, constipation, amenorrhea, dry and blotchy or sallow skin, alopecia, sleep disturbances, distorted self-image, anhedonia, and decreased libido. Paradoxically, the patient often exhibits extreme restlessness and vigor and may exercise avidly.

Depressive syndrome. Anorexia reflects anhedonia in this syndrome. Accompanying symptoms may include poor concentration, indecisiveness, delusions, menstrual irregularities, decreased libido, insomnia or hypersomnia, fatigue, mood swings, and gradual social withdrawal.

Neoplastic

Cancer. Chronic anorexia occurs, with possible weight loss, weakness, apathy, and cachexia.

Drugs

Anorexia results from use of amphetamines, chemotherapeutic agents, sympathomimetics such as ephedrine, and some antibiotics. It also signals digitalis toxicity.

Treatments

Radiation treatments can cause anorexia, possibly due to metabolic disturbances.

Maintenance of blood glucose levels by total parenteral nutrition may cause anorexia.

Clinical considerations

• The patient should be weighed.

• Diet and medical histories should be obtained.

• If the medical history does not reveal an organic basis for anorexia, psychological factors must be considered. For example, situational factors, such as a death in the family or problems at school or on the job, can lead to depression and subsequent loss of appetite.

• A physical examination should be performed, with signs of malnutrition noted.

• If the patient has signs of malnutrition, consistently refuses food, and has lost 7% to 10% of his body weight within the last month, the physician should be notified.

• Because the causes of anorexia are diverse, diagnostic procedures may include thyroid function studies, esophagography, upper GI series, gallbladder series, barium enema,

liver and kidney function tests, hormone assays, computed tomography scans, ultrasonography, and blood studies to assess nutritional status.

• Protein and caloric intake should be promoted by providing high-calorie snacks or frequent, small meals.

• The patient's family should be encouraged to supply his favorite foods to help stimulate his appetite.

• A 24-hour diet history should be taken daily.

• If the patient consistently exaggerates his food intake (a common occurrence in anorexia nervosa), strict calorie and nutrient counts should be maintained for the patient's meals.

• In severe malnutrition, supplemental nutritional support, such as total parenteral nutrition should be provided, as ordered.

Anosmia

Description

Anosmia is the absence of the sense of smell. Although usually an insignificant consequence of nasal congestion or obstruction, anosmia occasionally heralds a serious neural defect. Temporary anosmia can result from any condition that causes irritation and swelling of the nasal mucosa and obstructs the olfactory area in the nose, such as heavy smoking, rhinitis, or sinusitis. Permanent anosmia, on the other hand, usually indicates a lesion in the olfactory nerve pathway. Permanent or temporary anosmia can also result from inhalation of irritants, such as cocaine or acid fumes, that paralyze the nasal cilia. Anosmia may also be reported—without an identifiable organic cause—by patients suffering from hysteria, depression, or schizophrenia.

Anosmia is invariably perceived as bilateral; unilateral anosmia can occur but cannot be recognized by the patient. Because combined stimulation of taste buds and olfactory cells produces the sense of taste, anosmia is usually accompanied by ageusia, loss of the sense of taste.

Mechanism

The olfactory epithelium contains olfactory receptor cells, along with olfactory glands and sustentacular cells, both of which secrete mucus to keep the epithelial surface moist. The mucus covering the olfactory cells probably traps airborne odorous molecules, which then fit into the appropriate receptors on the cell surface. In response to this stimulus, the receptor cell then transmits an impulse along the olfactory nerve (cranial nerve I) to the olfactory area of the cortex, where it is interpreted. Any disruption along this transmission pathway, or any obstruction of the epithelial surface due to dryness or congestion, can cause anosmia.

Possible causes

Central nervous system

Anterior cerebral artery occlusion. Permanent anosmia may follow vascular damage involving the olfactory nerve.

Head trauma. Permanent anosmia may follow damage to the olfactory nerve.

Eyes, ears, nose, and throat

Lethal midline granuloma. Permanent anosmia accompanies this slowly progressive disease.

Nasal or sinus neoplasms. Anosmia may be permanent if the neoplasm destroys or displaces the olfactory nerve.

Polyps. Temporary anosmia occurs when multiple polyps obstruct nasal cavities.

Rhinitis. In common *acute viral rhinitis,* temporary anosmia occurs with nasal congestion; sneezing; watery or purulent nasal discharge; red, swollen nasal mucosa; dryness or a tickling sensation in the nasopharynx; headache; low-grade fever; and chills.

In *allergic rhinitis,* temporary anosmia accompanies nasal congestion; itching mucosa; pale, edematous turbinates; thin nasal discharge; sneezing; tearing; and headache.

In *atrophic rhinitis,* anosmia resolves with successful treatment of the disorder.

In *vasomotor rhinitis,* temporary anosmia is accompanied by chronic nasal congestion, watery nasal discharge, postnasal drip, sneezing, and pale nasal mucosa.

Septal fracture. Anosmia is usually temporary; sense of smell returns with septal repositioning.

Septal hematoma. Anosmia is temporary, resolving with repair of the nasal mucosa or absorption of the hematoma.

Sinusitis. Temporary anosmia may occur.

Endocrine

Diabetes mellitus. Insidious, permanent anosmia may occur.

Metabolic

Pernicious anemia. Anosmia may be temporary or permanent. It is accompanied by the classic triad of weakness; sour, pale tongue; and numbness and tingling in the extremities.

Environmental

Lead poisoning. Anosmia may be permanent or temporary, depending on the extent of damage to the nasal mucosa.

Drugs

Anosmia can result from prolonged use of nasal decongestants, which produces rebound nasal congestion. Occasionally, it results from naphazoline, a local decongestant that may cause paralysis of nasal cilia. It can also result from reserpine and, less commonly, amphetamines, phenothiazines, and estrogen, which cause nasal congestion.

Treatments

Permanent anosmia may result from radiation damage to the nasal mucosa or olfactory nerve following radiation therapy.

Temporary anosmia may result from damage to the olfactory nerve or nasal mucosa during nasal or sinus surgery. Permanent anosmia accompanies a permanent tracheostomy, which disrupts nasal breathing.

Clinical considerations

• A history should be obtained and a physical examination of nasal structures performed.

• The olfactory nerve (cranial nerve I) should be tested by having the patient identify common odors.

• If anosmia does not result from simple nasal congestion, diagnostic tests may be done, including sinus transillumination, skull X-ray, or computed tomography scan.

• If anosmia results from nasal congestion, local decongestants or antihistamines should be administered, as ordered, and a vaporizer or humidifier provided to prevent mucosal drying and to help thin purulent nasal discharge.

• The patient should be advised to avoid excessive use of local decongestants, which can lead to rebound nasal congestion.

• Although permanent anosmia usually doesn't respond to treatment, vitamin A given orally or by injection sometimes results in improvement.

Anuria

Description

Anuria is clinically defined as urine output of less than 75 ml daily. This sign indicates either urinary tract obstruction or acute renal failure. Fortunately, anuria rarely occurs—even in renal failure, the kidneys usually produce at least 75 ml of urine daily.

Because urine output is easily measured, anuria rarely goes undetected. However, without immediate treatment, anuria can rapidly cause uremia and other complications of urinary retention.

Possible causes

Cardiovascular

Vasculitis. This disorder occasionally produces anuria.

Genitourinary

Acute tubular necrosis. Prolonged (up to 2 weeks) anuria or, more commonly, oliguria is a common finding in this disorder. It precedes the onset of diuresis, which is heralded by polyuria.

Cortical necrosis (bilateral). This disorder is characterized by a sudden change from oliguria to anuria, along with gross hematuria, flank pain, and fever.

Glomerulonephritis (acute). This disorder produces anuria or oliguria.

Papillary necrosis (acute). Bilateral papillary necrosis produces anuria or oliguria.

Renal artery occlusion (bilateral). This disorder produces anuria or severe oliguria, often accompanied by severe, continuous upper abdominal and flank pain; nausea and vomiting; decreased bowel sounds; and fever up to 102° F. (39° C.).

Renal vein occlusion (bilateral). This disorder occasionally causes anuria.

Urinary tract obstruction. Severe obstruction can produce acute and sometimes total anuria, alternating with or preceded by burning and pain on urination, overflow incontinence or dribbling, increased urinary frequency and nocturia, voiding of small amounts, or altered urinary stream.

Hematologic

Hemolytic-uremic syndrome. Anuria often occurs in the initial stages of this disorder and may last from 1 to 10 days.

Drugs

Many classes of drugs can cause anuria or, more commonly, oliguria through their nephrotoxic effects. Antibiotics, especially the aminoglycosides, are the most commonly nephrotoxic. Adrenergic and anticholinergic drugs can cause anuria by affecting the nerves and muscles of micturition to produce urinary retention.

Diagnostic tests

Contrast media used in radiographic studies can cause nephrotoxicity, producing oliguria and, rarely, anuria.

Clinical considerations

After detecting anuria, the priorities are to determine if urine formation is occurring and to intervene appropriately:

• The physician should be notified.

• Catheterization should be anticipated to relieve any lower urinary tract obstruction and to check for residual urine.

• A complete history should be taken and an abdominal examination performed.

• If catheterization fails to initiate urine flow, diagnostic studies, such as ultrasonography, cystoscopy, retrograde pyelography, and renal scan, may be performed to detect possible obstruction higher in the urinary tract.

• If diagnostic tests reveal an obstruction, nephrostomy or ureterostomy tube insertion (to drain the urine) and surgery (to relieve the obstruction) should be anticipated.

• If diagnostic tests fail to reveal an obstruction, the patient will require further kidney function studies.

• While the diagnostic workup is being completed, the patient's vital signs and intake and output should be carefully monitored.

• The patient's daily fluid allowance should be restricted to 600 ml more than the previous day's total urine output.

• Foods and juices high in potassium and sodium should be restricted, and a balanced diet with controlled protein levels maintained.

• The patient's fluid intake and output and weight should be recorded daily.

Anxiety

Description

Anxiety, a subjective reaction to real or imagined threat, can best be described as a nonspecific feeling of uneasiness or dread. It may be mild, moderate, or severe. Mild anxiety may cause slight physical or psychological discomfort, whereas severe anxiety may be incapacitating or even life-threatening.

Everyone experiences anxiety from time to time—it is a normal response to actual danger, prompting the body (through stimulation of the sympathetic and parasympathetic nervous systems) to purposeful action. It is also a normal response to physical and emotional stress, which can be produced by virtually any illness. In addition, anxiety can be precipitated or exacerbated by many nonpathologic factors, including lack of sleep, poor diet, and excessive intake of caffeine or other stimulants. However, excessive, unwarranted anxiety may indicate an underlying psychological problem.

Possible causes

Central nervous system

Autonomic hyperreflexia (AHR). The earliest sign of AHR may be acute anxiety accompanied by severe headache and dramatic hypertension.

Postconcussion syndrome. This syndrome may produce chronic anxiety or periodic attacks of acute anxiety.

Respiratory

Adult respiratory distress syndrome. Acute anxiety occurs along with tachycardia, mental sluggishness, and, in severe cases, hypotension.

Asthma. In allergic asthma attacks, acute anxiety occurs with dyspnea, wheezing, productive cough, accessory muscle use, hyperresonant lung fields, diminished breath sounds, coarse rales, cyanosis, tachycardia, and diaphoresis.

Chronic obstructive pulmonary disease. Acute anxiety, dyspnea on exertion, cough, wheezing, rales, hyperresonant lung fields, tachypnea, and accessory muscle use characterize this disorder.

Hyperventilation syndrome. This disorder produces acute anxiety, pallor, circumoral and peripheral paresthesia, and, occasionally, carpopedal spasms.

Pneumonia. Acute anxiety may occur in pneumonia associated with hypoxemia.

Pneumothorax. Acute anxiety occurs in moderate-to-severe pneumothorax associated with profound respiratory distress.

Pulmonary edema. In this disorder, acute anxiety occurs with dyspnea, orthopnea, cough with frothy sputum, tachycardia, tachypnea, rales, ventricular gallop, hypotension, and thready pulse. The patient's skin may be cool, clammy, and cyanotic.

Pulmonary embolism. Acute anxiety is usually accompanied by dyspnea, tachypnea, chest pain, tachycardia, blood-tinged sputum, and low-grade fever.

Cardiovascular

Anaphylactic shock. Acute anxiety usually signals the onset of this shock state. It is accompanied by urticaria, angioedema, pruritus, and shortness of breath.

Angina pectoris. Acute anxiety may either precede or follow an attack of angina pectoris.

Cardiogenic shock. Acute anxiety occurs along with cool, pale, clammy skin, tachycardia, weak and thready pulse, tachypnea, ventricular gallop, rales, neck vein distention, decreased urine output, hypotension, narrowing pulse pressure, and peripheral edema.

Congestive heart failure. In this disorder, acute anxiety is frequently the first symptom of inadequate oxygenation.

Myocardial infarction. In this life-threatening disorder, acute anxiety commonly occurs with persistent, crushing, substernal pain that may radiate to the left arm, jaw, neck, or shoulder blades. It can be accompanied by shortness of breath, nausea, vomiting, diaphoresis, and cool, pale skin.

Endocrine

Hyperthyroidism. Acute anxiety may be an early sign of this disorder.

Hypoglycemia. Anxiety resulting from hypoglycemia is usually mild to moderate and associated with hunger, mild headache, palpitations, blurred vision, weakness, and diaphoresis.

Pheochromocytoma. Acute, severe anxiety accompanies this disorder's cardinal sign—persistent or paroxysmal hypertension.

Psychiatric

Affective disorder. In the depressive form of this disorder, chronic anxiety occurs with varying severity. The hallmark sign, though, is depression upon awakening, which abates over the course of the day.

Conversion disorder. Chronic anxiety is characteristic along with one or two specific somatic complaints that have no physiologic basis.

Hypochondriacal neurosis. Mild-to-moderate chronic anxiety occurs in this disorder. The patient tends to "physician hop" and is not reassured by any number of favorable physical examinations and laboratory test results.

Obsessive-compulsive disorders. Chronic anxiety occurs in these psychiatric disorders, which are characterized by recurrent, unshakable thoughts or impulses to perform ritualistic acts that the patient recognizes as irrational but cannot control. The patient's anxiety builds if he cannot perform these acts and diminishes after he does so.

Phobic disorder. In this disorder, chronic anxiety occurs with persistent fear of an object, activity, or situation that results in a compelling desire to avoid it.

Posttraumatic stress disorder. This disorder produces chronic anxiety of varying severity. It is accompanied by intrusive, vivid memories and thoughts of the traumatic event.

Somatization disorder. Most common in adolescents and young adults, this disorder is characterized by chronic anxiety and various somatic complaints that have no physiologic basis. Anxiety and depression may be prominent or hidden by dramatic, flamboyant, or seductive behavior.

Environmental

Rabies. Anxiety signals the beginning of the acute phase of this rare disorder. It is commonly accompanied by painful laryngeal spasms associated with difficulty swallowing and, as a result, hydrophobia.

Drugs

Many drugs cause anxiety, especially sympathomimetics and central nervous system stimulants. Tricyclic antidepressants may cause paradoxical anxiety.

Clinical considerations

If the patient displays acute, severe anxiety:

• Vital signs should be taken and the chief complaint explored. Because anxiety is a notoriously nonspecific symptom, this information will be needed to guide subsequent assessment and interventions. For example, if the patient's severe anxiety were accompanied by chest pain and shortness of breath, myocardial infarction might be suspected; interventions should be carried out, as appropriate.

• During the assessment, the patient should be reassured as much as possible—uncontrolled anxiety can alter vital signs and often exacerbate the causative disorder.

If the patient displays mild or moderate anxiety:

• A complete history should be taken and a physical examination performed, focusing on any complaints that may trigger or be aggravated by anxiety.

If the patient's anxiety is not accompanied by significant physical signs:

• A psychological basis should be suspected.

• The patient's level of consciousness should be assessed and his behavior observed.

• If appropriate the patient should be referred for psychiatric evaluation.

• Often supportive nursing care can do much to help relieve the patient's anxiety.

• A calm, quiet atmosphere should be provided and the patient made comfortable.

• The patient should be encouraged to freely express his feelings and concerns.

• Anxiety-reducing measures, such as distraction, relaxation techniques, or biofeedback, may be used.

Apathy

Description

Apathy is the absence or suppression of emotion or interest in the external environment and personal affairs. This indifference can result from many disorders—chiefly neurologic, psychological, respiratory, and renal—as well as from alcohol and drug use and abuse. It is associated with many chronic disorders that cause personality changes and depression. In fact, apathy may be an early indicator of a severe disorder, such as a brain tumor.

Aphasia
(Dysphasia)

Description

Aphasia is impaired expression or comprehension of written or spoken language. Depending on its severity, aphasia may slightly impede communication or may make it impossible. It can be classified as Broca's, Wernicke's, anomic, or global aphasia (see *Identifying Types of Aphasia,* p. 28). Anomic aphasia eventually resolves in more than 50% of patients, but global aphasia is irreversible.

The term *childhood aphasia* is sometimes mistakenly applied to children who fail to develop normal language skills but who are not considered mentally retarded or developmentally delayed. Aphasia refers solely to loss of previously developed communication skills.

Identifying Types of Aphasia

Type	Location of lesion	Clinical findings
Broca's aphasia (expressive aphasia)	Broca's area; usually in third frontal convolution of the left hemisphere	Patient's understanding of written and spoken language is slightly impaired, but his motor impairment causes nonfluent speech. His speech also displays word-finding difficulty, jargon, paraphasias (inaccurate, sometimes unintelligible sound/word substitutions or neologisms), limited vocabulary, and simple sentence construction. Also, the patient cannot repeat words or phrases.
Wernicke's aphasia (receptive aphasia)	Wernicke's area; usually in posterior/superior temporal lobe	Patient has difficulty understanding written and spoken language. He cannot repeat words or phrases or follow directions. His speech is fluent, but it contains paraphasias and tends to be rapid and rambling. Also, the patient has difficulty naming objects (anomia).
Anomic aphasia	Temporal-parietal area; may extend to angular gyrus, but sometimes poorly localized	Patient's understanding of written and spoken language is relatively unimpaired. His speech, though fluent, lacks meaningful content. Word-finding difficulty and circumlocution (roundabout sentence construction) are characteristic. Rarely, the patient also displays paraphasias.
Global aphasia	Broca's and Wernicke's areas	Patient has profoundly impaired receptive and expressive ability. He cannot repeat words or phrases and cannot follow directions. His occasional speech is marked by paraphasias or jargon.

Mechanism

Aphasia reflects disease or injury of the brain's language centers (see *Where Language Originates,* p. 30).

Possible causes

Central nervous system

Alzheimer's disease. In this degenerative disease, anomic aphasia may begin insidiously and then progress to Wernicke's and, finally, global aphasia.

Brain abscess. Any type of aphasia may occur in brain abscess. Usually, aphasia develops insidiously and may be accompanied by hemiparesis, ataxia, facial weakness, and signs of increased intracranial pressure (ICP).

Brain tumor. Anomic aphasia may be an early sign of this disorder. As the tumor enlarges, other aphasias may occur along with behavioral changes, memory loss, motor weakness, seizures, auditory hallucinations, and visual field deficits.

Cerebrovascular accident. The most common cause of aphasia, this disorder may produce Wernicke's, Broca's, or global aphasia.

Encephalitis. This disorder usually produces transient aphasia. Accompanying aphasia may be convulsions, confusion, stupor or coma, hemiparesis, asymmetrical deep tendon reflexes, positive Babinski's reflex, ataxia, myoclonus, nystagmus, ocular palsies, and facial weakness.

Head trauma. Any type of aphasia may accompany severe head trauma; typically, it occurs suddenly and may be transient or permanent, depending on the extent of brain damage.

Transient ischemic attack (TIA). This disorder can produce any type of aphasia. Usually, the aphasia occurs suddenly and resolves within 24 hours of the TIA.

Drugs

Heroin overdose can cause any type of aphasia.

Clinical considerations

If the patient *suddenly* develops aphasia:

• The physician should be notified immediately.

• The patient should be assessed for signs of increased ICP, such as pupillary changes, decreased level of consciousness, vomiting, seizures, bradycardia, widening pulse pressure, and irregular respirations.

• If signs of increased ICP are present, emergency interventions should be carried out.

• Emergency resuscitation equipment should be kept readily available to support respiratory and cardiac function, if necessary.

• Emergency surgery may be required.

   If the patient does not display signs of increased ICP, or if his aphasia has developed gradually:

• A complete history should be obtained and a thorough neurologic assessment performed. (The history should be obtained from the patient's family or friends if the patient's impairment prevents him from supplying information.)

• The examiner should keep in mind that the patient's aphasia may hinder the neurologic assessment. For example, assessing level of consciousness is often difficult because the patient's verbal responses may be unreliable. In addition, dysarthria (impaired articulation due to weakness or paralysis of the muscles necessary for speech) or speech apraxia (inability to voluntarily control the muscles of speech) may accompany aphasia.

• Diagnostic tests may include skull X-rays, computed tomography scan, angiography, and electroencephalography.

• Immediately after aphasia develops, the patient may become confused or disoriented. His sense of reality can be improved by frequently telling him what has happened, where he is and why, and the date.

• Later, periods of depression may be expected as the patient recognizes his handicap. Providing a relaxed, accepting environment with a minimum of distracting stimuli can help him to communicate.

• Sudden outbursts of profanity by the patient may occur. This common behavior usually reflects intense frustration with his impairment. Such outbursts must be dealt with as gently as possible to ease embarrassment.

• When speaking to the patient, the examiner must not assume that he understands. He may simply be interpreting subtle clues to meaning, such as social context, facial expressions, and gestures. To help avoid misunderstanding, simple phrases should be used and demonstration made to clarify verbal directions, when appropriate.

• Because aphasia is a *language* disorder, not an emotional or auditory one, the patient should be spoken to in a normal tone of voice.

• Necessary aids, such as eyeglasses or dentures, should be provided to facilitate communication.

• If appropriate, the patient should be referred to a speech pathologist early to help him cope with his aphasia.

• If the patient is unable to return to work, he should be referred to a social service agency.

Where Language Originates

Aphasia reflects damage to one or more of the brain's primary language centers, which, in most persons, are located in the left hemisphere. *Broca's area* lies next to the region of the motor cortex that controls the muscles necessary for speech, and presumably coordinates their movement. *Wernicke's area,* which helps control the content of speech and affects its auditory and visual comprehension, lies between Heschl's gyrus, the primary receiver of auditory stimuli, and the *angular gyrus,* a "way station" between the auditory and visual regions. Connecting Wernicke's and Broca's areas is a large nerve bundle, the *arcuate fasciculus,* which also helps control the content of speech and enables repetition.

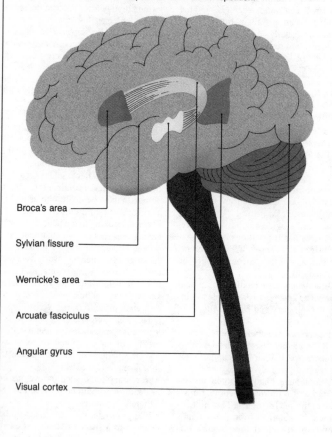

Broca's area

Sylvian fissure

Wernicke's area

Arcuate fasciculus

Angular gyrus

Visual cortex

Aphonia

Description
Aphonia is the inability to produce speech sounds. This sign may result from overuse of the vocal cords, disorders of the larynx or laryngeal nerves, psychological disorders, or muscle spasm.

Apnea

Description
Apnea is the cessation of spontaneous respiration. Occasionally, it is temporary and self-limiting, as occurs during Cheyne-Stokes and Biot's respirations. More often, though, it is a life-threatening emergency that requires immediate intervention to prevent death. Its most common causes include trauma, cardiac arrest, neurologic disease, aspiration of foreign objects, bronchospasm, and drug overdose.

Mechanism
Apnea usually results from one or more of six pathophysiologic mechanisms, each of which has numerous causes (see *Causes of Apnea*, p. 32).

Possible causes
Central nervous system
Brain stem dysfunction. Primary or secondary brain stem dysfunction can cause apnea by destroying the brain stem's ability to initiate respirations. Apnea may arise suddenly (as in trauma, hemorrhage, or infarction) or gradually (as in degenerative disease or tumor). It may be preceded by decreased level of consciousness and various motor and sensory deficits.
Respiratory
Airway obstruction. Occlusion or compression of the trachea, central airways, or smaller airways can cause sudden apnea by blocking airflow and producing acute respiratory failure.

Alveolar gas diffusion impairment. An occlusion at the alveolar-capillary membrane level or an accumulation of fluid within the alveoli themselves produces apnea by interfering with pulmonary gas exchange and producing acute respiratory failure. Apnea may arise suddenly, as in near-drowning and acute pulmonary edema, or more gradually, as in emphysema. It may be preceded by rales and labored respirations with accessory muscle use.

Pleural pressure gradient disruption. Conversion of normal negative pleural air pressure to positive pressure by chest wall injuries (such as flail chest) causes lung collapse, producing respiratory distress and, if untreated, apnea.

Pulmonary capillary perfusion decrease. Apnea can stem from obstructed pulmonary circulation, most commonly due to heart failure or lack of circulatory patency. It occurs suddenly in cardiac arrest, massive pulmonary embolism, and most cases of severe shock. In contrast, it occurs progressively in septic shock and pulmonary hypertension.

Respiratory muscle failure. Trauma or disease can disrupt the mechanics of respiration, causing sudden or gradual apnea.

Drugs
Central nervous system (CNS) depressants—such as narcotic analgesics, barbiturates, anesthetics, and alcohol—may cause hypoventilation and apnea. I.V. infusion of benzodiazepines, such as diazepam, may cause respiratory depression and apnea when given with other CNS depressants, especially in elderly or acutely ill patients. Neuromuscular blocking agents—such as curariform drugs (especially when given concomitantly with aminoglycosides) and anticholinesterase inhibitors—may produce sudden apnea due to respiratory muscle paralysis.

Causes of Apnea

Airway obstruction
- Airway edema
- Airway occlusion by tongue
- Airway occlusion by tumor
- Asthma
- Bronchospasm
- Chronic bronchitis
- Diffuse atelectasis
- Foreign body aspiration
- Hemothorax or pneumothorax
- Mucous plugging
- Obstructive sleep apnea
- Secretion retention
- Tracheal/bronchial rupture

Alveolar gas diffusion impairment
- Adult respiratory distress syndrome
- Diffuse pneumonia
- Emphysema
- Near-drowning
- Pulmonary edema
- Pulmonary fibrosis
- Secretion retention

Brain stem dysfunction
- Brain abscess
- Brain stem injury
- Brain tumor
- Cerebral hemorrhage
- Cerebral infarction

- Encephalitis
- Head trauma
- Hypoventilatory sleep apnea
- Increased intracranial pressure
- Meningitis
- Pontine/medullary hemorrhage or infarction
- Transtentorial herniation

Pleural pressure gradient disruption
- Flail chest
- Open chest wounds

Pulmonary capillary perfusion decrease
- Cardiac arrest
- Dysrhythmias
- Myocardial infarction
- Pulmonary embolism
- Pulmonary hypertension
- Shock

Respiratory muscle failure
- Amyotrophic lateral sclerosis
- Botulism
- Diphtheria
- Guillain-Barré syndrome
- Myasthenia gravis
- Phrenic nerve paralysis
- Rupture of the diaphragm
- Spinal cord injury

Clinical considerations
- When apnea is detected, the first priority is to establish and maintain a patent airway.
- Cardiopulmonary resuscitation should be initiated if spontaneous respirations do not occur with reestablishment of a patent airway and if a pulse is not palpated.

Once the patient's respiratory and cardiac status is stable:
- A history should be taken and a complete physical examination performed.
- The apneic patient's cardiac and respiratory status should be monitored closely to prevent further apneic episodes.

Apneustic respirations

Description
This irregular breathing pattern is characterized by prolonged, gasping inspiration and brief, inefficient expiration. It is an important localizing sign of severe brain stem damage.

Apneustic respirations must be differentiated from bradypnea and hyperpnea (disturbances in rate and depth, but not in rhythm), Cheyne-Stokes respirations (rhythmic alterations in rate and depth, followed by periods of apnea), and Biot's respirations (irregularly alternating periods of hyperpnea and apnea).

Mechanism

Involuntary breathing is primarily regulated by groups of neurons, or respiratory centers, in the medulla oblongata and the pons. In the medulla, neurons react to impulses from the pons and other areas to regulate respiratory rate and depth. In the pons, two respiratory centers regulate respiratory rhythm by interacting with the medullary respiratory center to smooth the transition from inspiration to expiration and back. The apneustic center in the pons stimulates inspiratory neurons in the medulla to precipitate inspiration. These inspiratory neurons, in turn, stimulate the pneumotaxic center in the pons to precipitate expiration. Destruction of neural pathways by pontine lesions disrupts regulation of respiratory rhythm, causing apneustic respirations.

Possible causes

Central nervous system

Pontine lesions. Apneustic respirations invariably result from extensive damage to the upper or lower pons, whether due to infarction, hemorrhage, herniation, severe infection, tumor, or trauma. Typically they are accompanied by profound stupor or coma; pinpoint midline pupils; ocular bobbing (a spontaneous downward jerk, followed by a slow drift up to midline); quadriplegia or, less commonly, hemiplegia with pupils pointing toward the affected side; a positive Babinski's reflex; negative oculocephalic and oculovestibular reflexes; and, possibly, decorticate posture.

Clinical considerations

- Adequate ventilation should be ensured as the first priority.
- The physician should be notified immediately and mechanical ventilation anticipated.

- Emergency equipment should be kept on hand and cardiopulmonary resuscitation initiated, if necessary.
- A brief history should be obtained from a family member or friend, if possible, and a neurologic assessment performed.
- Diagnostic tests may include electroencephalography and computed tomography.
- The patient's neurologic, respiratory, and arterial blood gas status should be monitored constantly.
- The physician should be notified immediately of prolonged apneic periods or signs of neurologic deterioration.

Apraxia

Description

Apraxia is the inability to perform purposeful movements in the absence of significant weakness, sensory loss, poor coordination, or lack of comprehension or motivation. This uncommon neurologic sign usually indicates a lesion in the cerebral cortex. Its onset, severity, and duration vary, depending on the location and extent of the lesion.

Apraxia is classified as *ideational, ideomotor,* or *kinetic,* depending on the stage at which voluntary movement is impaired (see *How Apraxia Interferes with Purposeful Movement,* p. 34). It can also be classified by type of motor or skill impairment. For example, *facial* and *gait* apraxia involve specific motor groups and are easily perceived. *Constructional* apraxia refers to the inability to copy simple drawings or patterns. *Dressing* apraxia refers to the inability to dress oneself correctly. *Callosal* apraxia refers to normal motor function on one side of the body accompanied by the inability to reproduce movements on the other side.

Possible causes

Central nervous system

Alzheimer's disease. This disorder sometimes causes gradual and irreversible ideomotor apraxia.

Brain abscess. Apraxia occasionally results from a large brain abscess but usually resolves spontaneously after the infection subsides. Typically, its type depends on the location of the abscess. The apraxia is accompanied by headache, fever, drowsiness, decreased mental acuity, aphasia, dysarthria, hemiparesis, focal or generalized seizures, and ocular disturbances such as nystagmus, decreased visual acuity, and unequal pupils.

Brain tumor. In this disorder, progressive apraxia may be preceded by decreased mental acuity, headache, dizziness, and seizures. It may occur with or directly after early signs of increased intracranial pressure, such as pupil changes. It may also occur with other localizing signs of the tumor, such as aphasia, visual field deficits, weakness, stiffness, and hyperreflexia in the extremities.

Cerebrovascular accident (CVA). This disorder commonly causes sudden onset of apraxia. Although apraxia often resolves spontaneously, it may persist after massive CVA.

Hepatic encephalopathy. This disorder may cause gradual onset of constructional apraxia, which may be reversible with treatment.

Treatments

Long-term hemodialysis occasionally causes a syndrome known as dialysis

---

How Apraxia Interferes with Purposeful Movement

Type of Apraxia	Description	Assessment Technique
Ideational apraxia	The patient can physically perform the steps required to complete a task but fails to remember the sequence in which they are performed.	The patient is asked to tie his shoelace. Typically, he will be able to grasp the shoelace, loop it, and pull on it. However, he will fail to remember the sequence of steps needed to tie a knot.
Ideomotor apraxia	The patient understands and can physically perform the steps required to complete a task but cannot formulate a plan to carry them out.	The patient is asked to wave or cross his arms. Typically, he will not respond. Later, he will be able to perform the gesture spontaneously.
Kinetic apraxia	The patient understands the task and formulates a plan but fails to set the proper muscles in motion.	The patient is asked to comb his hair. Typically, he will fail to move his arm and hand correctly to do so. However, he will be able to state that he needs to pick up the comb and draw it through his hair.

dementia or dialysis encephalopathy. In this syndrome, speech apraxia accompanies other speech deficits, seizures, and behavioral changes.

Clinical considerations

• A history should be obtained and a neurologic assessment performed. Signs of increased intracranial pressure should be noted during the assessment and emergency equipment kept nearby.

• Emergency interventions, as appropriate, should be carried out if the patient has seizure activity.

• When appropriate, the apraxia should be assessed further to help determine its type.

• Diagnostic studies may include computed tomography and a radionuclide brain scan.

• Because weakness, sensory deficits, confusion, and seizures may accompany apraxia, measures should be taken to ensure safety. For example, the patient with gait apraxia should be assisted in walking.

• The patient's apraxia should be explained to him, and he should be encouraged to participate in normal activities.

• To help him overcome his frustrations at being unable to perform routine tasks, each step in these tasks should be demonstrated and the patient given sufficient time to imitate each step.

• Complex directions should be avoided and the help of family members enlisted in rehabilitation.

• The patient should also be referred to a physical or occupational therapist, if appropriate.

Argyll Robertson pupil

Description

An Argyll Robertson pupil is a small, irregular pupil that constricts normally in accommodation for near vision, but poorly or not at all in response to light. Response to mydriatic drugs also is poor or absent. This condition may be unilateral or bilateral and most commonly results from chronic syphilitic meningitis or other forms of late syphilis.

Arthralgia

Description

Arthralgia is joint pain. This symptom may have no pathologic importance or may indicate such disorders as arthritis or systemic lupus erythematosus.

Asthenocoria

Description

Asthenocoria is slow dilation or constriction of the pupils in response to light changes. Photophobia may be present if constriction occurs slowly. Asthenocoria occurs in adrenal insufficiency.

Asterixis
(Liver flap, flapping tremor)

Description

Asterixis is a bilateral, coarse tremor characterized by rapid, nonrhythmic extensions and flexions. This elicited sign is most commonly observed in the wrists and fingers but also appears in the ankles, the corners of the mouth, the eyelids, and the tongue. Typically, it signals the onset of coma in end-stage hepatic, renal, and pulmonary disease.

To elicit asterixis, the examiner asks the patient to extend his arms, dorsiflex his wrists, and spread his fingers (or she may do this for him, if necessary). Briefly, she then observes for asterixis. Alternatively, if the patient has a decreased level of consciousness but can follow verbal commands, the examiner asks him to squeeze two of her fingers. Rapid clutching and unclutching indicates asterixis. Or the examiner may elevate the patient's leg off the bed and dorsiflex the foot, then briefly observe for asterixis in the ankle. If the patient can tightly close his eyes and mouth, the examiner observes for irregular, tremulous movements of the eyelids and corners of the mouth. If he can stick out his tongue, she observes for continuous quivering.

Possible causes
Central nervous system
Hepatic encephalopathy. This life-threatening disorder initially causes slight personality changes (disorientation, forgetfulness, slurred speech) and a slight tremor. This tremor progresses into asterixis—the hallmark of hepatic encephalopathy—and is accompanied by lethargy, aberrant behavior, and apraxia.
Respiratory
Severe respiratory insufficiency. Characterized by life-threatening respiratory acidosis, this disorder initially produces headache, restlessness, confusion, apprehension, and decreased reflexes. Eventually, the patient becomes somnolent and may demonstrate asterixis before slipping into coma.
Genitourinary
Uremic syndrome. This life-threatening disorder initially causes lethargy, somnolence, confusion, disorientation, behavior changes, and irritability. Eventually, though, signs and symptoms appear in diverse body systems. Asterixis is accompanied by stupor, paresthesias, muscle twitching, fasciculations, and foot drop.

Clinical considerations
• Because asterixis usually signals impending coma, neurologic and respiratory status should be monitored closely.
• Endotracheal intubation should be performed and ventilatory support provided, if necessary.

• Patient comfort should be maintained.
• Emotional support should be provided to the patient and his family.

Asynergy

Description
Asynergy is impaired coordination of muscles or organs that normally function harmoniously. This extrapyramidal symptom stems from disorders of the basal ganglia and cerebellum.

Ataxia

Description
Ataxia refers to incoordination and irregularity of voluntary, purposeful movements. It may be classified as cerebellar or sensory.

Cerebellar ataxia results from disease of the cerebellum and its pathways to and from the cerebral cortex, brain stem, and spinal cord. It causes gait, trunk, limb, and possibly speech disorders. *Sensory ataxia* results from impaired position sense (proprioception) caused by interruption of afferent nerve fibers in the peripheral nerves, posterior roots, posterior columns of the spinal cord, or medial lemnisci, or occasionally by a lesion in both parietal lobes. It causes gait disorders.

Ataxia also occurs in acute and chronic forms. *Acute ataxia,* usually cerebellar, may result from hemorrhage or a large tumor in the posterior fossa. In this life-threatening condition, the cerebellum may herniate downward through the foramen magnum behind the cervical spinal cord or upward through the tentorium upon the cerebral hemispheres. Herniation may also compress the brain stem. Acute ataxia may also result from drug toxicity or poisoning. *Chronic ataxia* can be progressive and, at times, can result from acute disease. It can also occur in metabolic and chronic degenerative neurologic disease.

Possible causes
Central nervous system
Behçet's disease. This rare, chronic meningitis causes cerebellar ataxia. It is accompanied by focal neurologic signs, such as cranial nerve palsy, mental disturbances, aphasia, and hemiparesis.

Cerebellar abscess. This disorder commonly causes limb ataxia on the side opposite the lesion, as well as gait and truncal ataxia.

Cerebellar hemorrhage. In this life-threatening disorder, ataxia usually occurs acutely but is transient. Unilateral or bilateral ataxia affects the trunk, gait, or limbs.

Cerebrovascular accident (CVA). In this life-threatening disorder, occlusions in the vertebrobasilar arteries cause infarction in the medulla, pons, or cerebellum that may lead to ataxia. The ataxia may occur at the onset of CVA and remain as a residual deficit. Worsening ataxia during the acute phase may indicate extension of the CVA. The ataxia may be accompanied by unilateral or bilateral motor weakness, possible altered level of consciousness, sensory loss, vertigo, nausea, vomiting, ocular motor palsy, and dysphagia.

Cranial trauma. This disorder rarely produces ataxia. Usually it is unilateral; bilateral ataxia suggests traumatic hemorrhage.

Diabetic neuropathy. Peripheral nerve damage caused by diabetes mellitus may cause sensory ataxia as well as extremity pain, slight leg weakness, skin changes, and bowel and bladder dysfunction.

Encephalomyelitis. This complication of measles, smallpox, chicken pox, or rubella, or of rabies or smallpox vaccination may damage cerebrospinal white matter. Rarely, it is accompanied by cerebellar ataxia.

Identifying Ataxia

Ataxia may be observed in the patient's speech, in the movements of his trunk and limbs, or in his gait.

In **speech ataxia,** a form of dysarthria, the patient typically speaks slowly and stresses usually unstressed words and syllables. Speech content is not affected.

In **truncal ataxia,** a disturbance in equilibrium, the patient cannot sit or stand without falling. Also, his head and trunk may bob and sway (titubation). If he is able to walk, his gait is reeling.

In **limb ataxia,** the patient loses the ability to gauge distance, speed, and power of movement, resulting in poorly controlled, variable, and inaccurate voluntary movements. He may move too quickly or too slowly, or his movements may break down into component parts, giving him the appearance of a puppet or a robot. Other effects include a coarse, irregular tremor in purposeful movement (but not at rest) and weak, flaccid muscles.

In **gait ataxia,** the patient's gait is wide-based, unsteady, and irregular. In cerebellar ataxia, the patient may stagger or lurch in zigzag fashion, turn with extreme difficulty, and lose his balance when his feet are together. In sensory ataxia, the patient moves abruptly and stomps or taps his feet. This occurs because he throws his feet forward and outward, then brings them down first on the heels, then on the toes. The patient also fixes his eyes on the ground, watching his steps. However, if he is unable to watch them, staggering worsens. When he stands with his feet together and eyes closed, he sways.

Friedreich's ataxia. This progressive familial disorder affects the spinal cord and cerebellum. It causes gait ataxia, followed by truncal, limb, and speech ataxia.

Guillain-Barré syndrome. Peripheral nerve involvement usually follows mild viral infection, rarely leading to sensory ataxia.

Hepatocerebral degeneration. Patients who survive hepatic coma are occasionally left with residual neurologic defects, including a mild cerebellar ataxia with a wide-based, unsteady gait. The ataxia may be accompanied by altered level of consciousness, dysarthria, rhythmic arm tremors, and choreoathetosis of the face, neck, and shoulders.

Hyperthermia. In this disorder, cerebellar ataxia occurs if the patient survives the coma and convulsions characteristic of the acute phase.

Multiple sclerosis. Nystagmus and cerebellar ataxia often occur in this disorder, but they are not always accompanied by limb weakness and spasticity. Speech ataxia (especially scanning) may occur, as well as sensory ataxia from spinal cord involvement. During remissions, ataxia may subside or even disappear. During exacerbations, it may worsen or even become permanent.

Olivopontocerebellar atrophy. This disease produces gait ataxia and, later, limb and speech ataxia.

Polyneuropathy. Carcinomatous and myelomatous polyneuropathy may occur before detection of the primary tumor in carcinoma, multiple myeloma, or Hodgkin's disease. Signs and symptoms include ataxia, severe motor weakness, muscle atrophy, and sensory loss in the limbs.

Posterior fossa tumor. Gait, truncal, or limb ataxia is an early sign of this tumor and may worsen as the tumor enlarges. It is accompanied by vomiting (the most common sign), headache, papilledema, vertigo, ocular motor palsy, decreased level of consciousness, and motor and sensory impairments.

Spinocerebellar ataxia. In this disorder, the patient may initially experience fatigue, followed by stiff-legged gait ataxia. Eventually, limb ataxia, dysarthria, static tremor, nystagmus, cramps, paresthesias, and sensory deficits occur.

Syringomyelia. This chronic degenerative disorder may cause a mixed spastic-ataxic gait.

Tabes dorsalis. This rare syndrome appears 25 to 30 years after syphilitic infection. Sensory ataxia, a major sign, is accompanied by paresthesia, sensory deficits, incontinence, impotence, trophic joint degeneration, optic atrophy, pupillary changes, and sharp, stabbing, and brief pain.

Cardiovascular

Polyarteritis nodosa. Acute or subacute polyarteritis may cause sensory ataxia.

Endocrine

Hypothyroidism. Rarely, cerebellar ataxia may occur as the chief sign in this disorder. It is accompanied by lethargy, constipation, cold intolerance, dry skin, menorrhagia, and other signs.

Hematologic

Porphyria. This disorder affects the sensory and, more frequently, the motor nerves, possibly leading to ataxia.

Metabolic

Pellagra. This rare disorder associated with niacin deficiency may cause sensory ataxia, photosensitive dermatitis, dementia, and diarrhea.

Wernicke's disease. The result of thiamine deficiency, this disease produces gait ataxia and, rarely, intention tremor or speech ataxia. In severe ataxia, the patient may be unable to stand or walk. Ataxia decreases with thiamine therapy.

Infectious diseases

Diphtheria. Within 4 to 8 weeks of the onset of symptoms, a life-threatening neuropathy can produce sensory ataxia.

Neoplastic

Metastatic carcinoma. Carcinoma that metastasizes to the cerebellum may cause gait ataxia accompanied by headache, dizziness, nystagmus, decreased level of consciousness, nausea, and vomiting.

Environmental

Poisoning. Chronic *arsenic* poisoning may cause sensory ataxia.

Drugs

Toxic levels of anticonvulsants, especially phenytoin, may result in gait ataxia. Toxic levels of anticholinergics and tricyclic antidepressants may also result in ataxia. Aminoglutethimide causes ataxia in about 10% of patients; however, this effect usually disappears 4 to 6 weeks after cessation of drug therapy.

Clinical considerations

• A neurologic assessment should be performed immediately, with special attention to signs of increased intracranial pressure and impending brain herniation.
• The physician should be notified of assessment findings.
• Emergency equipment should be kept close by.
  If the patient is not in distress:
• A history should be obtained.
• The type of ataxia should be identified. (See *Identifying Ataxia,* page 37.)
• The Romberg test may be performed to distinguish between cerebellar and sensory ataxia.
• Diagnostic tests may include laboratory studies, such as blood tests for toxic drug levels, and radiologic tests, such as computed tomography and brain scans.
• Ongoing care should focus on helping the patient adapt to his condition.
• The goals of rehabilitation should be promoted, and the patient's safety ensured in the hospital and home.
• The patient with progressive disease should be referred for counseling, if appropriate.

Athetosis

Description

Athetosis is an extrapyramidal sign characterized by slow, continuous, and twisting involuntary movements. Typically, these movements involve the face, neck, and distal extremities, such as the forearm, wrist, and hand. Facial grimaces, jaw and tongue movements, and occasional phonation are associated with neck movements. Athetosis worsens during stress and voluntary activity, may subside during relaxation, and may even disappear during sleep. Commonly a lifelong affliction, athetosis is sometimes difficult to distinguish from chorea (hence the term *choreoathetosis*). Typically, though, athetoid movements are slower than choreiform movements.

Athetosis most often begins during childhood, resulting from hypoxia at birth, kernicterus, or genetic disorders. In adults, athetosis most commonly results from vascular or neoplastic lesions, degenerative disease, or drug toxicity.

Possible causes

Central nervous system

Brain tumor. This disorder affects the basal ganglia, causing contralateral choreoathetosis and dystonia.

Calcification of the basal ganglia. This unilateral or bilateral disorder is characterized by choreoathetosis and rigidity. Usually, it arises in adolescence or early adult life.

Cerebral infarction. In this disorder, contralateral athetosis is accompanied by altered level of consciousness. The patient may also display contralateral paralysis of the face or limbs.

Hepatic encephalopathy. Episodic or persistent choreoathetosis occurs in the chronic stage of this encephalopathy. It is accompanied by cerebellar ataxia, myoclonus of the face and limbs, asterixis, dysarthria, and dementia.

Huntington's disease. In this hereditary degenerative disease, athetosis and chorea progressively develop in early or middle adult life. Accompanying signs and symptoms include dystonia, dysarthria, facial apraxia, rigidity, depression, and progressive mental deterioration leading to dementia.

Pick's disease. This rare degenerative disease occasionally causes mild athetosis accompanied by dementia (its chief sign) and dysphagia.

Metabolic

Wilson's disease. In this inherited metabolic disorder, choreoathetoid movements initially involve the fingers and hands and then spread to the arms, head, trunk, and legs.

Drugs

Toxic levels of levodopa and phenytoin may cause athetoid or choreoathetoid movements.

Phenothiazines and other antipsychotic drugs may also cause athetosis. The piperazine derivatives, such as acetophenazine and prochlorperazine, frequently cause it. The aliphatic phenothiazines, such as chlorpromazine and triflupromazine, occasionally cause it. A third derivative, the piperidine phenothiazines, such as thioridazine and piperacetazine, rarely cause it. Other antipsychotics—such as haloperidol, thiothixene, and loxapine—frequently cause athetosis.

Clinical considerations

• A complete history, including a family history, should be obtained and a neurologic assessment performed.

• Diagnostic tests may include urine and blood studies, lumbar puncture, electroencephalography, and computed tomography scan.

• Occasionally, athetosis can be prevented or treated (by decreasing body copper stores in Wilson's disease or by adjusting drug dosages). Typically, though, it has a lifelong impact on the patient's ability to carry out even routine activities; the patient must be given help in adapting to his condition.

• Assistive devices should be provided to help the patient carry out fine motor tasks.

• The patient should be encouraged in his rehabilitation program; swimming, stretching, and balance and gait exercises help maintain coordination, slow deterioration, and minimize antisocial behavior.

• The patient and his family should be encouraged to discuss their feelings about athetosis and its cause.

• The patient should be referred to a self-help group and appropriate support services, such as physical therapy, as necessary.

Aura

Description

An aura is a sensory or motor phenomenon that marks the initial stage of a seizure or the approach of a classic migraine headache. It may be classified as cognitive, affective, psychosensory, or psychomotor (see *Recognizing Types of Aura*).

Mechanism

When associated with a seizure, an aura stems from an irritable focus in the brain that spreads throughout the cortex.

The aura associated with classic migraine headache results from cranial vasoconstriction.

Possible causes

Central nervous system

Classic migraine headache. This disorder is preceded by a vague premonition and then, usually, a visual aura involving flashes of light. The aura develops over 10 to 30 minutes and may intensify until it completely obscures the patient's vision. Diagnostically important, it helps distinguish classic migraine from other types of headache. If the patient recognizes the aura as a warning sign, he may be able to prevent the headache by taking appropriate drugs.

Seizure. Although an aura was once considered a sign of impending seizure, it is now considered *an actual stage* of a seizure. Typically, it occurs seconds to minutes before the ictal phase. Its intensity, duration, and type depend on the origin of the irritable focus. For example, an aura of bitter taste often accompanies a frontal lobe lesion. Unfortunately, an aura is difficult to describe because the postictal phase of a seizure temporarily alters the patient's level of consciousness, impairing his memory of the event.

Clinical considerations

When an aura rapidly progresses to the ictal phase of a seizure:

• The seizure should be observed and the patient protected from harm.

• The physician should be notified.

When an aura heralds a classic migraine:

• The patient should be made as comfortable as possible and drugs administered, as ordered.

• Later, a thorough history of the migraines should be obtained.

• The patient should be advised to keep a diary of factors that precipitate each seizure or headache as well as associated symptoms to evaluate the effectiveness of drug therapy and recommended life-style changes. Measures to reduce stress frequently play a role here.

Autistic behavior

Description

Autistic behavior is exaggerated self-centered behavior marked by a lack of responsiveness to other people. It is characterized by highly personalized speech and actions that are not meaningful to an observer. For example, the patient may rock his body or repeat-

---

Recognizing Types of Aura

Determining whether an aura marks the patient's thought processes, emotions, or sensory or motor function frequently requires keen nursing assessment. An aura is typically difficult to describe and is only dimly remembered when associated with seizure activity. Among the types of aura the patient may experience are:

Cognitive Auras

Déjà vu (familiarity with unfamiliar events or environments)
Jamais vu (unfamiliarity with a known event)
Time standing still
Flashback of past events

Affective Auras

Fear
Paranoia
Other emotions

Psychosensory Auras

Visual: flashes of light, or scintillations
Olfactory: foul odors
Gustatory: acidic, metallic, or bitter tastes
Auditory: buzzing or ringing in the ears
Tactile: numbness or tingling
Vertigo

Psychomotor Auras

Automatisms (inappropriate, repetitive movements): lip smacking, chewing, swallowing, grimacing, picking at clothes, climbing stairs

---

edly bang his head against the floor or wall. Autistic behavior may occur in schizophrenic children and adults.

B

Babinski's reflex
(Extensor plantar reflex)

Description

Babinski's reflex—dorsiflexion of the great toe with extension and fanning of the other toes—is an abnormal reflex elicited by firmly stroking the sole of the foot. In some patients, this reflex can be triggered by noxious stimuli, such as pain, noise, or even bumping of the bed. It indicates corticospinal damage and helps differentiate neurologic and metabolic coma. Because the corticospinal tract is right- and left-sided, Babinski's reflex may occur unilaterally or bilaterally. It may also be temporary or permanent. A temporary Babinski's reflex commonly occurs during the postictal phase of a seizure, whereas a permanent Babinski's reflex occurs with irreparable corticospinal damage.

Babinski's reflex occurs normally in children under age 2 and reflects immaturity of the corticospinal tract.

Possible causes

Central nervous system

Amyotrophic lateral sclerosis. In this progressive motor neuron disorder, bilateral Babinski's reflex may occur with hyperactive deep tendon reflexes and spasticity.

Brain tumor. When it involves the corticospinal tract or the cerebellum, a brain tumor may produce Babinski's reflex unilaterally or bilaterally.

Cerebrovascular accident (CVA). Babinski's reflex varies with the site of the CVA. If the CVA involves the cerebrum, it produces unilateral Babinski's reflex accompanied by hemiplegia or hemiparesis, unilateral hyperactive deep tendon reflexes, hemianopia, and aphasia. If it involves the brain stem, it produces bilateral Babinski's reflex accompanied by bilateral weakness or paralysis, bilateral hyperactive deep tendon reflexes, cranial nerve dysfunction, incoordination, and unsteady gait.

Familial spastic paralysis. This disorder may produce bilateral Babinski's reflex accompanied by hyperactive deep tendon reflexes and progressive spasticity with ataxia and weakness.

Friedreich's ataxia. This disorder may produce bilateral Babinski's reflex.

Head trauma. Unilateral or bilateral Babinski's reflex may occur here—the result of primary corticospinal damage or secondary injury associated with increased intracranial pressure. Hyperactive deep tendon reflexes and spasticity commonly occur with Babinski's reflex. Occasionally, the patient also has weakness and incoordination.

Hepatic encephalopathy. Babinski's reflex occurs late in this disorder when the patient slips into a coma. It is accompanied by hyperactive reflexes and fetor hepaticus.

Meningitis. Bilateral Babinski's reflex commonly occurs in this infection. It is preceded by fever, chills, and malaise and accompanied by nausea and vomiting.

Eliciting Babinski's Reflex

To elicit Babinski's reflex, the examiner strokes the lateral aspect of the sole of the patient's foot with the thumbnail or another moderately sharp object. Normally, this elicits flexion of all toes (a negative Babinski's reflex), as shown at left. In a positive Babinski's reflex, the great toe dorsiflexes and the other toes fan out, as shown at right.

Negative Babinski's Reflex

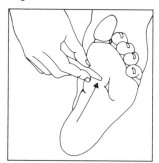

Positive Babinski's Reflex

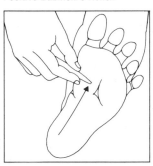

Multiple sclerosis (MS). In most patients with this demyelinating disorder, Babinski's reflex occurs bilaterally. It follows initial signs and symptoms of MS.

Spinal cord injury. In acute injury, spinal shock temporarily erases all reflexes. As shock resolves, Babinski's reflex occurs—unilaterally when injury affects only one side of the spinal cord (Brown-Séquard syndrome), bilaterally when injury affects both sides. Rather than signaling the return of neurologic function, this reflex confirms corticospinal damage.

Spinal cord tumor. In this disorder, bilateral Babinski's reflex occurs with variable loss of pain and temperature sensation, proprioception, and motor function.

Spinal paralytic poliomyelitis. Unilateral or bilateral Babinski's reflex occurs 5 to 7 days after the onset of fever in this disorder. It is accompanied by progressive weakness, paresthesias,

muscle tenderness, spasticity, irritability, and, later, atrophy.

Spinal tuberculosis. This disorder may produce bilateral Babinski's reflex accompanied by variable loss of pain and temperature sensation, proprioception, and motor function.

Syringomyelia. In this disorder, bilateral Babinski's reflex occurs with muscle atrophy and weakness that may progress to paralysis. It is accompanied by spasticity, ataxia, and, occasionally, deep pain.

Metabolic

Pernicious anemia. Bilateral Babinski's reflex occurs late in this disorder when vitamin B_{12} deficiency affects the central nervous system.

Environmental

Rabies. Bilateral Babinski's reflex—possibly elicited by nonspecific noxious stimuli alone—appears in the excitation phase of rabies. This phase occurs 2 to 10 days after the onset of prodromal symptoms, such as fever, malaise, and irritability. (These symptoms occur 30 to 40 days after an animal bite.) It is characterized by marked restlessness and extremely painful pharyngeal muscle spasms. Difficulty swallowing causes excessive drooling and hydrophobia in about 50% of affected patients. Seizures and hyperactive deep tendon reflexes may also occur.

Clinical considerations
• A complete neurologic assessment should be performed after a positive Babinski's reflex has been elicited and the physician should be notified of any changes in neurologic status.
• A computed tomography scan of the brain or spine, an angiogram or myelogram, or possibly a lumbar puncture may be done to clarify or confirm the cause of Babinski's reflex.
• Typically, Babinski's reflex is accompanied by incoordination, weakness, and spasticity, all of which increase the patient's risk of injury. Consequently, the patient should be assisted with activity, especially ambulation, and his environment kept hazard free.

Ballance's sign

Description
Ballance's sign is a fixed mass or area of dullness found by palpation and percussion of the left upper quadrant of the abdomen. It may indicate subcapsular or extracapsular hematoma following splenic rupture.

Ballet's sign

Description
Ballet's sign is ophthalmoplegia, or paralysis of the external ocular muscles. The patient displays no control of voluntary eye movement but has normal reflexive movement and pupillary light reflexes. This sign is an indicator of thyrotoxicosis.

Bárány's symptom

Description
Bárány's symptom is rotary nystagmus toward the irrigated side with warm water irrigation of the ear or rotary nystagmus away from the irrigated side with cold water irrigation. Absence of this symptom indicates labyrinthine dysfunction.

Barlow's sign

Description
Barlow's sign is an indicator of congenital dislocation of the hip, detected in the first 6 weeks of life. To elicit this sign, the examiner places the infant supine with the hips flexed 90° and the knees fully flexed. Then she places a palm over the infant's knee, with the thumb in the femoral triangle opposite the lesser trochanter, and the index finger over the greater trochanter. She then brings the hip into midabduction while gently exerting posterior and lateral pressure with the thumb and posterior and medial pressure with the palm. A click heard as the femoral head dislocates across the posterior lip of the acetabular socket indicates that Barlow's sign is present.

Barrel chest

Description
In barrel chest, the normal elliptical configuration of the chest is replaced by a rounded one in which the anteroposterior diameter enlarges to approximate the transverse diameter. The diaphragm is depressed and the sternum pushed forward with the ribs at-

tached in a horizontal, not angular, fashion. As a result, the chest appears continuously in the inspiratory position.

Typically a late sign of chronic obstructive pulmonary disease (COPD), barrel chest may go unnoticed by the patient because of its gradual development. In the elderly, senile kyphosis of the thoracic spine may be mistaken for barrel chest. However, unlike barrel chest, senile kyphosis lacks signs of pulmonary disease.

Mechanism

Barrel chest results from augmented lung volumes due to chronic airflow obstruction.

Possible causes

Respiratory
Asthma. Typically, barrel chest develops only in chronic asthma.
Chronic bronchitis. A late sign in chronic bronchitis, barrel chest is characteristically preceded by productive cough and exertional dyspnea.
Emphysema. In this form of COPD, barrel chest is also a late sign. Typically, the disorder begins insidiously, with dyspnea the predominant symptom.

Clinical considerations

• A respiratory assessment should be performed.
• Respiratory status should be monitored and the physician notified of changes.
• Chest X-rays and arterial blood gas determinations may be done.
• The patient should be advised to avoid bronchial irritants—especially cigarette smoke, which may exacerbate COPD; to notify the physician of purulent sputum production, which may indicate upper respiratory infection; and to rest between activities to minimize exertional dyspnea.
• To ease breathing, the patient should be advised to sit and lean forward, resting his hands on his knees to support the upper torso (tripod position). This position allows maximum diaphragmatic excursion, facilitating chest expansion.

Barré's pyramidal sign

Description

Barré's pyramidal sign is the inability to hold the lower legs still with the knees flexed. To detect this sign, the examiner places the patient prone and flexes his knees 90°. Then she asks him to hold his lower legs still. If he cannot maintain this position, this sign of pyramidal tract disease is present.

Barré's sign

Description

Barré's sign is delayed contraction of the iris, seen in mental deterioration.

Battle's sign

Description

Battle's sign is ecchymosis over the mastoid process of the temporal bone. It is often the only outward sign of basilar skull fracture. In fact, this type of fracture may go undetected by skull X-rays. If left untreated, it can be fatal because of associated injury to the nearby cranial nerves and brain stem as well as to blood vessels and the meninges.

Appearing behind one or both ears, Battle's sign is easily overlooked or even hidden by the patient's hair. Also, during emergency care of the trauma victim, it may be overshadowed by imminently life-threatening or more apparent injuries.

Mechanism

Force exerted on the head great enough to fracture the base of the skull causes Battle's sign by damaging supporting tissues of the mastoid area. Or the sign may result from seepage of blood from the fracture site to the mastoid.

Possible causes
Central nervous system

Basilar skull fracture. Battle's sign may be the only outward sign of this fracture. Or it may be accompanied by periorbital ecchymosis (raccoon eyes), conjunctival hemorrhage, nystagmus, ocular deviation, epistaxis, anosmia, a bulging tympanic membrane (from CSF or blood accumulation), visible fracture lines on the external auditory canal, tinnitus, hearing difficulty, facial paralysis, and vertigo.

Battle's sign usually develops 24 to 36 hours after the fracture and may persist for several days to weeks.

Clinical considerations
• Battle's sign should be reported to the physician immediately.
• A history should be obtained and a complete neurologic assessment performed.
• Skull X-rays and a computed tomography scan may be done to help confirm basilar skull fracture and to evaluate the severity of head injury.
• The patient's neurologic status should be monitored closely.

Beau's lines

Description
Beau's lines are transverse linear depressions on the fingernails. These lines may develop after any severe illness or toxic reaction. Other common causes include malnutrition, nail bed trauma, and coronary artery occlusion.

Beevor's sign

Description
Beevor's sign is upward movement of the umbilicus upon contraction of the abdominal muscles. To detect this sign, which is an indicator of paralysis of the lower recti abdominis muscles associated with lesions at T10, the examiner positions the patient supine, then asks him to sit up. This sign is present if the umbilicus moves upward.

Bell's sign

Description
Bell's sign is reflexive upward and outward deviation of the eyes that occurs when the patient attempts to close his eyes. It occurs on the affected side in Bell's palsy and indicates that the defect is supranuclear.

Bezold's sign

Description
Bezold's sign is swelling and tenderness of the mastoid area. Resulting from formation of an abscess beneath the sternocleidomastoid muscle, Bezold's sign indicates mastoiditis.

Biot's respirations

Description
A late and ominous sign of neurologic deterioration, Biot's respirations are characterized by breaths of equal volume interrupted by irregular periods of apnea. This rare breathing pattern may appear abruptly and reflects increased pressure on the medulla coinciding with brain stem herniation.

Bitot's spots

Description
Bitot's spots are white or foamy gray superficial spots, varying from a few

bubbles to a frothy white coating. Appearing on the conjunctiva at the lateral margin of the cornea, they are associated with vitamin A deficiency.

Blepharoclonus

Description
Blepharoclonus is excessive blinking of the eyes. This extrapyramidal sign occurs with disorders of the basal ganglia and cerebellum.

Blocking

Description
Blocking is a cognitive disturbance resulting in interruption of a stream of speech or thought. It usually occurs in midsentence or before completion of a thought. Generally, the patient is unable to explain the interruption. Blocking may occur in normal individuals but most commonly occurs in schizophrenics.

Blood pressure, decreased
(Hypotension)

Description
Decreased or low blood pressure refers to blood pressure inadequate to perfuse or oxygenate the body's tissues. Although commonly linked to shock, this sign may also result from cardiovascular, respiratory, neurologic, and metabolic disorders. Low blood pressure may be drug-induced or may accompany diagnostic tests—most often, those using contrast media. It may stem from stress or change of position—specifically, rising abruptly from a supine or sitting position to a standing position (postural hypotension).

Normal blood pressure varies considerably; what may qualify as low blood pressure for one person may be perfectly normal for another. Consequently, every blood pressure reading must be compared against the patient's baseline. Typically, a reading below 90/60 mm Hg or a drop of 30 mm Hg from the baseline is considered low blood pressure.

Mechanism
Low blood pressure can reflect an expanded intravascular space (as in vasodilatation), a reduced intravascular volume (as in dehydration and hemorrhage), or a decreased cardiac output (as in impaired cardiac muscle contractility). Because the body's pressure-regulating mechanisms are complex and interrelated, a combination of these factors usually contributes to low blood pressure.

Possible causes
Respiratory
Pulmonary embolism. This disorder causes sudden chest pain and dyspnea accompanied by cyanosis and, occasionally, fever. Low blood pressure occurs with narrowed pulse pressure and diminished Korotkoff sounds.
Cardiovascular
Anaphylactic shock. Following exposure to an allergen, such as penicillin or insect venom, a dramatic fall in blood pressure and narrowed pulse pressure signal this severe allergic reaction.

Cardiac contusion. In this disorder, low blood pressure occurs along with tachycardia and, at times, anginal pain and dyspnea.

Cardiac dysrhythmias. In dysrhythmias, blood pressure may fluctuate between normal and low readings.

Cardiac tamponade. An accentuated fall in systolic pressure (greater than 10 mm Hg) during inspiration, known as pulsus paradoxus, is characteristic in cardiac tamponade.

Cardiogenic shock. In this disorder, systolic pressure falls to less than 80 mm Hg, or 30 mm Hg less than the patient's baseline. Accompanying low blood pressure are narrowed pulse pressure, diminished Korotkoff sounds, peripheral cyanosis, and pale, cool, clammy skin.

Congestive heart failure. In this disorder, blood pressure may fluctuate between normal and low readings. However, a precipitous drop in blood pressure may signal cardiogenic shock.

Hypovolemic shock. In this disorder, systolic pressure falls to less than 80 mm Hg, or 30 mm Hg less than the patient's baseline. Accompanying it are diminished Korotkoff sounds, narrowed pulse pressure, and rapid, weak, and occasionally irregular pulse. Peripheral vasoconstriction causes cyanosis of the extremities and pale, cool, clammy skin.

Myocardial infarction. In this life-threatening disorder, blood pressure may be low or high. However, a precipitous drop in blood pressure may signal cardiogenic shock.

Neurogenic shock. The result of sympathetic denervation due to cervical injury or anesthesia, neurogenic shock produces low blood pressure and bradycardia. However, the patient's skin remains warm and dry because of cutaneous vasodilation and sweat gland denervation.

Septic shock. Initially, this disorder produces fever, chills, and rash. Low blood pressure, tachycardia, and tachypnea may also develop early, but the patient's skin remains warm. Later, low blood pressure becomes increasingly severe—less than 80 mm Hg, or 30 mm Hg less than the patient's baseline—and is accompanied by narrowed pulse pressure.

Vasovagal syncope. This transient attack is characterized by low blood pressure, pallor, cold sweats, nausea, and weakness.

Endocrine

Acute adrenal insufficiency. Postural hypotension is characteristic in this disorder. Accompanying it are fatigue, weakness, nausea, vomiting, abdominal discomfort, weight loss, fever, and tachycardia.

Diabetic ketoacidosis. Hypovolemia triggered by osmotic diuresis in hyperglycemia is responsible for low blood pressure in this disorder.

Hyperosmolar hyperglycemic nonketotic coma. This disorder decreases blood pressure—at times dramatically, if the patient loses significant fluid from diuresis.

Hematologic

Hypoxemia. In this condition, blood pressure may be alternately low and normal.

Drugs

Calcium channel blockers, diuretics, vasodilators, antihypertensives, general anesthetics, narcotic analgesics, monoamine oxidase inhibitors, antianxiety agents (such as benzodiazepines), tranquilizers, and most I.V. antiarrhythmics (especially bretylium tosylate) can cause low blood pressure.

Low blood pressure occurs infrequently in alcohol toxicity.

Diagnostic tests

Low blood pressure may be caused by a gastric acid stimulation test using histamine and X-ray studies using contrast media. The latter may trigger an allergic reaction, which causes low blood pressure.

Clinical considerations

If the patient's systolic pressure is less than 80 mm Hg or 30 mm Hg below his baseline:

• Shock should be suspected immediately and the physician notified.

• A quick assessment should be performed and appropriate emergency interventions initiated.

• An arterial catheter may be inserted for constant monitoring of blood pressure if it is extremely low.

If the patient's condition does not suggest an emergency:

• A history should be obtained and a physical examination performed.

• Diagnostic tests may include urinalysis; routine blood studies; EKG; and chest, cervical, and abdominal X-rays.

• Vital signs should be monitored frequently to determine if low blood pressure is constant or intermittent.

• Bed rest should be enforced, as ordered, and the patient assisted with activities, as necessary.

Blood pressure, increased

Description

Increased or elevated blood pressure is an intermittent or sustained increase in blood pressure exceeding 140/86 mm Hg. Elevated blood pressure strikes men more often than women and blacks twice as often as whites. By itself, this common sign is easily ignored by the patient; after all, he cannot see or feel it. However, its causes can be life-threatening.

Elevated blood pressure may develop suddenly or gradually. A sudden, severe rise in blood pressure (exceeding 200/120 mm Hg) indicates life-threatening hypertensive crisis. However, even a less dramatic rise may be equally significant if it heralds dissecting aortic aneurysm, increased intracranial pressure, eclampsia, or thyrotoxicosis.

Most commonly associated with essential hypertension, elevated blood pressure may also result from renal and endocrine disorders; treatments that affect fluid status, such as dialysis; and drug side effects. Ingestion of large amounts of certain foods, such as black licorice and cheddar cheese, may temporarily elevate blood pressure.

Unfortunately, elevated blood pressure may simply reflect inaccurate blood pressure measurement. However, careful measurement alone does not ensure a clinically useful reading. To be useful, each blood pressure reading must be compared to the patient's baseline. Also, serial readings may be necessary to establish elevated blood pressure.

Mechanism

See *Pathophysiology of Elevated Blood Pressure,* p. 50.

Possible causes

Central nervous system

Increased intracranial pressure (ICP). Initially, this condition causes increased respirations. Then, systolic pressure rises and pulse pressure widens.

Cardiovascular

Aortic aneurysm (dissecting). Initially, this life-threatening disorder causes a sudden rise in systolic pressure, but no change in diastolic pressure. However, this increase is short-lived; the body's ability to compensate fails, resulting in hypotension.

Atherosclerosis. Here, systolic pressure rises while diastolic pressure remains normal.

Hypertension. Essential hypertension develops insidiously and is characterized by a gradual increase in blood pressure from decade to decade. Except for this elevated blood pressure, the patient may be asymptomatic or he may complain of suboccipital headache, light-headedness, tinnitus, and fatigue. In *malignant hypertension,* diastolic pressure abruptly rises above 120 mm Hg, and systolic pressure may exceed 200 mm Hg.

Myocardial infarction. This life-threatening disorder may cause high or low blood pressure.

Renovascular stenosis. This disorder produces abruptly elevated systolic and diastolic pressure.

Endocrine

Aldosteronism (primary). This disorder causes elevated diastolic pressure, which may be accompanied by postural hypotension.

Pathophysiology of Elevated Blood Pressure

Blood pressure—the force blood exerts on vessels as it flows through them—depends on cardiac output, peripheral resistance, and blood volume. A brief review of its regulating mechanisms—nervous system control, capillary fluid shifts, kidney excretion, and hormonal changes—will help clarify how elevated blood pressure develops.

• *Nervous system control* involves the sympathetic division, chiefly baroreceptors and chemoreceptors, which promotes moderate vasoconstriction to maintain normal blood pressure. When this system responds inappropriately, increased vasoconstriction enhances peripheral resistance, resulting in elevated blood pressure.

• *Capillary fluid shifts* regulate blood volume by responding to arterial pressure. Increased pressure forces fluid into the interstitial space; decreased pressure allows it to be drawn back into the arteries by osmosis. However, this fluid shift may take several hours to adjust blood pressure.

• *Kidney excretion* also helps regulate blood volume by increasing or decreasing urine formation. Normally, an arterial pressure of about 60 mm Hg maintains urine output. When pressure drops below this reading, urine formation ceases, thereby increasing blood volume. Conversely, when arterial pressure exceeds this reading, urine formation increases, thereby reducing blood volume. Like capillary fluid shifts, this mechanism may take several hours to adjust blood pressure.

• *Hormonal changes* reflect stimulation of the kidney's renin-angiotensin system in response to low arterial pressure. This system effects vasoconstriction, which increases arterial pressure, and stimulates aldosterone release, which regulates sodium retention—a key determinant of blood volume.

Elevated blood pressure signals the breakdown or inappropriate response of these pressure-regulating mechanisms. Its associated signs and symptoms concentrate in the target organs and tissues illustrated here.

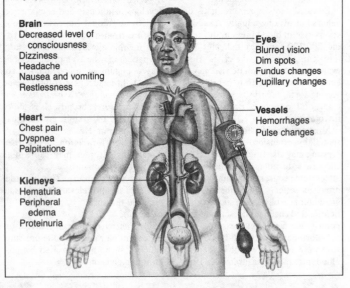

Brain
Decreased level of
     consciousness
Dizziness
Headache
Nausea and vomiting
Restlessness

Eyes
Blurred vision
Dim spots
Fundus changes
Pupillary changes

Heart
Chest pain
Dyspnea
Palpitations

Vessels
Hemorrhages
Pulse changes

Kidneys
Hematuria
Peripheral
   edema
Proteinuria

Cushing's syndrome. Twice as common in females as in males, this disorder causes elevated blood pressure and widened pulse pressure.

Pheochromocytoma. Paroxysmal or sustained elevated blood pressure characterizes pheochromocytoma and may be accompanied by postural hypotension.

Thyrotoxicosis. Accompanying elevated systolic pressure in this potentially life-threatening disorder are widened pulse pressure, tachycardia, bounding pulse, pulsations in the capillary nail beds, palpitations, weight loss, exophthalmos, an enlarged thyroid gland, weakness, diarrhea, fever (over 100° F. [37.2° C.]), and warm, moist skin.

Genitourinary
Polycystic kidney disease. Elevated blood pressure is typically preceded by flank pain.

Pyelonephritis (chronic). In some patients, this disorder produces no overt signs until severely elevated systolic and diastolic pressures develop.

Hematologic
Anemia. Accompanying elevated systolic pressure in this disorder are pulsations in the capillary beds, bounding pulse, tachycardia, systolic ejection murmur, pale mucous membranes, and, in sickle cell anemia, ventricular gallop and crackles.

Obstetrics-Gynecology
Preeclampsia/eclampsia. Potentially life-threatening to both mother and fetus, this disorder characteristically increases blood pressure. It is defined as a reading of 140/90 mm Hg or more in the first trimester, a reading of 130/80 mm Hg or more in the second or third trimester, an increase of 30 mm Hg above the patient's baseline systolic pressure, or an increase of 15 mm Hg above the patient's baseline diastolic pressure. Accompanying elevated blood pressure are generalized edema, sudden weight gain of 3 lb or more per week during the second or third trimester, severe frontal headache, blurred or double vision, decreased urinary output or oliguria, midabdominal pain, neuromuscular irritability, nausea, and possibly convulsions (eclampsia).

Drugs
Central nervous system stimulants (such as amphetamines), sympathomimetics, corticosteroids, oral contraceptives, monoamine oxidase inhibitors, and cocaine abuse can increase blood pressure.

Treatments
Kidney dialysis and *transplantation* cause transient elevation of blood pressure.

Clinical considerations
If sharply elevated blood pressure is detected:
• A rapid assessment should be performed to rule out life-threatening causes and the physician should be notified. If blood pressure exceeds 200/120 mm Hg, the patient is experiencing hypertensive crisis and requires prompt treatment.
• With less severely elevated blood pressure, emergency intervention may still be required.

After life-threatening causes of elevated blood pressure have been ruled out, or when the patient is stable:
• A complete history should be taken and a well-focused physical examination should be performed.
• Diagnostic tests may include routine blood tests, urinalysis, and radiographic studies (especially of the kidneys).
• The importance of long-term control of elevated blood pressure should be explained to the patient.
• The patient should be given clear medication instructions and told to adhere to them strictly.
• The patient should be assisted, as necessary, in altering his life-style to comply with his treatment regimen (which may include weight loss, dietary restrictions, exercise, and/or stress management).

• The patient should be taught to monitor his blood pressure at home, if appropriate.

Bonnet's sign

Description
Bonnet's sign is pain on adduction of the thigh, seen in sciatica.

Bowel sounds, absent
(Silent abdomen)

Description
Absent bowel sounds refers to the inability to hear any bowel sounds through a stethoscope after listening for at least 5 minutes in each abdominal quadrant.

Absent bowel sounds may be caused by mechanical or vascular obstructions or by neurogenic inhibition. Simple mechanical obstruction, resulting from adhesions, hernia, or tumor, causes loss of fluids and electrolytes and induces dehydration. Vascular obstruction cuts off circulation to the intestinal walls, leading to ischemia, necrosis, and shock. Neurogenic inhibition, affecting innervation of the intestinal wall, may result from infection, bowel distention, or trauma. It may also follow mechanical or vascular obstruction or metabolic derangement, such as hypokalemia.

Abrupt cessation of bowel sounds, when accompanied by abdominal pain, rigidity, and distention, signals a life-threatening crisis requiring immediate intervention. Absent bowel sounds following a period of hyperactivity are equally ominous and may indicate strangulation of a mechanically obstructed bowel.

Mechanism
Bowel sounds cease when mechanical or vascular obstruction or neurogenic inhibition halts peristalsis. When peristalsis halts, gas from bowel contents and fluid secreted from the intestinal walls accumulate and distend the lumen, leading to life-threatening complications such as perforation, peritonitis and sepsis, or hypovolemic shock.

Possible causes
Gastrointestinal
Complete mechanical intestinal obstruction. Absent bowel sounds follow a period of hyperactive bowel sounds in this potentially life-threatening disorder. This silence accompanies acute, colicky abdominal pain that arises in the quadrant of obstruction and may radiate to the flank or lumbar regions.
Mesenteric artery occlusion. In this life-threatening disorder, bowel sounds disappear after a brief period of hyperactive sounds.
Paralytic (adynamic) ileus. The cardinal sign of this potentially life-threatening disorder is absent bowel sounds.

Treatments
Bowel sounds are normally absent after *abdominal surgery*—the result of anesthetics and surgical manipulation.

Clinical considerations
If bowel sounds are not detected and the patient reports sudden, severe abdominal pain and cramping or exhibits severe abdominal distention:
• A brief history should be obtained and the physician notified.
• Emergency interventions should be initiated, if necessary, to decompress the bowel and to maintain adequate circulatory status.
• Surgery may be required to relieve an obstruction. If so, foods and fluids should be withheld and the patient prepared accordingly.
• Once mechanical obstruction and intraabdominal sepsis have been ruled out as causes of absent bowel sounds, drugs should be given, as ordered, to control pain and stimulate peristalsis.

If the patient's pain is not severe or accompanied by other life-threatening signs:

• A detailed medical and surgical history should be obtained and an abdominal assessment performed.

• Diagnostic tests, such as blood studies and X-rays, may be done to determine the cause of absent bowel sounds.

• If a nasogastric or intestinal tube has been left in place, appropriate care of the tube should be performed.

Bowel sounds, hyperactive

Description

Sometimes audible without a stethoscope, hyperactive bowel sounds are characterized as rapid, rushing, gurgling waves of sounds. They are higher in pitch and occur more frequently than normal sounds. They may stem from life-threatening bowel obstruction or gastrointestinal (GI) hemorrhage. However, hyperactive sounds may also stem from GI infection, inflammatory bowel disease (which usually follows a chronic course), food allergies, and stress.

Mechanism

Hyperactive bowel sounds reflect increased intestinal motility (peristalsis).

Possible causes
Gastrointestinal

Crohn's disease. Hyperactive bowel sounds usually arise insidiously.

Gastroenteritis. Hyperactive bowel sounds follow sudden nausea and vomiting and accompany "explosive" diarrhea.

GI hemorrhage. Hyperactive bowel sounds provide the most immediate indication of persistent bleeding.

Mechanical intestinal obstruction. Hyperactive bowel sounds occur simultaneously with cramping abdominal pain every few minutes in this potentially life-threatening disorder; bowel sounds may later become hypoactive and then disappear.

In *complete bowel obstruction*, hyperactive sounds are also accompanied by abdominal distention and constipation, although the bowel distal to the obstruction may continue to empty for up to 3 days.

Ulcerative colitis (acute). Hyperactive bowel sounds arise abruptly in this disorder. They are accompanied by bloody diarrhea, anorexia, abdominal pain, nausea, vomiting, fever, and tenesmus.

Immunologic

Food hypersensitivity. Hyperactive bowel sounds follow ingestion of allergenic foods.

Clinical considerations

• A brief history should be obtained and an abdominal examination completed.

• If the patient reports cramping abdominal pain or vomiting, the physician should be notified, vital signs taken, and bowel sounds monitored closely.

• If bowel sounds stop abruptly, emergency interventions should be initiated to decompress the bowel and relieve any obstruction.

• If life-threatening conditions have been ruled out, a detailed history should be obtained and a physical examination performed.

• Diagnostic tests may include endoscopy, barium X-rays, and stool analysis.

• Because stress often precipitates or aggravates bowel hyperactivity, the patient should be taught relaxation techniques, such as deep breathing, if appropriate.

Bowel sounds, hypoactive

Description

Hypoactive bowel sounds, detected by auscultation, are diminished in regularity, tone, or loudness from normal bowel sounds. In themselves, hypoactive bowel sounds do not herald an emergency; in fact, they are considered normal during sleep. However, they may portend the absence of bowel sounds, which can indicate a life-threatening disorder.

Hypoactive bowel sounds can also result from certain drugs and from abdominal surgery and irradiation.

Mechanism

Hypoactive bowel sounds result from decreased peristalsis, which, in turn, can result from a developing bowel obstruction. Such obstruction may be mechanical (as from hernia, tumor, or twisting), vascular (as from an embolism or thrombosis), or neurogenic (as from mechanical, ischemic, or toxic impairment of bowel innervation).

Possible causes

Gastrointestinal

Mechanical intestinal obstruction. Bowel sounds may become hypoactive after a period of hyperactivity.

Mesenteric artery occlusion. After a brief period of hyperactivity, bowel sounds become hypoactive and then quickly disappear, signifying a life-threatening crisis.

Paralytic (adynamic) ileus. Bowel sounds are hypoactive and may become absent.

Drugs

Certain classes of drugs reduce intestinal motility and thus produce hypoactive bowel sounds. These include opiates, such as codeine; anticholinergics, such as propantheline bromide; phenothiazines, such as chlorpromazine; and vinca alkaloids, such as vincristine. General or spinal anesthetics produce transient hypoactive sounds.

Treatments

Hypoactive bowel sounds and abdominal tenderness may occur following *irradiation of the abdomen*.

Hypoactive bowel sounds may occur after *surgical manipulation* of the bowel. Motility and bowel sounds in the small intestine usually resume in 24 hours; colonic bowel sounds in 3 to 5 days.

Clinical considerations

• A detailed medical and surgical history should be obtained and a careful abdominal examination performed.

• Diagnostic tests may include blood studies, X-rays, and endoscopy.

• The patient with hypoactive bowel sounds may require gastrointestinal suction and decompression, using a nasogastric or intestinal tube. If so, appropriate care should be given.

• Comfort measures should be provided.

• Bowel sounds should be monitored every 2 to 4 hours.

If bowel sounds suddenly cease:

• Vital signs should be taken and the physician notified.

• Emergency interventions should be anticipated to decompress the bowel and relieve obstruction.

Bozzolo's sign

Description

Bozzolo's sign is the pulsation of arteries in the nasal mucous membrane, seen occasionally with thoracic aortic aneurysms. To detect this sign, the examiner inspects both nostrils using a speculum and light.

Bradycardia

Description

Bradycardia refers to a heart rate of fewer than 60 beats/minute. It occurs normally in young adults, trained athletes, the elderly, and during sleep. It is also a normal response to vagal stimulation caused by coughing, vomiting, or straining during defecation. When bradycardia results from these causes, the heart rate rarely drops below 40 beats/minute. However, when it results from pathologic causes (such as cardiovascular disorders), the heart rate may be as slow as 1 beat/minute.

By itself, bradycardia is a nonspecific sign. However, in conjunction with such symptoms as chest pain, dizziness, and shortness of breath, it can signal a life-threatening disorder.

Possible causes

Central nervous system

Cervical spinal injury. Bradycardia may be transient or sustained, depending on the severity of injury. Its onset coincides with sympathetic denervation.

Increased intracranial pressure. Bradycardia occurs as a late sign of this condition along with rapid respirations, elevated systolic pressure, decreased diastolic pressure, and widened pulse pressure.

Cardiovascular

Cardiac dysrhythmia. Depending on the type and the patient's tolerance of dysrhythmia, bradycardia may be transient or sustained, and benign or life-threatening.

Cardiomyopathy. This potentially life-threatening disorder causes transient or sustained bradycardia.

Myocardial infarction (MI). Mild or severe bradycardia occurs in about 65% of patients with an inferior MI.

Endocrine

Hypothyroidism. This disorder causes severe bradycardia accompanied by fatigue, constipation, unexplained weight gain, and sensitivity to cold.

Environmental

Hypothermia. Bradycardia usually appears when core temperature drops below 89.6° (32° C.). It is accompanied by shivering, peripheral cyanosis, confusion leading to stupor, muscle rigidity, and bradypnea.

Drugs

Beta-adrenergic and calcium channel blockers, cardiac glycosides, topical miotics (such as pilocarpine), I.V. nitroglycerin, protamine sulfate, quinidine, and sympatholytics may cause transient bradycardia. Failure to take thyroid hormone replacements may cause bradycardia.

Treatments

Suctioning can induce hypoxia and vagal stimulation, causing bradycardia.
Cardiac surgery can cause edema or damage to conduction tissues, causing bradycardia.

Diagnostic tests

Cardiac catheterization and electrophysiologic studies can induce temporary bradycardia.

Clinical considerations

If the patient's condition suggests a life-threatening disorder:
• Vital signs should be taken quickly and the physician notified immediately.
• Cardiac monitoring should be initiated and appropriate emergency interventions anticipated, depending on the cause of bradycardia.
• Emergency equipment and medications should be kept nearby in case cardiac arrest occurs.

If the patient's bradycardia is not accompanied by untoward signs:
• A brief history should be obtained and a focused assessment performed to help pinpoint the cause of bradycardia.
• Diagnostic tests may include complete blood count; cardiac enzyme, serum electrolyte, blood glucose, and thyroid function tests; arterial blood gas and blood urea nitrogen levels; and a 12-lead EKG. If appropriate, 24-hour Holter monitoring may be initiated.
• Vital signs should be monitored continuously and the physician notified of any changes in cardiac rhythm.

Bradypnea

Description

Bradypnea is a pattern of regular respirations with a rate of fewer than 12 breaths/minute. Often preceding life-threatening apnea or respiratory arrest, this sign results from neurologic and metabolic disorders and drug overdose, which depress the brain's respiratory control centers.

Mechanism
Respiratory depression occurs when decreased cerebral perfusion inactivates respiratory center neurons, when changes in $PaCO_2$ and arterial blood pH affect chemoreceptor responsiveness, or when neuron responsiveness to $PaCO_2$ changes is reduced—for example, due to narcotic overdose.

Possible causes
Central nervous system
Increased intracranial pressure. A late sign of this life-threatening condition, bradypnea is preceded by decreased level of consciousness, deteriorated motor function, and fixed, dilated pupils. The triad of bradypnea, bradycardia, and hypertension is a classic sign of late medullary strangulation.
Respiratory
Respiratory failure. Bradypnea occurs in end-stage respiratory failure. Its accompanying signs include cyanosis, diminished breath sounds, tachycardia, mildly increased blood pressure, and decreased level of consciousness.
Endocrine
Diabetic keotacidosis. Bradypnea occurs late in severe, uncontrolled diabetes.
Gastrointestinal
Hepatic failure. Occurring in end-stage hepatic failure, bradypnea may be accompanied by coma, hyperactive reflexes, a positive Babinski's sign, fetor hepaticus, and other signs.
Genitourinary
Renal failure. Occurring in end-stage renal failure, bradypnea may be accompanied by convulsions, decreased level of consciousness, gastrointestinal bleeding, hypo- or hypertension, uremic frost, and diverse other signs.

Drugs
An overdose of narcotic analgesics and, less commonly, sedatives, barbiturates, phenothiazines, and other CNS depressants, can cause bradypnea. Use of any of these drugs with alcohol can also cause bradypnea.

Clinical considerations
• Depending on the degree of CNS depression, the patient with severe bradypnea may require constant stimulation to breathe. For example, if the patient appears excessively sleepy, an attempt to awaken him should be made and he should be instructed to breathe.
• Vital signs should be taken and the physician notified immediately.
• A rapid neurologic assessment should be performed.
• The patient should be placed on an apnea monitor and emergency equipment should be kept on hand to use in case respiratory arrest occurs.
• A brief history should be obtained.
• Diagnostic tests may include arterial blood gas and electrolyte studies, chest and skull X-rays, and computed tomography.
• Respiratory status should be monitored frequently.
• Ventilatory support should be kept readily available.

Braunwald sign

Description
Braunwald sign is the occurrence of a weak pulse rather than a strong pulse immediately after a premature ventricular contraction (PVC). To detect this sign, a PVC should be watched for during cardiac monitoring and the quality of the following pulse checked. Braunwald sign may indicate idiopathic hypertrophic subaortic stenosis.

Breast dimpling

Description

Breast dimpling is the puckering or retraction of skin on the breast. It results from the abnormal attachment of the skin to underlying tissue. This sign suggests an inflammatory or malignant mass beneath the surface of the skin and most often represents a late sign of breast cancer; benign lesions usually do not produce this effect. Dimpling most commonly affects women over age 40 but also occasionally occurs in males.

Because breast dimpling occurs over a mass or induration, the patient usually discovers other signs before becoming aware of dimpling. However, a thorough breast examination may reveal dimpling and may alert the patient and nurse to a breast problem.

Possible causes

Obstetrics-Gynecology

Breast abscess. Breast dimpling sometimes accompanies chronic breast abscess.

Breast cancer. Breast dimpling is an important but somewhat late sign of malignancy. A neoplasm that causes dimpling is usually close to the skin and at least 1 cm in diameter; it feels irregularly shaped and fixed to underlying tissue.

Fat necrosis. Breast dimpling from fat necrosis follows inflammation and trauma to fatty tissue of the breast.

Mastitis. Breast dimpling may signal bacterial mastitis, which most often results from duct obstruction and milk stasis during lactation. Heat, erythema, swelling, induration, pain, and tenderness usually accompany mastitis. Dimpling more likely occurs with diffuse induration than with a single hard mass. The skin on the breast may feel fixed to underlying tissue.

Clinical considerations

• A medical, reproductive, and family history should be obtained, with attention to factors that place the patient at a high risk for breast cancer.
• A thorough examination of the breasts and axillary lymph nodes should be performed.
• Diagnostic tests may include mammography, thermography, ultrasound, cytology of nipple discharge, and biopsy.
• Because any breast problem can arouse fears of mutilation, loss of sexuality, and death, the patient should be allowed to express her feelings.
• Breast self-examination should be discussed and taught when appropriate.

Breast nodule
(Breast lump)

Description

A frequently reported gynecologic sign, a breast nodule has two chief causes: benign breast disease and cancer. Benign breast disease, the leading cause of nodules, can stem from cyst formation in obstructed and dilated lactiferous ducts, hypertrophy or tumor formation in the ductal system, and inflammation or infection.

Although less than 20% of breast nodules are malignant, the clinical signs of breast cancer are not easily distinguished from those of benign breast disease. Breast cancer is a leading cause of death among women but can occur occasionally in men, with signs and symptoms mimicking those found in women. Thus, breast nodules in both sexes should always be evaluated.

A woman who is familiar with the feel of her breasts and performs monthly breast self-examination can detect a nodule 5 mm or less in size, considerably smaller than the 1-cm nodule that is readily detectable by an experienced examiner. However, a woman may not report a nodule because of fear of breast cancer.

Possible causes
Obstetrics-Gynecology
Adenofibroma. The extremely mobile or "slippery" feel of this benign neoplasm helps distinguish it from other breast nodules. The nodule usually occurs singly and characteristically feels firm, elastic, and round or lobular, with well-defined margins. It does not cause pain or tenderness, can vary from pinhead size to very large, often grows rapidly, and usually lies around the nipple or on the lateral side of the upper outer quadrant.

Areolar gland abscess. Tender, palpable abscesses on the periphery of the areola follow inflammation of the sebaceous glands of Montgomery. Fever may also be present.

Breast abscess. A localized, hot, tender, fluctuant mass with erythema and peau d'orange typifies *acute abscess.* In *chronic abscess,* the nodule is nontender, irregular, and firm and may feel like a thick wall of fibrous tissue. It is often accompanied by skin dimpling, peau d'orange, and nipple retraction and sometimes by axillary lymphadenopathy.

Breast cancer. A hard, poorly delineated nodule that is fixed to the skin or underlying tissue suggests breast cancer. Malignant nodules often cause breast dimpling, nipple deviation or retraction, or flattening of the nipple or breast contour. Forty to fifty percent of malignant nodules occur in the upper outer quadrant. Nodules usually occur singly, although satellite nodules may surround the main one.

Fat necrosis. This rare, benign mass mimics the poorly delineated nodule of breast cancer. The hard, indurated, and fibrotic nodule is usually fixed to overlying skin or underlying tissue.

Intraductal papilloma. The tiny nodules of this benign lesion usually resist palpation. Nodules large enough to be palpated usually occur singly, but they may be multiple and diffuse. Soft and poorly delineated, the nodules usually lie in the subareolar margin.

Mammary duct ectasia. The rubbery breast nodule in this menopausal or postmenopausal disorder usually lies under the areola. It is often accompanied by pain, itching, tenderness, and erythema of the areola; thick, sticky, multicolored nipple discharge; and nipple retraction. The skin overlying the mass may show bluish-green discoloration or edema (peau d'orange).

Mastitis. In this disorder, breast nodules feel firm and indurated or tender, flocculent, and discrete. Gentle palpation defines the area of maximum purulent accumulation.

Nipple adenoma. Although similar in symptoms to Paget's disease, adenomas rarely produce a deep-seated mass.

Paget's disease. This slow-growing intraductal carcinoma begins as a scaling, eczematoid nipple lesion. Later, the nipple becomes reddened and excoriated; complete destruction of the structure may result. The process extends along the skin as well as in the ducts, usually progressing to a deep-seated mass.

Proliferative breast disease. The most common cause of breast nodules, this fibrocystic condition produces smooth, round, slightly elastic nodules, which increase in size and tenderness just before menstruation. The nodules may occur in fine, granular clusters in both breasts or as widespread, well-defined lumps of varying sizes. A thickening of adjacent tissue may be palpable. Cystic nodules are mobile, which helps differentiate them from malignant ones. Because cystic nodules are not fixed to underlying breast tissue, they do not produce retraction signs, such as nipple deviation or dimpling.

Clinical considerations
• A complete history should be obtained, with special attention to fac-

tors that increase the patient's risk of breast cancer.

• A thorough breast examination should be performed.

• Diagnostic tests may include trans-illumination, mammography, thermography, needle aspiration or open biopsy of the nodule for tissue examination, and cytologic examination of nipple discharge.

• Procedures should be explained thoroughly to avoid alarming the patient unnecessarily.

• Emotional support should be provided and the patient encouraged to express her feelings.

• The patient should be taught how to perform breast self-examination until she overcomes her initial anxiety at discovering a nodule. Regular breast self-examination is especially important for women who have had a previous malignancy, who have a family history of breast cancer, who are nulliparous or had their first child after age 30, and who had an early menarche or late menopause.

Breast ulcer

Description

Appearing on the nipple, areola, or the breast itself, an ulcer indicates destruction of the skin and subcutaneous tissue. Usually, a breast ulcer is a late sign of cancer, appearing well after confirming diagnosis. However, it may be the presenting sign of breast cancer in men, who are more likely to dismiss earlier breast changes. Breast ulcer can also result from trauma, infection, or radiation.

Possible causes
Skin
Candida albicans *infection*. Severe *Candida* infection can cause maceration of breast tissue followed by ulceration.

Obstetrics-Gynecology
Breast cancer. A breast ulcer that fails to heal within a month usually indicates cancer. Ulceration along a mastectomy scar may indicate metastatic cancer; a nodule beneath the ulcer may be a late sign of a fulminating tumor.

Breast trauma. Tissue destruction with inadequate healing may produce breast ulcers.

Paget's disease. Bright red nipple excoriation can extend to the areola and ulcerate.

Treatments
After *radiation treatment*, the breasts appear sunburned. Subsequently, the skin ulcerates and the surrounding area becomes red and tender.

Clinical considerations

• A history should be obtained, with attention to factors that increase the patient's risk of breast cancer.

• A thorough breast examination should be performed.

• Diagnostic tests, such as ultrasonography, thermography, mammography, nipple discharge cytology, and breast biopsy may be done. If a *Candida* infection is suspected, skin or blood cultures should be obtained.

• Emotional support should be provided and the patient encouraged to express her feelings.

• Because breast ulcers become easily infected, the patient should be taught how to apply topical antifungal ointment or cream, as ordered.

• The patient should be instructed to keep the ulcer dry to reduce chafing, and to wear loose-fitting undergarments.

Breath odor, ammonia
(Uremic fetor)

Description

The odor of ammonia on the breath—described as urinous or "fishy" breath—typically occurs in end-stage chronic renal failure. This sign improves slightly after hemodialysis and persists throughout the disorder's course, but is not of great concern.

Ammonia breath odor reflects the long-term metabolic disturbances and biochemical abnormalities associated with uremia and end-stage chronic renal failure. Metabolic end products, blown off by the lungs, produce the ammonia odor, but a specific uremic toxin has not yet been identified. In animals, breath odor analysis has revealed toxic metabolites, such as dimethylamine and trimethylamine, which contribute to the "fishy" odor. The source of these amines, although still unclear, may be intestinal bacteria acting on dietary chlorine.

Breath odor, fecal

Description
Fecal breath odor may follow an episode of prolonged vomiting associated with long-standing intestinal obstruction or gastrojejunocolic fistula. It represents an important late diagnostic clue to a potentially life-threatening gastrointestinal disorder, since complete obstruction of any part of the bowel, if untreated, can cause death within hours from vascular collapse and shock.

Fecal breath odor may also occur in the patient with a nasogastric or intestinal tube. It is detected only while the underlying disorder persists and abates soon after its resolution.

Mechanism
Fecal breath odor accompanies fecal vomiting, which results when the obstructed or adynamic intestine attempts self-decompression by regurgitating its contents; vigorous peristaltic waves propel bowel contents backward into the stomach. When the stomach fills with intestinal fluid, further reverse peristalsis results in vomiting. The odor of feculent vomitus lingers in the mouth.

Possible causes
Gastrointestinal
Distal small-bowel obstruction. In late obstruction, nausea is present although vomiting may be delayed. Initially, vomitus is gastric contents, changing to bilious and then to fecal contents with resultant fecal breath odor.

Gastrojejunocolic fistula. In this disorder, symptoms may be variable and intermittent because of temporary plugging of the fistula. Fecal vomiting with resulting fecal breath odor may occur.

Large-bowel obstruction. Vomiting is usually absent at first, but fecal vomiting with resultant fecal breath odor occurs as a late sign. Typically, symptoms develop more slowly than in small-bowel obstruction.

Clinical considerations
• A brief history should be obtained and an abdominal examination performed.
• Vital signs should be monitored and the physician notified.
• Emergency interventions should be initiated, if necessary, to decompress the bowel and to maintain adequate circulatory status.
• Surgery may be required to relieve an obstruction; if so, the patient should be prepared accordingly.
• Diagnostic tests may include abdominal X-rays, barium enema, and proctoscopy.
• If a nasogastric tube has been left in place to decompress and rest the bowel, appropriate care of the tube should be provided.
• The patient should be encouraged to brush his teeth with a flavored mouthwash or to gargle with half-strength hydrogen peroxide to minimize the offensive breath odor.
• The patient should be assured that the fecal odor is temporary and will

abate after treatment of the underlying cause.

Breath odor, fruity

Description
Fruity breath odor results from respiratory elimination of excess acetone. This sign characteristically occurs in ketoacidosis—a potentially life-threatening condition that requires immediate treatment to prevent severe dehydration, irreversible coma, and death.

Breath sounds, absent or decreased

Description
Absent or decreased breath sounds may be defined as breath sounds that are inaudible (absent) or diminished in loudness (decreased), as detected by auscultation. This sign may reflect reduced airflow to a lung segment caused by a tumor, foreign body, mucous plug, or mucosal edema. It may also reflect hyperinflation of the lungs in emphysema or an asthmatic attack. Or it may reflect the presence of air or fluid in the pleural cavity from a pneumothorax, hemothorax, pleural effusion, atelectasis, or empyema. In an obese or extremely muscular patient, breath sounds may be diminished or inaudible because of increased thickness of the chest wall.

Broadbent's inverted sign

Description
Broadbent's inverted sign may be defined as pulsations on the left posterolateral chest wall during ventricular systole. To detect this sign, the examiner palpates the patient's chest with the fingers and palm over areas of visible pulsation while auscultating for ventricular systole. When she feels pulsations she notes their rate, rhythm, and intensity. This sign may indicate gross dilatation of the left atrium.

Broadbent's sign

Description
Broadbent's sign is visible retraction of the left posterior chest wall near the 11th and 12th ribs, occurring during systole. To detect this sign, the examiner inspects the chest wall while standing at the patient's right side. She then positions a strong light so that it casts rays tangential to the skin. While auscultating the heart, she watches for retraction of the skin and muscles and determines its timing in the cardiac cycle. Broadbent's sign may occur in extensive adhesive pericarditis.

Brudzinski's sign

Description
Brudzinski's sign is the flexion of the hips and knees in response to passive flexion of the neck. This sign is a common and important early indicator of life-threatening meningitis and subarachnoid hemorrhage. It can be elicited in children as well as in adults, although more reliable indicators of meningeal irritation exist for infants.

Normally, testing for Brudzinski's sign is not part of a routine examination, unless meningeal irritation is suspected. (See *Testing for Brudzinski's Sign*, p. 62.)

Mechanism
In meningitis and subarachnoid hemorrhage, meningeal irritation results from the pressure of blood or exudate collecting around the spinal nerve roots. Passive flexion of the neck stretches the nerve roots, causing pain

Testing for Brudzinski's Sign

If the examiner suspects meningeal irritation, she may elicit Brudzinski's sign as shown below.

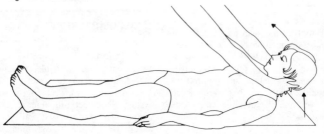

With the patient in a supine position, the examiner places her hands behind the patient's neck and lifts the patient's head toward her chest.

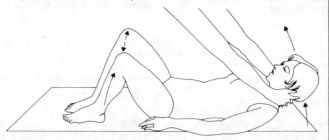

If the patient has meningeal irritation, she will flex her hips and knees in response to the passive neck flexion.

and involuntary flexion of the knees and hips.

Possible causes

Central nervous system

Bacterial meningitis. Brudzinski's sign can usually be elicited 24 hours after the onset of this life-threatening disorder.

Subarachnoid hemorrhage. Brudzinski's sign may be elicited within minutes after initial bleeding in this life-threatening disorder.

Musculoskeletal

Arthritis. In severe spinal arthritis, Brudzinski's sign can occasionally be elicited.

Clinical considerations

• Brudzinski's sign should be reported to the physician immediately.

• Because the patient with Brudzinski's sign is often critically ill, he requires constant intracranial pressure monitoring, frequent neurologic checks, and intensive assessment and monitoring of vital signs, intake and output, and cardiorespiratory status.

• Emergency equipment should be kept on hand.

• Diagnostic tests may include blood, urine, sputum, and cerebrospinal fluid cultures; computed tomography; cerebral angiography; and spinal X-rays.

Bruits

Description

Bruits are swishing sounds caused by turbulent blood flow. Often an indicator of life- or limb-threatening vascular disease, they are characterized by location, duration, intensity, pitch, and time of onset in the cardiac cycle. Loud bruits produce intensive vibration and a palpable *thrill*. A thrill, however, does not provide any further clue to the causative disorder or to its severity.

Bruits are most significant when heard over the abdominal aorta; the renal, carotid, femoral, popliteal, and subclavian arteries; and the thyroid gland. They are also significant when heard consistently despite changes in patient position and when heard during diastole.

Possible causes

Cardiovascular

Abdominal aortic aneurysm. A pulsating periumbilical mass accompanied by a systolic bruit over the aorta characterizes this disorder.

Abdominal aortic atherosclerosis. Loud systolic bruits in the epigastric and midabdominal areas are common.

Carotid artery stenosis. Systolic bruits can be heard over one or both carotid arteries.

Carotid cavernous fistula. Continuous bruits heard over the eyeballs and temples are characteristic, as are visual disturbances and protruding, pulsating eyeballs.

Peripheral arteriovenous fistula. A rough, continuous bruit with systolic accentuation may be heard over the fistula; in addition, a palpable thrill is often present.

Peripheral vascular disease. This condition characteristically produces bruits over the femoral artery and other arteries in the legs.

Renal artery stenosis. Systolic bruits commonly are heard over the abdominal midline and flank on the affected side.

Subclavian steal syndrome. In this syndrome, systolic bruits may be heard over one or both subclavian arteries as a result of narrowing of the arterial lumen.

Endocrine

Thyrotoxicosis. A systolic bruit is often heard over the thyroid gland.

Hematologic

Anemia. Increased cardiac output causes increased blood flow. In severe anemia, short systolic bruits may be heard over both carotid arteries.

Clinical considerations

- Because bruits can signal a life-threatening vascular disorder, a brief history should be taken, a rapid assessment performed, and the physician notified.
- Emergency interventions should be anticipated to prevent further vascular damage or to treat complications.
- Diagnostic tests may include blood studies, radiographs, an EKG, cardiac catheterization, and ultrasonography.
- Vital signs should be monitored frequently and the affected artery auscultated often to detect changes in the character of the bruit.
- Medications, such as vasodilators, anticoagulants, antiplatelets, or antihypertensives, should be administered, as ordered.

Buffalo hump

Description

Buffalo hump is an accumulation of cervicodorsal fat. It usually indicates hypercortisolism, or Cushing's syndrome. Hypercortisolism itself may result from adrenal carcinoma, adrenal adenoma, ectopic adrenocorticotropic hormone (ACTH) production, excessive pituitary secretion of ACTH (Cushing's disease), or long-term glucocorticoid therapy.

Buffalo hump does not help distinguish between the underlying causes of hypercortisolism, but it may help direct diagnostic testing.

Possible causes
Endocrine
Hypercortisolism. Buffalo hump varies in size depending on the severity of the disorder and the amount of weight gain. It is often accompanied by hirsutism, moon face, and truncal obesity with slender arms and legs.
Metabolic
Morbid obesity. The size of the buffalo hump depends on the amount of weight gain and the distribution of adipose tissue.
Drugs
Buffalo hump may result from excessive dosages of glucocorticoids, such as cortisone, hydrocortisone, and prednisone.

Clinical considerations
• A history should be obtained and a physical examination performed.
• Diagnostic tests to confirm the cause of hypercortisolism may include blood and urine studies; ultrasonography; computed tomography of the adrenal glands, abdomen, and skull; arteriography; chest X-rays; bronchography; and visual field testing.

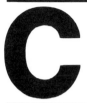

Café-au-lait spots

Description
Café-au-lait spots appear as flat, light brown, uniformly hyperpigmented macules on the skin surface. An important indicator of neurofibromatosis and other congenital melanotic disorders, they usually appear in childhood (most often before age 10) and can be differentiated from freckles and other benign birthmarks by their larger size (ranging from a few millimeters to 1.5 cm or larger) and more irregular shape. Although one to three spots may be a normal finding, the presence of café-au-lait spots usually indicates an underlying disorder.

Possible causes
Skin
Albright's syndrome. In this syndrome, café-au-lait spots are smaller (about 1 cm) and more irregularly shaped than those in neurofibromatosis. They may stop abruptly at the midline and seem to follow a dermatomal distribution. Usually, fewer than six spots appear, often unilaterally on the forehead, neck, and lower back. When they occur on the scalp, the hair overlying them may be more deeply pigmented.
Neurofibromatosis. The most common cause of café-au-lait spots, this disorder is characterized by six or more large, smooth-bordered spots.
Tuberous sclerosis. Mental retardation and seizures characteristically appear first, followed several years later by cutaneous facial lesions—multiple

café-au-lait spots, spherical areas of rough skin, and areas of yellow-red or depigmented nevi.

Clinical considerations
• A patient history, including family history, should be obtained and a thorough skin inspection performed.
• Diagnostic tests may include tissue biopsy and radiographic studies.
• Although café-au-lait spots require no treatment, emotional support should be provided to help the patient and his family cope with the underlying disorder.
• If appropriate, the patient should be advised to consider getting genetic counseling.

Capillary refill time, prolonged

Description
Capillary refill time is the duration required for color to return to the nail bed of a finger or toe after application of slight pressure, which causes blanching. This duration reflects the quality of peripheral vasomotor function. Normal capillary refill time is less than 3 seconds.

Prolonged refill time is not diagnostic of any disorder but must be evaluated along with other signs and symptoms. However, this sign usually signals obstructive peripheral arterial disease or decreased cardiac output.

Capillary refill time is typically tested during a routine cardiovascular assessment. It is not tested in suspected life-threatening disorders, because other, more characteristic signs and symptoms appear earlier.

Possible causes
Cardiovascular
Aortic aneurysm (dissecting). Capillary refill time is prolonged in the fingers and toes with a dissecting aneurysm in the thoracic aorta, and is prolonged in just the toes with a dissecting aneurysm in the abdominal aorta.

Aortic arch syndrome. Prolonged capillary refill time in the fingers occurs early in this syndrome.

Aortic bifurcation occlusion (acute). Prolonged capillary refill time in the toes is a late sign in this rare but usually fatal disorder.

Arterial occlusion (acute). Prolonged capillary refill time occurs early in the affected limb.

Buerger's disease. Capillary refill time is prolonged in the toes. If the disease affects the hands, prolonged capillary refill time may accompany painful fingertip ulcerations.

Cardiac tamponade. Prolonged capillary refill time represents a late sign of decreased cardiac output.

Peripheral arterial trauma. Any trauma to a peripheral artery that reduces distal blood flow also prolongs capillary refill time in the affected extremity.

Peripheral vascular disease. Prolonged capillary refill time in the affected extremities is a late sign.

Raynaud's disease. Capillary refill time is prolonged in the fingers, the usual site of this disease's characteristic episodic arterial vasospasm.

Shock. Prolonged capillary refill time appears late in almost all types of shock.

Musculoskeletal
Volkmann's contracture. Prolonged capillary refill time results from this contracture's characteristic vasospasm.

Enviromental
Hypothermia. Prolonged capillary refill time may appear early as a compensatory response.

Drugs
Drugs that cause vasoconstriction (particularly alpha-adrenergics) prolong capillary refill time.

Treatments
Prolonged capillary refill time can result from an *arterial line* or *umbilical line*, which can cause arterial hematoma and obstructed distal blood flow; or an *improperly fitting cast*, which constricts circulation.

Diagnostic tests
Cardiac catheterization can cause arterial hematoma or clot formation and prolonged capillary refill time.

Clinical considerations
• A brief medical history should be obtained, vital signs taken, and the vascular status of the affected limb assessed.

• Diagnostic tests may include arteriography and Doppler ultrasonography.

• Any changes in the patient's vital signs or level of consciousness or in the vascular status of the affected extremity (such as progressive cyanosis or pulse loss) should be reported to the physician.

Carpopedal spasm

Description
Carpopedal spasm is the violent, painful contraction of the muscles in the hands and feet. It is an important early sign of tetany, a potentially life-threatening condition characterized by increased neuromuscular excitation and sustained muscle contraction and commonly associated with hypocalcemia. Carpopedal spasm is usually accompanied by paresthesias of the fingers, toes, and perioral area; muscle weakness, twitching, and cramping;

Carpopedal Spasm

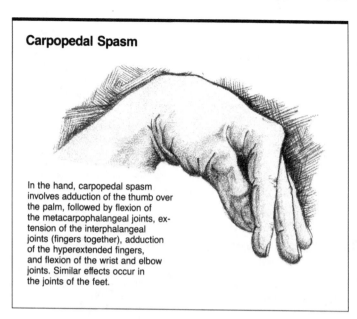

In the hand, carpopedal spasm involves adduction of the thumb over the palm, followed by flexion of the metacarpophalangeal joints, extension of the interphalangeal joints (fingers together), adduction of the hyperextended fingers, and flexion of the wrist and elbow joints. Similar effects occur in the joints of the feet.

hyperreflexia; chorea; fatigue; and palpitations. Positive Chvostek's and Trousseau's signs can be elicited.

Catatonia

Description
Catatonia is marked inhibition or excitation in motor behavior, occurring in psychotic disorders. *Catatonic stupor* refers to extreme inhibition of spontaneous activity or movement. *Catatonic excitement* refers to extreme psychomotor agitation.

Cat cry

Description
Occurring during infancy, this mewing, kittenlike sound is the primary indicator of cri du chat, or cat cry, syndrome. This syndrome affects 1 in 20,000 newborns, occurs more commonly in females, and causes profound mental retardation and, frequently, death before age 1. The chromosomal defect responsible (deletion of the short arm of chromosome 5) usually appears spontaneously, but may be inherited from a carrier parent. The characteristic cry is thought to result from abnormal laryngeal development.

Chaddock's sign

Description
Chaddock's *toe* sign is extension of the great toe and fanning of the other toes. To elicit this sign, the examiner strokes the side of the patient's foot just distal to the lateral malleolus. A positive sign indicates pyramidal tract disorders.

Chaddock's *wrist* sign is flexion of the wrist and extension of the fingers. To elicit this sign, the examiner strokes the ulnar surface of the patient's forearm near the wrist. A positive sign occurs on the affected side in hemiplegia.

Although Chaddock's sign signals pathology in children and adults, it is a normal finding in infants up to 7 months of age.

Cherry red spot

Description
Cherry red spot is an abnormal red circular area of the choroid, surrounded by an abnormal gray-white retina. It is viewed through the fovea centralis of the eye with an ophthalmoscope. A cherry red spot appears in infantile cerebral sphingolipidosis; for example, this spot appears in more than 90% of patients with Tay-Sachs disease.

Chest expansion, asymmetrical

Description
Asymmetrical chest expansion is the uneven extension of portions of the chest wall during inspiration. Asymmetrical expansion may develop suddenly or gradually and may affect one or both sides of the chest wall. It may occur as *delayed expiration* (chest lag); as *abnormal movement during inspiration* (for example, intercostal retractions, paradoxical movement, or chest-abdomen asynchrony); or as *unilateral absence of movement*. It most commonly results from pleural disorders, such as life-threatening hemothorax or tension pneumothorax. However, this sign can also result from musculoskeletal or neurologic disorders, airway obstruction, or trauma. Regardless of its underlying cause, asymmetrical chest expansion produces rapid and shallow or deep respirations that increase the work of breathing.

Mechanism
During normal respiration, the thorax uniformly expands upward and outward, then contracts downward and inward. When this process is disrupted, breathing becomes uncoordinated, causing asymmetrical chest expansion.

Possible causes
Central nervous system
Myasthenia gravis. Progressive loss of ventilatory muscle function produces chest-abdomen asynchrony that can lead to acute respiratory distress.
Respiratory
Bronchial obstruction. Life-threatening loss of airway patency may occur gradually or suddenly. Typically, lack of chest movement indicates complete obstruction; chest lag signals partial obstruction. If air is trapped in the chest, intercostal bulging during expiration and hyperresonance may be detected on percussion.
Flail chest. In this life-threatening injury to the ribs or sternum, the unstable portion of the chest wall collapses inward during inspiration and balloons outward during expiration (paradoxical movement).
Hemothorax. Typically resulting from trauma, this fulminating and life-threatening bleeding into the pleural space causes chest lag during inspiration.
Phrenic nerve dysfunction. In this disorder, the paralyzed hemidiaphragm fails to contract downward, causing asynchrony of the thorax and upper abdomen on the affected side during inspiration. Onset from trauma may be sudden; gradual onset may result from infection or spinal cord disease. If the patient has underlying pulmonary dysfunction that contributes to hyperventilation, his inability to breathe deeply or to cough effectively may cause atelectasis of the affected lung.
Pleural effusion. Chest lag at end-inspiration occurs gradually in this life-threatening accumulation of fluid,

blood, or pus in the pleural space. Usually, some combination of dyspnea, tachypnea, and tachycardia precedes chest lag; the patient may also have pleuritic pain that worsens with coughing or deep breathing.

Pneumonia. Depending on whether consolidation of fluid in the lungs develops unilaterally or bilaterally, asymmetrical chest expansion occurs as inspiratory chest lag or as chest-abdomen asynchrony.

Pneumothorax. Entrapment of air in the pleural space can cause chest lag at end-inspiration.

Pulmonary embolism. This acute, life-threatening disorder causes chest lag, sudden, stabbing chest pain, and tachycardia.

Musculoskeletal

Kyphoscoliosis. Abnormal curvature of both the anteroposterior thoracic spine (kyphosis) and the lateral spine (scoliosis) gradually compresses one lung and distends the other. This produces decreased chest wall movement on the compressed-lung side and ballooning of the intercostal muscles during inspiration on the opposite side.

Poliomyelitis. In this rare disorder, paralysis of the chest wall muscles and the diaphragm produces chest-abdomen asynchrony, fever, muscle pain, and weakness.

Treatments

Asymmetrical chest expansion can result from *pneumonectomy* and *surgical removal of several ribs.* Chest lag or absence of chest movement may also result from *intubation of a mainstem bronchus*—a serious complication typically due to incorrect insertion of an endotracheal tube or movement of the tube while it is in the trachea.

Clinical considerations

Traumatic injury to the patient's ribs or sternum, which can cause flail chest—a life-threatening emergency—should be suspected first.

• The physician should be notified and the unstable flail segment splinted with tape or sandbags.

• A rapid respiratory assessment should be performed and emergency interventions initiated for respiratory distress.

If flail chest has been ruled out and the patient is not experiencing respiratory distress:

• A history should be obtained and a thorough respiratory assessment performed.

• Diagnostic tests may include arterial blood gas studies and chest X-rays.

Chest pain

Description

This symptom most often results from disorders that affect thoracic or abdominal organs—the heart, pleurae, lungs, gallbladder, pancreas, or stomach. It is an important indicator of several acute and life-threatening cardiopulmonary and GI disorders. However, it can also result from musculoskeletal and hematologic disorders, anxiety, and drug therapy.

The cause of chest pain may be difficult to distinguish initially. Chest pain can arise suddenly or gradually. It can radiate to the arms, neck, jaw, or back. It can be steady or intermittent, mild or acute. And it can range in character from a sharp shooting sensation to a feeling of heaviness, fullness, or even indigestion. It can be provoked or aggravated by stress, anxiety, exertion, deep breathing, or eating certain foods.

Possible causes
Respiratory

Asthma. In a life-threatening asthmatic attack, diffuse and painful chest tightness arises suddenly along with a dry cough and mild wheezing, which progress to a productive cough, audible wheezing, and severe dyspnea.

Blastomycosis. Besides pleuritic chest pain, this disorder initially produces signs and symptoms that mimic those of viral upper respiratory infection.

Bronchitis. In its acute form, this disorder produces a burning chest pain or a sensation of substernal tightness.

Coccidioidomycosis. In this disorder, pleuritic chest pain occurs with a dry or slightly productive cough.

Interstitial lung disease. As this disease advances, the patient may have pleuritic chest pain along with progressive dyspnea, cellophane-type crackles, nonproductive cough, fatigue, weight loss, clubbing, or cyanosis.

Legionnaire's disease. This disorder produces pleuritic chest pain along with malaise, headache, and possibly diarrhea, anorexia, diffuse myalgias, and general weakness.

Lung abscess. Pleuritic chest pain develops insidiously in this disorder along with a pleural friction rub and a cough.

Lung cancer. The chest pain associated with lung cancer is often described as an intermittent aching felt deep within the chest. If the tumor metastasizes to the ribs or vertebrae, the pain becomes localized, continuous, and gnawing.

Nocardiosis. This disorder causes pleuritic chest pain with a cough.

Pleurisy. The chest pain of pleurisy arises abruptly and reaches maximum intensity within a few hours. It is sharp, even knifelike, usually unilateral, and located in the lower and lateral aspects of the chest. Deep breathing, coughing, or thoracic movement characteristically aggravates it.

Pneumonia. This disorder produces pleuritic chest pain that increases with deep inspiration and is accompanied by shaking chills and fever.

Pneumothorax. Spontaneous pneumothorax, a life-threatening disorder, causes sudden sharp chest pain that is severe, often unilateral, and rarely localized; it increases with chest movement. When it is located centrally and radiates to the neck, it may mimic myocardial infarction (MI). After the pain's onset, dyspnea and cyanosis progressively worsen.

Pulmonary actinomycosis. This disorder causes pleuritic chest pain with a cough that is initially dry but later produces purulent sputum.

Pulmonary embolism. This disorder produces a substernal pain or choking sensation. Typically, the patient first experiences sudden dyspnea with intense angina-like or pleuritic pain aggravated by deep breathing and thoracic movement.

Tuberculosis. In a patient with this disorder, pleuritic chest pain and fine crackles occur after coughing.

Cardiovascular

Angina. In *angina pectoris,* the patient may experience a feeling of tightness or pressure in the chest that he describes as pain or a sensation of indigestion or expansion. Usually, the pain occurs in the retrosternal region over a palm-sized or larger area. It may radiate to the neck, jaw, and arms—classically, to the inner aspect of the left arm. Anginal pain tends to begin gradually, build to its maximum, then slowly subside. Provoked by exertion, emotional stress, or a heavy meal, the pain typically lasts 2 to 10 minutes.

In *Prinzmetal's angina,* chest pain occurs when the patient is at rest—or it may awaken him.

Aortic aneurysm (dissecting). The chest pain associated with this disorder usually begins suddenly and is most severe at its onset. The patient describes an excruciating tearing, ripping, stabbing pain in his chest and neck that radiates to his upper back, abdomen, and lower back.

Cardiomyopathy. In hypertrophic cardiomyopathy, angina-like chest pain may be accompanied by dyspnea, a cough, dizziness, syncope, gallops, and murmurs.

Mediastinitis. This disorder produces severe retrosternal chest pain that radiates to the epigastrium, back, or shoulder and may worsen with breathing, coughing, or sneezing.

Mitral prolapse. Typically, the patient with a prolapsed mitral valve will experience sharp, stabbing precordial chest pain or precordial ache. The pain can last for seconds or for hours; it occasionally mimics the pain of ischemic heart disease.

Myocardial infarction (MI). The chest pain in MI lasts from 15 minutes to hours. Typically a crushing substernal pain, unrelieved by rest or nitroglycerin, it may radiate to the patient's left arm, jaw, neck, or shoulder blades.

Pericarditis. This disorder produces precordial or retrosternal pain aggravated by deep breathing, coughing, position changes, and occasionally by swallowing. Frequently, the pain is sharp or cutting and radiates to the shoulder and neck.

Pulmonary hypertension (primary). Angina-like pain develops late in this disorder, usually on exertion. The precordial pain may radiate to the neck but does not characteristically radiate to the arms.

Thoracic outlet syndrome. Often causing paresthesias along the ulnar distribution of the arm, this syndrome can be confused with angina. The patient usually experiences angina-like pain after lifting his arms above his head, working with his hands above his shoulders, or lifting a weight. The pain disappears immediately when he lowers his arms.

Gastrointestinal

Cholecystitis. This disorder typically produces abrupt epigastric or right upper quadrant pain, which may be sharp or intensely aching. The pain, either steady or intermittent, may radiate to the back.

Distention of the colon's splenic flexure. Central chest pain may radiate to the left arm in this disorder. The pain may be relieved by defecation or passage of flatus.

Esophageal spasm. In this disorder, substernal chest pain may last up to an hour or more and can radiate to the neck, jaw, arms, or back. It often mimics anginal pain—a squeezing or dull sensation.

Hiatal hernia. Typically, this disorder produces an angina-like sternal burning, ache, or pressure that may radiate to the left shoulder and arm. The discomfort often occurs after a meal when the patient bends over or lies down.

Pancreatitis. In its acute form, this disorder usually causes intense pain in the epigastric area that radiates to the back and worsens when the patient is supine.

Peptic ulcer. In this disorder, sharp and burning pain usually arises in the epigastric region. This pain characteristically arises hours after food intake, often occurring during the night. It lasts longer than angina-like pain and is relieved by food or antacids.

Musculoskeletal

Costochondritis. Pain and tenderness occur at the costochondral junctions, especially at the second costocartilage.

Muscle strain. Strained chest, arm, or shoulder muscles may cause a superficial and continuous ache or pulling sensation in the chest. Lifting, pulling, or pushing heavy objects may aggravate the discomfort.

Rib fracture. The chest pain due to fractured ribs is usually sharp, severe, and aggravated by inspiration, coughing, or pressure on the affected area.

Skin

Herpes zoster (shingles). The pain of pre-eruptive herpes zoster may mimic that of MI. Initially, the pain—characteristically unilateral—is sharp and shooting. About 4 or 5 days after its onset, small, red, nodular lesions erupt on the painful areas—usually the thorax, arms, and legs—and the chest pain becomes burning.

Hematologic

Sickle cell crisis. Chest pain associated with sickle cell crisis typically has a bizarre distribution. It may start as a vague pain, often located in the back, hands, or feet. As the pain worsens, it becomes generalized or localized to the abdomen or chest, causing severe pleuritic pain.

Immunologic

Chinese restaurant syndrome. This benign condition—a reaction to excessive ingestion of monosodium glutamate (a common additive in Chinese foods)—mimics the signs of acute MI. The patient may complain of retrosternal burning, ache, or pressure and a burning sensation over his arms, legs, and face; a sensation of facial pressure; shortness of breath; or tachycardia.

Psychiatric

Anxiety. Acute anxiety can produce intermittent, sharp, stabbing pain, often located in the left breast. This pain is not related to exertion and lasts only a few seconds, but the patient may experience a precordial ache or a sensation of heaviness that lasts for hours or days.

Drugs

Abrupt withdrawal of beta blockers can cause rebound angina in patients with coronary heart disease—especially those who have received high doses for a prolonged period.

Clinical considerations

• Vital signs should be taken, a brief history of the pain obtained, and the physician notified.

• Sudden, severe chest pain requires prompt evaluation and treatment since it may herald a life-threatening disorder.

• Appropriate assessment and interventions depend on the location and character of the pain as well as accompanying signs and symptoms.

• Cardiac monitoring should be initiated, emergency equipment kept close at hand, and emergency interventions anticipated to maintain adequate cardiopulmonary status.

• Vital signs should be monitored frequently.

• If chest pain is *not* severe, a complete history should be obtained and respiratory and cardiovascular assessments performed.

• Diagnostic tests may include an EKG, a lung scan, and blood studies.

• Because a patient with chest pain may deny his discomfort, the importance of reporting symptoms should be stressed to allow adjustment of his treatment.

• Emotional support and clear explanations should be provided to relieve anxiety, which may aggravate chest pain.

Cheyne-Stokes respirations

Description

The Cheyne-Stokes respirations pattern involves periodic breathing characterized by a waxing and waning period of hyperpnea alternating with a shorter period of apnea. This pattern can occur normally in people who live at high altitudes and in the elderly during sleep. Most often, though, it indicates increased intracranial pressure from a deep cerebral or brain stem lesion (usually bilateral), or a metabolic disturbance in the brain.

Cheyne-Stokes respirations always indicate a major change in the patient's condition—usually for the worse. For example, in a patient who has had head trauma or brain surgery, Cheyne-Stokes respirations may signal increasing intracranial pressure.

Possible causes

Central nervous system

Hypertensive encephalopathy. In this life-threatening disorder, severe hypertension precedes Cheyne-Stokes respirations.

Increased intracranial pressure (ICP). As ICP rises, Cheyne-Stokes is the first irregular respiratory pattern to occur. It is preceded by decreased level of consciousness and accompanied by hypertension, headache, vomiting, impaired or unequal motor movement, and visual disturbances (blurring, diplopia, photophobia, and pupillary changes.)

Cardiovascular

Heart failure. In left ventricular failure, Cheyne-Stokes respirations may occur with exertional dyspnea and orthopnea.

Stokes-Adams attacks. Cheyne-Stokes respirations may follow a Stokes-Adams attack—a syncopal episode associated with atrioventricular block.

Genitourinary

Renal failure. In end-stage chronic renal failure, Cheyne-Stokes respirations may occur along with bleeding gums, oral lesions, ammonia breath odor, and marked changes in every body system.

Drugs

Large doses of hypnotics, narcotics, or barbiturates can precipitate Cheyne-Stokes respirations.

Clinical considerations

• Vital signs should be taken and the physician notified immediately.
• Periods of hyperpnea and apnea should be timed for 3 or 4 minutes to evaluate respirations.
• A neurologic assessment should be performed.
• Emergency interventions should be anticipated to maintain airway patency and oxygenation.

Chills
(Rigors)

Description

Chills are extreme, involuntary muscle contractions with characteristic paroxysms of violent shivering and teeth-chattering. Commonly accompanied by fever, chills tend to arise suddenly, most often heralding the onset of infection. Certain diseases, such as pneumococcal pneumonia, produce only a single, shaking chill. Other diseases, such as malaria, produce intermittent chills with recurring high fever. Still others produce continuous chills for up to 1 hour, precipitating a high fever.

Chills can also result from lymphomas, transfusion reactions, and certain drugs. Of course, chills without fever occur as a normal response to exposure to cold.

Infants do not get chills because they have poorly developed shivering mechanisms.

Mechanism

Chills occur as a compensatory mechanism to generate body heat when the body feels cold. This feeling of cold may result from normal exposure to cold, or it may result from a resetting of the body's thermostat to a higher level, as occurs in fever.

Possible causes

Eyes, ears, nose, and throat

Otitis media. Acute suppurative otitis media produces chills accompanied by fever and severe, deep, and throbbing ear pain.

Sinusitis. In acute sinusitis, chills occur along with fever, headache, and pain, tenderness, and swelling over the affected sinuses.

Respiratory

Legionnaire's disease. Within 12 to 48 hours after onset of this disease, the patient suddenly develops chills and a high fever.

Lung abscess. Besides chills, this disorder causes sweating, pleuritic chest pain, dyspnea, clubbing, weakness, headache, malaise, anorexia, weight loss, and a cough that produces large amounts of purulent, foul-smelling, often bloody sputum.

Pneumonia. A single shaking chill usually heralds the sudden onset of pneumococcal pneumonia; other pneumonias characteristically cause intermittent chills.

Psittacosis. This disease typically begins with abrupt onset of chills, fever, headache, myalgias, epistaxis, and prostration.

Cardiovascular

Infective endocarditis. This infection produces abrupt onset of intermittent, shaking chills with fever.

Septic shock. Initially, septic shock produces chills, fever, and possibly nausea, vomiting, and diarrhea. The patient's skin is typically flushed, warm, and dry; his blood pressure is normal or slightly low; and he has tachycardia and tachypnea.

Gastrointestinal

Cholangitis. Charcot's triad—chills with spiking fever, abdominal pain, and jaundice—characterizes sudden obstruction of the common bile duct.

Hepatic abscess. Although this infection can occur insidiously, it most commonly arises abruptly, with chills, fever, nausea, vomiting, diarrhea, anorexia, and severe upper abdominal tenderness and pain that may radiate to the right shoulder.

Genitourinary

Pyelonephritis. In acute pyelonephritis, the patient develops chills, high fever, and possibly nausea and vomiting over several hours to days.

Renal abscess. This disorder initially produces sudden chills and fever.

Musculoskeletal

Septic arthritis. Chills and fever accompany the characteristic red, swollen, and painful joints this disorder causes.

Hematologic

Hemolytic anemia. In acute hemolytic anemia, fulminating chills occur with fever and abdominal pain.

Obstetrics-Gynecology

Pelvic inflammatory disease. This infection causes chills and fever with, typically, lower abdominal pain and tenderness; profuse, purulent vaginal discharge; or abnormal menstrual bleeding.

Puerperal or postabortal sepsis. Chills and high fever occur as early as 6 hours or as late as 10 days postpartum or postabortion.

Infectious diseases

Influenza. Initially, this disorder causes abrupt onset of chills, high fever, malaise, headache, myalgias, and nonproductive cough. Some patients may also suddenly develop rhinitis, rhinorrhea, laryngitis, conjunctivitis, hoarseness, and sore throat. Chills generally subside after the first few days, but intermittent fever, weakness, and cough may persist up to 1 week.

Lymphogranuloma venereum. Along with chills and lymphadenopathy, this disorder produces fever, headache, anorexia, myalgias, arthralgias, and weight loss. The primary genital lesion is a papule or small erosion, which precedes lymphatic involvement and heals spontaneously within a few days.

Malaria. The malarial paroxysm begins with a period of chills that lasts 1 to 2 hours. A high fever lasting 3 to 4 hours follows, and 2 to 4 hours of profuse diaphoresis complete the paroxysmal cycle. In benign malaria, the paroxysm may be interspersed with periods of well-being.

Miliary tuberculosis. In its acute form, this illness presents with intermittent chills, high fever, and night sweats.

Typhoid fever. This disorder may initially cause sudden chills and a sharply rising fever. More often, though, the patient's body temperature gradually increases for 5 to 7 days with accompanying chilliness or frank chills.

Neoplastic

Hodgkin's lymphoma. In some patients, this lymphoma produces a cyclical fever with intermittent chills. The patient characteristically experiences several days or weeks of fever and chills alternating with periods of no fever and no chills.

Infection

Gram-negative bacteremia. This infection causes sudden chills and fever. It also causes nausea, vomiting, diarrhea, and prostration.

Lymphangitis. Acute lymphangitis produces chills and other systemic symptoms, such as fever, malaise, and headache.

Environmental

Rocky Mountain spotted fever. This disorder begins with sudden onset of chills, fever, malaise, excruciating headache, and muscle, bone, and joint pain.

Snake bite. Most pit viper bites that result in envenomation cause chills, typically with fever.

Violin spider bite. The bite of this spider produces chills, fever, malaise, weakness, nausea, vomiting, and joint pain within 24 to 48 hours.

Drugs
Amphotericin B heads the list of common drugs associated with chills. However, I.V. bleomycin and intermittent administration of oral antipyretics can also cause chills.

Treatments
Infection at an I.V. insertion site can cause chills, high fever, and local redness, warmth, induration, and tenderness.

Hemolytic transfusion reactions may cause chills during the transfusion or immediately afterward. A *nonhemolytic febrile reaction* may also cause chills.

Clinical considerations
• Vital signs (rectal temperature) should be taken and a history obtained.
• Diagnostic tests may include samples of blood, sputum, or wound drainage for culture.
• Because chills are an involuntary response to an increased body temperature set by the hypothalamic thermostat, providing the patient with blankets will not stop his chills or shivering. However, room temperature should be kept consistent.
• Adequate hydration should be provided.

Chorea
(Choreiform movements)

Description
Chorea may be defined as brief, unpredictable bursts of rapid, jerky motion that interrupt normal coordinated movement. Chorea indicates dysfunction of the extrapyramidal system. Unlike tics, choreiform movements are seldom repetitive, but tend to appear purposeful despite their involuntary nature. Although any muscle can be affected, chorea most often involves the face, head, lower arms, and hands. It can affect both sides of the body or only one, but when it affects the face, both sides are always involved. Chorea may be aggravated by excitement or fatigue and may disappear during sleep. In some patients, it may be difficult to distinguish from athetosis (snakelike, writhing movements), although choreiform movements are generally more rapid than athetoid ones.

Possible causes
Central nervous system
Cerebral infarction. An infarction that involves the thalamic area produces unilateral or bilateral chorea.

Encephalitis. Chorea occurs in the recovery phase of this disorder.

Huntington's chorea. In this inherited disorder, chorea may be the first sign or may occur with intellectual decline that leads to emotional disturbances and dementia. The patient's movements tend to be choreoathetotic and may be accompanied by dysarthria, dystonia, prancing gait, dysphagia, and facial grimacing.

Gastrointestinal
Wilson's disease. Chorea is an early indicator of this disorder, along with dystonia affecting the arms and legs.

Environmental
Carbon monoxide poisoning. A patient who survives severe carbon monoxide poisoning may have neurologic sequelae, such as chorea, rigidity, dementia, impaired sensory function, masklike face, generalized seizures, and myoclonus.

Lead poisoning. In the later stages of lead poisoning, chorea occurs along with seizures, headache, memory lapses, and severe mental impairment.

Manganese poisoning. In miners who have been exposed to manganese dioxide for prolonged periods, chorea characteristically occurs with propulsive gait, dystonia, and rigidity.

Drugs
Phenothiazines (especially the piperazine derivatives), haloperidol, thiothixene, and loxapine frequently produce chorea. Metoclopramide, metyrosine, oral contraceptives, levo-

dopa, and phenytoin may also cause this sign.

Clinical considerations

• A complete medical and family history should be obtained and a physical examination performed to evaluate the severity of the chorea.

• Because the patient's movements are involuntary and increase his risk of severe injury, the side rails of the bed should be padded and sharp objects kept out of his environment.

• Physical activity and emotional distress should be minimized.

Chvostek's sign

Description

Chvostek's sign is an abnormal spasm of the facial muscles that is elicited by lightly tapping the patient's facial nerve near his lower jaw. This sign usually suggests hypocalcemia but can occur normally in about 25% of patients. Typically, it precedes other signs of hypocalcemia and persists until the onset of tetany. The degree of Chvostek's sign reflects the patient's

Eliciting Chvostek's Sign

To begin, the examiner tells the patient to relax his facial muscles. Then she stands directly in front of him and taps the facial nerve either just anterior to the earlobe and below the zygomatic arch or between the zygomatic arch and the corner of his mouth. A positive response varies from twitching of the lip at the corner of the mouth to spasm of all facial muscles, depending on the severity of hypocalcemia.

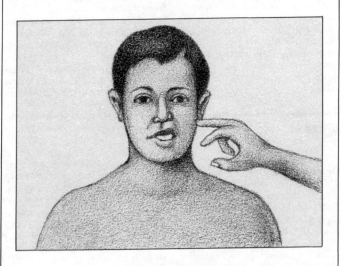

serum calcium level. The sign cannot be elicited during tetany because of strong muscle contractions.

Normally, eliciting Chvostek's sign is attempted only in patients with suspected hypocalcemic disorders. But because the parathyroid gland regulates calcium balance, Chvostek's sign may also be tested in patients before neck surgery, to provide a baseline.

Circumstantiality

Description
Circumstantiality is speech in which the main point is obscured by minute detail. Although the speaker may recognize his main point and return to it after many digressions, the listener may fail to recognize it. Circumstantiality commonly occurs in compulsive disorders, organic brain disorders, and schizophrenia.

Claude's hyperkinesis sign

Description
This sign reflects increased reflex activity of paretic muscles, elicited by painful stimuli.

Clavicular sign

Description
Clavicular sign is swelling, puffiness, or edema at the medial third of the right clavicle, most often seen in congenital syphilis.

Cleeman's sign

Description
Cleeman's sign is slight linear depression or wrinkling of the skin superior to the patella. It usually indicates a femoral fracture with overriding bone fragments.

Clenched fist sign

Description
This sign is present when the patient places a clenched fist against his chest. This gesture may be performed by patients with angina pectoris when they are asked to indicate the location of their pain. The patient's gesture conveys the constricting, oppressive quality of substernal pain.

Clicks

Description
Clicks are brief, high-frequency heart sounds auscultated during systole or diastole. *Ejection clicks* occur soon after the first heart sound. Presumably, they result from sudden distention of a dilated pulmonary artery or the aorta or from forceful opening of the pulmonic or aortic valves. Associated with increased pulmonary resistance and hypertension, they occur most commonly with septal defects or patent ductus arteriosus. To detect ejection clicks best, the examiner has the patient sit upright or lie down, then auscultates the heart with the diaphragm of the stethoscope.

Systolic clicks occur most often in mid- to late systole. They are characteristic of mitral valve prolapse. To detect systolic clicks, the examiner auscultates the heart over the mitral valve with the diaphragm of the stethoscope.

Clubbing

Description
Clubbing is the painless, usually bilateral increase in soft tissue around

Evaluating Clubbed Fingers

To quickly assess a patient's fingers for early clubbing, the examiner gently palpates the bases of the patient's nails. Normally, they will feel firm— but in early clubbing, nail bases will feel springy when palpated. To evaluate late clubbing, the examiner has the patient place the first phalanges of the forefingers together, as shown. Normal nail bases are concave and create a small, diamond-shaped space when the first phalanges are opposed (top). In late clubbing, however, the now-convex nail bases can touch without leaving a space (bottom).

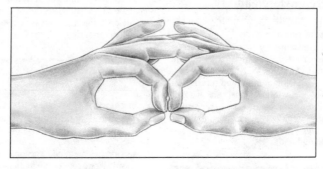

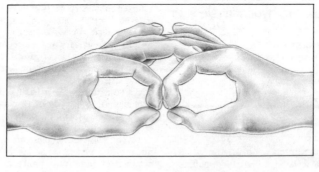

the terminal phalanges of the fingers or toes. A nonspecific sign of pulmonary and cyanotic cardiovascular disorders, it does not involve changes in the underlying bone. In early clubbing, the normal 160° angle between the nail and the nail base approximates 180°. As clubbing progresses, this angle widens and the base of the nail becomes visibly swollen. In late clubbing, the angle where the nail meets the now-convex nail base extends more than halfway up the nail.

Possible causes
Respiratory
Bronchiectasis. Clubbing occurs commonly in the late stage of this disorder.

Bronchitis. In chronic bronchitis, clubbing may occur as a late sign and is unrelated to the severity of the disease.

Emphysema. Clubbing occurs late in this disease.

Interstitial fibrosis. Clubbing occurs in almost all patients with advanced interstitial fibrosis.

Lung abscess. Initially, this disorder produces clubbing, which may reverse with resolution of the abscess.

Lung and pleural cancer. Clubbing occurs commonly in these diseases.

Cardiovascular

Congestive heart failure. Clubbing occurs as a late sign along with wheezing, dyspnea, and fatigue.

Endocarditis. In subacute infective endocarditis, clubbing may be accompanied by fever, anorexia, pallor, weakness, night sweats, fatigue, tachycardia, and weight loss.

Clinical considerations

• The extent of clubbing in both the fingers and the toes should be evaluated.

• The patient's plan of treatment should be reviewed periodically, since clubbing may resolve with correction of the underlying disorder.

Rare Causes of Clubbing

Clubbing is typically a sign of pulmonary or cardiovascular disease. But it can also result from certain hepatic and gastrointestinal disorders—such as cirrhosis, Crohn's disease, or ulcerative colitis. Clubbing occurs only rarely in these disorders, however, so first check for more common signs and symptoms. For example, a patient with *cirrhosis* usually experiences right upperquadrant pain and hepatomegaly. A patient with *Crohn's disease* typically has abdominal cramping and tenderness. And a patient with *ulcerative colitis* may have diffuse abdominal pain and blood-streaked diarrhea.

Codman's sign

Description

Codman's sign is pain resulting from the rupture of the supraspinatus tendon. The sign can be elicited by asking the patient to relax the arm on the affected side while the arm is abducted. Codman's sign is present if the deltoid muscle contracts and pain occurs when the arm is no longer supported.

Cogwheel rigidity

Description

Cogwheel rigidity is abnormal muscle rigidity that abates in a series of jerking movements when the muscle is passively stretched. The cardinal sign of Parkinson's disease, it may also be caused by certain drugs, for example phenothiazines and other antipsychotics (such as haloperidol, thiothixene, and loxapine). Metoclopramide and metyrosine infrequently cause cogwheel rigidity. This sign can be elicited by stabilizing the patient's forearm and then moving his hand through the range of motion. Cogwheel rigidity most often appears in the arms, but it can sometimes be elicited in the ankle. Both the patient and the examiner can see and feel these characteristic movements, thought to be a combination of rigidity and tremor.

Cold intolerance

Description

Cold intolerance is an increased sensitivity to cold temperatures. This symptom usually develops gradually and typically results from tumors or hormonal deficiency. In the elderly, though, it reflects normal age-related decreases in basal metabolic rate (BMR) and muscle mass.

Mechanism
Cold intolerance reflects damage to the body's temperature-regulating mechanism (located in the hypothalamus) or a decreased BMR.

Possible causes
Endocrine
Hypopituitarism. Clinical features usually develop slowly in this disorder and vary with its severity. Cold intolerance and shivering typically accompany cold, dry, and thin skin with a waxy pallor, and fine wrinkles around the mouth.
Hypothalamic lesion. A patient with hypothalamic damage may show unexplained fluctuations from cold intolerance to heat intolerance. Cold intolerance develops suddenly; the patient typically complains of feeling chilled, shivering, and wearing extra clothes to keep warm.
Hypothyroidism. Cold intolerance develops early in this disorder and progressively worsens.

Clinical considerations
• A history should be obtained and a physical examination performed.
• The patient's comfort level should be increased by regulating the room temperature and by providing extra clothing and blankets.
• With proper treatment, the patient can expect relief from this symptom.

Comolli's sign

Description
Comolli's sign is triangular swelling over the scapula that matches the shape of the scapula. This sign indicates scapular fracture.

Complementary opposition sign

Description
Complementary opposition sign is increased effort in lifting a paretic leg, demonstrated in the unaffected leg. To elicit this sign, the examiner positions the patient supine and places one hand under the heel of the unaffected leg. If the examiner feels downward pressure on the hand when the patient attempts to lift the paretic leg, the sign is present.

Compulsion

Description
Compulsion is stereotyped, repetitive behavior in which the individual recognizes the irrationality of his actions but is unable to stop them. These actions may be simple, mild, and uncomplicated (such as constant handwashing) or they may be dramatic, complex, and ritualized. Compulsion occurs in obsessive-compulsive disorders and occasionally in schizophrenia.

Confabulation

Description
Confabulation is fabrication to cover gaps in memory. It is most often seen in alcoholism and Korsakoff's syndrome.

Confusion

Description
Confusion is a mental state characterized by disorientation regarding time,

place, or person that causes bewilderment, perplexity, lack of orderly thought, and inability to choose or act decisively. Depending on its cause, confusion may arise suddenly or gradually and may be temporary or irreversible. Aggravated by stress and sensory deprivation, confusion often occurs in hospitalized patients—especially the elderly, in whom it may be mistaken for senility.

When severe confusion arises suddenly and the patient also has hallucinations and psychomotor hyperactivity, his condition is classified as *delirium*. Long-term, progressive confusion with deterioration of all cognitive functions is classified as *dementia*.

Confusion can result from hypoxemia due to pulmonary disorders. However, it can also have a metabolic, neurologic, cardiovascular, cerebrovascular, or nutritional origin or can result from a severe systemic infection or the effects of toxins, drugs, or alcohol. Confusion may signal worsening of an underlying and perhaps irreversible disease. It is often an early sign of fluid and electrolyte imbalance.

Possible causes
Central nervous system
Alzheimer's disease. This progressive brain disorder eventually produces severe and irreversible confusion along with memory loss and intellectual deterioration.

Brain tumor. In the early stages of brain tumor, confusion is usually mild and difficult to detect. As the tumor impinges on cerebral structures, however, the patient's confusion worsens.

Cerebrovascular disorders. These disorders produce confusion due to tissue hypoxia and ischemia. Confusion may be insidious and fleeting, as in a transient ischemic attack, or acute and permanent, as in cerebrovascular accident.

Head trauma. Concussion, contusion, and brain hemorrhage may produce confusion at the time of injury, shortly afterward, or months or even years afterward.

Infection. CNS infections, such as meningitis, cause varying degrees of confusion along with headache and nuchal rigidity.

Low perfusion states. Mild confusion is an early sign of decreased cerebral perfusion.

Metabolic encephalopathy. Both hyperglycemia and hypoglycemia can produce sudden onset of confusion. A patient with hypoglycemia may also experience transient delirium and seizures. Uremic and hepatic encephalopathies produce gradual confusion that may progress to seizures and coma.

Seizure disorders. Mild-to-moderate confusion may immediately follow any type of seizure. The confusion usually disappears within several hours.

Respiratory
Hypoxemia. Acute pulmonary disorders that result in hypoxemia produce confusion that can range from mild disorientation to delirium. Chronic pulmonary disorders produce persistent confusion.

Endocrine
Thyroid hormone disorders. Hyperthyroidism produces mild-to-moderate confusion along with nervousness, inability to concentrate, weight loss, flushed skin, and tachycardia. Hypothyroidism produces mild, insidious confusion and memory loss; weight gain; bradycardia; and fatigue.

Metabolic
Fluid and electrolyte imbalance. The extent of imbalance determines the severity of the patient's confusion.

Nutritional deficiencies. Inadequate dietary intake of thiamine, niacin, or vitamin B_{12} produces insidious, progressive confusion and possible mental deterioration.

Environmental

Heat stroke. This disorder causes pronounced confusion that gradually worsens as body temperature rises.

Heavy metal poisoning. Chronic ingestion or inhalation of heavy metals (such as lead, arsenic, mercury, and manganese) eventually produces confusion and, typically, weakness and drowsiness.

Hypothermia. Confusion may be an early sign of this disorder. As body temperature continues to drop, confusion progresses to stupor and coma.

Drugs

Large doses of CNS depressants produce confusion that can persist for several days after the drug is discontinued. Narcotic and barbiturate withdrawal also causes acute confusion, possibly with delirium. Other drugs that commonly cause confusion include lidocaine, digitalis, indomethacin, cycloserine, chloroquine, atropine, and cimetidine.

Alcohol intoxication causes confusion and stupor, and withdrawal may cause delirium and seizures.

Clinical considerations

• A history should be obtained with the help of family members and a physical examination performed.

• To protect himself and others, a confused patient should never be left unattended. Restraints should be used when necessary to ensure his safety.

• The patient's environment should be kept calm and quiet, and staff members should introduce themselves to the patient each time they enter the room.

• A calendar and clock should be kept nearby to help the patient remain oriented.

Conjunctival injection

Description

Conjunctival injection is nonuniform redness of the conjunctiva. This redness can be diffuse, localized, or pe-

ripheral—or it may encircle a clear cornea. It is a common ocular sign associated with inflammation.

Most often, conjunctival injection results from bacterial or viral conjunctivitis. But it can also signal a severe ocular disorder that, if untreated, may lead to permanent blindness. In particular, conjunctival injection is an early sign of trachoma—a leading cause of blindness in Third World countries and in American Indians living in the southwestern United States.

Conjunctival injection can also result from minor eye irritation due to inadequate sleep, overuse of contact lenses, environmental irritants, and excessive eye rubbing.

Mechanism

Conjunctival injection results from hyperemia, or increased infusion of blood to the area.

Possible causes

Eyes, ears, nose, and throat

Astigmatism. An uncorrected or poorly corrected astigmatism can produce diffuse conjunctival injection.

Blepharitis. This disorder produces diffuse conjunctival injection.

Conjunctival foreign bodies and abrasions. These conditions feature localized conjunctival injection with sudden, severe eye pain.

Conjunctivitis. Allergic, bacterial, fungal, or viral causes of conjunctivitis produce diffuse peripheral conjunctival injection but have different associated signs and symptoms.

Corneal abrasion. In this disorder, diffuse conjunctival injection is extremely painful—especially when the eyelids move over the abrasion.

Corneal erosion. Recurrent corneal erosion produces diffuse conjunctival injection.

Corneal ulcer. Bacterial, viral, and fungal corneal ulcers produce diffuse conjunctival injection that increases in the circumcorneal area.

Dacryoadenitis. In this disorder, the patient has large, diffuse conjunctival injection and complains of pain over the temporal part of the eye.

Episcleritis. Conjunctival injection is localized and raised and may be violet or purplish-pink in this disorder.

Glaucoma. In acute closed-angle glaucoma, conjunctival injection is typically circumcorneal.

Hyphema. Depending on the type and extent of traumatic injury, a hyphema produces diffuse conjunctival injection, possibly with lid and orbital edema.

Iritis. In acute iritis, marked conjunctival injection is located mainly around the cornea.

Keratoconjunctivitis sicca. This disorder produces severe diffuse conjunctival injection.

Ocular lacerations and intraocular foreign bodies. Diffuse conjunctival injection may be increased in the area of injury.

Ocular tumors. If a tumor is located in the orbit behind the globe, conjunctival injection may occur together with exophthalmos.

Scleritis. In this relatively rare disorder, conjunctival injection can be diffuse or localized over the area of the scleritis nodule.

Stevens-Johnson syndrome. This disorder produces diffuse conjunctival injection.

Uveitis. Diffuse conjunctival injection, which may be increased in the circumcorneal area, characterizes this disorder.

Environmental

Chemical burns. In this ocular emergency, diffuse conjunctival injection occurs, but severe pain is the most prominent symptom.

Clinical considerations

If conjunctival injection is due to a chemical splash:

• The eye(s) should be irrigated immediately with copious amounts of normal saline solution. Contact lenses, if present, should be removed first.

• Eyelids should be everted and fornices wiped with a cotton-tipped applicator to remove as much of the chemical as possible and to remove any foreign body particles.

• As soon as the patient's condition permits, a history should be obtained and an eye examination performed.

If conjunctival injection results from conjunctivitis (which is usually contagious):

• The affected eye(s) should not be touched.

• Hands must be washed before and after administration of eye medication or other treatments.

Conjunctival paleness

Description

Conjunctival paleness is the lack of color in the tissues inside the eyelid. Although the conjunctiva is a transparent mucous membrane, the portion lining the eyelids normally appears pink or red because it overlies the vasculature of the inner lid. This sign indicates anemia.

Constipation

Description

Constipation is defined as small, infrequent, and difficult bowel movements. Because normal bowel movements can vary in frequency from twice a day to once every 3 days, constipation must be determined in relation to the patient's normal elimination pattern. Constipation may be a minor annoyance or, uncommonly, a sign of a life-threatening disorder, such as acute intestinal obstruction or mesenteric artery ischemia. Untreated, constipation can lead to headache, anorexia, and abdominal discomfort, and can adversely affect the patient's lifestyle and well-being.

Mechanism

Most often, constipation occurs when the urge to defecate is suppressed and the muscles associated with bowel movements remain contracted. Because the autonomic nervous system controls bowel movements—by sensing rectal distention from fecal contents and by stimulating the external sphincter—any factor that influences this system may cause bowel dysfunction. (See *How Habits and Stress Cause Constipation*.)

Possible causes

Central nervous system

Multiple sclerosis. This disorder can produce constipation along with many other signs and symptoms of sensory and motor disturbances.

Spinal cord lesion. Constipation may occur in this disorder, depending on the level of the lesion.

Endocrine

Diabetic neuropathy. This neuropathy produces episodic constipation or diarrhea.

Hypothyroidism. This disorder causes early and insidious onset of constipation.

Gastrointestinal

Anal fissure. A crack or laceration in the lining of the anal wall can cause acute constipation—usually due to the patient's fear of the severe tearing or burning pain associated with bowel movements.

Anorectal abscess. In this disorder, constipation occurs together with severe, throbbing, localized pain and tenderness at the abscess site.

Cirrhosis. In the early stages of cirrhosis, the patient has constipation along with nausea, vomiting, and a dull pain in the right upper quadrant.

Crohn's disease. Although most patients with this disorder experience diarrhea, some develop chronic constipation due to strictures.

Diverticulitis. In this disorder, constipation occurs together with left lower quadrant pain and tenderness.

Hemorrhoids. Thrombosed hemorrhoids cause constipation as the patient tries to avoid the severe pain of defecation.

Hepatic porphyria. Abdominal pain—which may be severe, colicky, localized, or generalized—precedes constipation in hepatic porphyria.

Intestinal obstruction. Constipation associated with this disorder varies in severity and onset with the location and extent of the obstruction. In partial obstruction, constipation may alternate with leakage of liquid stool. In complete obstruction, obstipation may occur. Constipation can be the earliest sign of partial colon obstruction, but it usually occurs later if the level of the obstruction is more proximal.

Irritable bowel syndrome. Usually, this common syndrome produces chronic constipation, although some patients may have intermittent, watery diarrhea and others may complain of alternating constipation and diarrhea.

Mesenteric artery ischemia. This life-threatening disorder produces sudden constipation with failure to expel stool or flatus.

Ulcerative colitis. In chronic ulcerative colitis, constipation may occur—but bloody diarrhea with pus and/or mucus is the hallmark of this disorder.

Ulcerative proctitis. This disorder produces acute constipation with tenesmus. The patient feels an intense urge to defecate but is unable to do so. Instead, he may eliminate mucus, pus, or blood.

Metabolic

Hypercalcemia. In this disorder, constipation usually occurs along with anorexia, nausea, vomiting, and polyuria.

Drugs

Constipation often results from use of codeine, meperidine, methadone, and morphine. Less frequently, it may be due to hydrocodone, hydromorphone, levorphanol, oxycodone, oxymorphone, or pentazocine.

How Habits and Stress Cause Constipation

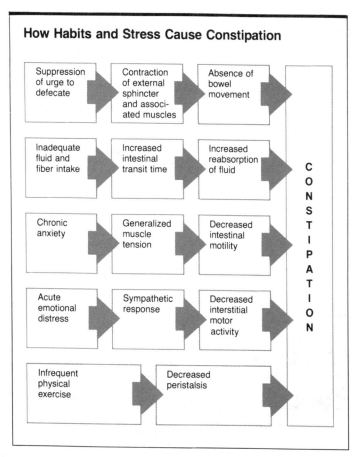

Constipation may result from drugs other than narcotic analgesics. These include vinca alkaloids, polystyrene sodium sulfonate, antacids containing aluminum or calcium, anticholinergics, and drugs with anticholinergic effects (such as tricyclic antidepressants). Constipation may also result from excessive use of laxatives or enemas.

Treatments
Constipation can result from *rectoanal surgery,* which may traumatize nerves, and *abdominal irradiation,* which may cause intestinal stricture.

Diagnostic tests
Constipation can result from retention of barium given during certain GI studies.

Clinical considerations
• A history should be obtained and a physical examination performed.
• Diagnostic tests include proctosigmoidoscopy, barium enema, plain abdominal films, and an upper GI series.
• Unless contraindicated, laxatives and enemas should be given, as ordered.

• An oil retention enema should be given, as ordered, to soften fecal material before removal of impacted feces.
• The patient should be encouraged to get adequate exercise and to include plenty of fluids and fiber in his diet.

Conversion

Description
Conversion is a type of hysterical neurosis in which emotional conflicts are repressed and converted into sensory, motor, or visceral symptoms having no underlying organic cause. Causal factors include a conscious or unconscious desire to escape from or avoid an unpleasant situation or a responsibility or to obtain sympathy or some other secondary gain.

Coopernail sign

Description
Coopernail sign is the presence of ecchymoses on the perineum, scrotum, or labia. This sign indicates pelvic fracture.

Corneal reflex, absent

Description
Absent corneal reflex refers to a condition in which neither eyelid closes when the cornea of one eye is touched. (When the corneal reflex is present, it serves as a protective mechanism causing eyelid closure when the cornea is touched.) (See *Eliciting the Corneal Reflex*.)

Mechanism
The site of the afferent fibers for the corneal reflex is in the ophthalmic

Eliciting the Corneal Reflex

To elicit the corneal reflex, the examiner has the patient turn the eyes away from her to avoid involuntary blinking during the procedure. Then she approaches the patient from the opposite side, out of the line of vision, and brushes the cornea lightly with a fine wisp of sterile cotton. She repeats the procedure on the other eye.

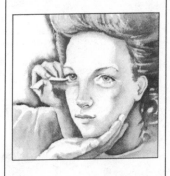

branch of the trigeminal nerve (cranial nerve V); the efferent fibers are located in the facial nerve (cranial nerve VII). Unilateral or bilateral absence of the corneal reflex may result from damage to these nerves.

Possible causes
Central nervous system
Acoustic neuroma. This tumor affects the trigeminal nerve, causing a diminished or absent corneal reflex.
Bell's palsy. A common cause of diminished or absent corneal reflex, this disorder causes paralysis of cranial nerve VII.
Brain stem infarction or injury. Absent corneal reflex can occur on the side opposite the lesion when infarction or injury affects cranial nerve V or VII,

or their connection in the central trigeminal tract.

Guillain-Barré syndrome. In this polyneuropathic disorder, a diminished or absent corneal reflex accompanies ipsilateral loss of facial muscle control.

Trigeminal neuralgia (tic douloureux). A diminished or absent corneal reflex may stem from a superior maxillary lesion that affects the ophthalmic branch.

Clinical considerations

• Artificial tears should be used regularly to lubricate the eye and prevent it from drying.

• The cornea of the affected eye should be covered with a shield to protect the eye from injury.

• Diagnostic tests include cranial X-rays or a computed tomography scan.

Corrigan's pulse

Description

Corrigan's pulse is a bounding pulse in which a great surge is felt followed by a sudden and complete absence of force or fullness in the artery. The sign may be detected by holding the patient's hand above his head and palpating the carotid artery. Corrigan's pulse occurs in aortic insufficiency, severe anemia, patent ductus arteriosus, coarctation of the aorta, and systemic arteriosclerosis.

Costovertebral angle tenderness

Description

Costovertebral angle (CVA) tenderness refers to tenderness to percussion over one or two angles that outline a space over the kidneys (see *Eliciting C.V.A. Tenderness*, p. 88). A patient

who does not have this symptom will perceive a thudding, jarring, or pressurelike sensation when tested, but no pain. This elicited symptom indicates sudden distention of the renal capsule. It almost always accompanies unelicited, dull, constant flank pain in the CVA just lateral to the sacrospinalis muscle and below the 12th rib. This associated pain typically travels anteriorly in the subcostal region toward the umbilicus.

Mechanism

A patient with a disorder that distends the renal capsule will experience intense pain as the renal capsule stretches and stimulates the afferent nerves, which emanate from the spinal cord at levels T11 through L2 and innervate the kidney.

Possible causes

Genitourinary

Calculi. Infundibular and ureteropelvic junction calculi produce CVA tenderness and flank pain.

Perirenal abscess. Causing exquisite CVA tenderness, this disorder may also produce severe unilateral flank pain.

Pyelonephritis (acute). This disorder is perhaps the most common cause of CVA tenderness.

Renal artery occlusion. In this disorder, the patient experiences flank pain as well as CVA tenderness.

Renal vein occlusion. The patient with this disorder has CVA tenderness and flank pain.

Clinical considerations

• A history should be obtained and a physical examination performed.

• Diagnostic tests include intravenous pyelography, renal arteriography, and computed tomography.

• Vital signs and fluid intake and output should be monitored.

• Analgesics should be administered, as ordered, to alleviate pain.

Eliciting C.V.A. Tenderness

To elicit CVA tenderness, the examiner has the patient sit upright facing away from her or has him lie prone. Placing the palm of her left hand over the left costovertebral angle, she then strikes the back of her left hand with the ulnar surface of her right fist, as shown. She repeats this percussion technique over the right CVA. A patient with CVA tenderness will experience intense pain.

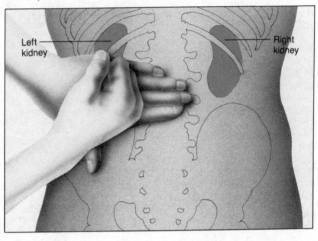

Left kidney

Right kidney

Cough, barking

Description
A barking cough is a resonant, brassy, harsh-sounding cough. It is part of a complex of signs and symptoms that characterize croup syndrome—a group of pediatric disorders marked by varying degrees of respiratory distress. Croup syndrome is most common in boys and most prevalent in winter, and it may recur in the same child. Because infants' and children's airways are smaller in diameter than adults', pediatric patients can rapidly develop airway occlusion—a life-threatening emergency.

Mechanism
A barking cough results from edema of the larynx and surrounding tissue.

Possible causes
Respiratory
Aspiration of foreign body. Partial obstruction of the upper airway first produces sudden hoarseness, then a barking cough and inspiratory stridor.
Epiglottitis. Typically, this life-threatening disorder arises during the night, heralded by barking cough and high fever. The cough may progress to severe respiratory distress. Total airway occlusion may occur within 2 to 5 hours.
Laryngotracheobronchitis (acute). A barking cough, hoarseness, and inspi-

ratory stridor occur if this viral infection descends into the laryngotracheal area.

Spasmodic croup. Acute spasmodic croup usually occurs during sleep with abrupt onset of a barking cough that awakens the child. Fever is absent.

Clinical considerations

• A quick respiratory assessment should be performed and the physician notified of findings.

• The examiner should determine if the child had been playing with a small object that he may have aspirated.

• Preparations should be made for endotracheal intubation or tracheotomy if necessary.

• A lateral neck X-ray may be done to visualize any epiglottal edema; a chest X-ray may also be done, to rule out lower respiratory tract infection.

• Depending on the child's age and his degree of respiratory distress, a mist tent, oxygen hood, or bedside humidifier may be used.

Cough, nonproductive

Description

A nonproductive cough is a noisy, forceful expulsion of air from the lungs that does not yield sputum or blood. It is one of the most common complaints of patients with respiratory disorders.

Coughing is a necessary protective mechanism that clears airway passages. However, a nonproductive cough is not only ineffective but can also cause damage—such as airway collapse or rupture of alveoli or blebs. And a nonproductive cough that later becomes productive is a classic sign of progressive respiratory disease.

Cough may occur once or several times, as in a paroxysm of coughing, and can worsen by becoming more frequent. An acute cough has a sudden onset and may be self-limiting; a cough

that persists beyond 1 month is considered chronic and often results from cigarette smoking.

Mechanism

The cough reflex generally occurs when mechanical, chemical, thermal, inflammatory, or psychogenic stimuli activate cough receptors. External pressure—for example, from subdiaphragmatic irritation or a mediastinal tumor—can also induce a cough. So can voluntary expiration of air, which occasionally occurs as a nervous habit.

Possible causes

Eyes, ears, nose, and throat

Sinusitis (chronic). This disorder can cause a chronic nonproductive cough due to postnasal drip.

Respiratory

Airway occulsion. Partial occlusion of the upper airway produces sudden onset of dry, paroxysmal coughing.

Asthma. An attack often occurs at night and starts with a nonproductive cough and mild wheezing; this progresses to severe dyspnea, audible wheezing, chest tightness, and cough that produces thick mucus.

Atelectasis. As lung tissue deflates, it stimulates cough receptors, causing a nonproductive cough.

Bronchitis (chronic). This disorder starts with a nonproductive, hacking cough that later becomes productive.

Bronchogenic carcinoma. The earliest indicators of this disorder can be a chronic nonproductive cough, dyspnea, and vague chest pain.

Common cold. This disorder generally starts with a nonproductive, hacking cough.

Hypersensitivity pneumonitis. In this disorder, acute nonproductive coughing, fever, dyspnea, and malaise usually occur 5 to 6 hours after exposure to an antigen.

Interstitial lung disease. A patient with this disorder has a nonproductive cough and progressive dyspnea.

Laryngeal tumor. Mild, nonproductive cough is an early sign of this disorder, along with minor throat discomfort and hoarseness.

Laryngitis. In its acute form, this disorder causes a nonproductive cough with localized pain (especially during swallowing or speaking) as well as fever and malaise.

Legionnaire's disease. After a prodrome of malaise, headache, and possibly diarrhea, anorexia, diffuse myalgias, and general weakness, this disease causes a nonproductive cough that later becomes productive of mucoid, nonpurulent, possibly bloody sputum.

Lung abscess. This disorder typically begins with nonproductive coughing, weakness, dyspnea, and pleuritic chest pain.

Mediastinal tumor. A large mediastinal tumor produces a nonproductive cough, dyspnea, and retrosternal pain.

Pneumonia. Bacterial pneumonia usually starts with a nonproductive, hacking, painful cough that rapidly becomes productive.

In *mycoplasma pneumonia,* a nonproductive cough arises 2 to 3 days after onset of malaise, headache, and sore throat. The cough can be paroxysmal, causing substernal chest pain.

Viral pneumonia causes a nonproductive, hacking cough and gradual onset of malaise, headache, anorexia, and low-grade fever.

Psittacosis. Initially, this disorder causes a dry, hacking cough that later becomes productive of small amounts of blood-streaked mucoid sputum.

Pulmonary edema. Initially, this disorder causes dry cough. As the condition becomes more severe, coughing produces a frothy, bloody sputum.

Sarcoidosis. In this disorder, a nonproductive cough is accompanied by dyspnea, substernal pain, and malaise.

Tracheobronchitis (acute). Initially, this disorder produces a dry cough that later becomes productive as secretions increase.

Cardiovascular

Aortic aneurysm (thoracic). This disorder causes associated respiratory symptoms, including a brassy cough with dyspnea, hoarseness, and wheezing.

Gastrointestinal

Esophageal achalasia. In this disorder, regurgitation produces a dry cough. The patient may also have recurrent pulmonary infections and dysphagia.

Esophageal cysts. This disorder is typically asymptomatic, but it occasionally causes a nonproductive cough as well as dyspnea, dysphagia, cyanosis, and pressurelike chest pain.

Esophageal diverticula. The patient with this disorder has a nocturnal nonproductive cough, regurgitation, dyspepsia, and dysphagia.

Esophageal occlusion. Immediate nonproductive coughing and gagging characterize this disorder.

Esophagitis with reflux. This disorder often causes a nonproductive nocturnal cough due to regurgitation while the patient is recumbent.

Diagnostic tests

Pulmonary function tests and bronchoscopy may stimulate cough receptors and trigger coughing.

Clinical considerations

• A history should be obtained and a respiratory assessment performed.

• The physician should be notified of signs or symptoms of respiratory distress or airway obstruction, and emergency equipment should be kept readily available.

• Diagnostic tests include a lung scan, bronchoscopy, pulmonary function tests, and a chest X-ray.

• Treatment of a nonproductive cough depends on the underlying cause and may include administration of bronchodilators or antitussives and use of a humidifier.

Cough, productive

Description

A productive cough is a sudden, forceful, noisy expulsion of air from the lungs that contains sputum or blood (or both). It can occur as a single cough or as paroxysmal coughing.

Usually due to a cardiovascular or respiratory disorder, productive coughing often results from an acute or chronic infection causing inflammation, edema, and increased mucous production in the airways. However, this sign can also result from inhalation of antigenic or irritating substances or foreign bodies. The most common cause of chronic productive coughing is cigarette smoking, which produces brownish, mucoid sputum.

Many patients minimize or overlook chronic productive coughing or accept it as normal. Such patients may not seek medical attention until an associated problem develops—such as dyspnea, hemoptysis, chest pain, weight loss, or recurrent respiratory infections. The delay can have serious consequences, because productive coughing is associated with several life-threatening disorders and can also herald airway occlusion from excessive secretions.

Mechanism

A cough can be voluntarily induced, although it is usually a reflexive response to stimulation of cough receptors by mechanical, chemical, thermal, inflammatory, or psychogenic stimuli.

Possible causes

Respiratory

Actinomycosis. This disorder begins with a cough that produces purulent sputum.

Aspiration pneumonitis. This disorder causes coughing productive of pink, frothy, possibly purulent sputum.

Asthma. A severe asthmatic attack, which can be life-threatening, may produce mucoid, tenacious sputum and mucous plugs. Such an attack typically starts with a dry cough and mild wheezing, then progresses to severe dyspnea, audible wheezing, chest tightness, and productive cough.

Bronchiectasis. The chronic cough of this disorder produces copious, mucopurulent sputum that has characteristic layering (top, frothy; middle, clear; bottom, dense with purulent particles).

Bronchitis (chronic). This disorder causes a cough that may be nonproductive initially. Eventually, however, it produces mucoid sputum that becomes purulent. Secondary infection can also cause mucopurulent sputum, which may become blood-tinged and foul-smelling. The coughing, which may be paroxysmal during exercise, most often occurs when the patient is recumbent or rises from sleep.

Common cold. When this disorder causes productive coughing, the sputum is mucoid or mucopurulent. Early indications of the common cold include a dry, hacking cough.

Legionnaire's disease. Initially, the cough is dry and nonproductive, but may progress to become productive of scant mucoid, nonpurulent, possibly blood-streaked sputum.

Lung abscess (ruptured). The cardinal sign of ruptured lung abscess is coughing that produces copious amounts of purulent, foul-smelling, possibly blood-tinged sputum.

Lung cancer. One of the earliest signs of bronchogenic carcinoma is a chronic cough that produces small amounts of purulent (or mucopurulent), blood-streaked sputum. In a patient with bronchioalveolar cancer, however, coughing produces large amounts of frothy sputum.

Nocardiosis. This disorder causes a productive cough (with purulent, thick, tenacious, and possibly blood-tinged sputum) and fever that may last several months.

North American blastomycosis. In this chronic disorder, coughing is dry and hacking or productive of bloody or purulent sputum.

Pneumonia. Bacterial pneumonias initially produce a dry cough that becomes productive. Rust-colored sputum occurs in pneumococcal pneumonia; "brick red" or "currant jelly" sputum in *Klebsiella* pneumonia; salmon-colored sputum in staphylococcal pneumonia; or mucopurulent sputum in streptococcal pneumonia.

Mycoplasma pneumonia may cause a cough that produces scant, blood-flecked sputum. Most common, however, is a nonproductive cough that starts 2 to 3 days after the onset of malaise, headache, fever, and sore throat. Paroxysmal coughing causes substernal chest pain.

Psittacosis. As this disorder progresses, the characteristic hacking cough, nonproductive at first, may later produce a small amount of mucoid, blood-streaked sputum.

Pulmonary coccidioidomycosis. This disorder causes a nonproductive or slightly productive cough.

Pulmonary edema. When severe, this life-threatening disorder causes coughing productive of frothy, bloody sputum.

Pulmonary embolism. This life-threatening disorder causes a cough that may be nonproductive or may produce blood-tinged sputum.

Pulmonary emphysema. This disorder causes minimal chronic productive cough with scant, mucoid, translucent, grayish–white sputum that can become mucopurulent.

Pulmonary tuberculosis. This disorder causes a mild-to-severe productive cough along with hemoptysis. Sputum may be scant and mucoid or copious and purulent.

Silicosis. Productive cough with mucopurulent sputum is the earliest sign of this disorder.

Tracheobronchitis. Inflammation initially causes a nonproductive cough that later—following onset of chills, sore throat, slight fever, muscle and back pain, and substernal tightness—

becomes productive as secretions increase. Sputum is mucoid, mucopurulent, or purulent.

Drugs
Expectorants, of course, increase productive coughing. These include ammonium chloride, calcium iodide, guaifenesin, iodinated glycerol, potassium iodide, and terpin hydrate.

Treatments
Intermittent positive pressure breathing (IPPB) and *incentive spirometry* often loosen secretions and cause or increase productive cough.

Diagnostic tests
Bronchoscopy and pulmonary function tests may increase productive coughing.

Clinical considerations
• A history should be obtained when the patient's condition permits and a respiratory assessment performed.

• The physician should be notified of signs or symptoms of respiratory distress or airway obstruction and emergency equipment kept readily available.

• Diagnostic tests include sputum analysis, chest X-ray, bronchoscopy, a lung scan, and pulmonary function tests.

• Usually, a productive cough should not be suppressed because retention of sputum may interfere with alveolar aeration or impair pulmonary resistance to infection. An expectorant, mucolytic agent, bronchodilator, or antibiotic should be administered, if ordered.

• Treatment of a productive cough depends on the underlying cause and may include respiratory therapy, supplemental oxygen, humidification of air, and increased fluid intake.

Cowen's sign

Description
Cowen's sign is a jerky consensual pupillary light reflex. This sign is elicited by shining light in one eye and ob-

serving for consensual dilatation or constriction in the opposite eye.

Crackles
(Rales, crepitations)

Description

Crackles are nonmusical clicking or rattling noises heard during auscultation of breath sounds. They usually occur during inspiration and recur constantly from one respiratory cycle to the next. They can be unilateral or bilateral, moist or dry. They are characterized by their pitch, loudness, occurrence during the respiratory cycle, location, and persistence.

Crackles indicate abnormal movement of air through fluid-filled airways. They can be irregularly dispersed, as in pneumonia, or localized, as in bronchiectasis. A few basilar crackles can be heard in normal lungs after prolonged shallow breathing. These normal crackles clear with a few deep breaths. Usually, though, crackles indicate the degree of an underlying illness. When crackles result from a generalized disorder, they usually occur in the less distended and more dependent areas of the lungs, such as the lung bases when the patient is standing. Crackles from air passing through inflammatory exudate may not be audible if the involved portion of the lung is not being ventilated because of shallow respirations.

Possible causes

Respiratory

Adult respiratory distress syndrome (ARDS). A life-threatening disorder, ARDS causes diffuse, fine-to-coarse crackles usually heard in the dependent portions of the lungs.

Asthma. A severe attack usually occurs at night or during sleep, causing dry, whistling crackles.

Bronchiectasis. In this disorder, persistent, coarse crackles are heard over the affected area of the lung. They are accompanied by a chronic cough that produces copious amounts of mucopurulent sputum.

Bronchitis (chronic). This disorder causes coarse crackles that are usually heard at the lung bases.

Interstitial fibrosis of the lungs. In this disorder, cellophane-like crackles can be heard over all lobes.

Legionnaire's disease. This disorder produces diffuse moist crackles and cough productive of scant mucoid, nonpurulent, possibly blood-streaked sputum.

Lung abscess. This disorder produces fine-to-medium and moist inspiratory crackles.

Pneumonia. Bacterial pneumonia produces diffuse fine crackles. *Mycoplasma pneumonia* produces medium-to-fine crackles together with a nonproductive cough. *Viral pneumonia* causes gradually developing, diffuse crackles.

Psittacosis. As this disorder progresses, diffuse fine crackles may be heard.

Pulmonary edema. Moist, bubbling crackles on inspiration are one of the first signs of this life-threatening disorder.

Pulmonary embolism. This life-threatening disorder can cause fine-to-coarse crackles and a cough that may be dry or productive of blood-tinged sputum.

Pulmonary tuberculosis. In this disorder, fine crackles occur after coughing.

Sarcoidosis. This disorder produces fine, bibasilar, end-inspiratory crackles and (rarely) wheezes.

Silicosis. This disorder produces end-inspiratory, fine crackles heard at the lung bases.

Tracheobronchitis. In its acute form, this disorder produces moist or coarse crackles along with a productive cough.

Environmental

Chemical pneumonitis. In acute chemical pneumonitis, diffuse, fine-to-coarse, moist crackles accompany a productive cough with purulent sputum.

Clinical considerations

• A history should be obtained when the patient's condition permits and a respiratory assessment performed.

• The physician should be notified of signs or symptoms of respiratory distress or airway obstruction and emergency equipment should be kept readily available.

• Diagnostic tests include chest X-rays, a lung scan, and sputum analysis.

• As ordered, treatment measures, such as increasing fluid intake and humidifying the air to liquefy secretions and relieve mucous membrane inflammation, should be carried out.

Crepitation, bony
(Bony crepitus)

Description

Bony crepitation is a palpable vibration or an audible crunching sound that results when one bone grates against another. It often results from a fracture. Or it can happen when bones that have been stripped of their protective articular cartilage grind against each other as they articulate—for example, in advanced arthritic or degenerative joint disorders.

Although eliciting bony crepitation can help confirm a diagnosis, it can also cause further soft tissue, nerve, or vessel injury. Also, rubbing fractured bone ends together can convert closed fracture into an open one if a bone end penetrates the skin. Therefore, after initial detection of crepitation in a patient with a fracture, subsequent elicitation of this sign should be avoided.

Possible causes
Musculoskeletal

Closed fracture. Bony crepitation typically occurs with this injury and helps confirm the diagnosis.

Osteoarthritis. In advanced cases of this disorder, joint crepitation may be elicited during range-of-motion testing.

Rheumatoid arthritis. In advanced cases of this disorder, bony crepitation is heard when the affected joint is rotated.

Clinical considerations

• If a fracture is suspected, the patient should be prepared for X-rays of the affected area.

• The neurovascular status of the affected area should be assessed frequently.

• The affected part should be kept immobilized and elevated until treatment is begun.

• Analgesics should be given, as ordered, to relieve pain.

Crepitation, subcutaneous
(Subcutaneous crepitus)

Description

Subcutaneous crepitation is the crackling sound heard on palpation of the skin when bubbles of air or other gases are trapped in subcutaneous tissue. The bubbles feel like small, unstable nodules that are not painful, even though subcutaneous crepitation is often associated with painful disorders. Usually, the affected tissue is visibly edematous—this can lead to life-threatening airway occlusion if the edema affects the neck or upper chest.

Mechanism

The air or gas bubbles enter the tissues through open wounds, from the action of anaerobic microorganisms, or from traumatic or spontaneous rupture or perforation of pulmonary or gastrointestinal organs.

Possible causes
Eyes, ears, nose, and throat

Orbital fracture. This fracture allows air from the nasal sinuses to escape into subcutaneous tissue, causing subcutaneous crepitations of the eyelid and orbit.

Respiratory
Pneumothorax. Severe pneumothorax produces subcutaneous crepitation in the upper chest and neck.
Rupture of the trachea or major bronchus. This life-threatening injury produces abrupt subcutaneous crepitation of the neck and anterior chest wall.
Gastrointestinal
Rupture of the esophagus. A ruptured esophagus usually produces subcutaneous crepitation in the neck, chest wall, or supraclavicular fossa, although this sign does not always occur.
Infection
Gas gangrene. Subcutaneous crepitation over the skin near the wound is the hallmark of this rare but often fatal infection.
Treatments
Mechanical ventilation and *intermittent positive pressure breathing* can rupture alveoli, producing subcutaneous crepitation. If air escapes into the tissue in the area of the incision during *thoracic surgery,* subcutaneous crepitation can occur.
Diagnostic tests
Endoscopic tests, such as bronchoscopy, can cause rupture or perforation of respiratory or GI organs, producing subcutaneous crepitation.

Clinical considerations
• The patient's vital signs should be monitored frequently for evidence of respiratory distress because excessive edema from subcutaneous crepitation in the neck and upper chest can cause airway obstruction.
• The area of subcutaneous crepitation should be reassessed frequently for increased size.

Crossed extensor reflex

Description
Crossed extensor reflex is the extension of one leg in response to stimulation of the opposite leg; a normal reflex in newborn infants. It is me-

diated at the spinal cord level and should disappear after 6 months of age. This sign may be elicited by placing the infant in a supine position with his legs extended. The medial aspect of the thigh is tapped just above the patella. The infant should respond by extending and adducting the opposite leg and fanning the toes of that foot. Persistence of this reflex beyond 6 months of age indicates anoxic brain damage. Its appearance in a child signals a central nervous system lesion or injury.

Crowing respirations

Description
Crowing respirations are slow, deep inspirations accompanied by a high-pitched crowing sound. These respirations are the characteristic whoop of the paroxysmal stage of pertussis.

Cruveilhier's sign

Description
Cruveilhier's sign is a swelling in the groin associated with inguinal hernia. This sign may be elicited by asking the patient to flex one knee slightly while the examiner inserts the index finger in the inguinal canal on the same side. With the finger inserted as deeply as possible, the patient is asked to cough. If a hernia is present, a mass of tissue that subsequently withdraws will be felt.

Cry, high-pitched
(Cerebral cry)

Description
A high-pitched cry is a brief, sharp, piercing vocal sound produced by a neonate or infant. Whether acute or chronic, this cry is a late sign of increased intracranial pressure (ICP).

However, the acute onset of a high-pitched cry demands emergency treatment to prevent permanent brain damage or death.

Any change in the volume of one of the brain's components—brain tissue, cerebrospinal fluid, and blood—may cause increased ICP. In the neonate, increased ICP may result from intracranial bleeding associated with birth trauma or from congenital malformation, such as craniostenosis and Arnold-Chiari syndrome. In the infant, increased ICP may result from meningitis or head trauma.

Cullen's sign

Description
Cullen's sign is the presence of irregular, bluish hemorrhagic patches on the skin around the umbilicus and occasionally around abdominal scars. Cullen's sign indicates massive hemorrhage after trauma or rupture in such disorders as duodenal ulcer, ectopic pregnancy, abdominal aneurysm, gallbladder or common bile duct obstruction, or acute hemorrhagic pancreatitis. Usually, Cullen's sign appears gradually; blood travels from a retroperitoneal organ or structure to the periumbilical area, where it diffuses through subcutaneous tissues. It may be difficult to detect in a dark-skinned patient. The extent of discoloration depends on the extent of bleeding. In time, the bluish discoloration fades to greenish yellow and then yellow before disappearing.

Cyanosis

Description
Cyanosis is a bluish or bluish-black discoloration of the skin and mucous membranes. It may develop abruptly or gradually and can be classified as central or peripheral, although the two types may exist together.

Central cyanosis reflects inadequate oxygenation of systemic arterial blood caused by right-to-left cardiac shunting or pulmonary disease, or by hematologic disorders. It may occur anywhere on the skin and also on the mucous membranes of the mouth, lips, and conjunctiva.

Peripheral cyanosis reflects sluggish peripheral circulation caused by vasoconstriction, reduced cardiac output, or vascular occlusion. It may be widespread or may occur locally in one extremity; however, it does not affect mucous membranes. Typically, peripheral cyanosis appears on exposed areas, such as the fingers, nail beds, feet, nose, and ears.

Although cyanosis is an important sign of cardiovascular and pulmonary disorders, it is not always an accurate gauge of oxygenation. Several factors contribute to its development: hemoglobin concentration and oxygen saturation, cardiac output, and PO_2. Cyanosis is usually undetectable until the oxygen saturation of hemoglobin falls below 80%. Severe cyanosis is quite obvious, whereas mild cyanosis is more difficult to detect—even in natural, bright light. In dark-skinned patients, cyanosis is most apparent in the mucous membranes and nail beds.

A transient, nonpathologic cyanosis may result from environmental factors. For example, peripheral cyanosis may result from cutaneous vasoconstriction following brief exposure to cold air or water. Central cyanosis may result from reduced PO_2 at high altitudes.

Mechanism
Cyanosis is the result of an excessive concentration of unoxygenated hemoglobin in the blood.

Possible causes
Respiratory
Bronchiectasis. This disorder produces chronic central cyanosis. (Its classic sign, though, is chronic pro-

ductive cough with copious, foul-smelling, mucopurulent sputum or hemoptysis.)

Chronic obstructive pulmonary disease (COPD). Chronic central cyanosis occurs with this disorder and may be aggravated by exertion.

Lung cancer. This disorder causes chronic central cyanosis accompanied by fever, weakness, weight loss, anorexia, dyspnea, chest pain, hemoptysis, and wheezing.

Pneumonia. In this disorder, acute central cyanosis is usually preceded by fever, shaking chills, cough with purulent sputum, rales and rhonchi, and pleuritic chest pain that is exacerbated by deep inspiration.

Pneumothorax. A cardinal sign of pneumothorax, acute central cyanosis is accompanied by sharp chest pain that is exacerbated by movement, deep breathing, and coughing; asymmetrical chest wall expansion; and shortness of breath.

Pulmonary edema. In this disorder, acute central cyanosis occurs with dyspnea; orthopnea; frothy, blood-tinged sputum; tachycardia; tachypnea; dependent rales; ventricular gallop; cold, clammy skin; hypotension; weak, thready pulse; and confusion.

Pulmonary embolism. Acute central cyanosis occurs when a large embolus causes significant obstruction of the pulmonary circulation.

Cardiovascular

Arteriosclerotic occlusive disease (chronic). In this disorder, peripheral cyanosis occurs in the legs whenever they are in a dependent position.

Buerger's disease. In this disorder, exposure to cold initially causes the feet to become cold, cyanotic, and numb; later, they redden, become hot, and tingle. Intermittent claudication of the instep is characteristic; it is aggravated by exercise and relieved by rest.

Congestive heart failure. Acute or chronic cyanosis may occur. Typically, it is a late sign and may be central, peripheral, or both. In left heart failure, central cyanosis occurs with

tachycardia, fatigue, dyspnea, cold intolerance, orthopnea, cough, ventricular or atrial gallop, bibasilar rales, and diffuse apical impulse. In right heart failure, peripheral cyanosis occurs with fatigue, peripheral edema, ascites, jugular vein distention, and hepatomegaly.

Deep-vein thrombosis. In this disorder, acute peripheral cyanosis occurs in the affected extremity associated with tenderness, painful movement, edema, warmth, and prominent superficial veins. Also, Homans' sign can be elicited.

Peripheral arterial occlusion (acute). This disorder produces acute cyanosis of one arm or leg or, occasionally, of both legs. The cyanosis is accompanied by sharp or aching pain that worsens when the patient moves.

Raynaud's disease. In this disorder, exposure to cold or stress causes the fingers or hands first to blanch and turn cold, then to become cyanotic, and finally to redden with return of normal temperature.

Shock. In this disorder, acute peripheral cyanosis develops in the hands and feet, which may also be cold, clammy, and pale.

Hematologic

Methemoglobinemia. Whether the result of toxicity or heredity, this disorder produces chronic central cyanosis.

Polycythemia vera. Chronic central cyanosis, often marked by a ruddy complexion, is characteristic in this chronic myeloproliferative disorder.

Clinical considerations

• A history should be obtained and a physical examination performed.

• The physician should be notified of signs or symptoms of respiratory distress or shock, and emergency equipment should be kept readily available.

• Arterial blood gas analysis and complete blood count may be ordered to determine the cause of cyanosis.

• Supplemental oxygen should be administered, if ordered, to relieve shortness of breath and decrease cyanosis.

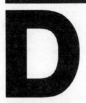

D

Dalrymple's sign

Description
Dalrymple's sign is the presence of abnormally wide palpebral fissures associated with retraction of the upper eyelids. To detect this sign, the examiner has the patient focus his gaze on a fixed point or close his eyes. The examiner may observe infrequent blinking and noticeable restriction of lid movement. The patient may not be able to close his eyes completely. Dalrymple's sign indicates thyrotoxicosis.

Darier's sign

Description
Darier's sign is the whealing and itching of the skin upon rubbing the macular lesions of urticaria pigmentosa (mastocytosis). To elicit this sign, the pigmented macules are vigorously rubbed with the blunt end of a pen or a similar blunt object. The appearance of pruritic, red, palpable wheals around the macules—a positive Darier's sign—follows the release of histamine when mast cells are irritated.

Dawbarn's sign

Description
Dawbarn's sign is pain on palpation of the acromial process in acute subacromial bursitis. To elicit this sign,

the patient's shoulder is palpated while his arm hangs at his side and as he abducts it. If palpation causes pain that disappears on abduction, Dawbarn's sign is present.

Decerebrate posture
(Decerebrate rigidity, abnormal extensor reflex)

Description
Decerebrate posture is characterized by adduction and extension of the arms, with the wrists pronated and the fingers flexed. The legs are stiffly extended, with plantar flexion of the feet. In severe cases, the back is acutely arched (opisthotonos). Usually, decerebrate posture heralds neurologic deterioration. It indicates upper brain stem damage, which may result from primary lesions such as infarction, hemorrhage, or tumor; metabolic encephalopathy; head injury; or brain stem compression associated with increased intracranial pressure (ICP).

Decerebrate posture may be elicited by noxious stimuli or may occur spontaneously. It may be unilateral or bilateral. In concurrent brain stem and cerebral damage, decerebrate posture may affect only the arms, while the legs may remain flaccid. Or decerebrate posture may affect one side of the body and decorticate posture the other (see *Comparing Decerebrate and Decorticate Postures,* p. 100). The two postures may also alternate as the patient's neurologic status fluctuates. Generally, the duration of each posturing episode correlates with the severity of brain stem damage.

Possible causes
Central nervous system
Brain stem infarction. When this primary lesion produces coma, decerebrate posture may also be elicited.

Brain stem tumor. In this disorder, decerebrate posture is a late sign that accompanies coma.

Cerebral lesion. Whether the etiology is trauma, tumor, abscess, or infarction, any cerebral lesion that increases ICP may also produce decerebrate posture. Typically, this posture is a late sign.

Hepatic encephalopathy. A late sign in this disorder, decerebrate posture occurs with coma resulting from increased ICP and ammonia toxicity.

Hypoglycemic encephalopathy. Characterized by extremely low blood glucose levels, this disorder may produce decerebrate posture and coma.

Hypoxic encephalopathy. Severe hypoxia may produce decerebrate posture—the result of brain stem compression associated with anaerobic metabolism and increased ICP.

Pontine hemorrhage. Typically, this life-threatening disorder rapidly leads to decerebrate posture with coma.

Posterior fossa hemorrhage. This subtentorial lesion causes decerebrate posture.

Diagnostic tests
Rarely, certain neurologic tests may cause decerebrate posture. In this category are *lumbar puncture, cisternography,* and *pneumoencephalography*—which may increase ICP, leading to brain stem compression.

Clinical considerations
• The physician should be notified immediately.

• An artificial airway should be inserted and emergency equipment kept readily available.

• Vital signs, neurologic signs, and ICP should be assessed and monitored.

• A history should be obtained from family members and a neurologic assessment performed.

• Diagnostic tests include skull X-rays, computed tomography scan, cerebral angiography, digital subtraction angiography, electroencephalography, brain scan, and ICP monitoring.

Decorticate posture
(Decorticate rigidity, abnormal flexor response)

Description
A sign of corticospinal damage, decorticate posture is characterized by adduction and flexion of the arms, with the wrists and fingers flexed on the chest. The legs are extended and internally rotated, with plantar flexion of the feet. This posture may occur unilaterally or bilaterally. Most often, it results from cerebrovascular accident (CVA) or head injury. It may be elicited by noxious stimuli or may occur spontaneously. The intensity of the required stimulus, the duration of the posture, and the frequency of spontaneous episodes vary with the severity of cerebral injury.

Although a serious sign, decorticate posture carries a more favorable prognosis than decerebrate posture. However, if the causative disorder extends lower in the brain stem, decorticate posture may progress to decerebrate posture. (See *Comparing Decerebrate and Decorticate Postures,* p. 100.)

Possible causes
Central nervous system
Brain abscess. Decorticate posture may occur in this infection.

Brain tumor. This disorder may produce decorticate posture that is usually bilateral—the result of increased intracranial pressure (ICP) associated with tumor growth.

Comparing Decerebrate and Decorticate Postures

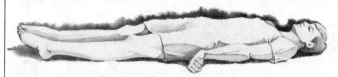

Decerebrate posture results from damage to the upper brain stem. In this posture, the arms are adducted and extended, with the wrists pronated and the fingers flexed. The legs are stiffly extended, with plantar flexion of the feet.

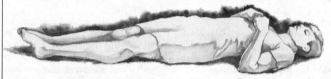

Decorticate posture results from damage to one or both corticospinal tracts. In this posture, the arms are adducted and flexed, with the wrists and fingers flexed on the chest. The legs are stiffly extended and internally rotated, with plantar flexion of the feet.

Cerebrovascular accident (CVA). Typically, a CVA involving the cerebral cortex produces unilateral decorticate posture, also called spastic hemiplegia.

Head injury. Decorticate posture may be among the variable features of this disorder, depending on the site and severity of head injury.

Clinical considerations

• The physician should be notified immediately.
• An artificial airway should be inserted and emergency equipment kept readily available.
• Neurologic status, vital signs, and ICP should be assessed and monitored.
• A history should be obtained from family members and a neurologic assessment performed.

Deep tendon reflexes, hyperactive

Description

A hyperactive deep tendon reflex (DTR) is an abnormally brisk muscle contraction in response to a sudden stretch induced by sharply tapping the muscle's tendon of insertion. This elicited sign may be graded as brisk (+ + +) or hyperactive (+ + + +).

Normally, a DTR operates via the reflex arc, which is governed by the corticospinal tract. Sharply tapping a tendon initiates a sensory (afferent) impulse that travels along a peripheral nerve to a spinal nerve and then to the spinal cord. The impulse enters the spinal cord through the posterior root, synapses with a motor (efferent) neuron in the anterior horn on the same side of the spinal cord, and then is transmitted through a motor nerve fiber back to the muscle. When the impulse crosses the neuromuscular junction, the muscle contracts, completing the reflex arc.

A corticospinal lesion above the level of the reflex arc being tested may result in a hyperactive DTR. Abnormal neuromuscular transmission at the end of the reflex arc may also cause a hyperactive DTR. For example, deficiency of calcium or magnesium may cause a hyperactive DTR because these electrolytes regulate neuromuscular excitability.

Hyperactive DTRs frequently accompany other neurologic findings but usually lack specific diagnostic value. An exception is hypocalcemia, in which hyperactive DTRs are an early, cardinal sign. Hyperreflexia may be a normal sign in neonates. After age 6, reflex responses are similar to those of adults.

Possible causes
Central nervous system
Amyotrophic lateral sclerosis. This disorder produces generalized hyperactive DTRs.

Brain tumor. A cerebral tumor causes hyperactive DTRs on the side opposite the lesion.

Cerebrovascular accident (CVA). Any CVA that affects the origin of the corticospinal tracts causes sudden onset of hyperactive DTRs on the side opposite the lesion.

Hepatic encephalopathy. Generalized hyperactive DTRs occur late and are followed by a positive Babinski's reflex, fetor hepaticus, and coma.

Multiple sclerosis. Typically, hyperactive DTRs are preceded by weakness and paresthesia in one or both arms or legs.

Spinal cord lesion. Incomplete spinal cord lesions cause hyperactive DTRs below the level of the lesion. In a trau-

matic lesion, hyperactive DTRs follow resolution of spinal shock. In a neoplastic lesion, hyperactive DTRs gradually replace normal DTRs.
Metabolic
Hypocalcemia. This disorder may produce sudden or gradual onset of generalized hyperactive DTRs with paresthesia, muscle twitching and cramping, positive Chvostek's and Trousseau's signs, carpopedal spasm, and tetany.

Hypomagnesemia. This disorder results in gradual onset of generalized hyperactive DTRs accompanied by muscle cramps, hypotension, tachycardia, paresthesia, ataxia, tetany, and possible convulsions.
Obstetrics–Gynecology
Preeclampsia. Occurring in pregnancy of at least 20 weeks' duration, preeclampsia may cause gradual onset of generalized hyperactive DTRs.
Infection
Tetanus. In this disorder, sudden onset of generalized hyperactive DTRs accompanies tachycardia, diaphoresis, low-grade fever, painful and involuntary muscle contractions, trismus (lock-jaw), and risus sardonicus.
Environmental
Hypothermia. Mild hypothermia (90° to 94° F., 32.2° to 34.4° C.) produces generalized hyperactive DTRs.

Clinical considerations
Diagnostic tests include serum calcium and magnesium, spinal X-rays, computed tomography, lumbar puncture, and myelography.

Deep tendon reflexes, hypoactive

Description
A hypoactive deep tendon reflex (DTR) is an abnormally diminished muscle contraction in response to a sudden stretch induced by sharply tapping the muscle's tendon of insertion.

It may be graded as minimal (+) or absent (0).

Normally, a DTR operates via the reflex arc, which is governed by the corticospinal tract. Sharply tapping a tendon initiates a sensory (afferent) impulse that travels along a peripheral nerve to a spinal nerve and then to the spinal cord. The impulse enters the spinal cord through the posterior root, synapses with a motor (efferent) neuron in the anterior horn on the same side of the spinal cord, and then is transmitted through a motor nerve fiber back to the muscle. When the impulse crosses the neuromuscular junction, the muscle contracts, completing the reflex arc.

A hypoactive DTR may result from damage to the reflex arc involving the specific muscle, the peripheral nerve, the nerve roots, or the spinal cord at that level. Hypoactive DTRs are an important sign of many disorders, especially when they appear with other neurologic signs and symptoms.

Possible causes

Central nervous system
Botulism. In this disorder, generalized hypoactive DTRs accompany progressive descending muscle weakness.
Eaton-Lambert syndrome. This disorder produces generalized hypoactive (but not absent) DTRs.
Guillain-Barré syndrome. This disorder causes bilateral hypoactive DTRs that progress rapidly from hypotonia to areflexia in several days.
Peripheral neuropathy. Characteristic in end-stage diabetes mellitus, renal failure, and alcoholism, peripheral neuropathy results in progressive hypoactive DTRs.
Spinal cord lesions. Spinal cord injury or complete transection produces spinal shock, resulting in hypoactive DTRs (areflexia) below the level of the lesion.
Syringomyelia. Permanent bilateral hypoactive DTRs occur early in this slowly progressive disorder.

Tabes dorsalis. This progressive disorder results in bilateral hypoactive DTRs in the legs and, occasionally, the arms.
Musculoskeletal
Polymyositis. In this disorder, hypoactive DTRs accompany muscle weakness, pain, stiffness, spasms, and, possibly, increased size or atrophy. These effects are usually temporary; their location varies with the affected muscles.
Drugs
Barbiturates and paralyzing drugs, such as pancuronium and curare, may cause hypoactive DTRs.

Clinical considerations
• A history should be obtained and a physical examination performed.
• The patient should be assisted with activities of daily living and his safety ensured.

Delbet's sign

Description
Delbet's sign is the presence of adequate collateral circulation to the distal portion of a limb associated with aneurysmal occlusion of the main artery. To detect this sign, pulses, color, and temperature in the affected limb are checked. If pulses are absent but color and temperature are normal, Delbet's sign is present.

Delirium

Description
Delirium is an acute organic mental disorder characterized by confusion, disorientation, restlessness, clouding of the consciousness, incoherence, fear, anxiety, excitement, and often illusions, hallucinations, and, sometimes, delusions. Typically, delirium develops suddenly and lasts for a short period. It is a common effect of drug

and alcohol abuse, metabolic disorders, and high fever. Delirium may also follow head trauma or seizure.

Delusion

Description
Delusion is a persistent false belief held despite invalidating evidence. A *delusion of grandeur,* which may occur in schizophrenia and bipolar disorders, refers to an exaggerated belief in one's importance, wealth, or talent. The patient may take a powerful figure, such as Napoleon, as his persona. In a *paranoid delusion,* which may occur in schizophrenia and paranoid disorders, the patient believes that he or someone close to him is the victim of an attack, harrassment, or conspiracy. In a *somatic delusion,* which may occur in psychotic disorders, the patient believes that his body is diseased or distorted.

Demianoff's sign

Description
Demianoff's sign is lumbar pain caused by stretching the sacrolumbalis muscle. To elicit this sign, the examiner has the patient lie in a supine position with legs extended, then raises the extended leg. Lumbar pain that prevents lifting the leg high enough to form a 10° angle to the table is a positive Demianoff's sign and occurs in lumbago.

Denial

Description
Denial is an unconscious defense mechanism used to ward off distressing feelings, thoughts, wishes, or needs. Denial occurs in normal and pathologic mental states. In terminal illness, it represents the first stage of the response to dying.

Depersonalization

Description
Depersonalization is a perception of the self as strange or unreal. For example, a person may report feeling as if he is observing himself from a distance. This symptom occurs in patients with schizophrenia and depersonalization disorders and in normal individuals during periods of great stress or anxiety.

Depression

Description
Depression defies easy definition, often eluding diagnosis and treatment. Its character, intensity, and duration vary from periodic bouts of "the blues" to persistent thoughts of suicide.

Depression can be classified as mild, moderate, or severe. *Mild depression* is transient and characterized by downheartedness, sadness, and dejection. *Moderate depression* is marked by noticeably disturbed thought processes, impaired communication and socialization, and sensory dysfunction. These factors intensify in *severe depression:* The patient may appear withdrawn, expressionless, or unaffected by his surroundings, and may exhibit delusional thinking, dramatic sensory dysfunction, and limited or agitated motor activity.

Depression is more common in women than men and is especially prevalent among adolescents.

Possible causes
Organic disorders
Various organic disorders and chronic illnesses produce mild, moderate, or severe depression. Among these are *metabolic and endocrine disorders,*

such as hypothyroidism, hyperthyroidism, and diabetes; *infectious diseases,* such as influenza, hepatitis, and encephalitis; *degenerative diseases,* such as Alzheimer's disease, multiple sclerosis, and multi-infarct dementia; and *neoplastic disorders,* such as cancer of the pancreas.

Psychiatric disorders

Affective disorders are often characterized by abrupt mood swings from depression to elation (mania) or by prolonged episodes of either mood. Severe depression may last for weeks. More moderate depression occurs in *cyclothymic disorders* and usually alternates with moderate mania. Moderate depression that is more or less constant over a 2-year period often results from *dysthymic disorders.* In addition, *chronic anxiety disorders,* characterized by obsessive-compulsive behavior, may cause depression.

Drugs

Various drugs cause depression as a side effect. Among the more common are barbiturates; antineoplastic agents, such as asparaginase; anticonvulsants, such as diazepam; and antiarrhythmics, such as disopyramide. Other depression-inducing drugs include centrally acting antihypertensives, such as reserpine (common in high dosages), methyldopa, and clonidine; beta-adrenergic blockers, such as propranolol; levodopa; indomethacin; cycloserine; corticosteroids; and oral contraceptives.

Alcohol intoxication or withdrawal often produces depression.

Clinical considerations

• A history should be obtained and a physical examination performed to determine if the cause of depression is organic or psychiatric.

• The patient's suicide potential should be evaluated and steps taken to ensure his safety.

• The patient should be given help in setting realistic goals.

• Feelings of self-worth should be promoted by encouraging the patient to assert his opinions and make decisions.

• The patient should be encouraged to acknowledge his angry feelings and express them safely.

• The patient should be encouraged to participate in activities he can succeed in and to engage in constructive problem solving, to help overcome feelings of hopelessness.

• Feelings of competency should be fostered by focusing on past situations in which the patient achieved success.

• Drugs should be administered, as ordered.

Desault's sign

Description

Desault's sign is an alteration of the arc made by the greater trochanter upon rotation of the femur. It is seen in fracture of the intracapsular region of the femur. In this fracture, the greater trochanter rotates only on the axis of the femur, making a much smaller arc than it does upon normal rotation of the femur in the capsule of the hip joint.

Diaphoresis

Description

Diaphoresis is profuse sweating. At times, diaphoresis can amount to more than 1 liter of sweat per hour. This sign represents an autonomic nervous system response to physical or psychogenic stress, or to fever or high environmental temperature. When caused by stress, diaphoresis may be generalized or limited to the palms, soles, and forehead. When caused by fever or high environmental temperature, it is usually generalized.

Usually, diaphoresis begins abruptly and may be accompanied by other autonomic system signs, such as tachycardia and increased blood pressure.

However, it varies with age because sweat glands function immaturely in the infant and are less active in the elderly. As a result, these age-groups may fail to display diaphoresis associated with its common causes.

Intermittent diaphoresis may accompany chronic disorders characterized by recurrent fever; isolated diaphoresis may mark an episode of acute pain or fever. Night sweats may characterize intermittent fever because body temperature tends to return to normal between 2 and 4 a.m. before rising again.

When caused by excessive external temperature, diaphoresis is a normal response. Acclimatization usually requires several days of exposure to high temperatures; during this process, diaphoresis helps maintain normal body temperature. Diaphoresis also commonly occurs during menopause. It is preceded by a sensation of intense heat (a hot flash). Other causes include exercise or exertion that accelerates metabolism, creating internal heat, and mild-to-moderate anxiety that helps initiate the fight-or-flight response.

Mechanism
The mechanism differs depending on whether it is a sympathetic or parasympathetic reaction (see *Diaphoresis—A Physiologic Response,* page 106).

Possible causes
Central nervous system
Autonomic hyperreflexia. Occurring after resolution of spinal shock in spinal cord injury above T6, hyperreflexia causes profuse diaphoresis, pounding headache, blurred vision, and dramatically elevated blood pressure. Diaphoresis occurs above the level of the injury, especially on the forehead, and is accompanied by flushing.
Eyes, ears, nose, and throat
Ménière's disease. Characterized by severe vertigo, tinnitus, and hearing

loss, this disorder may also cause diaphoresis.
Respiratory
Empyema. Pus accumulation in the pleural space leads to drenching night sweats and fever.
Lung abscess. Drenching night sweats are common in this disorder.
Pneumonia. Intermittent, generalized diaphoresis accompanies fever and chills in pneumonia.
Tuberculosis. Although often asymptomatic in primary infection, this disorder may cause night sweats, low-grade fever, fatigue, weakness, anorexia, and weight loss.
Cardiovascular
Congestive heart failure. Typically, diaphoresis follows fatigue, dyspnea, orthopnea, and tachycardia in left heart failure and neck vein distention and dry cough in right heart failure.
Infective endocarditis (subacute). Generalized night sweats occur early in this disorder.
Myocardial infarction. Usually, diaphoresis accompanies acute, substernal, radiating chest pain in this life-threatening disorder.
Endocrine
Acromegaly. In this slowly progressive disorder, diaphoresis is a sensitive gauge of disease activity, which involves hypersecretion of growth hormone and increased metabolic rate.
Hypoglycemia. Rapidly induced hypoglycemia may cause diaphoresis accompanied by irritability, tremors, hypotension, blurred vision, tachycardia, hunger, and loss of consciousness.
Pheochromocytoma. This disorder commonly produces diaphoresis. (Its cardinal sign, though, is persistent or paroxysmal hypertension.)
Thyrotoxicosis. This disorder commonly produces diaphoresis.
Gastrointestinal
Liver abscess. Signs and symptoms vary, depending on the extent of the abscess. Common findings include diaphoresis, right upper quadrant pain, weight loss, fever, chills, nausea, vomiting, and signs of anemia.

Diaphoresis—A Physiologic Response

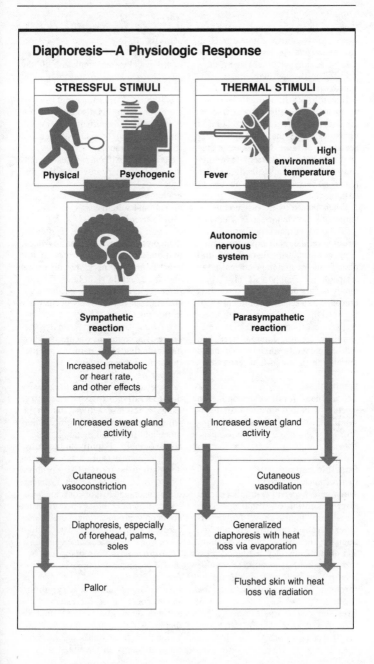

Immunologic

Acquired immunodeficiency syndrome. Night sweats may be an early feature.

Psychiatric

Anxiety disorders. Acute anxiety characterizes panic, while chronic anxiety characterizes phobias, conversion disorders, obsessions, and compulsions. Whether acute or chronic, anxiety may cause diaphoresis. The diaphoresis is most dramatic on the palms, soles, and forehead.

Neoplastic

Hodgkin's disease. Especially in the elderly, early features of Hodgkin's disease may include night sweats, fever, fatigue, pruritus, and weight loss.

Immunoblastic lymphadenopathy. Resembling Hodgkin's disease but rarer, this disorder causes episodic diaphoresis.

Environmental

Envenomation. Depending on the type of snake bite, neurotoxic effects may include diaphoresis.

Heat exhaustion. Initially, this condition causes profuse diaphoresis, fatigue, weakness, and anxiety.

Malaria. Profuse diaphoresis marks the third stage of the malarial paroxysm. It is preceded by chills (first stage) and high fever (second stage).

Pesticide poisoning. Among the toxic effects of pesticides are diaphoresis, nausea, vomiting, diarrhea, blurred vision, miosis, and excess lacrimation and salivation.

Relapsing fever. Profuse diaphoresis marks resolution of the crisis stage in this disorder.

Tetanus. This disorder commonly causes profuse sweating accompanied by low-grade fever, tachycardia, and hyperactive deep tendon reflexes.

Drugs

Sympathomimetics, certain antipsychotics, thyroid hormone, and antipyretics may cause diaphoresis. Aspirin and acetaminophen poisoning also cause this sign.

Withdrawal from alcohol and narcotic analgesics may cause generalized diaphoresis, dilated pupils, tachycardia, tremors, and altered mental status (confusion, delusions, hallucinations, agitation).

Treatments

After partial gastrectomy, *dumping syndrome* may occur. Dumping syndrome results from rapid emptying of gastric contents into the small intestine and occurs soon after eating. This syndrome causes diaphoresis, palpitations, profound weakness, epigastric distress, nausea, and explosive diarrhea.

Clinical considerations

If *hypoglycemia* is the suspected cause of diaphoresis:

• The physician should be notified immediately.

• Vital signs should be taken.

• The blood glucose level should be determined.

• I.V. glucose should be administered, as ordered.

• Emergency equipment should be kept readily available.

If *heatstroke* is the suspected cause of diaphoresis:

• Vital signs should be taken and a normal or subnormal temperature noted.

• The patient should be placed in a cool room and his clothing removed. A fan may be used to direct cool air over the body.

• An I.V. line should be started for fluid and electrolyte replacement.

• The patient should be observed frequently for signs and symptoms of shock.

If *myocardial infarction* or *congestive heart failure* is the suspected cause of diaphoresis:

• The patient should be connected to a cardiac monitor.

• A patent airway should be ensured and supplemental oxygen administered, as ordered.

• An I.V. line should be started.

• Emergency equipment should be kept readily available.

If a life-threatening cause of diaphoresis has been ruled out:

• A history should be obtained and a physical examination performed.

• Diagnostic tests include blood tests, cultures, chest X-rays, immunologic studies, biopsy, computed tomography scan, and audiometry.

• After an episode of diaphoresis, the patient's face and body should be sponged and wet clothes and sheets changed. Skin folds in the groin, axillae, and under pendulous breasts should be dusted with cornstarch or powder to prevent skin irritation.

• Fluid and electrolytes should be replaced, as ordered.

• The patient's room temperature should be kept moderate to prevent additional diaphoresis.

Diarrhea

Description
Diarrhea is an increase in the frequency and fluidity of bowel movements compared to the patient's normal bowel habits. Usually a chief sign of intestinal disorders, it varies in severity and may be acute or chronic.

Acute diarrhea may result from acute infection, stress, fecal impaction, or the effects of drugs. Chronic diarrhea may result from chronic infection, obstructive and inflammatory bowel disease, malabsorption syndrome, certain endocrine disorders, and the effects of gastrointestinal surgery. Periodic diarrhea may result from food allergy or from ingestion of spicy or high-fiber foods or caffeine. The fluid and electrolyte imbalances diarrhea produces may precipitate life-threatening dysrhythmias or hypovolemic shock.

Mechanism
One or more pathophysiologic mechanisms may contribute to diarrhea (see *What Causes Diarrhea*).

Possible causes
Endocrine
Thyrotoxicosis. In this disorder, diarrhea is accompanied by nervousness, tremor, diaphoresis, weight loss despite increased appetite, dyspnea, palpitations, tachycardia, an enlarged thyroid, heat intolerance, and possibly exophthalmos.

Gastrointestinal
Crohn's disease. This recurring inflammatory disorder produces diarrhea accompanied by hyperactive bowel sounds, abdominal pain with guarding and tenderness, and nausea.

Intestinal obstruction. Partial intestinal obstruction increases intestinal motility, resulting in diarrhea.

Irritable bowel syndrome. Diarrhea alternates with constipation or normal bowel function.

Ischemic bowel disease. In this life-threatening disorder, bloody diarrhea occurs with abdominal pain.

Lactose intolerance. Diarrhea occurs within several hours of ingesting milk or milk products with this disorder.

Large-bowel neoplasms. In this disorder, bloody diarrhea alternates with pencil-thin stools.

Malabsorption syndrome. Occurring after meals, diarrhea is accompanied by steatorrhea, abdominal distention, and muscle cramps.

Pseudomembranous enterocolitis. This life-threatening disorder produces copious watery or bloody diarrhea that rapidly precipitates signs of shock.

Ulcerative colitis. The hallmark of this disorder is recurrent bloody diarrhea with pus or mucus.

Infection
Acute viral, bacterial, and protozoal infections. These infections cause the sudden onset of extremely watery diarrhea.

Chronic tuberculosis and fungal and parasitic infections. These infections cause less severe but more persistent diarrhea and possibly passage of blood and mucus.

What Causes Diarrhea

Ingestion of poorly absorbable material, such as bulk-forming laxatives	Local lymphatic or venous obstruction	Stimulation of mucosal intracellular enzymes (cyclic AMP) by bacterial toxins or other factors	Disrupted integrity of small intestinal mucosa	Increased intestinal motility
Excess osmotic load in small intestine	Increased intravascular and intracellular hydrostatic pressure	Active transport of electrolytes into small intestine	Impaired intestinal absorption	Decreased intestinal absorption
Increased fluid drawn into and retained in the small intestine	Altered permeability of intestinal mucosa	Excess fluid in small intestine	Excess fluid in small intestine	Excess fluid in small intestine
	Passive secretion of fluid and electrolytes into small intestine			

Diarrhea

Neoplastic
Carcinoid syndrome. In this disorder, severe diarrhea occurs with abdominal cramps.
Environmental
Lead poisoning. Alternating diarrhea and constipation occur here.
Drugs
Many antibiotics, such as ampicillin, cephalosporins, tetracyclines, and clindamycin, cause diarrhea. Other drugs that may cause diarrhea include magnesium-containing antacids, colchicine, guanethidine, lactulose, dantrolene, ethacrynic acid, mefenamic acid, methotrexate, metyrosine, and, in high doses, digitalis and quinidine. Laxative abuse can cause acute or chronic diarrhea.
Treatments
Gastrectomy, gastroenterostomy, and *pyloroplasty* may produce diarrhea.
   High-dose radiation therapy may produce enteritis associated with diarrhea.

Clinical considerations

• If diarrhea is profuse, the patient should be observed for signs and symptoms of shock.

• A history should be obtained and a physical examination performed.

• Diagnostic tests include blood studies, stool cultures, X-rays, and endoscopy.

• Fluid and electrolytes should be replaced, as ordered.

• Fluid intake and output should be monitored. Liquid stool volume should be measured and recorded.

• The patient's perineum should be cleansed thoroughly after each bowel movement and ointment applied to prevent skin breakdown.

Diplopia

Description

Diplopia is double vision—seeing one object as two. Orbital lesions, the effects of surgery, or impaired function of cranial nerves that supply extraocular muscles (oculomotor, CN III; trochlear, CN IV; abducens, CN VI) may cause this symptom.

Diplopia usually begins intermittently or affects near or far vision exclusively. It can be classified as monocular or binocular. More common binocular diplopia may result from ocular deviation or displacement, extraocular muscle palsies, or psychoneurosis. It may also follow retinal surgery. Monocular diplopia may result from an early cataract, retinal edema or scarring, iridodialysis, subluxated lens, a poorly fitting contact lens, or uncorrected refractive error. Diplopia may also occur in hysteria or malingering.

In young children, the brain rapidly compensates for double vision by suppressing one image, so diplopia is a rare complaint. School-age children who complain of double vision require a careful examination to rule out serious disorders, such as brain tumor.

Mechanism

Diplopia occurs when extraocular muscles fail to work together, causing images to fall on noncorresponding parts of the retinas.

Possible causes

Central nervous system

Brain tumor. In this disorder, diplopia may be an early symptom.

Cerebrovascular accident. Diplopia characterizes this life-threatening disorder when it affects the vertebrobasilar artery.

Encephalitis. Initially, this disorder may cause a brief episode of diplopia and eye deviation.

Head injury. This potentially life-threatening disorder may cause diplopia, depending on the site and extent of the injury.

Intracranial aneurysm. This life-threatening disorder initially produces diplopia and eye deviation, perhaps accompanied by ptosis and a dilated pupil on the affected side.

Multiple sclerosis. Diplopia is commonly an early symptom in this disorder. It is usually accompanied by blurred vision and paresthesias.

Myasthenia gravis. Initially, this disorder produces diplopia and ptosis that worsen throughout the day.

Ophthalmoplegic migraine. Occurring most often in young adults, this disorder results in diplopia that persists for days after the headache.

Eyes, ears, nose, and throat

Cavernous sinus thrombosis. This disorder may produce diplopia and limited eye movement.

Orbital blowout fracture. This fracture usually causes monocular diplopia affecting the upward gaze. However, with marked periorbital edema, diplopia may affect other directions of gaze.

Orbital cellulitis. Inflammation of the orbital tissues and eyelids causes sudden diplopia.

Orbital tumors. Enlarging tumors can cause diplopia.

Endocrine
Diabetes mellitus. Among the long-term effects of this disorder may be diplopia—the result of isolated third cranial nerve palsy. Typically, diplopia begins suddenly and may be accompanied by pain.

Thyrotoxicosis. Diplopia occurs when exophthalmos characterizes the disorder.

Environmental
Botulism. Hallmark signs are diplopia, dysarthria, dysphagia, and ptosis.

Drugs
Diplopia is a common symptom of *alcohol intoxication*.

Treatment
Fibrosis associated with eye surgery may restrict eye movement, resulting in diplopia.

Clinical considerations
• A history should be obtained and a physical examination peformed.
• The patient's environment should be kept uncluttered and hazard free.
• In severe diplopia, the patient should be given assistance with ambulation.
• Vital signs and neurologic status should be monitored if an acute neurologic disorder is suspected.

Discharge, eye

Description
Eye discharge refers to the excretion from the eye of any substance other than tears. It can come from the tear sac, punctum, meibomian glands, or canaliculi. This sign may occur in one or both eyes, producing scant-to-copious discharge. The discharge may be purulent, frothy, mucoid, cheesy, or ropey. Sometimes, discharge can be expressed by applying pressure to the tear sac, punctum, meibomian glands, or canaliculus.

Eye discharge commonly results from inflammatory and infectious eye disorders but may also result from certain systemic disorders. Because this sign may accompany a disorder that threatens vision, it must be assessed and treated immediately.

Possible causes
Eyes, ears, nose, and throat
Canaliculitis. This uncommon, chronic disorder causes scant purulent discharge, usually from one eye's lower canaliculus.

Conjunctivitis. Four types of conjunctivitis may cause eye discharge with redness and hyperemia.

In *allergic conjunctivitis,* bilateral ropey discharge is accompanied by itching and tearing.

Bacterial conjunctivitis causes moderate purulent discharge that may form sticky crusts on the eyelids during sleep.

Fungal conjunctivitis produces copious, thick, purulent discharge that makes eyelids crusty and sticky.

Inclusion conjunctivitis causes scant mucoid discharge—especially in the morning—in both eyes, accompanied by pseudoptosis and conjunctival follicles.

Corneal ulcers. Both bacterial and fungal ulcers produce copious, purulent, unilateral eye discharge.

Dacryoadenitis. This disorder may cause moderate purulent discharge.

Dacryocystitis. Lacrimal sac infection may produce scant but continuous purulent discharge that is easily expressed from the tear sac.

Herpes zoster ophthalmicus. This disorder yields moderate-to-copious serous eye discharge accompanied by excessive tearing.

Keratoconjunctivitis sicca. Better known as dry eye syndrome, this disorder typically causes excessive, continuous mucoid discharge and insufficient tearing.

Meibomianitis. This disorder may produce continuous frothy eye discharge. The application of pressure on the meibomian glands yields a soft, foul-smelling, cheesy yellow discharge.

Orbital cellulitis. Although exophthalmos is the most obvious sign of this disorder, unilateral purulent eye discharge may also be present.

Trachoma. A bilateral eye discharge occurs in this disorder.

Skin

Erythema multiforme major (Stevens-Johnson syndrome). A purulent discharge characterizes this disorder.

Pemphigus. This rare disorder may cause thick, mucuslike discharge. Initially, it may cause unilateral or bilateral conjunctivitis that is unrelieved by treatment, followed by entropion and, occasionally, corneal ulceration.

Psoriasis vulgaris. Usually, psoriasis vulgaris causes substantial mucous discharge in both eyes, accompanied by redness. The characteristic lesions it produces on the eyelids may extend into the conjunctiva, causing irritation, excessive tearing, and a foreign-body sensation.

Clinical considerations

• A history should be obtained and an eye examination performed.

• Diagnostic tests include culture and sensitivity studies.

• Warm soaks should be applied to soften crusts on the patient's eyelids and eyelashes.

• Clean gloves should be worn to protect the caregiver from infection during dressing removal, eye treatments, and eye medication administration if the eye condition is contagious.

• If the eye condition is contagious, the patient should be told to avoid touching the affected eye to prevent cross-contamination of the unaffected eye.

Discharge, nipple

Description

Nipple discharge can occur spontaneously or can be elicited by nipple stimulation. It is characterized as intermittent or constant, unilateral or bilateral, and by color, consistency, and composition. Its incidence increases with age and parity. This sign rarely occurs (but is more likely to be pathologic) in men and in nulligravid, regularly menstruating women. It is relatively common and often normal in parous women. A thick, grayish discharge—benign epithelial debris from inactive ducts—can often be elicited in middle-aged parous women. Colostrum, a thin, yellowish or milky discharge, often occurs in the last weeks of pregnancy.

Nipple discharge can signal serious underlying disease, particularly when accompanied by other breast changes. Significant causes include endocrine disorders, cancer, certain drugs, and blocked lactiferous ducts. (See *Eliciting Nipple Discharge.*)

Possible causes

Endocrine

Hypothyroidism. This disorder occasionally causes galactorrhea (a white or grayish milky discharge).

Prolactin-secreting pituitary tumor. Bilateral galactorrhea may occur with this tumor.

Obstetrics-Gynecology

Breast abscess. This disorder, most common in lactating women, may produce a thick, purulent discharge from a cracked nipple or infected duct.

Breast cancer. This may cause bloody, watery, or purulent discharge from a normal appearing nipple.

Choriocarcinoma. Galactorrhea may result from this highly malignant neoplasm, whch can follow pregnancy.

Intraductal papilloma. Unilateral serous, serosanguineous, or bloody nipple discharge is the predominant sign of this disorder. Discharge may be intermittent or profuse and constant, and can often be stimulated by gentle pressure around the areola.

Mammary duct ectasia. A thick, sticky, grayish discharge may be the first sign of this disorder; it may be bilateral and is usually spontaneous.

Paget's disease. Serous or bloody discharge emits from denuded skin on the

Eliciting Nipple Discharge

If the patient has a history or evidence of nipple discharge, the examiner can try to elicit this sign by positioning the patient supine and gently squeezing the nipple between the thumb and index finger. The examiner should also palpate the entire areolar surface, as shown below, and watch for discharge through the areolar ducts.

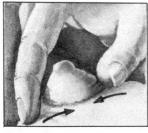

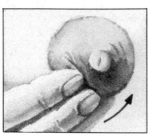

Environmental
Trauma. Bilateral galactorrhea can result from trauma to the breasts.
Drugs
Galactorrhea can be caused by psychotropic agents, particularly phenothiazines and tricyclic antidepressants; some antihypertensives (reserpine and methyldopa); oral contraceptives; cimetidine; metoclopramide; and verapamil.
Treatment
Chest wall surgery may stimulate the thoracic nerves, causing intermittent bilateral galactorrhea.

Clinical considerations
• A history should be obtained and a physical examination performed.
• Diagnostic tests include tissue biopsy (if a breast lump is found), cytologic study of discharge, mammography, ultrasonography, transillumination, and serum prolactin.
• The examiner should clearly explain the nature and origin of the nipple discharge.

Discharge, urethral

Description
This excretion from the urinary meatus may be purulent, mucoid, or thin; sanguineous or clear; and scant or profuse. It usually develops suddenly, most commonly in men with a prostate infection. In children, urethral discharge indicates sexual abuse.

nipple, which is red, intensely itchy, and possibly eroded or excoriated.
Proliferative (fibrocystic) breast disease. This benign disorder occasionally causes bilateral clear, purulent, or bloody discharge.
Infectious diseases
Herpes zoster. This virus can stimulate the thoracic nerves, causing bilateral, spontaneous, intermittent galactorrhea.

Possible causes
Genitourinary
Prostatitis. Acute prostatitis is characterized by purulent urethral discharge. *Chronic prostatitis,* although often asymptomatic, may produce a persistent urethral discharge that is thin, milky or clear, and sometimes sticky. The discharge appears at the meatus after a long interval between voidings, as in the morning.

Reiter's syndrome. In this self-limiting syndrome that most commonly affects males, urethral discharge and other signs of acute urethritis occur 1 to 2 weeks after sexual contact. Arthritic and ocular symptoms and skin lesions usually develop within several weeks.

Urethral neoplasm. This rare cancer is sometimes heralded by painless urethral discharge that is initially opaque and gray. Later, the discharge becomes yellowish and blood-tinged.

Urethritis. This inflammatory disorder, which is often sexually transmitted (as in gonorrhea), commonly produces scant or profuse urethral discharge that is either thin and clear, mucoid, or thick and purulent.

Clinical considerations

• A history should be obtained and a physical examination performed to determine the cause of urethral discharge.

• A urethral discharge specimen should be obtained for culture and sensitivity studies, as ordered.

• The patient with *acute* prostatitis should be told to discontinue sexual activity until acute symptoms subside. However, the patient with *chronic* prostatitis should be encouraged to engage regularly in sexual activity.

• The patient should be told that taking hot sitz baths several times daily, increasing fluid intake, voiding frequently, and avoiding ingestion of caffeine, tea, and alcohol will relieve symptoms.

Discharge, vaginal

Description

Common in women of childbearing age, physiologic vaginal discharge is mucoid, clear or white, nonbloody, and odorless. Produced by the cervical mucosa and, to a lesser degree, by the vulvar glands, this discharge may oc-

casionally be scant or profuse without pathologic significance. However, a marked increase in discharge or a change in discharge color, odor, or consistency can signal disease. Often, the abnormal discharge stems from altered estrogen production. However, it may also result from infection, sexually transmitted disease, reproductive tract disease, fistulas, and certain drugs. In addition, the prolonged presence of a foreign body, such as a tampon or diaphragm, in the vagina can cause excessive mucus production, as can irritation from frequent douching, feminine hygiene products, contraceptive products, bubble baths, and colored or perfumed toilet papers.

Possible causes

Obstetrics-Gynecology

Atrophic vaginitis. In this disorder, a thin, scant, white vaginal discharge is present.

Candidiasis. Infection with *Candida albicans* causes a profuse, white, curd-like discharge with a yeasty, sweet odor. Onset is abrupt, usually just before menses. Exudate may be lightly attached to the labia and vaginal walls and is often accompanied by vulvar redness and edema.

Chancroid. This rare, sexually transmitted disease produces a mucopurulent, foul-smelling discharge.

Chlamydia infection. This infection causes a yellow, mucopurulent, odorless or acrid vaginal discharge.

Endometritis. A scant, serosanguineous discharge with a foul odor can result from bacterial invasion of the endometrium.

Gardnerella vaginitis. This infection (by *Gardnerella vaginalis,* formerly called *Hemophilus vaginalis*) causes a thin, foul-smelling, green or grayish white discharge. It adheres to the vaginal walls and can be easily wiped away, leaving healthy-looking tissue.

Genital warts. Characteristic vulvar lesions can cause a profuse, mucopurulent vaginal discharge, which may be foul-smelling if the warts are infected.

Gonorrhea. Although 80% of women with gonorrhea are asymptomatic, others have a yellow or green, foul-smelling discharge that can be expressed from Bartholin's or Skene's ducts.

Gynecologic cancer. Endometrial or cervical cancer produces a chronic, watery, bloody or purulent vaginal discharge that may be foul-smelling.

Herpes simplex (genital). A copious, mucoid discharge results from this disorder.

Trichomoniasis. This infection can cause a foul-smelling discharge, which may be frothy, greenish yellow, and profuse or thin, white, and scant.

Drugs
Estrogen-containing drugs, including oral contraceptives, can cause increased mucoid vaginal discharge. Antibiotics, such as tetracycline, can predispose the patient to vaginal infection and discharge.

Treatments
Irradiation of the reproductive tract can cause a watery, odorless vaginal discharge.

Clinical considerations

• A history should be obtained and a physical examination performed.

• Vaginal discharge specimens should be obtained for testing, as ordered.

If the patient has a vaginal infection:

• She should be told to continue taking the prescribed medication even if her symptoms clear or she menstruates.

• She should be advised to avoid intercourse until her symptoms clear, and then to have her partner use condoms until she completes her course of medication.

• If appropriate, she should be advised to douche with a solution of 5 tablespoons of white vinegar to 2 quarts of warm water to help relieve her discomfort.

Disorientation

Description
Disorientation is an inaccurate perception of time, place, or identity. Disorientation may occur in organic brain disorders, cerebral anoxia, and drug and alcohol intoxication. It occurs occasionally after prolonged, severe stress.

Distention, abdominal

Description
Abdominal distention refers to increased abdominal girth—the result of increased intraabdominal pressure forcing the abdominal wall outward. Distention may be mild or severe, depending on the amount of pressure. It may be localized or diffuse and may occur gradually or suddenly. Acute abdominal distention may signal life-threatening peritonitis or acute bowel obstruction.

Abdominal distention does not always signal pathology. For example, in anxious patients or those with digestive distress, localized distention in the left upper quadrant can result from aerophagia—the unconscious swallowing of air. Generalized distention can result from ingestion of fruits or vegetables with large amounts of unabsorbable carbohydrates, such as legumes, or from abnormal food fermentation by microbes.

Mechanism
Abdominal distention results from accumulation of fluid or gas (or both) within the lumen of the gastrointestinal (GI) tract or peritoneal cavity. Both fluid and gas are normally present in the GI tract, but not in the peritoneal cavity. However, if fluid and gas are unable to

pass freely through the GI tract, abdominal distention occurs. In the peritoneal cavity, distention may reflect acute bleeding, accumulation of ascitic fluid, or air from perforation of an abdominal organ.

Possible causes
Cardiovascular
Congestive heart failure (CHF). Generalized abdominal distention caused by ascites is confirmed by shifting dullness and a fluid wave. Accompanying the distention are the hallmarks of CHF: peripheral edema, jugular vein distention, dyspnea, and tachycardia.

Gastrointestinal
Abdominal cancer. Generalized abdominal distention may occur when the cancer—most often, an ovarian or pancreatic tumor—produces ascites. Shifting dullness and a fluid wave accompany distention.

Abdominal trauma. When brisk internal bleeding accompanies trauma, abdominal distention may be acute and dramatic.

Cirrhosis. In this disorder, ascites causes generalized distention and is confirmed by a fluid wave, shifting dullness, and a puddle sign. Umbilical eversion and caput medusae (dilated veins around the umbilicus) are common.

Gastric dilatation (acute). Left upper quadrant distention is characteristic in acute gastric dilatation.

Irritable bowel syndrome. This disorder may produce intermittent, localized distention—the result of periodic intestinal spasms.

Large-bowel obstruction. Dramatic abdominal distention is characteristic in this life-threatening disorder; in fact, loops of the large bowel may become visible on the abdomen. Constipation precedes the distention and, in fact, may be the only symptom for days.

Mesenteric artery occlusion (acute). In this life-threatening disorder, abdominal distention usually occurs several hours after the sudden onset of severe, colicky periumbilical pain that later becomes constant and diffuse.

Paralytic ileus. This disorder produces generalized distention with a tympanic percussion note.

Peritonitis. In this life-threatening disorder, abdominal distention may be localized or generalized, depending on the extent of peritonitis. Fluid accumulates first within the peritoneal cavity and then within the bowel lumen, causing a fluid wave and shifting dullness. Typically, distention is accompanied by sudden and severe abdominal pain that worsens with movement, rebound tenderness, and abdominal rigidity. The skin over the patient's abdomen may appear taut.

Small-bowel obstruction. Abdominal distention is characteristic in this life-threatening disorder. It is most pronounced in late obstruction, especially in the distal small bowel.

Toxic megacolon (acute). This life-threatening complication of infectious or ulcerative colitis produces dramatic abdominal distention that usually develops gradually.

Genitourinary
Bladder distention. Various disorders cause bladder distention, which in turn causes lower abdominal distention. Slight dullness on percussion above the symphysis indicates mild bladder distention. A palpable, smooth, rounded, fluctuant suprapubic mass suggests severe distention; a fluctuant mass extending to the umbilicus indicates extremely severe distention.

Nephrotic syndrome. This may produce massive edema, causing generalized abdominal distention with a fluid wave and shifting dullness.

Obstetrics-Gynecology
Ovarian cysts. Typically, large ovarian cysts produce lower abdominal distention accompanied by umbilical eversion. Because they are thin-walled and fluid-filled, these cysts produce a fluid wave and shifting dullness—signs that mimic ascites.

Clinical considerations

If abdominal distention is accompanied by pain, abdominal rigidity, and abnormal bowel sounds:

• The patient should be assessed for signs of hypovolemia, such as pallor, diaphoresis, hypotension, and a rapid, thready pulse.

• The physician should be notified immediately and emergency interventions begun.

• Oxygen should be administered and an I.V. line started, as ordered.

• A nasogastric tube should be inserted, as ordered.

• The patient should be reassured and prepared for surgery, if necessary.

If abdominal distention does not suggest an acute condition:

• A history should be obtained and a physical examination performed.

• Diagnostic tests include abdominal X-rays, endoscopy, laparoscopy, ultrasonography, computed tomography, or possibly paracentesis.

• The patient should be positioned comfortably, using pillows for support. If appropriate, he should be assisted onto his left side to help flatus escape, or, if he has ascites, the head of the bed should be elevated to ease breathing.

• If the patient has an obstruction or ascites, food and fluid restrictions should be enforced and explained.

Distention, bladder

Description

Bladder distention is the abnormal enlargement of the bladder. It results from an inability to excrete urine, causing its accumulation. Distention can result from mechanical and anatomic obstructions, neuromuscular disorders, and drugs. Relatively common in all ages and both sexes, it occurs most frequently in older men with prostate disorders, leading to urine retention.

Typically, bladder distention occurs gradually, but occasionally its onset may be sudden. Gradual distention usually remains asymptomatic until stretching of the bladder produces discomfort. Acute distention produces perineal fullness, pressure, and pain. If severe distention is not corrected promptly by catheterization or massage, the bladder rises within the abdomen, its walls become thin, and the risk of rupture increases.

Bladder distention is aggravated by intake of caffeine, alcohol, large quantities of fluid, and diuretics.

Possible causes

Central nervous system

Multiple sclerosis. In this neuromuscular disorder, urinary retention and bladder distention result from interruption of upper motor neuron control of the bladder.

Spinal neoplasms. Disrupting upper neuron control of the bladder, spinal neoplasms cause neurogenic bladder and resultant distention.

Endocrine

Diabetes mellitus. If this disorder affects the autonomic nervous system, it may cause neurogenic bladder, leading to urinary retention and bladder distention.

Genitourinary

Benign prostatic hypertrophy. In this disorder, bladder distention gradually develops as the prostate enlarges. Occasionally, its onset is acute.

Bladder calculi. This disorder may produce bladder distention, but more often it produces pain as its only symptom.

Bladder neoplasms. By blocking the urethral orifice, neoplasms can cause bladder distention.

Prostatic neoplasms. This disorder eventually causes bladder distention in up to 25% of patients.

Prostatitis. In *acute prostatitis,* bladder distention occurs rapidly along with perineal discomfort and fullness.

In *chronic prostatitis,* bladder distention usually occurs gradually.

Urethral calculi. In this disorder, urethral obstruction leads to bladder distention.

Urethral stricture. This disorder results in urinary retention and bladder distention.

Drugs

Parasympatholytics, ganglionic blockers, sedatives, anesthetics, and opiates can produce urinary retention and bladder distention.

Treatments

Use of an *indwelling urethral catheter* can result in urinary retention and bladder distention. While the catheter is in place, inadequate drainage due to kinked tubing or an occluded lumen may lead to urinary retention. After removal of the catheter, irritation may cause edema, blocking urine outflow.

Clinical considerations

• If the patient has *severe distention,* an indwelling urethral catheter should be inserted, as ordered, to help relieve discomfort and prevent bladder rupture.

• If the distention is not severe, a history should be obtained and a physical examination performed.

• Diagnostic tests include endoscopy and radiologic studies.

• The patient's vital signs and the extent of bladder distention should be monitored.

• The patient should be encouraged to change positions to alleviate discomfort and analgesics given, if ordered.

If the patient does not require immediate urethral catheterization, the normal voiding process should be encouraged through the following measures:

• Privacy should be provided and the patient instructed to assume a normal voiding position.

• The patient should be taught to perform Valsalva's maneuver.

• A sitz bath or warm tub bath should be provided to promote relaxation.

• Water should be run in the sink to stimulate the desire to urinate.

Dizziness

Description

Dizziness is a sensation of imbalance or faintness, sometimes associated with giddiness, weakness, confusion, and blurred or double vision. Usually, episodes of dizziness are brief; they may be mild or severe with abrupt or gradual onset. Dizziness may be aggravated by standing up quickly and alleviated by lying down and by rest.

Dizziness may occur in anxiety, in respiratory and cardiovascular disorders, and in postconcussion syndrome. It is a key symptom in certain serious disorders such as hypertension and vertebrobasilar artery insufficiency.

Dizziness is often confused with vertigo—a sensation of revolving in space or of surroundings revolving about oneself. However, unlike dizziness, vertigo is often accompanied by nausea, vomiting, nystagmus, staggering gait, and tinnitus or hearing loss. Dizziness and vertigo may occur together, as in postconcussion syndrome.

Mechanism

Typically, dizziness results from inadequate blood flow and oxygen supply to the cerebrum and spinal cord.

Possible causes

Central nervous system

Postconcussion syndrome. Occurring 1 to 3 weeks after head injury, this syndrome is marked by dizziness, headache, emotional lability, alcohol intolerance, fatigue, anxiety, and possibly vertigo. Dizziness and other symptoms are intensified by mental or physical stress. The syndrome may persist for years, but symptoms eventually abate.

Transient ischemic attack. Lasting from a few seconds to 24 hours, an attack frequently signals impending stroke and may be triggered by turning the head to the side. Dizziness of varying severity occurs during an attack.

Respiratory

Emphysema. Dizziness may follow exertion or the chronic, productive cough in this disorder.

Hyperventilation syndrome. Episodes of hyperventilation cause dizziness that usually lasts a few minutes; however, if these episodes occur frequently, dizziness may persist between them.

Cardiovascular

Cardiac dysrhythmias. Dizziness lasts for several minutes or longer with this disorder, before it resolves spontaneously or initiates fainting.

Carotid sinus hypersensitivity. Brief episodes of dizziness that usually terminate in fainting are characteristic. These episodes are precipitated by stimulation of one or both carotid arteries by wearing a tight collar, movement of the patient's head, or other seemingly minor sensations or actions.

Hypertension. In this disorder, dizziness may initiate fainting or a stroke. However, it may also be relieved by rest.

Orthostatic hypotension. This condition produces dizziness that may terminate in fainting or disappear with rest.

Hematologic

Anemia. Typically, this disorder causes dizziness that is aggravated by postural changes or exertion.

Psychiatric

Generalized anxiety disorder. This disorder produces continuous dizziness that may intensify as the disorder worsens.

Panic disorder. Dizziness accompanies acute attacks of panic in this disorder.

Drugs

Antianxiety drugs, central nervous system depressants, narcotics, decongestants, antihistamines, antihypertensives, and vasodilators frequently cause dizziness.

Clinical considerations

If *hypertension* is the suspected cause of dizziness:

• Vital signs should be taken and the physician notified if diastolic pressure exceeds 100 mm Hg.

• An I.V. line should be started for administration of antihypertensive medication.

• If the patient has been taking antihypertensive medication, the time of the last dose should be determined.

If the patient has normal blood pressure:

• A history should be obtained and a physical examination performed.

• Diagnostic tests include blood studies, arteriography, computed tomography, electroencephalography, and magnetic resonance imaging.

• If the patient is hyperventilating, he should be told to breathe and rebreathe into cupped hands or a paper bag.

• If the patient experiences dizziness in an upright position, he should be told to lie down and to rest, then rise slowly.

• The patient should be assisted with activities of daily living and his safety ensured, as needed.

Doll's eye sign, absent
(Negative oculocephalic reflex)

Description

An ominous indicator of brain stem dysfunction, absent doll's eye sign is detected by rapid, but gentle, turning of the patient's head from side to side. The eyes remain fixed in midposition, instead of moving laterally toward the side opposite the direction the head is turned. Usually, this sign cannot be elicited in the conscious patient because he voluntarily controls eye movements. *Important:* Eliciting this sign in a patient with suspected cervical spine injury is contraindicated.

Absent doll's eye sign indicates injury to the midbrain, pons, and cranial nerves III, VI, and VIII. Typically, it accompanies coma caused by lesions of the cerebellum and brain stem. When it is detected in deep coma, absent doll's eye sign is a mark of brain death.

A variant of absent doll's eye sign that develops gradually is known as abnormal doll's eye sign: conjugate eye movement is lost, so that one eye may move laterally while the other remains fixed or moves in the opposite direction. Usually, an abnormal doll's eye sign accompanies metabolic coma or increased intracranial pressure. The associated brain stem dysfunction may be reversible or may progress to deeper coma with absent doll's eye sign.

Normally, doll's eye sign is absent for the first 10 days after birth, and it may be irregular until age 2. After that, this sign reliably indicates brain stem function.

Possible causes
Central nervous system
Brain stem infarction. This infarction causes absent doll's eye sign with coma.
Brain stem tumors. Absent doll's eye sign accompanies coma with this disorder.
Central midbrain infarction. Accompanying absent doll's eye sign are coma, Weber's syndrome, contralateral ataxic tremor, nystagmus, and pupillary abnormalities.
Cerebellar lesion. Whether associated with abscess, hemorrhage, or tumor, a cerebellar lesion that progresses to coma may also cause an absent doll's eye sign.
Pontine hemorrhage. Absent doll's eye sign and coma develop within minutes in this life-threatening disorder.
Posterior fossa hematoma. A subdural hematoma at this location typically causes absent doll's eye sign and coma.
Drugs
Barbiturates may produce severe central nervous system depression, resulting in coma and absent doll's eye sign.

Clinical considerations
• The physician should be notified.
• Cold caloric testing may be done to confirm absent doll's eye sign.

Dorendorf's sign

Description
Dorendorf's sign is fullness at the supraclavicular groove. This sign may occur in an aneurysm of the aortic arch.

Drooling

Description
Drooling is the flow of saliva from the mouth. It may stem from facial muscle paralysis or weakness that prevents mouth closure, from neuromuscular disorders or local pain that causes dysphagia, or less commonly from the effects of drugs or toxins that induce salivation. Drooling may be scant or copious (up to 1 liter daily) and may cause circumoral irritation. Because it signals an inability to handle secretions, drooling warns of potential aspiration.

Mechanism
Drooling results from a failure to swallow or retain saliva, or from excess salivation.

Possible causes
Central nervous system
Acoustic neuroma. When this malignant tumor involves the facial nerve, it produces facial weakness or paralysis with constant scant-to-copious drooling.
Amyotrophic lateral sclerosis. Brain stem involvement in this degenerative disorder weakens muscles of the face and tongue, resulting in constant scant-to-copious drooling.
Bell's palsy. In this disorder, constant drooling accompanies sudden onset of facial hemiplegia.

Cerebrovascular accident (CVA). Facial paralysis associated with CVA results in scant-to-copious drooling.

Guillain-Barré syndrome. The hallmark of this polyneuritis is ascending muscle weakness that typically starts in the legs and extends to the arms and face within 24 to 72 hours. Facial diplegia and dysphagia set the stage for scant-to-copious drooling.

Myasthenia gravis. Facial and pharyngeal muscle weakness in this disorder causes scant-to-copious drooling.

Myotonic dystrophy. Facial weakness and a sagging jaw account for constant drooling in this disorder.

Paralytic poliomyelitis. When this infection involves the brain stem, it may produce facial paralysis and dysphagia, resulting in scant-to-copious drooling.

Parkinson's disease. In this degenerative disorder, drooling occurs because saliva is not directed to the back of the mouth.

Seizures (generalized). This tonic-clonic muscular reaction causes excessive salivation and frothing at the mouth accompanied by loss of consciousness and cyanosis. In the unresponsive postictal state, the patient may also drool.

Eyes, ears, nose, and throat

Glossopharyngeal neuralgia. Drooling may accompany the sharp paroxysms of pain that characterize this rare disorder.

Ludwig's angina. In this disorder, moderate-to-copious drooling stems from dysphagia and local swelling of the floor of the mouth, causing tongue displacement.

Peritonsillar abscess. Severe sore throat causes dysphagia with moderate-to-copious drooling with this abscess.

Retropharyngeal abscess. This disorder causes painful swallowing, resulting in moderate-to-copious drooling. The patient complains of a lump in his throat that he cannot swallow and of dyspnea when he is sitting that disappears when he lies down.

Gastrointestinal

Achalasia. Progressively severe dysphagia may cause copious drooling late in this disorder. When the patient lies down, food and saliva in the dilated esophagus flow back to the pharynx and mouth, resulting in drooling. Coughing or choking and aspiration may follow regurgitation.

Esophageal tumor. In this disorder, copious and persistent drooling is typically preceded by weight loss and progressively worsening dysphagia.

Metabolic

Hypocalcemia. The chief feature of this disorder is tetany, characterized by muscle twitching, cramps, and convulsions; carpopedal spasm; and a positive Chvostek's sign. Moderate-to-copious drooling may accompany the resultant dysphagia.

Infectious diseases

Diphtheria. In this infection, moderate drooling results from dysphagia associated with sore throat.

Environmental

Envenomation. Some snake bites trigger excess salivation, resulting in drooling. The drooling is accompanied by other neurotoxic effects.

Pesticide poisoning. Toxic effects of pesticides may include excess salivation with drooling.

Rabies. When this acute central nervous system infection advances to the brain stem, it produces drooling, or "foaming at the mouth." Drooling stems from excessive salivation, facial palsy, and/or extremely painful pharyngeal spasms that prohibit swallowing.

Tetanus. This acute infection may produce scant-to-copious drooling associated with dysphagia.

Drugs

Excess salivation caused by drugs such as clonazepam, ethionamide, and haloperidol may result in drooling.

Clinical considerations

• A history should be obtained and a physical examination performed.

• The patient should be assessed for signs and symptoms of aspiration and emergency equipment should be kept readily available.

• The patient should be positioned upright or on his side to prevent aspiration.

• Suctioning should be performed as needed to prevent aspiration.

• To help the patient cope with drooling, a covered container should be provided to collect secretions, decrease odor, and prevent possible transmission of infection.

• Tissues should be kept within the patient's reach and a towel should be draped across the patient's chest at mealtime.

• Good oral hygiene should be encouraged.

• Exercises to help strengthen facial muscles should be taught, if appropriate.

Duchenne's sign

Description
Duchenne's sign is inward movement of the epigastrium during inspiration. This may indicate diaphragmatic paralysis or accumulation of fluid in the pericardium.

Dugas' sign

Description
Dugas' sign is an indicator of a dislocated shoulder. To detect this sign, the examiner asks the patient to place the hand of the affected side on his opposite shoulder and to move his elbow toward his chest. The inability to perform this maneuver—a positive Dugas' sign—indicates dislocation.

Duroziez's sign

Description
Duroziez's sign—an indicator of aortic insufficiency—is a double murmur heard over a large peripheral artery. To detect this sign, the examiner auscultates the area over the femoral artery while alternately compressing the vessel proximally and then distally. If the examiner hears a systolic murmur with proximal compression and a diastolic murmur with distal compression, Duroziez's sign is present.

Dysarthria

Description
Dysarthria is poorly articulated speech characterized by slurring and a labored, irregular rhythm. It may be accompanied by nasal voice tone caused by palate weakness. Whether it occurs abruptly or gradually, dysarthria is usually evident in ordinary conversation. It is confirmed by asking the patient to produce a few simple sounds and words, such as "ba," "sh," and "cat." However, dysarthria is occasionally confused with aphasia, which involves loss of the ability to produce or comprehend speech.

Degenerative neurologic disorders commonly cause dysarthria. In fact, dysarthria is a chief sign of olivopontocerebellar degeneration. It may also result from ill-fitting dentures.

Mechanism
Dysarthria results from damage to the brain stem that affects cranial nerves IX, X, or XI.

Possible causes
Central nervous system
Alcoholic cerebellar degeneration. This disorder commonly causes chronic, progressive dysarthria.
Amyotrophic lateral sclerosis. Dysarthria occurs when this disorder affects the bulbar nuclei. It may worsen as the disease progresses.
Brain stem cerebrovascular accident (CVA). This CVA is characterized by bulbar palsy, resulting in the triad of dysarthria, dysphonia, and dysphagia.

The dysarthria is most severe at the onset of stroke; it may lessen or disappear with rehabilitation.

Cerebral CVA. A massive bilateral CVA causes pseudobulbar palsy. Bilateral weakness produces dysathria that is most severe at the onset of the stroke.

Multiple sclerosis. When demyelination affects the brain stem and cerebellum, the patient displays dysarthria accompanied by nystagmus, blurred or double vision, dysphagia, ataxia, and intention tremor. These signs and symptoms worsen and subside with exacerbation and remission of the disorder.

Myasthenia gravis. This neuromuscular disorder causes dysarthria associated with nasal voice tone. Typically, the dysarthria worsens during the day.

Olivopontocerebellar degeneration. Dysarthria, a major sign, accompanies cerebellar ataxia and spasticity.

Parkinson's disease. This disorder produces dysarthria and low-pitched monotonic speech.

Shy-Drager syndrome. Characterized by chronic orthostatic hypotension, this syndrome eventually causes dysarthria.

Cardiovascular

Basilar artery insufficiency. This disorder causes random, brief episodes of bilateral brain stem dysfunction, resulting in dysarthria.

Environmental

Botulism. The hallmark of this disorder is acute cranial nerve dysfunction causing dysarthria, dysphagia, diplopia, and ptosis.

Poisoning. Chronic manganese or mercury poisoning causes progressive dysarthria.

Drugs

Usually, dysarthria occurs at the start of anticonvulsant therapy but then disappears. Ingestion of large doses of barbiturates may also cause dysarthria.

Clinical considerations

• A history should be obtained with the help of family members and a physical examination performed.

• The patient should be encouraged to speak slowly so that he can be understood.

• The patient should be given ample time to express himself and encouraged to use gestures when necessary.

Dysdiadochokinesia

Description

Dysdiadochokinesia is difficulty in stopping one movement and starting another. This extrapyramidal sign occurs with disorders of the basal ganglia and cerebellum.

Dysmenorrhea

Description

Dysmenorrhea is painful menstruation. It affects over 50% of menstruating women. It is the leading cause of lost time from school and work among women of childbearing age. Dysmenorrhea may involve sharp, intermittent pain or dull, aching pain. Usually, it is characterized by mild-to-severe cramping or colicky pain in the pelvis or lower abdomen that may radiate to the thighs and lower sacrum. This pain may precede menstruation by several days or may accompany it. The pain gradually subsides as bleeding tapers off.

Dysmenorrhea may be idiopathic, as in premenstrual syndrome and primary dysmenorrhea. It commonly results from endometriosis and other pelvic disorders. It may also result from structural abnormalities, such as an imperforate hymen. Stress and poor health may aggravate dysmenorrhea, whereas rest and mild exercise may relieve it. Intrauterine devices may cause severe cramping and heavy menstrual flow.

Possible causes
Obstetrics-Gynecology
Adenomyosis. In this disorder, endometrial tissue invades the myometrium, resulting in severe dysmenorrhea with pain radiating to the back or rectum.

Cervical stenosis. This structural disorder causes dysmenorrhea and scant menstrual flow.

Endometriosis. Typically, this disorder produces steady, aching pain that begins before menses and peaks at the height of menstrual flow. However, the pain may also occur between menstrual periods. It may arise at the endometrial deposit site or may radiate to the perineum or rectum.

Pelvic inflammatory disease. Chronic infection produces dysmenorrhea.

Premenstrual syndrome (PMS). Usually, PMS follows an ovulatory cycle. As a result, it is rare during the first 12 months of menses, which may be anovulatory. The cramping pain usually begins with menstrual flow and persists for several hours or days, diminishing with decreasing flow.

Primary (idiopathic) dysmenorrhea. Increased prostaglandin secretion intensifies uterine contractions, apparently causing mild-to-severe spasmodic cramping pain in the lower abdomen, which radiates to the sacrum and inner thighs. Cramping abdominal pain peaks a few hours before menses.

Right ovarian vein syndrome. Intermittent flank pain occurs before and early in menses, accompanied by signs of ureteral obstruction, such as chills, fever, costovertebral angle tenderness, and pyuria.

Uterine leiomyomas. Tumors may cause lower abdominal pain that worsens with menses. The pain may be constant or intermittent.

Uterine prolapse. Displacement of the uterus may produce dysmenorrhea and chronic lower back pain.

Clinical considerations
• A history should be obtained and a pelvic examination performed.
• A heating pad should be placed over the abdomen, as needed, to relieve pain caused by idiopathic dysmenorrhea. This therapy reduces abdominal muscle tension and increases blood flow.
• Effleurage, a light circular massage with the fingertips, may also be performed to provide relief.
• Other comfort measures should be suggested, such as drinking warm beverages, taking a warm shower, performing waist-bending and pelvic-rocking exercises, and walking.
• Treatment may include the use of oral contraceptives and prostaglandin inhibitors.

Dyspareunia

Description
Dyspareunia is painful or difficult coitus. Although most sexually active women occasionally experience mild dyspareunia, persistent or severe dyspareunia is cause for concern. Dyspareunia may occur with attempted penetration or during or after coitus. It may stem from friction of the penis against perineal tissue or from jarring of deeper adnexal structures. The location of pain helps determine its cause.

Dyspareunia frequently accompanies pelvic disorders. However, it may also result from diminished vaginal lubrication associated with aging, the effects of drugs, and psychological factors—most notably, fear of pain or injury. A fear-pain-tension cycle may become established in which repeated painful coitus conditions the patient to anticipate pain, causing fear that prevents sexual arousal and adequate vaginal lubrication. Contraction of the pubococcygeus muscle also occurs, making penetration still more difficult and traumatic. Other psychological factors include guilt feelings about sex, fear of pregnancy or of injury to the fetus during pregnancy, and anxiety caused by a disrupted sexual relationship or by a new sexual partner. Inadequate vaginal lubrication associated with insufficient foreplay and mental or physical fatigue may also cause dyspareunia.

Dyspareunia may also stem from use of some spermicidal jellies, douches, and vaginal creams and deodorants that cause irritation and edema. An ill-fitting diaphragm may produce cramps with intercourse. An incorrectly placed intrauterine device may cause dyspareunia during orgasm.

Possible causes

Genitourinary
Cystitis. Vulvar pain may occur during coitus.

Obstetrics-Gynecology
Atrophic vaginitis. In postmenopausal and lactating women, decreased estrogen secretion may lead to inadequate vaginal lubrication and dyspareunia, which intensifies as intercourse continues.

Bartholinitis. This inflammatory disorder may produce throbbing pain during intercourse accompanied by vulvar tenderness.

Cervicitis. This inflammatory disorder causes pain with deep penetration. It may also cause dull, lower abdominal pain.

Condylomata acuminata. These warty growths occur on the vulva, vaginal and cervical walls, and perianal area. They may bleed, itch, and become tender during and after intercourse.

Endometriosis. This disorder causes intense pain during deep penetration, which jars endometrial deposits on the ovaries or cul-de-sac. Aching pain may also occur with gentle thrusting or during a pelvic examination. The pain is usually bilateral in the lower abdomen, although it may be worse on one side. It may be relieved by changing coital positions.

Herpes genitalis. This sexually transmitted disease causes pain during intercourse, due to friction against lesions on the labia, vulva, vagina, or perianal skin.

Occlusive or rigid hymen. In this condition, dyspareunia may prevent penetration.

Ovarian cyst or tumor. In this disorder, lower abdominal pain accompanies deep penetration during intercourse.

Pelvic inflammatory disease. Deep penetration causes the most severe pain. It is unrelieved by changing coital positions. Uterine tenderness may also occur with gentle thrusting or during a pelvic examination.

Uterine prolapse. Sharp or aching pain occurs with uterine prolapse when the penis strikes the descended cervix.

Vaginitis. Infection produces dyspareunia along with vulvar pain, burning, and itching during and for several hours following coitus. These symptoms may be aggravated by sexual arousal aside from intercourse.

Treatment
If an *episiotomy scar* constricts the vaginal introitus or narrows the vaginal barrel, the patient may experience perineal pain with coitus.

Radiation therapy for pelvic cancer may cause pelvic and vaginal scarring, resulting in dyspareunia.

Clinical considerations
• A history should be obtained and a pelvic examination performed.
• As appropriate, the patient should be advised to apply vaginal lubricants before intercourse, to attempt different coital positions, to increase foreplay time, or to perform Kegel exercises to reduce muscle tension.

• An antimicrobial or anti-inflammatory agent should be administered, if ordered and needed.

Dyspepsia

Description

Dyspepsia is an uncomfortable fullness after meals that is associated with nausea, belching, heartburn, and possibly cramping and abdominal distention. Frequently aggravated by spicy, fatty, or high-fiber foods and by excess caffeine consumption, dyspepsia indicates impaired digestive function.

Dyspepsia results from gastrointestinal (GI) disorders and, to a lesser extent, from cardiac, pulmonary, and renal disorders and the effects of drugs. This symptom may also result from emotional upset and overly rapid eating or improper chewing. Usually, it occurs a few hours after eating and lasts for a variable period of time. Its severity depends on the amount and type of food eaten and on GI motility. Additional food or antacids may relieve the discomfort.

Possible causes
Respiratory
Pulmonary embolus. Sudden dyspnea characterizes this potentially fatal disorder; however, dyspepsia may occur as an oppressive, severe, substernal discomfort.
Pulmonary tuberculosis. Vague dyspepsia may occur, along with anorexia, malaise, and weight loss.
Cardiovascular
Congestive heart failure. Common in right heart failure, transient dyspepsia may be accompanied by chest tightness and a constant ache or sharp pain in the right upper quadrant.
Gastrointestinal
Cholelithiasis. Heavy or greasy meals can precipitate dyspepsia with bloating, flatulence, nausea, vomiting, belching, and biliary colic.

Cirrhosis. Dyspepsia in this chronic disorder varies in intensity and duration and is relieved by antacids.
Duodenal ulcer. A primary symptom of duodenal ulcer, dyspepsia ranges from a vague feeling of fullness or pressure to a boring or aching sensation in the middle or right epigastrium. It usually occurs 1½ to 3 hours after eating and is relieved by food or antacids. The pain may awaken the patient at night with heartburn and water brash (fluid regurgitation).
Gastric dilatation (acute). Epigastric fullness is an early symptom of this painless, yet life-threatening, disorder.
Gastric ulcer. Typically, dyspepsia and heartburn after eating occur early in this disorder.
Gastritis (chronic). In this disorder, dyspepsia is relieved by antacids and aggravated by spicy foods or excessive caffeine.
GI neoplasms. These neoplasms usually produce chronic dyspepsia.
Hepatitis. Dyspepsia occurs in two of the three stages in hepatitis. The preicteric phase produces moderate-to-severe dyspepsia, fever, malaise, arthralgia, coryza, myalgia, nausea, vomiting, an altered sense of taste or smell, and hepatomegaly. Jaundice then marks the onset of the icteric phase, along with continued dyspepsia and anorexia, irritability, and severe pruritus. As jaundice clears, the dyspepsia and other GI effects also diminish.
Pancreatitis (chronic). A feeling of fullness or dyspepsia is usually accompanied by severe continuous or intermittent epigastric pain that radiates to the back or through the abdomen.
Genitourinary
Uremia. Of the many GI complaints associated with this condition, dyspepsia may be the earliest and most important.
Drugs
Nonsteroidal anti-inflammatory drugs, especially aspirin, commonly cause dyspepsia. Diuretics, antibiotics, antihypertensives, and many other drugs

can cause dyspepsia, depending on the patient's tolerance of the dosage.

Treatments

After GI or other surgery, *postoperative gastritis* can cause dyspepsia, which usually disappears in a few weeks.

Clinical considerations

• A history should be obtained and a physical examination performed.

• Food or antacids may relieve dyspepsia. Treatment may include dietary changes and the use of antacids between meals.

• Drugs that cause dyspepsia should be administered after meals, if possible.

• Rest should be promoted and a calm environment provided to reduce stress-related dyspepsia.

• Endoscopy may be performed to determine the cause of dyspepsia.

Dysphagia

Description

Dysphagia is difficulty swallowing. It is a common symptom that is usually easy to localize. It may be constant or intermittent. Among the factors that interfere with swallowing are severe pain, obstruction, abnormal peristalsis, impaired gag reflex, and excessive, scanty, or thick oral secretions.

Dysphagia is the most common—and sometimes the *only*—symptom of esophageal disorders. However, it may also result from oropharyngeal, respiratory, neurologic, and collagen disorders and the effects of toxins and treatments. Dysphagia increases the risk of choking and aspiration and may lead to malnutrition and dehydration.

Mechanism

Dysphagia is classified as phase 1, 2, or 3 by the phase of swallowing it affects (see *Classifying Dysphagia by Phases of Swallowing,* page 128).

Possible causes

Central nervous system

Amyotrophic lateral sclerosis. Dysphagia occurs with this disorder, particularly if the brain stem is involved.

Bulbar paralysis. Phase 1 dysphagia occurs along with drooling, difficulty chewing, dysarthria, and nasal regurgitation. Dysphagia, which occurs for both solids and liquids, is painful and progressive.

Myasthenia gravis. Fatigue and progressive muscle weakness characterize this disorder and account for painless phase 1 dysphagia and possibly choking. Typically, dysphagia follows ptosis and diplopia.

Parkinson's disease. Usually a late symptom, phase 1 dysphagia is painless but progressive and may cause choking.

Eyes, ears, nose, and throat

Laryngeal carcinoma (extrinsic). Phase 2 dysphagia and dyspnea develop late in this disorder.

Laryngeal nerve damage. Often the result of radical neck surgery, superior laryngeal nerve damage may produce painless phase 2 dysphagia.

Oral cavity tumor. Painful phase 1 dysphagia develops along with hoarseness and ulcerating lesions.

Pharyngitis (chronic). This condition causes painful phase 2 dysphagia for solids and liquids. Rarely serious, it is accompanied by a dry sore throat, cough, and thick mucus in the throat.

Respiratory

Airway obstruction. Life-threatening upper airway obstruction is marked by signs of respiratory distress, such as crowing and stridor. Phase 2 dysphagia occurs with gagging and dysphonia. When hemorrhage obstructs the trachea, dysphagia is usually painless and rapid in onset. When inflammation causes the obstruction, dysphagia may be painful and develop slowly.

Cardiovascular

Progressive systemic sclerosis. Typically, dysphagia is preceded by Ray-

Classifying Dysphagia by Phases of Swallowing

Swallowing occurs in three distinct phases and dysphagia can be classified by the phase that it affects. Each phase suggests a specific pathology for dysphagia.

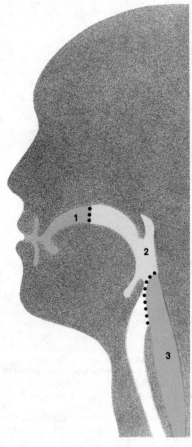

Phase 1

Swallowing begins in the *transfer phase* with chewing and moistening of food with saliva. The tongue presses against the hard palate to transfer the chewed food to the back of the throat; the fifth cranial nerve then stimulates the swallowing reflex. Phase 1 dysphagia typically results from a neuromuscular disorder.

Phase 2

In the *transport phase,* the soft palate closes against the pharyngeal wall to prevent nasal regurgitation. At the same time, the larynx rises and the vocal cords close to keep food out of the lungs; breathing stops momentarily as the throat muscles constrict to move food into the esophagus. Phase 2 dysphagia usually indicates spasm or carcinoma.

Phase 3

Peristalsis and gravity work together in the *entrance phase* to move food through the esophageal sphincter and into the stomach. Phase 3 dysphagia results from lower esophageal narrowing by diverticula, esophagitis, and other disorders.

naud's phenomenon in this disorder. The dysphagia may be mild at first and described as a feeling of food sticking behind the breastbone.

Gastrointestinal

Achalasia. Most common in patients age 20 to 40, this disorder produces phase 3 dysphagia for solids and liquids. The dysphagia develops gradually and may be precipitated or exacerbated by stress. Occasionally, it is preceded by esophageal colic. Regurgitation of undigested food, especially at night, may cause wheezing, coughing, or choking as well as halitosis.

Dysphagia lusoria. The only symptom of this congenital anomaly is phase 3 dysphagia for solids, which may not occur until late adulthood.

Esophageal carcinoma. Phase 2 and 3 dysphagia is the earliest and most common symptom of esophageal carcinoma. Typically, this painless, progressive symptom is accompanied by rapid weight loss. As carcinoma advances, dysphagia becomes painful and constant.

Esophageal compression (external). Most often caused by a dilated carotid or aortic aneurysm, this rare condition causes phase 3 dysphagia as the primary symptom.

Esophageal diverticulum. This disorder causes phase 3 dysphagia when the enlarged diverticulum obstructs the esophagus.

Esophageal leiomyoma. This relatively rare benign tumor may cause phase 3 dysphagia with retrosternal pain.

Esophageal obstruction by foreign body. Sudden onset of phase 2 or 3 dysphagia, gagging, coughing, and esophageal pain characterize this potentially life-threatening condition.

Esophageal spasm. The two most striking symptoms of this disorder are phase 2 dysphagia for solids and liquids and dull or squeezing substernal chest pain. Frequently, the pain is relieved by drinking a glass of water. It may last up to an hour and may radiate to the neck, arm, back, or jaw.

Esophagitis. Corrosive esophagitis, resulting from ingestion of alkalies or acids, causes severe phase 3 dysphagia.

Monilial esophagitis causes phase 2 dysphagia, sore thorat, and possibly retrosternal pain on swallowing.

In *reflux esophagitis,* phase 3 dysphagia is a late symptom that usually accompanies stricture development.

Gastric carcinoma. Infiltration of the cardia or esophagus by gastric carcinoma causes phase 3 dysphagia.

Hiatal hernia. This common disorder causes phase 3 dysphagia with retrosternal or substernal chest pain.

Lower esophageal ring. Narrowing of the lower esophagus may cause an attack of phase 3 dysphagia that may recur several weeks or months later. During the attack, the patient complains of a foreign body in the lower esophagus—a sensation that may be relieved by drinking water or vomiting.

Mediastinitis. Varying with the extent of esophageal perforation, mediastinitis can cause insidious or rapid onset of phase 3 dysphagia.

Plummer-Vinson syndrome. Also known as sideropenic dysphagia, this syndrome causes phase 3 dysphagia for solids in some women with severe iron deficiency anemia.

Musculoskeletal

Systemic lupus erythematosus. This disorder may cause progressive phase 2 dysphagia.

Metabolic

Hypocalcemia. Although tetany is its primary sign, severe hypocalcemia may cause neuromuscular irritability, producing phase 1 dysphagia.

Infectious diseases

Syphilis. Rarely, tertiary-stage syphilis causes ulceration and stricture of the upper esophagus, resulting in phase 3 dysphagia. The dysphagia may be accompanied by regurgitation after meals and heartburn that is aggravated by lying down or bending over.

Environmental

Botulism. This type of food poisoning causes phase 1 dysphagia and dysuria, usually within 36 hours of toxin ingestion.

Lead poisoning. Painless, progressive dysphagia may result from lead poisoning.

Rabies. Severe phase 2 dysphagia for liquids results from painful pharyngeal muscle spasms occurring late in this rare, life-threatening disorder. In fact, the patient may become dehydrated and possibly apneic. Dysphagia also causes drooling, and in 50% of patients, it is responsible for hydrophobia.

Tetanus. About 1 week after receiving a puncture wound, phase 1 dysphagia usually develops.

Treatments

When directed against oral cancer, *radiation therapy* may cause scant salivation and temporary dysphagia.

Recent tracheostomy may also cause temporary dysphagia.

Clinical considerations

• If the patient suddenly complains of dysphagia and displays signs of respiratory distress (dyspnea and stridor) an airway obstruction should be suspected and the Heimlich maneuver performed.

• If the patient does not have signs of airway obstruction, a history should be obtained and a physical examination performed.

• Diagnostic tests include endoscopy, esophageal manometry, the acid perfusion test, and the esophageal acidity test.

• The risk of choking and aspiration at mealtime should be minimized by assisting the patient to an upright position with his neck flexed forward.

• Sticky foods, such as bananas and peanut butter, should be avoided.

• The patient should be instructed to consume solids separately from liquids, which are harder to swallow.

• If the patient has decreased saliva production, food should be moistened with a little liquid.

• If the patient has a weak or absent cough reflex, tube feedings or esophageal drips of special formulas should be given, as ordered.

Dysphonia

Description

Dysphonia is hoarseness or difficulty in producing voice sounds. This sign may reflect disorders of the larynx or laryngeal nerves, overuse or spasm of the vocal cords, or central nervous system disorders, such as Parkinson's disease. It may also occur at puberty.

Dyspnea

Description

Dyspnea is the sensation of difficult or uncomfortable breathing. Usually, it is reported as shortness of breath. Its severity varies greatly but is often unrelated to the severity of the underlying cause. Dyspnea may arise suddenly or slowly and may subside rapidly or persist for years.

Most people normally experience dyspnea when they overexert themselves, and its severity depends on their physical condition. In the healthy person, dyspnea is quickly relieved by rest. Pathologic causes of dyspnea include pulmonary, cardiac, neuromuscular, and allergic disorders. In addition, anxiety may cause shortness of breath.

Possible causes

Central nervous system

Amyotrophic lateral sclerosis. Also known as Lou Gehrig's disease, this disorder causes slow onset of dyspnea that worsens with time.

Guillain-Barré syndrome. Usually following a fever and upper respiratory infection, this syndrome causes slowly worsening dyspnea.

Myasthenia gravis. This neuromuscular disorder causes bouts of dyspnea as the respiratory muscles weaken. With myasthenic crisis, acute respiratory distress may occur, with shallow respiration and tachypnea.

Respiratory

Adult respiratory distress syndrome. This life-threatening form of noncardiogenic pulmonary edema usually produces acute dyspnea as the first complaint.

Aspiration of a foreign body. Acute dyspnea marks this life-threatening condition, along with paroxysmal intercostal, suprasternal, and substernal retractions.

Asthma. Acute dyspneic attacks occur in this chronic disorder.

Emphysema. This chronic disorder gradually causes progressive exertional dyspnea.

Flail chest. Sudden dyspnea results from multiple rib fractures, along with paradoxical chest movement, severe chest pain, hypotension, tachypnea, tachycardia, and cyanosis.

Interstitial fibrosis. Besides dyspnea, this disorder causes chest pain, dry cough, rales, weight loss and, possibly, cyanosis and pleural friction rub.

Lung cancer. Dyspnea that develops slowly and progressively worsens occurs with late-stage cancer.

Pleural effusion. Dyspnea develops slowly and becomes progressively worse with this disorder. Initially, a pleural friction rub occurs, accompanied by pleuritic pain that worsens with coughing or deep breathing.

Pneumonia. Dyspnea occurs suddenly, usually accompanied by fever, shaking chills, pleuritic chest pain that worsens with deep inspiration, and a productive cough.

Pneumothorax. This life-threatening disorder causes acute dyspnea unrelated to the severity of pain.

Pulmonary edema. Often preceded by signs of congestive heart failure, such as distended neck veins and orthopnea, this life-threatening disorder causes acute dyspnea.

Pulmonary embolism. Acute dyspnea usually accompanied by sudden pleuritic chest pain characterizes this life-threatening disorder.

Cardiovascular

Cardiac dysrhythmias. In dysrhythmias, acute or gradual dyspnea can result from decreased cardiac output.

Congestive heart failure. Dyspnea usually develops gradually with this condition.

Cor pulmonale. Chronic dyspnea begins gradually with exertion and progressively worsens until it occurs even at rest.

Myocardial infarction. Sudden dyspnea occurs with crushing substernal chest pain that may radiate to the back, neck, jaw, and arms.

Shock. Dyspnea arises suddenly and worsens progressively in this life-threatening disorder.

Infection

Sepsis. This potentially fatal disorder gradually causes dyspnea along with chills and sudden fever.

Hematologic

Anemia. Usually, dyspnea develops gradually in this disorder.

Infectious diseases

Poliomyelitis (bulbar). Dyspnea develops gradually and progressively worsens.

Tuberculosis. Dyspnea commonly occurs with chest pain, crackles, and productive cough.

Environmental

Inhalation injury. Dyspnea may develop suddenly or gradually over several hours, following inhalation of chemicals or hot gases.

Clinical considerations

If dyspnea is acute:

• A quick respiratory assessment should be performed and the physician notified of signs and symptoms of acute respiratory distress.

• The patient should be placed in a high Fowler's position, clothing loosened, and oxygen administered, as ordered.

• An I.V. line should be started and cardiac monitoring begun, if ordered.

• If the patient has a pneumothorax, chest tube insertion should be anticipated.

• A calm, confident manner should be maintained and the patient reassured throughout his care.

• EKG monitoring should be performed, as needed, to detect and correct cardiac dysrhythmias.

• Treatment may include the use of bronchodilators, antiarrhythmics, diuretics, and analgesics to dilate bronchioles.

If dyspnea does not reflect an emergency situation:
• A history should be obtained and a physical examination performed.
• Diagnostic tests include arterial blood gas analysis, pulmonary function studies, and chest X-rays.
• The patient should be placed in a high Fowler's or forward leaning position to facilitate breathing.

Dystonia

Description

Dystonia is characterized by slow involuntary movements of large muscle groups of the limbs, trunk, and neck. This extrapyramidal sign may involve flexion of the foot, hyperextension of the legs, extension and pronation of the arms, arching of the back, and extension and rotation of the neck (spasmodic torticollis). It is typically aggravated by walking and emotional stress and relieved by sleep. It may be intermittent—lasting just a few minutes—or continuous and painful. Occasionally, it causes permanent contractures, resulting in a grotesque posture. Although dystonia may be hereditary or idiopathic, it results more often from extrapyramidal disorders or drugs.

Possible causes

Central nervous system
Alzheimer's disease. Dystonia is a late sign of this disorder.
Dystonia musculorum deformans. Prolonged, generalized dystonia is the hallmark of this disorder, which usually develops in childhood and worsens with age.
Hallervorden-Spatz disease. This degenerative disease causes dystonic trunk movements accompanied by choreoathetosis, ataxia, myoclonus, and generalized rigidity.
Huntington's chorea. Dystonic movements mark the preterminal stage of Huntington's chorea.

Olivopontocerebellar atrophy. Ataxia, an early sign in this rare disorder, slowly progresses to dystonia.
Parkinson's disease. Dystonic spasms are common in this disorder.
Pick's disease. Dystonia appears as a late sign in this rare disorder, which resembles Alzheimer's disease.
Supranuclear ophthalmoplegia (Steele-Richardson-Olszewski syndrome). This rare disorder affects mainly the middle-aged, causing intermittent dystonia with extreme neck flexion or extension.
Wilson's disease. Progressive dystonia and chorea of the arms and legs mark this disorder.
Drugs
All three types of phenothiazines may cause dystonia. Piperazine phenothiazines, such as acetophenazine and carphenazine, produce this sign most frequently; aliphatics, such as chlorpromazine, cause it less often; and piperidines rarely cause it.

Haloperidol, loxapine, and other antipsychotics usually produce acute facial dystonia. Antiemetic doses of metoclopramide, excessive doses of L-dopa, and metyrosine can also cause facial dystonia.

Clinical considerations

• A history should be obtained and a neurologic assessment performed.
• The patient should be encouraged to get adequate sleep and to avoid stress and active range-of-motion exercises.
• If dystonia is severe, the patient's bed rails should be raised and his environment kept uncluttered to protect him from injury.

Dysuria

Description

Dysuria is painful or difficult urination. It is often accompanied by urinary frequency, urgency, or hesitancy. Usually, this symptom reflects lower urinary tract infection—a common disorder, especially in women.

Dysuria results from lower urinary tract irritation or inflammation, which stimulates nerve endings in the bladder and urethra. The pain's onset provides clues to its cause: for example, pain just *before* voiding usually indicates bladder irritation or distention, while pain at the *start* of urination typically results from bladder outlet irritation. Pain at the *end* of voiding may signal bladder spasms.

Possible causes
Gastrointestinal
Appendicitis. Occasionally, this disorder causes dysuria that persists throughout voiding and is accompanied by bladder tenderness.
Diverticulitis. Inflammation near the bladder may cause dysuria throughout voiding.
Genitourinary
Bladder tumor. In this predominantly male disorder, dysuria throughout voiding is a late symptom.
Cystitis. Dysuria throughout voiding is common in all types of cystitis, as are urinary frequency, nocturia, straining to void, and hematuria. *Bacterial cystitis* is the most common cause of dysuria in women. In *chronic interstitial cystitis,* the dysuria is accentuated at the end of voiding. In *tubercular cystitis,* the patient may also have urinary urgency, flank pain, fatigue, and anorexia. In *viral cystitis,* severe dysuria occurs with gross hematuria, urinary urgency, and fever.
Paraurethral gland inflammation. Dysuria throughout voiding occurs with this disorder.
Prostatitis. Acute prostatitis commonly causes dysuria throughout or toward the end of voiding. In *chronic prostatitis,* urethral narrowing causes dysuria throughout voiding.
Pyelonephritis (acute). More common in females, this disorder causes dysuria throughout voiding.

Urethral syndrome. Occurring in women, this syndrome mimics urethritis. Dysuria throughout voiding may occur with urinary frequency, diminished urinary stream, suprapubic aching and cramping, tenesmus, and low back and unilateral flank pain.
Urethritis. Primarily found in males, this infection causes dysuria throughout voiding.
Urinary obstruction. Outflow obstruction by urethral strictures or calculi produces dysuria throughout voiding.
Musculoskeletal
Reiter's syndrome. In this male disorder, dysuria occurs 1 to 2 weeks after sexual contact.
Obstetrics-Gynecology
Vaginitis. Characteristically, dysuria occurs throughout voiding as urine touches inflamed or ulcerated labia.
Environmental
Chemical irritants. Dysuria may result from irritating substances such as bubble bath salts and feminine deodorants; it is usually most intense at the end of voiding.
Drugs
Dysuria can result from monoamine oxidase inhibitors. Metyrosine can also cause transient dysuria.

Clinical considerations
• A history should be obtained and a physical examination performed.
• Diagnostic tests include urinalysis, urine culture and sensitivity studies, kidney-ureter-bladder radiography or computed tomography scan, and cystoscopy.
• As needed, warm sitz baths should be administered to provide relief for perineal discomfort and to facilitate urination.

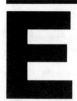

Earache
(Otalgia)

Description

Usually, earache results from disorders of the external and middle ear associated with infection, obstruction, or trauma. Its severity ranges from a feeling of fullness or blockage to deep, boring pain; at times, it may be difficult to localize precisely. This common symptom may be intermittent or continuous and may develop suddenly or gradually. If untreated, an earache may progress to permanent hearing loss or even to death in disorders such as malignant otitis externa or extradural abscess.

Possible causes

Eyes, ears, nose, and throat

Cerumen impaction. Impacted cerumen (earwax) may cause a plugged, blocked, or full sensation in the ear.

Chondrodermatitis nodularis chronica helicis. This disorder produces small, painful, indurated areas along the auricle's upper rim.

Extradural abscess. Severe earache accompanied by persistent ipsilateral headache, malaise, and recurrent mild fever characterizes this serious complication of middle ear infection.

Furunculosis. Infected hair follicles in the outer ear canal may produce severe, localized ear pain associated with a pus-filled furuncle (boil). The pain is aggravated by jaw movement and relieved by rupture or incision of the furuncle.

Mastoiditis (acute). This bacterial infection causes a dull ache behind the ear accompanied by low-grade fever and thick, purulent discharge in the external canal.

Ménière's disease. This inner ear disorder can produce a sensation of fullness in the affected ear.

Middle ear tumor. Deep, boring ear pain and facial paralysis are late signs of a malignant tumor.

Myringitis bullosa. This rare viral infection causes sudden, severe ear pain that radiates over the mastoid and lasts for up to 48 hours.

Perichondritis. This infection may cause ear pain accompanied by warmth and tenderness in the outer ear.

Petrositis. The result of acute otitis media, this infection produces deep ear pain with headache and pain behind the eye.

Temporomandibular joint infection. Typically unilateral, this infection produces ear pain that is referred from the jaw joint. The pain is aggravated by pressure on the joint with jaw movement; commonly, it radiates to the temporal area or the entire side of the head.

Skin

Keratosis obturans. Mild ear pain occurs in this disorder, along with otorrhea and tinnitus.

Infection

Herpes zoster oticus (Ramsay Hunt syndrome). This disorder causes burning or stabbing ear pain, often associated with ear vesicles.

Otitis externa. Earache characterizes both types of otitis externa. *Acute otitis externa* begins with mild-to-moderate ear pain that occurs with tragus manipulation. *Malignant otitis externa* abruptly causes ear pain that is aggravated by moving the auricle or tragus. *Otitis media (acute)*. This middle ear inflammation may be serous or suppurative. *Acute serous otitis media* may cause a feeling of fullness in the ear, hearing loss, and a vague sensation of top-heaviness. Severe, deep, throbbing ear pain and fever that may reach 102° F. (38.9° C.) characterize *acute suppurative otitis media*. The pain increases steadily over several hours or days and may be aggravated by pressure on the mastoid antrum. Rupture releases purulent drainage and relieves the pain.

Environmental
Barotrauma (acute). Earache associated with this trauma ranges from mild pressure to severe pain.

Ear canal obstruction by an insect. An insect lodged in the ear canal may cause severe pain and distressing noise.

Frostbite. Prolonged exposure to cold may cause burning or tingling pain in the ear, followed by numbness.

Clinical considerations
• A history should be obtained and an ear examination performed.
• An ear discharge specimen should be obtained, as ordered, for culture and sensitivity studies.
• Analgesics should be administered and heat applied, as ordered, to relieve discomfort.

Echolalia

Description
In an adult, echolalia is the repetition of another's words or phrases with no comprehension of their meaning. This sign occurs in schizophrenia and frontal lobe disorders.

Echolalia in a child is an imitation of sounds or words produced by others.

Echopraxia

Description
Echopraxia is the repetition of another's movements with no comprehension of their meaning. This sign may occur in catatonic schizophrenia and certain neurologic disorders.

Ectropion

Description
Ectropion is the eversion of the eyelid. It may affect the lower eyelid or both lids, exposing the palpebral conjunctiva. If the lacrimal puncta are everted, the eye cannot drain properly, and tearing occurs. Ectropion may occur gradually as part of aging but may also occur with injury or paralysis of the facial nerve.

Edema, generalized
(Anasarca)

Description
Generalized edema is the excessive accumulation of interstitial fluid throughout the body. It is a common sign in severely ill patients, and its severity varies widely; slight edema may be difficult to detect, especially if the patient is obese, while massive edema is immediately apparent.

Typically, generalized edema is chronic and progressive. It may result from cardiac, renal, endocrine, or hepatic disorders; severe burns; malnutrition; or the effects of certain drugs and treatments. Common factors responsible for edema are hypoalbuminemia and excess sodium ingestion or retention. Also, cyclic edema associated with increased aldosterone secretion may occur in premenopausal women.

Edema may be pitting or nonpitting. To differentiate between the two, a finger is pressed against a swollen area for five seconds and then quickly removed. In *pitting edema*, pressure forces fluid into the underlying tissues, causing an indentation that slowly fills. The severity of pitting edema is determined by estimating the indentation's depth in centimeters: 1 + (1 cm), 2 + (2 cm), 3 + (3 cm), or 4 + (4 cm). In *nonpitting edema*, pressure leaves no indentation because fluid has coagulated in the tissues. Typically, the skin feels unusually firm.

Mechanism

Normally, the lymphatic system transports excess interstitial fluid back to the intravascular space. Edema results when this balance is upset by increased capillary permeability, lymphatic obstruction, persistently increased capillary hydrostatic pressure, decreased plasma osmotic or interstitial fluid pressure, or dilation of precapillary sphincters.

Possible causes

Cardiovascular

Congestive heart failure. Severe, pitting generalized edema may follow leg edema late in this disorder. The edema may improve with exercise or elevation of the limbs.

Pericardial effusion. Generalized pitting edema may be most prominent in the arms and legs.

Pericarditis (chronic constrictive). Resembling right heart failure, this disorder usually begins with pitting edema of the arms and legs that may progress to generalized edema.

Endocrine

Myxedema. In this severe form of hypothyroidism, nonpitting generalized edema is accompanied by dry, waxy, pale skin.

Gastrointestinal

Cirrhosis. Progressive anasarca is a late sign of this chronic disorder.

Protein-losing enteropathy. Progressive, pitting generalized edema occurs in this disorder.

Genitourinary

Nephrotic syndrome. Pitting generalized edema characterizes this syndrome. In severe cases, anasarca develops—increasing body weight by up to 50%.

Renal failure. In *acute renal failure*, generalized pitting edema occurs as a late sign. In *chronic renal failure*, though, generalized edema is less likely; its severity depends on the degree of fluid overload.

Metabolic

Malnutrition. Anasarca in this disorder may mask dramatic muscle wasting.

Immunologic

Angioneurotic edema. Recurrent attacks of acute, painless, pitting edema affect the skin and mucous membranes, especially those of the respiratory tract.

Infection

Septic shock. A late sign of this life-threatening disorder, generalized edema typically develops rapidly. The edema is pitting and moderately severe.

Environmental

Burns. Edema and associated tissue damage vary with the severity of the burn. Severe generalized edema (4 +) may occur within 2 days of a major burn, while localized edema may occur with a less severe burn.

Drugs

Any drug that causes sodium retention may aggravate or cause generalized edema. Some examples are antihypertensives, corticosteroids, androgenic and anabolic steroids, estrogens, and nonsteroidal anti-inflammatory agents such as phenylbutazone, ibuprofen, and naproxen.

Treatments

I.V. saline administration or *internal feedings* may cause sodium and fluid overload, resulting in generalized edema.

Clinical considerations

If the patient has severe edema along with signs and symptoms of cardiac failure or pulmonary congestion:

• The physician should be notified immediately.

• The patient should be placed in Fowler's position to promote lung expansion, unless he is hypotensive.

• Oxygen and I.V. diuretics should be administered, as ordered.

• Emergency equipment should be kept readily available.

If the patient has no signs or symptoms of cardiac failure or pulmonary congestion:

• A history should be obtained and a physical examination peformed.

• Diagnostic tests include serum electrolyte and albumin levels, urinalysis, X-rays, echocardiography, or electrocardiography.

• The patient should be positioned with his limbs above heart level to promote drainage and periodically repositioned to avoid pressure sores.

• If the patient develops dyspnea, his limbs should be lowered, the head of the bed elevated, and oxygen administered, as ordered.

• Reddened areas, especially where dependent edema has formed (back, sacrum, hips, buttocks) should be massaged regularly. Skin breakdown in these areas can be prevented by placing a pressure mattress, lamb's wool pad, or flotation ring on the patient's bed.

• Treatment may include fluid and sodium restriction, and diuretic and I.V. albumin administration.

• Fluid intake and output should be measured and the patient weighed daily.

Edema, arm

Description

The result of excess interstitial fluid in the arm, this edema may be unilateral or bilateral and may develop gradually or abruptly. It may be aggravated by immobility and alleviated by arm elevation and exercise. Commonly, it results from trauma, venous disorders, toxins, and treatments.

Edema may be pitting or nonpitting. To differentiate between the two, a finger is pressed against a swollen area for five seconds and then quickly removed. In *pitting edema*, pressure forces fluid into the underlying tissues, causing an indentation that slowly fills. The severity of pitting edema is determined by estimating the indentation's depth in centimeters: $1+$ (1 cm), $2+$ (2 cm), $3+$ (3 cm), or $4+$ (4 cm). In *nonpitting edema*, pressure leaves no indentation because fluid has coagulated in the tissues. Typically, the skin feels unusually firm.

Mechanism

Normally, the lymphatic system transports excess interstitial fluid back to the intravascular space. Edema results when this balance is upset by increased capillary permeability, lymphatic obstruction, persistently increased capillary hydrostatic pressure, decreased plasma osmotic or interstitial fluid pressure, or dilation of precapillary sphincters.

Possible causes

Cardiovascular

Superior vena cava syndrome. Usually, bilateral arm edema progresses slowly and is accompanied by facial and neck edema. Dilated veins mark these edematous areas.

Thrombophlebitis. This disorder may cause arm edema, pain, and warmth.

Immunologic

Allergic reaction. Edema of the arm may indicate a local, allergic response to an allergen, such as a medication or bee sting venom.

Environmental

Arm trauma. Shortly after a crushing-type injury, severe edema may affect the entire arm.

Burns. Two days or less after injury, arm burns may cause mild-to-severe edema, pain, and tissue damage.

Envenomation. Initially, envenomation by snakes, aquatic animals, or insects may cause edema around the bite or sting that quickly spreads to the entire arm.

Treatments

Localized arm edema may result from *infiltration of an I.V.* catheter into the interstitial tissue. A *radical* or *modified radical mastectomy* that disrupts lymphatic drainage may cause edema of the entire arm. Also, *radiation therapy* for breast cancer may produce arm edema immediately after treatment or months later.

Clinical considerations

• A history should be obtained and a physical examination performed.

• A pneumatic cuff may be used to alternate venous compression.

• Warm compresses should be applied, as ordered.

• The affected arm(s) should be elevated about 6″ above heart level.

• Anticoagulants and analgesics should be administered, as ordered.

Edema, facial

Description

Facial edema refers to localized swelling—around the eyes, for instance—or more generalized facial swelling that may extend to the neck and upper arms. Occasionally painful, this sign may develop gradually or abruptly. At times, it precedes onset of peripheral or generalized edema. Mild edema may be difficult to detect; the patient or someone who is familiar with the patient's appearance may report it before it is noticed during assessment. It may result from venous, inflammatory, and certain systemic disorders; trauma; allergy; malnutrition; or the effects of drugs, tests, and treatments.

Mechanism

Normally, the lymphatic system transports excess interstitial fluid back to the intravascular space. Edema results when this balance is upset by increased capillary permeability, lymphatic obstruction, persistently increased capillary hydrostatic pressure, decreased plasma osmotic or interstitial fluid pressure, or dilation of precapillary sphincters.

Possible causes

Central nervous system

Melkersson's syndrome. Facial edema—especially of the lips—is one of three characteristic signs of this rare disorder, along with facial paralysis and folds in the tongue.

Eyes, ears, nose, and throat

Cavernous sinus thrombosis. This rare disorder may begin with unilateral edema that quickly progresses to bilateral edema of the forehead, base of the nose, and eyelids.

Chalazion. A chalazion causes localized swelling and tenderness of the affected eyelid, accompanied by a small red lump on the conjunctival surface.

Conjunctivitis. This inflammation causes eyelid edema, excessive tearing, and itchy, burning eyes.

Corneal ulcers (fungal). Red, edematous eyelids occur in this disorder.

Dacryoadenitis. Severe periorbital swelling characterizes this disorder.

Dacryocystitis. Lacrimal sac inflammation causes prominent eyelid edema and constant tearing.

Frontal sinus carcinoma. This rare disorder causes cheek edema on the affected side.

Herpes zoster ophthalmicus (shingles). In this disorder, edematous and red eyelids are usually accompanied by excessive tearing and a serous discharge.

Hordeolum (stye). Typically, localized eyelid edema occurs with a hordeolum.

Orbital cellulitis. Sudden onset of periorbital edema marks this inflammatory disorder.

Peritonsillar abscess. This complication of tonsillitis may cause unilateral facial edema.

Rhinitis (allergic). In this disorder, red and edematous eyelids are accompanied by paroxysmal sneezing, itchy nose and eyes, and profuse, watery rhinorrhea.

Sinusitis. Frontal sinusitis causes edema of the forehead and eyelids. *Maxillary sinusitis* produces edema in the maxillary area.

Trachoma. In this disorder, edema affects the eyelid and conjunctiva and is accompanied by eye pain, excessive tearing, photophobia, and eye discharge.

Cardiovascular
Superior vena cava syndrome. This disorder gradually produces facial and neck edema accompanied by thoracic or neck vein distention.

Endocrine
Myxedema. This disorder eventually causes generalized facial edema.

Genitourinary
Nephrotic syndrome. Often the first sign of nephrotic syndrome, periorbital edema precedes dependent and abdominal edema.

Musculoskeletal
Dermatomyositis. Periorbital edema and heliotropic rash develop gradually in this rare disease.

Osteomyelitis. When this disorder affects the frontal bone, it may cause forehead edema, as well as fever, chills, headache, and cool, pallid skin.

Metabolic
Malnutrition. Severe malnutrition causes facial edema followed by swelling of the feet and legs.

Immunologic
Allergic reaction. Facial edema may characterize both local allergic reactions and anaphylaxis. In life-threatening *anaphylaxis,* angioneurotic facial edema may occur with urticaria and flushing.

Obstetrics-Gynecology
Preeclampsia. Edema of the face, hands, and ankles is an early sign of this disorder of pregnancy.

Infection
Trichinosis. This relatively rare disorder causes sudden onset of eyelid edema with fever (102° to 104° F., or 38.9° to 40° C.), conjunctivitis, muscle pain, itching and burning skin, sweating, skin lesions, and delirium.

Environmental
Facial burns. These may cause extensive edema that impairs respiration.

Facial trauma. In this disorder, edema depends on the type of injury. For example, contusion may cause localized edema, whereas nasal or maxillary fracture causes more generalized edema.

Drugs
Long-term use of glucocorticoids may produce facial edema. Any drug that causes an allergic reaction (aspirin, antipyretics, penicillin, and sulfa preparations, for example) may have the same effect.

Treatments
Cranial, nasal, or *jaw surgery* may cause facial edema, as may a *blood transfusion* that causes an allergic reaction.

Diagnostic tests
An allergic reaction to *contrast media* used in radiologic tests may produce facial edema.

Clinical considerations
If facial edema is associated with burns or if the patient reports recent exposure to an allergen:

• A quick respiratory assessment should be performed.

• The physician should be notified of signs or symptoms of respiratory distress.

• Preparations should be made for tracheal intubation, cricothyroidotomy, or tracheotomy.

• Oxygen should be administered, as ordered.

If respiratory distress does not accompany facial edema:

• A history should be obtained and a physical examination performed.

• Cold compresses should be applied, as ordered.

• The head of the bed should be elevated to decrease edema.
• Pain medication should be administered or medicated cream applied, if ordered.

Edema, leg

Description

This edema results when excess interstitial fluid accumulates in one or both legs. It may affect just the foot and ankle or extend to the thigh. This common sign may be slight or dramatic, pitting or nonpitting.

Leg edema may result from venous disorders, trauma, and certain bone and cardiac disorders that disturb normal fluid balance. However, several nonpathologic mechanisms may also cause it. For example, prolonged sitting, standing, or immobility may cause bilateral orthostatic edema. Usually, this pitting edema affects the foot and disappears with rest and leg elevation. Increased venous pressure late in pregnancy may also cause ankle edema.

Edema may be pitting or nonpitting. To differentiate between the two, a finger is pressed against a swollen area for five seconds and then quickly removed. In *pitting edema*, pressure forces fluid into the underlying tissues, causing an indentation that slowly fills. The severity of pitting edema is determined by estimating the indentation's depth in centimeters: $1+$ (1 cm), $2+$ (2 cm), $3+$ (3 cm), or $4+$ (4 cm). In *nonpitting edema*, pressure leaves no indentation because fluid has coagulated in the tissues. Typically, the skin feels unusually firm.

Mechanism

Normally, the lymphatic system transports excess interstitial fluid back to the intravascular space. Edema results when this balance is upset by increased capillary permeability, lymphatic obstruction, persistently increased capillary hydrostatic pressure, decreased plasma osmotic or interstitial fluid pressure, or dilation of precapillary sphincters.

Possible causes

Cardiovascular

Congestive heart failure. Bilateral leg edema is an early sign in right heart failure.

Phlegmasia cerulea dolens. Severe unilateral leg edema and cyanosis may spread to the abdomen and flank in this rare form of venous thrombosis.

Thrombophlebitis. Both deep and superficial vein thrombosis may cause sudden onset of unilateral mild-to-moderate edema.

Venous insufficiency (chronic). Unilateral or bilateral leg edema occurs and is moderate to severe in this disorder. Initially, the edema is soft and pitting; later, it becomes hard as tissues thicken.

Musculoskeletal

Osteomyelitis. When this bone infection affects the lower leg, it usually produces localized, mild-to-moderate edema, which may spread to the adjacent joint. Typically, edema follows fever, localized tenderness, and pain that increases with leg movement.

Environmental

Burns. Two days or less after injury, leg burns may cause mild-to-severe edema, pain, and tissue damage.

Envenomation. Mild-to-severe localized edema may develop suddenly at the site of a bite or sting.

Leg trauma. Mild-to-severe localized edema may form around the trauma site.

Treatments

Infiltration of an I.V. site can cause leg edema.

Diagnostic tests

Venography is a rare cause of leg edema.

Clinical considerations

• A history should be obtained and a physical examination performed.

• Antiembolism stockings may be used to promote venous return.
• A zinc-gelatin compression boot (Unna's boot) may be ordered to help reduce edema.
• Unless contraindicated, walking or leg exercises should be encouraged.
• The patient should be encouraged to elevate his legs and to avoid prolonged sitting or standing.
• Fluid intake and output, daily weight, and leg circumference should be measured and recorded, as ordered.

Parry-Romberg syndrome. This syndrome produces enophthalmos and, possibly, irises of different color.
Metabolic
Dehydration. Mild-to-severe enophthalmos may accompany severe dehydration.

Clinical considerations
• A history should be obtained and an eye examination performed.
• Vital signs and pupillary response to light should be monitored, as ordered.

Enophthalmos

Description
Enophthalmos is the backward displacement of the eye into the orbit. This sign may develop suddenly or gradually. It may be severe or mild enough to go unnoticed by the patient. Most often, enophthalmos results from trauma. It may also result from severe dehydration and eye disorders. In the elderly, senile atrophy of orbital fat may produce physiologic enophthalmos.

Because enophthalmos allows the upper lid to droop over the sunken eye, it is often mistaken for ptosis. However, exophthalmometry can differentiate these signs.

Possible causes
Eyes, ears, nose, and throat
Greig's syndrome (craniofacial dystosis). Typically, enophthalmos is accompanied by an abnormally wide distance between the pupils in this syndrome.
Orbital fracture. Here, enophthalmos may not be apparent until edema subsides. The affected eyeball is displaced down and in, and is surrounded by ecchymosis.
Parinaud's syndrome. In this form of ophthalmoplegia, enophthalmos is accompanied by nystagmus when the patient tries to look up.

Entropion

Description
Entropion is the inversion of the eyelid. It typically affects the lower lid but may also affect the upper lid. The eyelashes may touch and irritate the cornea. Most commonly associated with aging, entropion may also stem from chemical burns, mechanical injuries, spasm of the orbicularis muscle, pemphigoid, Stevens-Johnson syndrome, and trachoma.

Enuresis

Description
Usually, enuresis refers to nighttime urinary incontinence in a girl over age 5 or a boy over age 6. Rarely, this sign may continue into adulthood. It is most common in boys and may be classified as primary or secondary. *Primary enuresis* describes the child who has never achieved bladder control; *secondary enuresis* describes the child who achieved bladder control for at least 3 months but has lost it.

Among factors that may contribute to enuresis are delayed development of detrusor muscle control, unusually deep or sound sleep, organic disorders such as urinary tract infection or obstruction, and psychological stress. Probably the most important factor,

Helping a Child Have Dry Nights

Although no single treatment for bed-wetting is always effective, following these recommendations can help a child achieve bladder control.

• Restrict the child's fluid intake—especially of cola drinks—after supper.

• Make sure the child urinates before bedtime. In addition, wake him once during the night to go to the bathroom.

• Reward the child after each dry night with praise and encouragement.

• Keep a progress chart, marking each dry night with a sticker. Reward a certain number of consecutive dry nights with a book, small toy, or special activity.

• Always give the child emotional support. Never punish him if he wets the bed, but reassure him that he will learn to achieve bladder control. Remember that most children simply "outgrow" bed-wetting. However, periods of wet and dry nights will occur before the child develops a constant pattern of dryness.

psychological stress commonly results from the birth of a sibling, the death of a parent or loved one, or premature, rigorous toilet training. The child may be too embarrassed or ashamed to discuss his enuresis, which intensifies psychological stress and makes enuresis more likely—thus creating a vicious cycle.

Possible causes
Genitourinary
Detrusor muscle hyperactivity. Involuntary detrusor muscle contractions may cause primary or secondary enuresis associated with urinary urgency, frequency, and incontinence.

Urinary tract infection. In children, most urinary tract infections produce secondary enuresis.
Urinary tract obstruction. Although daytime incontinence occurs more frequently, this disorder may produce primary or secondary enuresis.

Clinical considerations
• A history should be obtained from both the parent(s) and the child and a physical examination performed.

• If the child has detrusor muscle hyperactivity, bladder training may be used to help control enuresis.

• The Enuretone device may be recommended for the child over age 8. This moisture-sensitive device fits in the child's mattress and triggers an alarm when it becomes wet. The alarm wakes the child immediately, conditioning him to avoid bed-wetting.

• Emotional support should be provided for the child and his family and the parents encouraged to accept and support the child.

• The parents should be given suggestions for managing enuresis at home. (See *Helping a Child Have Dry Nights.*)

Epicanthal folds

Description
Epicanthal folds are vertical skin folds that partially or fully obscure the inner canthus of the eye. These folds may make the eyes appear crossed, since the pupil lies closer to the inner canthus than to the outer canthus. Epicanthal folds are a normal characteristic in many young children and Orientals. They also occur as a familial trait in other ethnic groups, and as an acquired trait in aging. However, the presence of epicanthal folds along with oblique palpebral fissures in non-Oriental children indicates Down's syndrome.

Epistaxis

Description

Epistaxis is bleeding from the nose. It can be spontaneous or induced from the front or back of the nose. Most nosebleeds occur in the anterior-inferior nasal septum (Kiesselbach's plexus), but they may also occur at the point where the inferior turbinates meet the nasopharynx. Usually unilateral, they may seem bilateral when blood runs from the bleeding side behind the nasal septum and out the opposite side. Epistaxis ranges from mild oozing to severe—possibly life-threatening—blood loss.

A rich supply of fragile blood vessels makes the nose particularly vulnerable to bleeding. Air moving through the nose can dry and irritate the mucous membranes, forming crusts that bleed when removed; dry mucous membranes are also more susceptible to infections, which can produce epistaxis as well. Trauma is another common cause of epistaxis. Additional causes include hematologic, coagulation, renal, and GI disorders, and certain drugs and treatments.

In children, a foreign body that causes nasal trauma is the most common cause of epistaxis. Nose-picking is also a common cause.

Possible causes

Eyes, ears, nose, and throat

Juvenile angiofibroma. This rare disorder usually occurs in males and is characterized by severe recurrent epistaxis and nasal obstruction.

Maxillofacial injury. With this type of injury, a pumping arterial bleed usually causes severe epistaxis.

Nasal fracture. Bilateral epistaxis is accompanied by nasal swelling, periorbital ecchymoses and edema, pain, nasal deformity and displacement, and crepitation of the nasal bones.

Nasal tumors. Blood may ooze from the nose when a tumor disrupts the nasal vasculature. Benign tumors usually bleed when touched, but malignant tumors produce spontaneous unilateral epistaxis.

Orbital floor fracture. This type of trauma may damage the maxillary sinus mucosa and—on rare occasions—cause epistaxis.

Sinusitis (acute). In this disorder, a bloody or blood-tinged nasal discharge may become purulent and copious after 24 to 48 hours.

Respiratory

Sarcoidosis. An oozing epistaxis may occur in this disorder.

Cardiovascular

Hypertension. If severe, hypertension can produce extreme epistaxis, usually in the posterior nose, with pulsation above the middle turbinate.

Gastrointestinal

Biliary obstruction. This disorder produces bleeding tendencies, including epistaxis.

Cirrhosis. In this disorder, epistaxis is a late sign that occurs with a tendency to bleed in other areas.

Hepatitis. When this disorder interferes with the clotting mechanism, epistaxis and abnormal bleeding tendencies can result.

Genitourinary

Glomerulonephritis (chronic). This disorder insidiously produces nosebleeds.

Renal failure. Chronic renal failure is more likely than acute renal failure to cause epistaxis and a tendency to bruise easily.

Musculoskeletal

Skull fracture. Depending on the type of fracture, epistaxis can be direct—when blood flows directly down the nares—or indirect—when blood drains through the eustachian tube and into the nose.

Hematologic

Aplastic anemia. This disorder develops insidiously, eventually producing nosebleeds as well as other bleeding problems.

Coagulation disorders. Such disorders as hemophilia and thrombocytopenic purpura can cause epistaxis along with other bleeding problems.

Hereditary hemorrhagic telangiectasia (Rendu-Osler-Weber disease). This disease causes frequent, sometimes daily, epistaxis, as well as hemoptysis and GI bleeding.

Leukemia. In *acute leukemia,* sudden epistaxis is accompanied by a high fever and other abnormal bleeding.

In *chronic leukemia,* epistaxis is a late sign that may be accompanied by other abnormal bleeding.

Polycythemia vera. Spontaneous epistaxis is a common sign of polycythemia vera.

Metabolic

Scurvy. This disorder causes capillary fragility that leds to epistaxis.

Immunologic

Systemic lupus erythematosus (SLE). Commonly affecting women under age 50, SLE causes oozing epistaxis.

Infectious diseases

Infectious mononucleosis. Blood may ooze from the nose in this disorder.

Influenza. When influenza affects the capillaries, a slow, oozing nosebleed results.

Syphilis. Epistaxis occurs most frequently in tertiary syphilis as posterior septum ulcerations produce a foul, bloody nasal discharge.

Typhoid fever. Oozing epistaxis and dry cough are common.

Environmental

Barotrauma. Commonly seen in airline passengers and scuba divers, barotrauma may cause severe, painful epistaxis when the patient has an upper respiratory infection.

Chemical irritants. Some chemicals, including phosphorus, sulfuric acid, ammonia, printer's ink, and chromates, irritate the nasal mucosa, producing epistaxis.

Drugs

Anticoagulants, such as coumarin, and anti-inflammatories, such as aspirin, can cause epistaxis.

Treatments

Rarely, epistaxis results from *facial* and *nasal surgery,* including septoplasty, rhinoplasty, Caldwell-Luc, antrostomy, and *sinus procedures,* as well as *orbital decompression* and *dental extraction.*

Clinical considerations

If epistaxis is severe:

• Vital signs should be taken.

• The physician should be notified of any signs or symptoms of hypovolemic shock.

• Unless nasal fracture is suspected, the nares should be pinched closed to try to control bleeding.

• The hypovolemic patient should be instructed to lie down and turn his head to the side to prevent blood from draining down the back of his throat, which could cause aspiration or vomiting of swallowed blood. Or, if the patient is not hypovolemic, he should be instructed to sit upright and tilt his head forward.

• An I.V. line should be started and airway patency monitored.

• Emergency equipment should be kept readily available.

• Anterior or posterior nasal packing is inserted if other measures to control bleeding fail.

If epistaxis is not severe:

• A history should be obtained and a physical examination performed.

• Diagnostic tests include a complete blood count, prothrombin and activated partial thromboplastin time measurements, and X-rays.

• The patient should be monitored for signs and symptoms of hypovolemic shock.

• Cotton impregnated with a vasoconstrictor and local anesthetic may be inserted into the patient's nose if external pressure does not control bleeding.

• Humidified oxygen should be administered, as ordered.

Erben's reflex

Description
Erben's reflex is slowing of the pulse when the head and trunk are forcibly bent forward. It may indicate vagal excitability.

Erb's sign

Description
In tetany, Erb's sign is increased irritability of motor nerves, detected by electromyography. Erb's sign also refers to dullness on percussion over the sternum's manubrium in acromegaly.

Eructation

Description
Eructation is belching. Depending on the cause, it may vary in duration and intensity. Occasionally, this sign results from GI disorders. More often, though, it results from aerophagia—the unconscious swallowing of air—or from ingestion of gas-producing food. Eructation may relieve associated symptoms, most notably nausea, heartburn, or dyspepsia.

Mechanism
Eructation occurs when gas or acidic fluid rises from the stomach, producing a characteristic sound.

Possible causes
Gastrointestinal
Abdominal lymphadenopathy. The result of infectious or neoplastic disorders, enlarged abdominal lymph nodes may cause belching and other digestive effects.

Gastric outlet obstruction. Eructation is a common complication of duodenal ulcer disease.
Hiatal hernia. In this disorder, eructation occurs after eating and is accompanied by heartburn, regurgitation of sour-tasting fluid, and abdominal distention.
Peptic ulcer. This common disorder may cause eructation.
Superior mesenteric artery syndrome (acute). Eructation and halitosis are late signs of this uncommon syndrome. Typically, the eructation occurs after eating and is accompanied by regurgitation.

Clinical considerations
• A history should be obtained and a physical examination performed.
• The patient should be encouraged to lie in a side-lying or knee-chest position to help relieve eructation.
• The patient should be advised not to chew gum or smoke, to prevent aerophagia.
• The patient should be instructed to eliminate gas-producing foods from the diet.

Erythema
(Erythroderma)

Description
Erythema is redness or inflammation of the skin or mucous membranes. It may be localized or generalized and may occur suddenly or gradually. Skin color can range from bright red in acute conditions to pale violet or brown in chronic problems. Erythema must be differentiated from purpura, which causes redness from bleeding into the skin. When pressure is applied directly to the skin, erythema blanches momentarily, but purpura does not. Erythema can result from trauma and tissue damage as well as from changes

in supporting tissues, which increase vessel visibility.

Mechanism
Erythema results from dilatation and congestion of superficial capillaries.

Possible causes
Cardiovascular
Raynaud's disease. Typically, the skin on hands and feet blanches and cools after exposure to cold or stress. Later, it becomes warm and purplish red.

Thrombophlebitis. Although this disorder is sometimes asymptomatic, it can produce erythema over the inflamed vein.

Gastrointestinal
Liver disease (chronic). Any chronic liver disease, such as cirrhosis, can cause local vasodilation and palmar erythema.

Musculoskeletal
Lupus erythematosus. Both discoid and systemic lupus erythematosus can produce a characteristic butterfly rash. This erythematous eruption may range from a blush with swelling to a scaly, sharply demarcated, macular rash with plaques that may spread to the forehead, chin, ears, chest, and other sun-exposed parts of the body.

Rheumatoid arthritis. In a flare-up of this disorder, erythema over the affected joints occurs with heat, swelling, pain, and stiffness.

Skin
Candidiasis. When this fungal infection affects the skin, it produces erythema and a scaly, papular rash under the breasts and at the axillae, neck, umbilicus, and groin.

Dermatitis. Erythema commonly occurs with this family of inflammatory disorders. In *atopic dermatitis*, erythema and intense pruritus precede the development of small papules that may redden, weep, scale, and lichenify.

Contact dermatitis occurs after exposure to an irritant. It quickly produces erythema and vesicles, blisters, or ulcerations on exposed skin.

In *seborrheic dermatitis*, erythema appears with dull red or yellow lesions.

Dermatomyositis. This disorder, most common in women over age 50, produces a dusky lilac rash on the face, neck, upper torso, and nail beds.

Erysipelas. This infection suddenly causes rosy or crimson swollen lesions, mainly on the head and neck.

Erythema annulare centrifugum. Small pink infiltrated papules appear on the trunk, buttocks, and inner thighs, slowly spreading at the margins and clearing in the center.

Erythema marginatum rheumaticum. Associated with rheumatic fever, this disorder causes erythematous lesions that are superficial, flat, and slightly hardened. They shift, spread rapidly, and may last for hours or days, recurring after a time.

Erythema multiforme. Often occurring in the spring and fall, *erythema multiforme major* (Stevens-Johnson syndrome) produces sudden hivelike erythema with blisters, and pathognomonic petechial or "iris" lesions that usually appear symmetrically and bilaterally on the face, hands, and feet. Erythema is characteristically preceded by blisters on the lips, tongue, and buccal mucosa; a thick, gray film over the mucous membranes; increased salivation; and an extremely sore throat.

With *erythema multiforme minor*, erythematous macules and papules, purpura, and occasional blisters occur.

Erythema nodosum. Sudden bilateral eruption of tender erythematous nodules characterizes this disorder. These firm, round, protruding lesions usually appear in crops on the shins, knees, and ankles but may occur on the buttocks, arms, calves, and trunk as well.

Intertrigo. In this disorder, skin friction usually causes symmetrical erythema that may be accompanied by soreness or itching. Typically, erythema occurs in skin folds, such as in the groin; in severe cases, the skin may

Drugs and Erythema

Drug-induced erythema should be suspected in any patient who develops this sign within one week of starting a medication. Erythematous lesions can vary in size, shape, type, or amount, but they almost always appear suddenly and symmetrically on the trunk and inner arms. Some drugs that can produce them include:

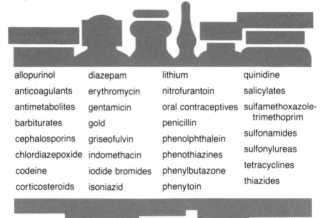

allopurinol	diazepam	lithium	quinidine
anticoagulants	erythromycin	nitrofurantoin	salicylates
antimetabolites	gentamicin	oral contraceptives	sulfamethoxazole-trimethoprim
barbiturates	gold	penicillin	
cephalosporins	griseofulvin	phenolphthalein	sulfonamides
chlordiazepoxide	indomethacin	phenothiazines	sulfonylureas
codeine	iodide bromides	phenylbutazone	tetracyclines
corticosteroids	isoniazid	phenytoin	thiazides

Some of these—particularly barbiturates, oral contraceptives, phenolphthalein, phenylbutazone, salicylates, sulfonamides, and tetracycline—can cause a "fixed" drug eruption. With this reaction, lesions can appear in any body part and flake off after a few days, leaving a brownish purple pigmentation. Repeated drug administration causes the original lesions to recur and new ones to develop.

---

become bright red with erosion and maceration.

Polymorphous light eruption (PLE). PLE produces erythema, vesicles, plaques, and multiple small papules on sun-exposed areas.

Psoriasis. Silvery white scales over a thickened erythematous base usually affect the elbows, knees, chest, scalp, and intergluteal folds.

Rosacea. Scattered erythema across the center of the face characterizes this disorder initially.

Immunologic

Allergic reactions. Foods, drugs, chemicals, and other allegens can cause a mild-to-severe allergic reaction and erythema. A *localized allergic reaction* also produces hivelike eruptions and edema.

Anaphylaxis, a life-threatening condition, produces relatively sudden erythema in the form of urticaria.

Obstetrics-Gynecology

Toxic shock syndrome. This disorder, which usually affects young women, causes sudden, diffuse erythema in the form of a macular rash.

Infectious diseases

Rubella. Typically, flat solitary lesions join to form a blotchy pink erythematous rash that spreads rapidly to the trunk and extremities in this disorder.

Environmental

Burns. With *thermal burns,* erythema and swelling appear first, possibly followed by deep or superficial blisters and other signs of damage that depend on the severity of the burn. *Burns from ultraviolet rays,* such as sunburn, cause delayed erythema and tenderness on exposed areas of the skin.

Frostbite. First-degree frostbite turns the affected body part a lifeless gray, followed by an intense bluish red flush on rewarming.

Drugs

Many drugs commonly cause erythema. (See *Drugs and Erythema,* p. 147.)

Treatments

Radiation therapy may produce dull erythema and edema within 24 hours. As the erythema fades, the skin becomes light brown and mildly scaly. In addition, any treatment that causes an allergic reaction, such as a blood transfusion, can cause erythema.

Clinical considerations

If erythema occurs suddenly and progresses:

• Anaphylactic shock should be suspected.

• Vital signs should be taken.

• The physician should be notified immediately of signs or symptoms of respiratory distress.

• Emergency equipment should be kept readily available.

If erythema is not associated with anaphylaxis:

• A history should be obtained and a physical examination performed.

• Diagnostic tests include a skin biopsy to detect cancerous lesions, cultures to identify infectious organisms, and sensitivity studies to confirm allergies.

• Fluid and electrolyte levels should be monitored and replaced, as needed and ordered.

• Medications should be withheld until the cause of the erythema has been identified, as ordered.

• Antibiotics, analgesics, antihistamines, topical or systemic corticosteroids, and medicated or soothing baths should be administered, if ordered.

• Erythematous limbs should be elevated above heart level to reduce erythema.

Escherich's sign

Description

Escherich's sign is the contraction of the lips, tongue, and masseters, occurring in tetany. To elicit Escherich's sign, the examiner percusses the inner surface of the lips or the tongue and observes for contraction.

Euphoria

Description

Euphoria is a feeling of great happiness or well-being. When euphoria does not accompany enlightening experiences or superb achievements, it may reflect bipolar disorders, organic brain disease, or use of such drugs as heroin, cocaine, and amphetamines.

Ewart's sign

Description

Ewart's sign is bronchial breathing heard on auscultation of the lungs and dullness heard on percussion below the angle of the left scapula. These compression signs commonly occur in pericardial effusion.

Exophthalmos
(Proptosis)

Description

Exophthalmos is the abnormal protrusion of one or both eyeballs. It may result from hemorrhage, edema, or inflammation behind the eye; extraocular muscle relaxation; or space-occupying intraorbital lesions. This sign may occur suddenly or gradually, causing mild-to-dramatic protrusion. Occasionally, the affected eye also pulsates.

Usually, exophthalmos is easily observed. However, lid retraction may mimic exophthalmos even though protrusion is absent. Similarly, ptosis in one eye may make the other eye appear exophthalmic by comparison. An exophthalmometer can differentiate these signs by measuring ocular protrusion.

Possible causes
Eyes, ears, nose, and throat
Cavernous sinus thrombosis. Usually, this disorder causes sudden onset of pulsating, unilateral exophthalmos.

Dacryoadenitis. Unilateral, slowly progressive exophthalmos is the most common sign of dacryoadenitis.

Foreign body in the eye. Although rare, exophthalmos may accompany other signs and symptoms of ocular trauma, such as eye pain, redness, and tearing.

Hemangioma. Most common in young adults, this orbital tumor produces progressive exophthalmos, which may be mild or severe, unilateral or bilateral.

Lacrimal gland tumor. Exophthalmos usually develops slowly in one eye, causing its downward displacement toward the nose.

Lymphangioma. Hemorrhage of this congenital tumor causes unilateral or bilateral exophthalmos, among other signs.

Ocular tuberculosis. Occasionally, this rare disease causes progressive exophthalmos.

Optic nerve meningioma. Usually, this tumor produces unilateral exophthalmos and a swollen temple.

Orbital cellulitis. Often the result of sinusitis, this ocular emergency causes sudden onset of unilateral exophthalmos, which may be mild or severe.

Orbital choristoma. A common sign of this benign tumor, progressive exophthalmos may be associated with diplopia and blurred vision.

Orbital emphysema. Air leaking from the sinus into the orbit usually causes unilateral exophthalmos.

Orbital pseudotumor. Progressive unilateral exophthalmos characterizes this uncommon disorder.

Scleritis (posterior). Gradual onset of mild-to-severe unilateral exophthalmos is common in conjunction with scleritis.

Endocrine
Thyrotoxicosis. Although a classic sign of this disorder, exophthalmos is absent in many patients. It is usually bilateral, progressive, and severe.

Hematologic
Leukemia. When leukemia causes intraorbital hemorrhage, mild-to-moderate bilateral exophthalmos and lacrimal gland enlargement also result.

Neoplastic
Hodgkin's disease. In this disorder, unilateral exophthalmos may develop gradually, along with eyelid edema, diplopia, and a palpable eyelid mass.

Clinical considerations
- A history should be obtained and a physical examination performed.
- A slit-lamp examination may be ordered.
- Because exophthalmos usually makes the patient self-conscious, privacy and emotional support should be provided, as necessary.
- Artificial tears may be administered, if ordered, to lubricate the eye(s).

Extensor thrust reflex

Description
Extensor thrust reflex is extension of the leg upon stimulation of the sole of the foot. A normal reflex in newborn infants, it is mediated at the spinal cord level and should disappear after 6 months of age.

To elicit the extensor thrust reflex, the examiner places the infant supine with the leg flexed, then stimulates the sole. If the extensor thrust reflex is present, the leg will slowly extend. In premature infants, this reflex may be weak. Its persistence beyond age 6 months indicates anoxic brain damage. Its recurrence in a child signals a central nervous system lesion or injury.

Extinction

Description
In *neurology*, extinction is the inability to perceive one of two stimuli presented simultaneously. To detect this sign, the examiner simultaneously stimulates two corresponding areas on opposite sides of the body. Extinction is present if the patient fails to perceive one sensation.

In *neurophysiology*, extinction is the loss of excitability of a nerve, synapse, or nervous tissue in response to stimuli that were previously adequate.

In *psychology*, extinction is the disappearance of a conditioned reflex resulting from lack of reinforcement.

Extrapyramidal signs and symptoms

Description
Extrapyramidal signs and symptoms are movement and posture disturbances characteristically resulting from disorders of the basal ganglia and cerebellum. These disturbances include asynergy, ataxia, athetosis, blepharoclonus, chorea, dysarthria, dysdiadochokinesia, dystonia, muscle rigidity and spasticity, myoclonus, spasmodic torticollis, and tremors.

Fabere sign

Description
Fabere sign is pain produced by maneuvers used in Patrick's test. It indicates an arthritic hip. The name is an acronym for maneuvers used to elicit the sign: flexion, abduction, external rotation, and extension. To detect fabere sign, the examiner places the patient supine and asks him to flex the thigh and knee of the affected leg. Then she has him externally rotate the leg and place the lateral malleolus on the patella of the opposite leg. If the patient experiences pain when his knee is depressed, fabere sign has been detected.

Fajersztajn's crossed sciatic sign

Description
In sciatica, Fajersztajn's crossed sciatic sign is pain on the affected side caused by lifting the extended opposite leg. To elicit this sign, the examiner places the patient supine and has him flex his unaffected hip while keeping the knee extended. Flexion at the hip will cause pain on the affected side by stretching the irritated sciatic nerve.

Fan sign

Description
A component of Babinski's reflex, this sign refers to the spreading apart of the patient's toes after firmly stroking his foot.

Fasciculations

Description
Fasciculations are minor local muscle contractions. These contractions cause visible dimpling or wavelike twitching of the skin but are not strong enough to produce joint movement. They occur irregularly at frequencies ranging from once every several seconds to two or three times per second; infrequently, myokymia—continuous, rapid fasciculations that cause a rippling effect—may occur. Because fasciculations are brief and painless, they often go undetected or are ignored.

Benign, nonpathologic fasciculations are common and normal. They often occur in tense, anxious, or overtired persons and typically affect the eyelid, thumb, or calf. However, fasciculations may also indicate a severe neurologic disorder, most notably a diffuse motor neuron disorder that causes loss of control over muscle fiber discharge. They are also an early sign of pesticide poisoning.

Mechanism

Fasciculations represent the spontaneous discharge of a muscle fiber bundle innervated by a single motor nerve filament.

Possible causes

Central nervous system

Amyotrophic lateral sclerosis. Coarse fasciculations usually begin in the small muscles of the hands and feet, then spread to the forearms and legs.

Bulbar palsy. Fasciculations of the face and tongue commonly appear early.

Guillain-Barré syndrome. Fasciculations may occur, but the dominant neurologic sign is muscle weakness, which typically begins in the legs and spreads quickly to the arms and face.

Herniated disk. Fasciculations of the muscles innervated by compressed nerve roots may be widespread and profound, but the overriding symptom is severe low back pain that may radiate unilaterally to the leg.

Poliomyelitis (spinal paralytic). Coarse fasciculations, usually transient but occasionally persistent, accompany progressive muscle weakness, spasms, and atrophy.

Spinal cord tumors. Fasciculations may develop, along with muscle atrophy and cramps, asymmetrically at first and then bilaterally as cord compression progresses.

Syringomyelia. Fasciculations may occur along with Charcot's joints, deep aching pain, areflexia, and muscle atrophy.

Environmental

Pesticide poisoning. Ingestion of organophosphate or carbamate pesticides commonly produces acute onset of long, wavelike fasciculations and muscle weakness that rapidly progresses to flaccid paralysis.

Clinical considerations

If onset is acute:

• Pesticide poisoning should be suspected.

• Pesticide poisoning, although uncommon, represents a medical emergency requiring prompt and vigorous intervention. A poison control center should be called to obtain information regarding appropriate medical treatment.

If the patient is not in severe distress:

• A history should be obtained and a neurologic assessment performed.

• The patient's life-style should be explored, and stress at home, on the job, or at school noted.

• Diagnostic tests may include spinal X-rays, myelography, computed tomography, and electromyography with nerve conduction velocity tests.

Fatigue

Description

Fatigue is a feeling of excessive tiredness, lack of energy, or exhaustion accompanied by a strong desire to rest or sleep. This common symptom is distinct from weakness, which involves the muscles, but may occur with it.

Fatigue represents a normal and important response to physical overexertion, prolonged emotional stress, and sleep deprivation. However, it can also be a nonspecific symptom of a psychological or physiologic disorder. Fatigue that worsens with activity and improves with rest usually indicates a physical disorder; the opposite pattern, a psychological disorder. Also associated with psychological disorders are fatigue lasting longer than 4 months, constant fatigue that is unrelieved by rest, and transient exhaustion that quickly gives way to bursts of energy.

Fatigue without an organic cause occurs normally during accelerated growth phases in preschool-age and prepubescent children. However, psychological causes of fatigue must be considered; for instance, a depressed child may try to escape problems at home or school by taking refuge in sleep. The possibility of drug abuse, particularly of hypnotics and tranquilizers, should also be considered.

Mechanism
Fatigue resulting from a physical disorder reflects both hypermetabolic and hypometabolic states in which nutrients needed for cellular energy and growth are lacking because of overly rapid depletion, impaired replacement mechanisms, insufficient hormone production, or inadequate nutrient intake or metabolism.

Possible causes
Central nervous system
Myasthenia gravis. The cardinal symptoms of this disorder are easy fatigability and muscle weakness, which worsen with exertion and abate with rest.

Respiratory
Chronic obstructive pulmonary disease. The earliest and most persistent symptoms of this disease are progressive fatigue and dyspnea.

Restrictive lung disease. Chronic fatigue may accompany characteristic signs: dyspnea, cough, and rapid, shallow respirations.

Cardiovascular
Congestive heart failure (CHF). Persistent fatigue and lethargy characterize this disorder. Fatigue may be a very early sign of CHF—one that is often overlooked.

Myocardial infarction (MI). Fatigue can be severe, but is typically overshadowed by chest pain. Fatigue may also be a predictive sign of MI, occurring up to 2 weeks before the onset of chest pain and infarction.

Valvular heart disease. All types of valvular heart disease commonly produce progressive fatigue and a cardiac murmur.

Endocrine
Adrenocortical insufficiency. Mild fatigue, the hallmark of this disorder, initially appears after exertion and stress but later becomes more severe and persistent.

Diabetes mellitus. Fatigue, the most common symptom in this disorder, may begin insidiously or abruptly.

Hypercortisolism. This disorder typically causes fatigue, related in part to accompanying sleep disturbances.

Hypopituitarism. Fatigue, lethargy, and weakness usually develop slowly.

Hypothyroidism. Fatigue begins early, along with forgetfulness, cold intolerance, weight gain, and constipation.

Thyrotoxicosis. In this disorder, fatigue may occur with characteristic signs and symptoms.

Gastrointestinal
Cirrhosis. Severe fatigue typically occurs late in this disorder, accompanied by weight loss, bleeding tendencies, jaundice, hepatomegaly, ascites, dependent edema, severe pruritus, and decreased level of consciousness.

Genitourinary
Renal failure. Acute renal failure commonly causes sudden fatigue, drowsiness, and lethargy. In *chronic renal failure,* insidious fatigue and lethargy are accompanied by marked changes in all body systems.

Musculoskeletal
Rheumatoid arthritis. Fatigue, weakness, and anorexia precede localized articular signs and symptoms.

Systemic lupus erythematosus. Fatigue usually occurs along with generalized aching, malaise, low-grade fever, headache, and irritability.

Hematologic
Anemia. Fatigue following mild activity is often the first symptom of this disorder.

Metabolic
Malnutrition. Easy fatigability commonly occurs in protein-calorie malnutrition, along with lethargy and apathy.

Psychiatric
Anxiety. Chronic, unremitting anxiety invariably produces fatigue, often characterized as nervous exhaustion.

Depression. Persistent fatigue, unrelated to exertion, nearly always accompanies chronic depression.

Neoplastic

Cancer. Unexplained fatigue is often the earliest sign of cancer.

Infection

Chronic infection. Fatigue is often the most prominent symptom—and sometimes the only one. Low-grade fever and weight loss may accompany symptoms that reflect the type and location of infection.

Acute infection. Brief fatigue typically accompanies headache, anorexia, arthralgia, chills, high fever, and such infection-specific signs as cough, vomiting, or diarrhea in acute infection.

Drugs

Fatigue may result from various drugs, notably antihypertensives and sedatives. In cardiac glycoside therapy, it may indicate toxicity.

Treatments

Most types of surgery cause temporary fatigue, probably due to the combined effects of hunger, anesthesia, and sleep deprivation.

Clinical considerations

• A complete medical and psychiatric history should be obtained and a physical examination performed.

• The pattern of the fatigue should be especially noted.

• Diagnostic tests will depend on the patient's history and physical findings, and may include blood and urine studies and X-rays to help determine the cause.

• No matter what is causing the patient's fatigue, the patient may need advice on how to alter his life-style to achieve a balanced diet, a program of regular exercise (within prescribed limits), and adequate rest.

• The patient should be counseled about setting priorities, maintaining a reasonable schedule, and developing good sleep habits.

• Stress management techniques should be taught as appropriate.

• If fatigue results from organic illness, the patient should be given help in determining what activities he must accomplish, which of these he may

need help with, and how to pace himself to ensure sufficient rest.

• The patient should be told that chronic fatigue can often be reduced by alleviating pain, which may interfere with rest, or nausea, which may lead to malnutrition.

• If needed, the patient should be referred to a community health nurse or housekeeping service.

• If fatigue results from a psychogenic cause, the patient should be referred for psychological counseling.

Fetor hepaticus

Description

Fetor hepaticus is a distinctive musty-sweet breath odor that characterizes the final, comatose stage of hepatic encephalopathy—a life-threatening complication of severe liver disease. The odor results from inability of the damaged liver to metabolize and detoxify mercaptans produced by bacterial degradation of methionine, a sulfurous amino acid. These substances circulate in the blood, are expelled by the lungs, and flavor the breath.

Fever
(Pyrexia)

Description

Fever is an abnormal elevation of body temperature above 98.6° F. (37° C.) resulting from disease. This common sign can arise from disorders affecting virtually every body system. As a result, fever in the absence of other signs usually has little diagnostic significance. Persistent high fever, though, represents an emergency.

Fever can be classified as low (oral reading of 99° to 100.4° F., or 37.2° to 38° C.), moderate (100.5° to 104° F., or 38° to 40° C.), or high (above 104° F.). Fever over 108° F. (42.2° C.) causes unconsciousness and, if sustained, leads to permanent brain damage.

Fever can be classified as remittent, intermittent, sustained, or relapsing. *Remittent fever*, the most common type, is characterized by daily temperature fluctuations above the normal range. *Intermittent fever* is characterized by a daily temperature drop into the normal range, then a rise back to above normal. An intermittent fever that fluctuates widely, typically producing chills and sweating, is called *hectic* or *septic fever*. *Sustained fever* involves persistent temperature elevation with little fluctuation. *Relapsing fever* consists of alternating feverish and afebrile periods.

Further classification involves duration—either brief (less than 3 weeks) or prolonged. Prolonged fevers include fever of unknown origin, a classification used when careful examination fails to detect an underlying cause.

Infants and young children experience higher and more prolonged fevers, more rapid temperature increases, and greater temperature fluctuations than older children and adults.

Mechanism

Fever results from an imbalance between the elimination and the production of heat. Specifically, body temperature is regulated by the hypothalamic thermostat, which has a specific set point under normal conditions. Fever can result from a resetting of this set point or from an abnormality in the thermoregulatory system itself.

Possible causes

Immune complex dysfunction

When present, fever usually remains low, although moderate elevations may accompany erythema multiforme. Fever may be remittent or intermittent, as in acquired immunodeficiency syndrome (AIDS) or systemic lupus erythematosus, or sustained, as in polyarteritis. As one of several vague prodromal complaints (such as fatigue, anorexia, and weight loss), fever produces nocturnal diaphoresis.

Infectious and inflammatory disorders

Fever ranges from low (in Crohn's disease and ulcerative colitis) to extremely high (in bacterial pneumonia). It may be remittent, as in infectious mononucleosis and otitis media; hectic, as in lung abscess, influenza, and endocarditis; sustained, as in meningitis; or relapsing, as in malaria. Fever may arise abruptly, as in toxic shock syndrome and Rocky Mountain spotted fever, or insidiously, as in mycoplasmal pneumonia. In hepatitis, fever may represent a disease prodrome; in appendicitis, it follows the acute stage. Its sudden late appearance with tachycardia, tachypnea, and confusion heralds life-threatening septic shock in peritonitis and gram-negative bacteremia.

Neoplasms

Primary neoplasms and metastases can produce prolonged fever of varying elevations. For instance, acute leukemia may present insidiously with low fever, pallor, and bleeding tendencies, or more abruptly with high fever, frank bleeding, and prostration. Occasionally, Hodgkin's lymphoma produces Pel-Ebstein fever, an irregularly relapsing fever.

Thermoregulatory dysfunction

Sudden onset of fever that rises rapidly and remains as high as 107° F. (41.7° C.) typically occurs in life-threatening disorders such as heatstroke, thyroid storm, and malignant hyperthermia, and with lesions of the central nervous system. Low or moderate fever appears with dehydration.

Drugs

Fever and skin rash commonly result from hypersensitivity to antifungals, sulfonamides, penicillins, cephalosporins, tetracyclines, barbiturates, phenytoin, quinidine, iodides, phenolphthalein, methyldopa, procainamide, and some antitoxins. Fever can accompany chemotherapy, especially with bleomycin, vincristine, and asparaginase. It can result from drugs that impair sweating, such as anticholinergics, phenothiazines, and monoamine oxidase inhibitors. Fever can also stem from toxic doses of salicylates, amphetamines, and tricyclic antidepressants.

Inhalant anesthetics and muscle relaxants can trigger malignant hyperthermia in patients with this inherited trait.

Treatments

After surgery, remittent or intermittent low fever may occur for several days. Transfusion reactions characteristically produce abrupt onset of fever and chills.

Diagnostic tests

Immediate or delayed fever infrequently follows radiographic tests that use contrast medium.

Clinical considerations

If fever exceeds 106° F. (41.1° C.):
• The physician should be notified immediately.
• The patient's other vital signs should be taken and his level of consciousness assessed.
• Rapid cooling measures should be initiated and antipyretic drugs administered, as ordered.

If fever is only mild to moderate:
• A history should be obtained and a physical examination performed.
• Diagnostic tests will vary depending on the patient's history and physical findings, but may include blood and urine tests, such as a complete blood count and cultures, as well as X-rays.
• The patient's temperature should be monitored frequently.
• Fluid and nutritional intake should be increased, as ordered.
• During administration of prescribed antipyretic drugs, resultant chills and diaphoresis can be minimized by following a regular dosage schedule.
• Patient comfort should be promoted by maintaining a stable room temperature and providing frequent changes of bedding and clothing.

Flatulence

Description

Flatulence is a sensation of gaseous abdominal fullness that can result from GI disorders, abdominal surgery, and excessive intake of certain foods. It can also stem from stress and can be accompanied by belching, discomfort, and excessive passage of flatus. Although usually not a serious symptom, flatulence and accompanying expulsion of flatus may cause the patient embarrassment and discomfort.

Mechanism

Flatulence reflects slowed intestinal motility, which hampers the passage of gas; excessive swallowing of air (aerophagia), often brought on by stress; or increased intraluminal gas production due to an excess of fermentable substrates, such as digested, unabsorbed carbohydrates and proteins.

Possible causes
Gastrointestinal

Cholecystitis. Both acute and chronic cholecystitis commonly produce flatulence with frequent passage of flatus. Accompanying colicky pain in the right upper quadrant becomes persistent and severe in an acute attack.

Cholelithiasis. Complaints of flatulence and belching are common in this disorder.

Cirrhosis. Typically, flatulence develops early and insidiously, along with anorexia, dyspepsia, nausea, vomiting, diarrhea or constipation, dull right upper quadrant pain, hepatomegaly, and splenomegaly.

Colon cancer. Obstruction of the colon by a tumor may cause flatulence; acute obstruction also produces abdominal distention and tympany on percussion.

Crohn's disease. Flatulence accompanies other acute inflammatory signs and symptoms that mimic appendicitis: right lower quadrant pain, cramps, and tenderness; diarrhea; low-grade fever; nausea; and melena.

Irritable bowel syndrome. Effects include chronic flatulence, belching, and excessive flatus.

Malabsorption syndromes. This group of syndromes may cause flatulence.

Metabolic

Lactose intolerance. Flatulence, cramping abdominal pain, and possibly diarrhea develop within several hours of ingesting dairy products.

Treatments

After abdominal surgery, the return of peristalsis after postoperative paralytic ileus causes gas accumulation in hypomotile areas, producing flatulence.

Clinical considerations

• A history should be obtained and an abdominal assessment performed.

• Diagnostic tests may include blood tests, stool analysis, upper GI series, barium enema, and endoscopy.

• To aid expulsion of excessive flatus, the examiner should position the patient on his left side; to prevent gas buildup, frequent repositioning, ambulation, and normal fluid intake should be encouraged, as permitted.

• If these measures are not effective, a rectal tube should be inserted to relieve flatus or enemas, suppositories, antiflatulents, or anticholinergics should be administered as ordered.

• As appropriate, the patient should be provided with a dietary plan that excludes gaseous foods.

Flexor withdrawal reflex

Description

Flexor withdrawal reflex describes flexion of the knee upon stimulation of the sole of the foot; a normal reflex in newborn infants, it is mediated at the spinal cord level and should disappear after 6 months of age.

To elicit this reflex, the examiner places the infant supine with his legs extended, and pinches the sole of his foot. Normally, an infant younger than 6 months of age will respond with slow, uncontrolled flexion of the knee. This reflex may be weak in premature infants. Its persistence beyond age 6 months may indicate anoxic brain damage. Its recurrence signals a central nervous system lesion or injury.

Flight of ideas

Description

This term describes continuous, often seemingly pressured speech with abrupt changes of topic. In contrast with *looseness of association*, a listener can discern the connection between topics based on word similarities or sounds. This sign characteristically occurs in the manic phase of a bipolar disorder.

Fontanelle, bulging

Description

A bulging fontanelle refers to a widened, tense, markedly pulsating anterior fontanelle. In a normal infant, the anterior fontanelle, or "soft spot," is flat, soft yet firm, and well demarcated against surrounding skull bones. (The posterior fontanelle, if not fused at birth, usually closes by age 2 months.) Subtle pulsations may be visible, reflecting the arterial pulse. A bulging fontanelle is a cardinal sign of potentially life-threatening increased intracranial presure, a medical emergency. Since prolonged coughing, crying, or lying down can cause transient, physiologic bulging, the infant's head should be observed and palpated while he is upright and relaxed to detect pathologic bulging.

Fontanelle, depressed

Description
A depressed fontanelle refers to depression of the anterior fontanelle below the surrounding bony ridges of the skull. It is a sign of dehydration. A common disorder of infancy and early childhood, dehydration can result from insufficient intake, but typically reflects excessive fluid loss from severe vomiting or diarrhea. It may also reflect insensible water loss, pyloric stenosis, or tracheoesophageal fistula. In *mild dehydration* (5% weight loss), the anterior fontanelle appears slightly depressed. *Moderate dehydration* (10% weight loss) causes slightly more pronounced fontanelle depression, along with gray skin with poor turgor, dry mucous membranes, and decreased urine output. *Severe dehydration* (15% or greater weight loss) may result in a markedly depressed fontanelle, along with extremely poor skin turgor, parched mucous membranes, marked oliguria, lethargy, and signs of shock.

Footdrop

Description
Footdrop is plantar flexion of the foot with the toes bent toward the instep. A characteristic and important sign of certain peripheral nerve or motor neuron disorders, it may also stem from prolonged immobility when inadequate support, improper positioning, or infrequent passive exercise produces shortening of the Achilles' tendon. Unilateral footdrop can result from compression of the common peroneal nerve against the head of the fibula.

Footdrop can range in severity from slight to complete, depending on the extent of muscle weakness or paralysis. It develops slowly in progressive muscle degeneration, or suddenly in spinal cord injury.

Mechanism
Footdrop results from weakness or paralysis of the dorsiflexor muscles of the foot and ankle.

Possible causes
Central nervous system
Cerebrovascular accident. Unilateral footdrop often appears with arm and leg weakness or paralysis. Other effects depend on the site and severity of vascular damage.

Guillain-Barré syndrome. Unilateral or bilateral footdrop and steppage gait may result from profound muscle weakness. This weakness usually begins in the legs and extends to the arms and face within 72 hours. It can progress to total motor paralysis with respiratory failure.

Herniated lumbar disk. Footdrop and steppage gait may result from leg muscle weakness and atrophy. However, the most pronounced symptom is severe low back pain, which may radiate to the buttocks, legs, and feet, usually unilaterally.

Multiple sclerosis. Footdrop may develop suddenly or slowly, producing steppage gait; it typically fluctuates in severity with this disorder's cycle of periodic exacerbation and remission.

Myasthenia gravis. Footdrop and related limb weakness are common manifestations of this disorder, which is often heralded by weak eye closure, ptosis, and diplopia.

Peroneal nerve trauma. Footdrop may occur suddenly, but it is temporary, resolving with the release of peroneal nerve compression.

Poliomyelitis. Unilateral or bilateral footdrop may develop, producing a steppage gait.

Polyneuropathy. Footdrop and steppage gait may accompany muscle weakness, which usually affects distal areas of the extremities and can progress to flaccid paralysis.

Spinal cord trauma. Unilateral or bilateral footdrop can occur suddenly and may be permanent. In the ambulatory patient, it also produces steppage gait.

Musculoskeletal

Peroneal muscle atrophy. Bilateral footdrop, ankle instability, and steppage gait occur early in this chronic disorder. Foot, peroneal, and ankle dorsiflexor muscles are affected first.

Clinical considerations

• A history should be obtained and a neurologic assessment performed.

• Diagnostic tests may include electromyography to evaluate nerve damage.

• The patient may be referred to a physical therapist for gait retraining and possible in-shoe splints or leg braces to maintain correct foot alignment for walking and standing.

Foot malposition, congenital

Description

Foot malposition refers to anomalous positioning of the foot, present at birth in roughly 0.4% of infants. It may reflect the fetal position of comfort, neuromuscular disease, or malformation of a joint or connective tissue. To assess this sign, the examiner observes the resting infant's foot to determine the position of comfort, then observes the foot during spontaneous activity. Using gentle passive maneuvers, the examiner then determines the full range of motion of the foot and ankle.

Fränkel's sign

Description

Fränkel's sign is excessive range of passive motion at the hip joint in tabes dorsalis. This excessive motion stems from decreased tone in the surrounding muscles.

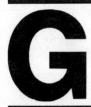

G

Gag reflex, abnormal
(Pharyngeal reflex, abnormal)

Description
An abnormal gag reflex is one that is either decreased or absent. The gag reflex—a protective mechanism that prevents aspiration of food, fluid, and vomitus—normally can be elicited by touching the posterior wall of the oropharynx with a tongue depressor or by suctioning the throat. Prompt elevation of the palate, constriction of the pharyngeal musculature, and a sensation of gagging indicate a normal gag reflex.

An abnormal gag reflex interferes with the ability to swallow and, more importantly, increases susceptibility to life-threatening aspiration. An impaired gag reflex can result from any lesion affecting its mediators—cranial nerves IX (glossopharyngeal) and X (vagus) or the pons or medulla. It can also occur in coma or temporarily as a result of anesthesia.

Possible causes
Central nervous system
Basilar artery occlusion. This disorder may suddenly diminish or obliterate the gag reflex.
Brain stem glioma. This lesion causes gradual loss of the gag reflex.
Bulbar palsy. Loss of the gag reflex reflects temporary or permanent paralysis of muscles supplied by cranial nerves IX and X.

Wallenberg's syndrome. Paresis of the palate and an impaired gag reflex usually develop within hours to days of thrombosis.
Drugs
General and local (throat) anesthesia can produce temporary loss of the gag reflex.

Clinical considerations
• A history should be taken and neurologic and respiratory assessments performed.
• Diagnostic studies may include computed tomography, electroencephalography, lumbar puncture, and arteriography.
• Oral intake should be stopped to prevent aspiration and tube feedings instituted, as ordered.
• Suction equipment should be kept close at hand in case aspiration occurs.
• If the gag reflex is merely slightly decreased, puréed foods may be given with supervision.

Gait, bizarre
(Hysterical gait)

Description
A bizarre gait is an abnormal gait that has no obvious organic basis; rather, it is produced unconsciously by a person with a somatoform disorder (hysterical neurosis) or consciously by a malingerer. The gait has no consistent pattern. It may mimic an organic impairment, but characteristically has a more theatrical or bizarre quality with

key elements missing—such as spastic gait without hip circumduction, or leg "paralysis" with normal reflexes and motor strength. Its manifestations may include wild gyrations, exaggerated stepping, leg dragging, or mimicking an unusual walk, such as that of a tight-rope walker.

Possible causes
Psychiatric
Conversion disorder. In this rare somatoform disorder, bizarre gait usually develops suddenly after severe stress and is not accompanied by other symptoms. The patient typically shows indifference toward his impairment.
Malingering. In this rare cause of bizarre gait, the patient may also complain of headache and chest and back pain.
Somatization disorder. Bizarre gait is one of many possible somatic complaints.

Clinical considerations
• A history should be obtained and a neurologic assessment performed to rule out an organic cause of the abnormal gait.

• Appropriate referrals should be made for psychiatric counseling.

Gait, propulsive
(Festinating gait)

Description
Propulsive gait is an abnormal gait characterized by a stooped, rigid posture—the patient's head and neck are bent forward, his flexed, stiffened arms are held away from the body, his fingers are extended, and his knees and hips are stiffly bent. During ambulation, this posture results in a forward shifting of the body's center of gravity and consequent impairment of balance, causing increasingly rapid, short, shuffling steps with involuntary acceleration (festination) and lack of control over forward motion (propul-

sion) or backward motion (retropulsion). (See *Identifying Gait Abnormalities,* p. 163.)

Propulsive gait is a cardinal sign of advanced Parkinson's disease, resulting from progressive degeneration of the ganglia, which are primarily responsible for smooth muscle movement. Because this sign develops gradually and its accompanying effects are often wrongly attributed to aging, propulsive gait often goes unnoticed or unreported until severe disability results.

Possible causes
Central nervous system
Parkinson's disease. The characteristic and permanent propulsive gait begins early as a shuffle. As the disease progresses, the gait slows.
Environmental
Carbon monoxide poisoning. Propulsive gait often appears several weeks after acute carbon monoxide intoxication.
Manganese poisoning. Chronic overexposure to manganese can cause an insidious, usually permanent, propulsive gait.
Drugs
Propulsive gait and possibly other extrapyramidal effects can also result from use of phenothiazines, other antipsychotics (notably haloperidol, thiothixene, and loxapine), and, infrequently, metoclopramide and metyrosine. Such effects are usually temporary, disappearing within 1 to 2 weeks after cessation of therapy.

Clinical considerations
• A history should be obtained.

• Because of his gait and associated motor impairment, the patient may have problems performing activities of daily living; consequently, the patient should be assisted as needed but encouraged to maintain independence and self-reliance.

• The patient and his family should be instructed to allow plenty of time for daily activities, especially walking, be-

cause he is particularly susceptible to falls due to festination and poor balance.
• The patient should be encouraged to maintain ambulation; for safety reasons, he should be assisted while walking, especially if he is on unfamiliar or uneven ground.
• The patient may be referred to a physical therapist for exercise therapy and gait retraining.

Gait, scissors

Description
A scissors gait is an abnormal gait in which the patient's legs flex slightly at the hips and knees, giving the appearance of crouching. With each step, his thighs adduct and his knees hit or cross in a scissorslike movement. His steps are short, regular, and laborious, as if he were wading through waist-deep water. His feet may be plantar-flexed and turned inward (equinovarus position), with a shortened Achilles' tendon—as a result, he walks on his toes or the balls of his feet and may scrape his toes on the ground. Resulting from spastic hemiparesis (diplegia), a scissors gait affects both legs and has little or no effect on the arms.

Possible causes
Central nervous system
Cerebrovascular accident. Rarely, scissors gait develops during the late recovery stage of bilateral occlusion of the anterior cerebral artery.
Multiple sclerosis. Progressive scissors gait usually develops gradually, with infrequent remissions.
Spinal cord trauma. Scissors gait may develop during recovery from partial spinal cord compression, particularly with injury below C6.
Spinal cord tumor. Scissors gait can develop gradually from a thoracic or lumbar tumor.
Syphilitic meningomyelitis. Scissors gait appears late in this disorder and may improve with treatment.

Syringomyelia. Scissors gait usually occurs late, along with analgesia and thermanesthesia, muscle atrophy and weakness, and Charcot's joints.
Gastrointestinal
Hepatic failure. Scissors gait may appear several months before the onset of hepatic encephalopathy.
Musculoskeletal
Cervical spondylosis with myelopathy. Scissors gait develops in the late stages of this degenerative disease and steadily worsens.
Metabolic
Pernicious anemia. Scissors gait sometimes occurs as a late sign in untreated anemia.

Clinical considerations
• Because of the sensory loss associated with scissors gait, meticulous skin care should be provided to prevent skin breakdown and decubiti formation.
• As appropriate, the patient should be referred to a physical therapist for gait retraining and for possible in-shoe splints or leg braces to maintain proper foot alignment for standing and walking.

Gait, spastic
(Hemiplegic gait)

Description
Spastic gait is a stiff, foot-dragging walk caused by unilateral leg muscle hypertonicity. It indicates focal damage to the corticospinal tract. The affected leg becomes rigid, with a marked decrease in flexion at the hip and knee and possibly plantar flexion and equinovarus deformity of the foot. Because the patient's leg doesn't swing normally at the hip or knee, his foot tends to drag or shuffle, scraping his toes on the ground. To compensate, the pelvis of the affected side tilts upward in an attempt to lift the toes, causing the patient's leg to abduct and circumduct. In addition, arm swing is hindered on the same side as the affected leg.

Identifying Gait Abnormalities

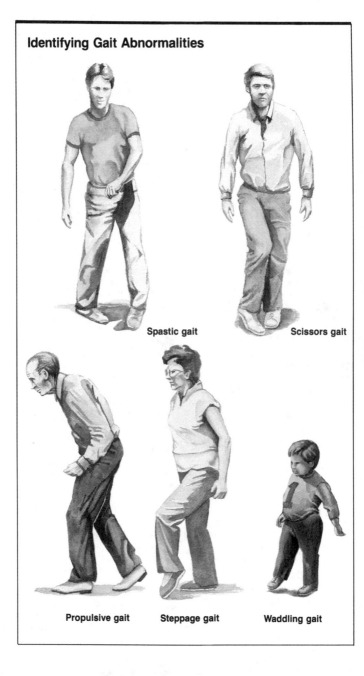

Spastic gait

Scissors gait

Propulsive gait

Steppage gait

Waddling gait

Spastic gait usually develops after a period of flaccidity (hypotonicity) in the affected leg. Once the gait develops, it's usually permanent—regardless of the cause.

Possible causes
Central nervous system
Brain abscess. In this disorder, spastic gait usually develops slowly after a period of muscle flaccidity and fever.

Brain tumor. Depending on the site and type of tumor, spastic gait usually develops gradually and worsens over time.

Cerebrovascular accident. Spastic gait usually appears after a period of muscle weakness and hypotonicity on the affected side.

Head trauma. Spastic gait typically follows the acute stage of head trauma.

Multiple sclerosis. Spastic gait begins insidiously and follows this disorder's characteristic cycle of remission and exacerbation. The gait, as well as other signs and sysmptoms, often worsens in warm weather or after a warm bath or shower.

Clinical considerations
● Because leg muscle contractures are commonly associated with spastic gait, daily exercise—both active and passive—should be encouraged.

● As appropriate, the patient may be referred to a physical therapist for gait retraining and possible in-shoe splints or leg braces to maintain proper foot alignment for standing and walking.

● The patient may have poor balance and a tendency to fall to the paralyzed side; consequently, assistance should be provided during ambulation. The patient may need a cane or a walker.

Gait, steppage
(Equine gait, prancing gait)

Description
Steppage gait is an abnormal gait that typically results from footdrop caused by weakness or paralysis of pretibial and peroneal muscles, usually from lower motor neuron lesions. Footdrop causes the foot to hang with the toes pointing down, causing the toes to scrape the ground during ambulation. To compensate, the hip rotates outward and the hip and knee flex in an exaggerated fashion to lift the advancing leg off the ground. The foot is thrown forward and the toes hit the ground first, producing an audible slap. The rhythm of the gait is usually regular, with even steps and normal upper body posture and arm swing.

Steppage gait can be unilateral or bilateral and permanent or transient, depending on the site and type of neural damage.

Possible causes
Central nervous system
Guillain-Barré syndrome. Typically occurring after recovery from the acute stage of this disorder, steppage gait can be mild or severe, and unilateral or bilateral; it is invariably permanent.

Herniated lumbar disk. Unilateral steppage gait and footdrop commonly occur with late-stage weakness and atrophy of leg muscles.

Multiple sclerosis. Steppage gait and footdrop typically fluctuate in severity with this disorder's cycle of periodic exacerbation and remission.

Peroneal nerve trauma. Temporary ipsilateral steppage gait occurs suddenly, but resolves with the release of peroneal nerve pressure.

Poliomyelitis. Steppage gait, usually permanent and unilateral, often develops after the acute stage. It's typically preceded by fever, asymmetrical muscle weakness, coarse fasciculations, paresthesias, hypoactive or absent deep tendon reflexes, and permanent muscle paralysis and atrophy.

Polyneuropathy. Diabetic polyneuropathy is a rare cause of bilateral steppage gait, which appears as a late but permanent effect. It is preceded by burning pain in the feet and accompanied by leg weakness, sensory loss, and skin ulcers.

In *polyarteritis nodosa with polyneuropathy,* unilateral or bilateral steppage gait is a late finding.

In *alcoholic polyneuropathy,* steppage gait appears 2 to 3 months after onset of vitamin B deficiency. The gait may be bilateral, and it resolves with treatment of the deficiency.

Spinal cord trauma. In the ambulatory patient, spinal cord trauma may cause steppage gait.

Musculoskeletal

Peroneal muscle atrophy. Bilateral steppage gait and footdrop begin insidiously in this disorder. Foot, peroneal, and ankle dorsiflexor muscles are affected first.

Clinical considerations

• The patient with steppage gait may tire rapidly when walking because of the extra effort he must expend to lift his feet off the ground. And when he tires, he may stub his toes, causing a fall. To prevent this, the patient must be helped to recognize his exercise limits and encouraged to get adequate rest.

• If appropriate, the patient may be referred to a physical therapist, for gait retraining and possible application of in-shoe splints or leg braces to maintain foot alignment.

Gait, waddling

Description

Waddling gait is a distinctive ducklike walk. It is an important sign of muscular dystrophy, spinal muscle atrophy, or, rarely, congenital hip displacement. It may be present when the child begins to walk or may appear only later in life. The gait results from deterioration of the pelvic girdle muscles—primarily the gluteus medius, hip flexors, and hip extensors. Weakness in these muscles hinders stabilization of the weight-bearing hip during

walking, causing the opposite hip to drop and the trunk to lean toward that side in an attempt to maintain balance. Typically, the legs assume a wide stance and the trunk is thrown back to further improve stability, exaggerating lordosis and abdominal protrusion. In severe cases, leg and foot muscle contractures may cause equinovarus deformity of the foot combined with circumduction or bowing of the legs.

Possible causes
Musculoskeletal

Congenital hip dysplasia. Bilateral hip dislocation produces waddling gait with lordosis and pain.

Muscular dystrophy. In *Duchenne's muscular dystrophy,* waddling gait gradually appears at ages 3 to 4 and becomes pronounced by age 6. The gait worsens as the disease progresses, until the child loses the ability to walk and becomes wheelchair-bound—usually by age 12.

In *Becker's muscular dystrophy,* waddling gait typically becomes apparent in late adolescence, slowly worsens during the 3rd decade, and culminates in total loss of ambulation. In *facioscapulohumeral muscular dystrophy,* waddling gait appears late, after muscle wasting has spread downward from the face and shoulder girdle to the pelvic girdle and legs.

Spinal muscle atrophy. In *Kugelberg-Welander disease,* waddling gait occurs early and usually progresses slowly, with loss of ambulation occurring up to 20 years later.

In *Werdnig-Hoffmann disease,* waddling gait typically begins when the child learns to walk. The gait progressively worsens, culminating in complete loss of ambulation by adolescence.

Clinical considerations

• A complete medical and family history should be obtained from the family if the child is young and a neurologic examination performed.

Identifying Gower's Sign

To check for Gower's sign, the examiner places the patient supine and asks him to rise. A positive Gower's sign—an inability to lift the trunk without using the hands and arms to brace and push—indicates pelvic muscle weakness, as occurs in muscular dystrophy and spinal muscle atrophy.

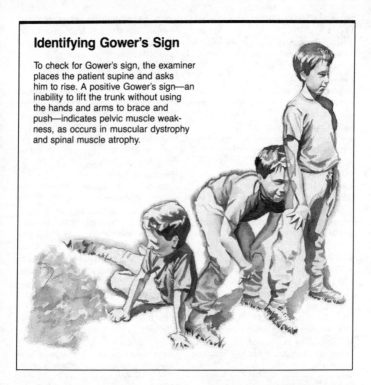

• To determine the extent of pelvic girdle and leg muscle weakness, the patient should be assessed for Gower's sign. (See *Identifying Gower's Sign*.)

• Daily passive and active muscle stretching exercises should be performed for both the arms and legs. If possible, the patient should be instructed to walk at least 3 hours each day (with leg braces, if necessary) to maintain muscle strength, reduce contractures, and delay further gait deterioration.

• The patient and his family should be cautioned against long, unbroken periods of bed rest, which accelerate muscle deterioration.

• A balanced diet should be provided to maintain energy levels and prevent obesity.

• Because of the grim prognosis associated with muscular dystrophy and spinal muscle atrophy, emotional support should be provided for the patient and his family.

• As indicated, the patient should be referred to a local Muscular Dystrophy Association chapter.

Galant reflex

Description
Galant reflex is movement of the pelvis toward the stimulated side when the back is stroked laterally to the spinal column. Normally present at birth, this reflex disappears by age 2 months. To elicit this reflex, the examiner places the infant prone on the examining table or on her hand. Then, using a pin or a finger, she strokes the back laterally to the midline. Normally, the infant

responds by moving the pelvis toward the stimulated side, indicating integrity of the spinal cord from T1 to S1. The absence, irregularity, or asymmetry of this reflex may indicate a spinal cord lesion.

Galeazzi's sign

Description
Galeazzi's sign reflects unequal leg lengths in an infant, seen in congenital dislocation of the hip. To detect this sign, the examiner places the infant supine on a flat, hard surface. She flexes the knees and hips 90° and compares the heights of the knees. With dislocation of the hip, the knee will be lower and the femur will appear shortened on the affected side.

Gallop, atrial
(S₄)

Description
An atrial or presystolic gallop (S_4) is an extra heart sound that is heard or often palpated immediately before the first heart sound. This low-pitched sound is best heard with the bell of the stethoscope pressed lightly against the cardiac apex. Some clinicians say an S_4 has the cadence of the "Ten" in Tennessee (Ten = S_4; nes = S_1; see = S_2).

Typically, this gallop results from hypertension, conduction defects, valvular disorders, and other cardiac abnormalities. Occasionally, it helps differentiate angina from other causes of chest pain.

Usually, an S_4 originates from left atrial contraction, is heard at the apex, and does not vary with inspiration. It may also originate from right atrial contraction. Here it is best heard at the lower left sternal border and intensifies with inspiration.

An S_4 seldom occurs in normal hearts; however, it may occur in the elderly, in athletes with physiologic hypertrophy of the left ventricle, or during pregnancy because of augmented ventricular filling.

Mechanism
Atrial gallop results from abnormally forceful atrial contraction caused by augmented ventricular filling or by decreased left ventricular compliance.

Possible causes
Respiratory
Pulmonary embolism. This life-threatening disorder causes a right-sided S_4 that is usually heard along the lower left sternal border with a loud pulmonic closure sound.
Cardiovascular
Angina. An intermittent S_4 is characteristic here, occurring during an anginal attack and disappearing when it subsides. This gallop may be accompanied by a paradoxical S_2 or a new murmur.

Aortic insufficiency (acute). This disorder causes an S_4 accompanied by a soft, short diastolic murmur along the left sternal border. S_2 may be soft or absent. Sometimes, a soft, short mid-systolic murmur may be heard over the second right intercostal space.

Aortic stenosis. This disorder usually causes an S_4, especially when valvular obstruction is severe. Auscultation reveals a harsh, crescendo-decrescendo, systolic ejection murmur that is loudest at the right sternal border near the second intercostal space.

Atrioventricular (AV) block. First-degree AV block may cause an S_4 accompanied by a faint first heart sound (S_1). In *second-degree AV block*, an S_4 is easily heard. An S_4 is also common in *third-degree AV block.* It varies in intensity with S_1 and is loudest when atrial systole coincides with early, rapid ventricular filling during diastole.

Cardiomyopathy. In this disorder, an S_4 becomes progressively louder with

Interpreting Heart Sounds

Detecting subtle variations in heart sounds requires concentration and practice. Learning to recognize normal heart sounds makes the abnormal gallops more obvious.

Heart sound and its cause	Auscultation tips
First heart sound (S$_1$) Vibrations associated with mitral and tricuspid valve closure	Best heard with the diaphragm of the stethoscope at the apex (mitral area)
Second heart sound (S$_2$) Vibrations associated with aortic and pulmonic valve closure	Best heard with the diaphragm of the stethoscope in the aortic area with the patient sitting or supine
Ventricular gallop (S$_3$) Vibrations produced by rapid blood flow into the ventricles	Best heard through the bell of the stethoscope at the apex with the patient in the left lateral position. May be visible and palpable during early diastole at the midclavicular line between the fourth and fifth intercostal spaces
Atrial gallop (S$_4$) Vibrations produced by an increased resistance to sudden, forceful ejection of atrial blood	Best heard through the bell of the stethoscope at the apex with the patient in the left semilateral position. May be visible in late diastole at the midclavicular line between the fourth and fifth intercostal spaces. May also be palpable in the midclavicular area with the patient in the left lateral decubitus position.
Summation gallop Vibrations produced in middiastole by simultaneous ventricular and atrial gallops, usually caused by tachycardia	Best heard through the bell of the stethoscope at the apex with the patient in the left lateral position. May be louder than S$_1$ or S$_2$. May be visible and palpable during diastole.

Timing and cadence

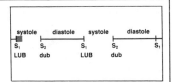

systole	diastole	systole	diastole	
S₁	S₂	S₁	S₂	S₁
LUB	dub	LUB	dub	

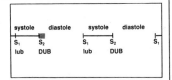

systole	diastole	systole	diastole	
S₁	S₂	S₁	S₂	S₁
lub	DUB	lub	DUB	

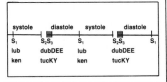

systole	diastole	systole	diastole	
S₁	S₂S₃	S₁	S₂S₃	S₁
lub	dubDEE	lub	dubDEE	
ken	tucKY	ken	tucKY	

systole	diastole	systole	diastole	
S₁	S₂	S₄S₁	S₂	S₄S₁
		DEElub	dub	DEElub
		TENnes	see	TENnes

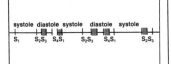

systole	diastole	systole	diastole	systole
S₁	S₂S₃ S₄S₁	S₂S₃	S₄S₁	S₂S₃

advancing disease. However, in some patients, it may become faint or occasionally disappear.

Hypertension. One of the earliest findings in systemic arterial hypertension is an S₄.

Mitral insufficiency. In acute mitral insufficiency, auscultation may reveal an S₄ accompanied by an S₃, a harsh holosystolic murmur that's heard best at the apex or over the precordium.

Mitral stenosis. When associated with a normal sinus rhythm, mitral stenosis commonly causes an S₄. Cardinal findings include a loud apical first sound and an opening snap with a diastolic murmur heard at the apex.

Myocardial infarction (MI). An S₄ is a classic sign of life-threatening MI; in fact, it may persist even after the infarction heals.

Endocrine

Thyrotoxicosis. An S₄ and an S₃ may be auscultated in thyroid hormone overproduction.

Hematologic

Anemia. In this disorder, an S₄ may accompany increased cardiac output.

Clinical considerations

If an S₄ is detected in a patient with chest pain:

• Myocardial ischemia should be suspected and the physician notified immediately.

• Vital signs should be taken and a rapid cardiac assessment performed.

• An EKG should be obtained and cardiac monitoring instituted.

• Emergency interventions should be carried out, as ordered and needed, depending on the patient's status and cardiac rhythm.

• Diagnostic tests may include EKG and echocardiography, cardiac catheterization, and possibly a lung scan.

Gallop, ventricular
(S₃)

Description

A ventricular gallop is an extra heart sound associated with rapid ventricular filling in early diastole. Usually

---

Summation Gallop: Two Gallops in One

When atrial and ventricular gallops occur simultaneously, they produce a short, low-pitched sound known as a summation gallop. This relatively uncommon gallop occurs during middiastole (between S_2 and S_1) and is best heard with the bell of the stethoscope pressed lightly against the cardiac apex. It may be louder than either S_1 or S_2 and may cause visible apical movement during diastole.

A summation gallop may result from tachycardia or from delayed or blocked atrioventricular (AV) conduction. Tachycardia shortens ventricular filling time during diastole, causing it to coincide with atrial contraction. When heart rate slows, the summation gallop is replaced by separate atrial and ventricular gallops, producing a quadruple rhythm much like the canter of a horse. Delayed AV conduction also brings atrial contraction closer to ventricular filling, creating a summation gallop. Most commonly, a summation gallop results from congestive heart failure and dilated congestive cardiomyopathy; it may also accompany other cardiac disorders. Occasionally, it signals further cardiac deterioration. For example, consider the hypertensive patient with a chronic atrial gallop who develops tachycardia and a superimposed ventricular gallop. If this patient abruptly displays a summation gallop, heart failure is the likely cause.

---

palpable, this low-frequency sound occurs about 0.15 second after the second heart sound (S_2). It may originate in either the left or right ventricle. A right-sided gallop usually sounds louder on inspiration and is best heard along the lower left sternal border or over the xiphoid region. A left-sided gallop usually sounds louder on expiration and is best heard at the apex.

Ventricular gallops are easily overlooked because they are usually faint. Fortunately, certain techniques make their detection more likely. These include auscultating in a quiet environment; examining the patient in the supine, left lateral, and semi-Fowler's positions; and having the patient cough or raise his legs to augment the sound.

A physiologic ventricular gallop occurs in children and young adults; however, most people lose this third heart sound by age 40. This gallop may also occur during the third trimester of pregnancy. Although the physiologic S_3 has the same timing as the pathologic S_3, its intensity waxes and wanes with respiration. It is also heard more faintly if the patient is sitting or standing.

Mechanism

A pathologic ventricular gallop may be one of the earliest signs of ventricular failure. It may result from one of two mechanisms: rapid deceleration of blood entering a stiff, noncompliant ventricle or rapid acceleration of blood associated with increased flow into the ventricle. The gallop's intensity correlates with the patient's prognosis. Usually, the louder the gallop, the more ominous the prognosis. A gallop that persists despite therapy is also more significant.

Possible causes
Cardiovascular

Aortic insufficiency. Both acute and chronic aortic insufficiency may produce an S_3. Typically, *acute aortic insufficiency* also causes an S_4 and a soft, short diastolic murmur over the left sternal border. S_2 may be soft or absent. At times, a soft, short midsystolic murmur may be heard over the second right intercostal space.

Chronic aortic insufficiency produces an S_3 and a high-pitched blowing, decrescendo diastolic murmur that is best heard over the second or third right intercostal space or the left sternal border. An Austin Flint murmur—an apical, rumbling, middle-to-late diastolic murmur—may also occur.

Cardiomyopathy. A ventricular gallop is characteristic. When accompanied by pulsus alternans and altered first and second heart sounds, this gallop usually signals advanced heart disease.

Congestive heart failure (CHF). A cardinal sign of CHF is a ventricular gallop. When it is loud and accompanied by sinus tachycardia, this gallop may indicate severe heart failure.

Mitral insufficiency. Both acute and chronic mitral insufficiency may produce a ventricular gallop. In *acute mitral insufficiency,* auscultation may also reveal an early or holosystolic decrescendo murmur at the apex, an S_4, and a widely split second heart sound.

In *chronic mitral insufficiency,* a progressively severe ventricular gallop is typical. Auscultation will also reveal a holosystolic, blowing, high-pitched apical murmur.

Endocrine

Thyrotoxicosis. This disorder may produce ventricular and atrial gallops.

Clinical considerations

• A history should be obtained and a cardiovascular assessment performed.

• Diagnostic tests may include echocardiography, gated blood pool imaging, and cardiac catheterization.

• The patient should be monitored closely and any changes in status reported to the physician.

• Oxygen, diuretics, and other drugs, such as digitalis, should be administered, as ordered, to prevent pulmonary edema.

Genital lesions, female

Description

Female genital lesions are cutaneous lumps, nodules, papules, vesicles, or ulcers. Resulting from benign or malignant tumors, dystrophies, dermatoses, or infection, they can appear anywhere on the vulva and may go undetected until a gynecologic examination. Usually, however, the patient notices lesions because of associated symptoms, such as pruritus, dysuria, or dyspareunia.

Possible causes

Skin

Basal cell carcinoma. Occurring most often in postmenopausal women, this nodular tumor has a central ulcer and a raised, rolled border. Typically asymptomatic, the tumor may occasionally cause pruritus, bleeding, discharge, and a burning sensation.

Dermatoses (systemic). Psoriasis, seborrheic dermatitis, and other skin conditions may produce vulvar lesions.

Herpes zoster. This viral infection may produce vulvar lesions, although other areas are more commonly affected. Small, red nodular lesions erupt on painful erythematous areas. The lesions quickly evolve into vesicles or pustules, which dry and form scabs about 10 days later.

Malignant melanoma. This disorder causes irregular, pigmented vulvar lesions that enlarge rapidly. Lesions may ulcerate and bleed.

Pediculosis pubis. This parasitic infection produces erythematous vulvar papules with pruritus and skin irritation. Pubic lice nits are visible on pubic hair with magnification.

Squamous cell carcinoma. Invasive carcinoma occurs primarily in postmenopausal women and may produce vulvar pruritus and a vulvar lump. As the tumor enlarges, it may encroach on the vagina, anus, and urethra. *Carcinoma in situ* occurs most often in premenopausal women, producing a vulvar lesion that may be white or red, raised, well defined, moist, crusted, and isolated.

Obstetrics-Gynecology

Benign cysts. Epidermal inclusion cysts, the most common vulvar cysts, appear primarily on the labia majora and are usually round and asymptomatic. *Bartholin's duct cysts* are usually tense, nontender, and palpable. They appear on the posterior labia minora and may cause minor discomfort during intercourse or, when large, difficulty with intercourse or even walking. *Bartholin's abscess,* infection of a Bartholin's duct cyst, causes gradual pain and tenderness and possibly vulvar swelling, redness, and deformity.

Benign vulvar tumors. Cystic or solid benign vulvar tumors are usually asymptomatic.

Granuloma inguinale. Initially, a single painless macule or papule appears on the vulva, ulcerating into a raised, beefy-red lesion with a granulated, friable border. Other painless and possibly foul-smelling lesions may occur on the labia, vagina, or cervix. These become infected and painful, and regional lymph nodes enlarge and may become tender.

Herpes simplex (genital). In this disorder, fluid-filled vesicles appear on the cervix and, possibly, on the vulva, labia, perianal skin, vagina, or mouth. The vesicles, initially painless, may rupture and develop into extensive, shallow, painful ulcers, with redness, marked edema, and tender inguinal lymph nodes.

Hyperplastic dystrophy. Vulvar lesions may be well delineated or poorly defined; localized or extensive; and red, brown, white, or both red and white. However, intense pruritus, possibly with vulvar pain and dyspareunia, is the cardinal symptom. In *lichen sclerosus,* a type of vulvar dystrophy, vulvar skin has a parchmentlike appearance. Fissures may develop between the clitoris and urethra or other vulvar areas.

Infectious diseases

Chancroid. This rare, sexually transmitted disease causes painful vulvar lesions.

Genital warts. This sexually transmitted disease produces painless warts on the vulva, vagina, and cervix. Warts start as tiny red or pink swellings that grow (sometimes to 4", or 10 cm) and become pedunculated. Multiple swellings with a cauliflower appearance are common.

Gonorrhea. Vulvar lesions may develop along with pruritus, a burning sensation, pain, and a greenish yellow vaginal discharge, but most patients are asymptomatic.

Lymphogranuloma venereum. This bacterial infection commonly presents with a single, painless papule or ulcer on the posterior vulva that heals in a few days. Inguinal lymphadenopathy develops about 2 weeks later.

Molluscum contagiosum. This viral infection produces raised vulvar papules that are 1 to 2 mm in diameter and have a white core. Pruritic lesions may also appear on the face, eyelids, breasts, and inner thighs.

Syphilis. Chancres, the primary vulvar lesions of this sexually transmitted disease, may appear on the vulva, vagina, or cervix 10 to 90 days after initial contact. Usually painless, they start as papules that then erode, with indurated, raised edges and clear bases. Condylomata lata, highly contagious secondary vulvar lesions, are raised, gray, flat-topped, and often ulcerated.

Viral disease (systemic). Varicella, measles, and other systemic viral diseases may produce vulvar lesions.

Clinical considerations

• A history should be obtained and a pelvic examination performed.

• Diagnostic tests may include a culture and a biopsy of the lesion(s). A VDRL (Venereal Disease Research Laboratory) blood sample for test will be drawn.

- Systemic antibiotics, antiviral agents, topical corticosteroids, topical testosterone, or an antipruritic agent should be administered, as ordered.
- Sitz baths should be given to relieve crusting and itching.
- Changes in the lesion(s) should be reported.
- If the patient has a sexually transmitted disease, she should be encouraged to inform her sexual partners and persuade them to be treated.
- The patient should be advised to avoid sexual contact until the lesions are no longer contagious.

Genital lesions, male

Description

Male genital lesions include warts, papules, ulcers, scales, and pustules. These common lesions may be painful or painless, singular or multiple. They may be limited to the genitalia or may also occur elsewhere on the body.

Genital lesions may result from infection, neoplasms, parasites, allergy, or the effects of drugs. Often, these lesions profoundly affect the patient's self-image. In fact, he may hesitate to seek medical attention, fearing malignancy or sexually transmitted disease. Unfortunately, self-treatment may alter the lesions, making differential diagnosis especially difficult.

Possible causes
Genitourinary

Balanitis and balanoposthitis. Typically, balanitis (glans infection) and posthitis (prepuce infection) occur together (balanoposthitis), causing painful ulceration on the glans, foreskin, or penile shaft. Ulceration is usually preceded by 2 to 3 days of prepuce irritation and soreness, followed by foul discharge and edema. The patient may then develop features of acute infection, such as fever with chills, malaise, and dysuria. Without treatment,

the ulcers may deepen and multiply. Eventually, the entire penis and scrotum may become gangrenous, resulting in life-threatening sepsis.

Bowen's disease. This painless, premalignant lesion commonly occurs on the penis or scrotum but may also appear elsewhere. It appears as a brownish red, raised, scaly, indurated plaque, which may ulcerate at its center.

Penile cancer. Usually, this cancer produces a painless, ulcerative lesion or enlarging "wart" on the glans or foreskin. It may be accompanied by localized pain, though, if the foreskin becomes unretractable.

Skin

Candidiasis. When this infection involves the anogenital area, it produces erythematous, weepy, circumscribed lesions, usually under the prepuce. Sometimes, vesicles and pustules also develop.

Erythroplasia of Queyrat. This premalignant lesion may occur on the penis, glans, or corona. Typically, it appears as a red, raised, indurated plaque, which may have an ulcerated center.

Folliculitis and furunculosis. Hair follicle infection may cause red, sharply pointed lesions that are tender and swollen with central pustules. If folliculitis progresses to furunculosis, these lesions become hard, painful nodules that may gradually enlarge and rupture, discharging pus and necrotic material. Rupture relieves the pain, but erythema and edema may persist for days or weeks.

Fournier's gangrene. In this life-threatening cellulitis, the scrotum suddenly becomes tense, swollen, painful, red, warm, and glossy. As gangrene develops, the scrotum also becomes moist.

Leukoplakia. This precancerous disorder is characterized by white, scaly patches on the glans and prepuce accompanied by skin thickening and occasionally fissures.

Lichen planus. Small, polygonal, violet papules develop on the glans penis in this disorder. Usually, they are shiny and less than 3 cm in diameter and have milky striations. They may be linear or coalesce into plaques. Occasionally, oral lesions precede genital lesions. Also, lesions may affect the lower back, ankles, and lower legs.

Pediculosis pubis. This parasitic infestation is characterized by erythematous, itching papules in the pubic area and around the anus, abdomen, and thigh.

Psoriasis. Red, raised, scaly plaques typically affect the scalp, chest, knees, elbows, and lower back. When they occur on the groin or on the shaft and glans of the penis, the plaques are usually redder and lack the characteristic silver scale.

Scabies. Mites burrow under the skin in this disorder, possibly causing crusted lesions on the glans and shaft of the penis and on the scrotum. Lesions may also occur on the wrists, elbows, axillae, and waist. Usually, they are threadlike and 1 to 10 cm long and have a swollen nodule or red papule that contains the mite.

Seborrheic dermatitis. Initially, this disorder causes erythematous, scaling papules that enlarge to form annular plaques. These pruritic plaques may affect the glans and shaft of the penis, scrotum, and groin as well as the scalp, chest, eyebrows, back, axillae, and umbilicus.

Tinea cruris. Also called "jock itch," this fungal infection usually causes sharply defined, slightly raised, scaling patches on the inner thigh or groin and, less commonly, on the scrotum and penis. Pruritus may be severe.

Immunologic

Urticaria. This common allergic reaction is characterized by intensely pruritic hives, which may appear on the genitalia, especially on the foreskin or shaft of the penis. These distinct, raised, evanescent wheals are surrounded by an erythematous flare.

Infectious diseases

Chancroid. In this sexually transmitted disease, one or more lesions erupt, usually on the groin, inner thigh, or penis. Within 24 hours, the lesion changes from a reddened area to a small papule. (A similar papule may erupt on the tongue, lip, breast, or umbilicus.) It then becomes an inflamed pustule that rapidly ulcerates. This painful—usually deep—ulcer bleeds easily and commonly has a purulent gray or yellow exudate covering its base. Rarely more than 2 cm in diameter, it is typically irregular in shape.

Herpes simplex (genital). Caused by herpesvirus Type II, this infection produces fluid-filled vesicles on the glans penis, foreskin, or penile shaft and, occasionally, on the mouth or anus. Usually painless at first, these vesicles may rupture and become extensive, shallow, painful ulcers accompanied by redness, marked edema, and tender, inguinal lymph nodes. If the vesicles recur in the same area, the patient will usually feel localized numbness and tingling before they erupt. Typically, associated inflammation is less marked.

Genital warts. Most common in uncircumcised, sexually active males, genital warts initially develop on the subpreputial sac, urethral meatus, and less commonly on the penile shaft and then spread to the perineum and the perianal area. These painless warts start as tiny red or pink swellings that may grow to 4″ (10 cm) and become pendunculated. Multiple swellings are common, giving the warts a cauliflower appearance. Infected warts are also malodorous.

Granuloma inguinale. Initially, this rare, chronic venereal infection causes a single, painless macule or papule on the external genitalia that ulcerates and becomes a raised, beefy-red lesion with a granulated, friable border. Then other painless lesions may erupt and blend together on the glans penis, foreskin, or penile shaft. Sometimes lesions develop on the nose, mouth, or pharynx, too. Eventually, these lesions become infected, foul-smelling, and painful and may be accompanied by pseudobuboes, fever, weight loss, malaise, and signs of anemia, such as weakness. Later, lesions are marked by fibrosis, keloidal scarring, and depigmentation.

Lymphogranuloma venereum. One to three weeks after sexual exposure, this disorder may produce a penile erosion or papule that heals rapidly and spontaneously; in fact, it often goes unnoticed. A few days or weeks later, the inguinal and subinguinal nodes enlarge, becoming painful, fluctuant masses. If these nodes become infected, they rupture and form sinus tracts, discharging a thick, yellow, granular secretion. Eventually, a scar or chronic indurated mass forms in the inguinal area.

Syphilis. Two to four weeks after exposure to *Treponema pallidum,* one or more primary lesions, or chancres, may erupt on the genitalia; occasionally, they also erupt elsewhere on the body. The chancre usually starts as a small, red, fluid-filled papule and then erodes to form a painless, firm, indurated, shallow ulcer with a clear base or, less commonly, a hard papule. This lesion gradually involutes and disappears. Painless, unilateral regional lymphadenopathy is also typical.

Drugs

Phenolphthalein, barbiturates, and certain broad-spectrum antibiotics, such as tetracycline and sulfonamides, may cause a fixed drug eruption and a bright red to purplish genital lesion.

Clinical considerations

• A history should be obtained (with any self-treatment of the lesion[s] noted) and an examination of the lesion(s) performed.

• Diagnostic tests may include a culture and a biopsy of the lesion(s).

• A blood sample for a VDRL (Venereal Disease Research Laboratory test) will be drawn.

• A heat lamp may be used to dry moist lesions; sitz baths may be used to relieve crusting and itching.

• Systemic antibiotics, antiviral agents, topical corticosteroids, topical testosterone, or an antipruritic agent should be administered, as ordered.

• Changes in the lesion(s) should be reported.

• If the patient has a sexually transmitted disease, he should be encouraged to inform his sexual partners and persuade them to be treated.

• The patient should be advised to avoid sexual contact until the lesions are no longer contagious.

Gifford's sign

Description

Gifford's sign is resistance to everting the upper eyelid, seen in thyrotoxicosis. To detect this sign, the examiner attempts to raise and evert the eyelid over a blunt object.

Glabella reflex

Description

The glabella reflex is persistent blinking in response to repeated light tapping on the forehead between the eyebrows. This reflex occurs in Parkinson's disease, presenile dementia, and diffuse tumors of the frontal lobes.

Goldthwait's sign

Description

Goldthwait's sign is pain elicited by maneuvers of the leg, pelvis, and lower back to differentiate irritation of the sacroiliac joint from irritation of the lumbosacral or sacroiliac articulation. To elicit this sign, the examiner positions the patient supine and places one hand under the small of his back. With the other hand, she raises the patient's leg. Pain occurring with this movement suggests sacroiliac joint irritation. If the patient does not have pain, the examiner places her hand under his lower back and applies pressure. Pain occurring with this maneuver suggests irritation of the lumbosacral or sacroiliac articulation.

Gower's sign

Description
In an adult, Gower's sign is irregular contraction of the iris, occurring when the eye is illuminated. This sign can be detected in certain stages of tabes dorsalis.

In a child, Gower's sign is the characteristic maneuver used to rise from the floor or a low sitting position to compensate for proximal muscle weakness in Duchenne's or Becker's muscular dystrophy. (See "Gait, waddling.")

Grasp reflex

Description
The grasp reflex is flexion of the fingers when the palmar surface is touched, and of the toes when the plantar surface is touched.

In an infant, this reflex develops at approximately 26 to 28 weeks gestational age but may be weak until term. The absence, weakness, or asymmetry of this reflex during the neonatal period may indicate paralysis, central nervous system depression, or injury. To elicit this reflex, a finger is placed in each of the infant's palms. His reflexive grasping should be symmetrical and strong enough at term to allow him to be lifted. Flexion of the toes is elicited by gently touching the ball of the foot.

In an adult, the grasp reflex is an abnormal finding, indicating a disorder of the premotor cortex.

Grasset's phenomenon

Description
Grasset's phenomenon is the inability to raise both legs simultaneously, even though each can be raised separately. In an adult, this phenomenon occurs in incomplete organic hemiplegia. To elicit it, the examiner places the patient supine and lifts and supports the affected leg. Then she attempts to lift the opposite leg. In Grasset's phenomenon, the unaffected leg will drop—the result of an upper motor neuron lesion.

In an infant, this sign is normally present until 5 to 7 months of age.

Grey Turner's sign

Description
Grey Turner's sign is a bruiselike discoloration of the skin of the flanks. This sign appears 6 to 24 hours after onset of retroperitoneal hemorrhage in acute pancreatitis.

Grief

Description
Grief may be defined as deep anguish or sorrow typically felt upon the loss of a loved one, a job, a goal, or an ideal. In patients with terminal illness, grief may precede acceptance of dying. Unlike depression, grief proceeds in stages and often resolves with the passage of time.

Griffith's sign

Description
Griffith's sign is lagging motion of the lower eyelids during upward rotation of the eyes, seen in thyrotoxicosis. To

detect this sign, the patient is asked to focus on a steadily rising point, such as a moving finger. If the lower lid doesn't follow eye motion smoothly, this sign is present.

Grunting respirations

Description
Grunting respirations are characterized by a deep, low-pitched grunting sound at the end of each breath. These respirations are a chief sign of respiratory distress in infants and children. They may be soft and heard only on auscultation, or loud and clearly audible without a stethoscope. Typically, the intensity of grunting respirations reflects the severity of respiratory distress.

Grunting respirations indicate intrathoracic disease with lower respiratory involvement. Although they may also occur in adults with severe respiratory distress, they are not as common. Whether they occur in children or adults, grunting respirations demand immediate medical attention.

Mechanism
The grunting sound coincides with closure of the glottis—an effort to increase end-expiratory pressure in the lungs and prolong alveolar gas exchange, thereby enhancing ventilation and perfusion.

Possible causes
Respiratory
Respiratory distress syndrome. The result of lung immaturity in a premature infant (<37 weeks gestation), this syndrome initially causes audible expiratory grunts along with intercostal, subcostal, or substernal retractions; tachycardia; and tachypnea. Later, as respiratory distress tires the infant, apnea or irregular respirations replace the grunting.

Staphylococcus aureus pneumonia. Life-threatening bacterial pneumonia primarily affects infants under age 1 and often follows upper respiratory infections or colds. It causes grunting respirations accompanied by high fever, tachypnea, productive cough, anorexia, and lethargy.

Cardiovascular
Congestive heart failure. A late sign of left ventricular failure, grunting respirations accompany increasing pulmonary edema.

Clinical considerations
• A rapid respiratory assessment should be performed to evaluate the severity of the respiratory distress; the physician should be notified immediately.

• Vital signs should be taken.

• Emergency intervention should be anticipated to maintain an open airway and adequate oxygenation.

• Emergency equipment should be kept on hand in case respiratory distress worsens.

• When the child is stable, a history should be obtained from the parents.

• Diagnostic tests may include blood studies for arterial blood gas analysis and culture, and chest X-rays.

• Respiratory status should be monitored closely and inhalation therapy with bronchodilators or antimicrobials begun, as ordered. Chest physical therapy (CPT) should follow.

• CPT should be scheduled before meals to help prevent severe or spasmodic coughing and resultant vomiting. Optimally, CPT should be grouped with other treatments or activities, such as bathing, to ensure regular 2- to 4-hour rest periods.

• All procedures should be explained, and emotional support provided to the parents.

Guilland's sign

Description
Guilland's sign is quick, energetic flexion of the hip and knee in response to pinching the contralateral quadri-

ceps muscle. This sign indicates meningeal irritation.

Gums, bleeding
(Gingival bleeding)

Description
Bleeding gums usually result from dental disorders or, less often, from blood dyscrasias or the effects of certain drugs. Physiologic causes of this common sign include pregnancy, which can produce gum swelling in the first or second trimester (pregnancy epulis); atmospheric pressure changes, which most commonly affect divers and aviators; and oral trauma.

Bleeding may range from slight oozing to life-threatening hemorrhage. It may be spontaneous or may follow trauma. Occasionally, direct pressure can control it.

Possible causes
Eyes, ears, nose, and throat
Giant cell epulis. This pedunculated granuloma occurs on the gums or alveolar process in front of the molars. It is dark red and vascular, resembling a surface ulcer. Gums bleed easily with slight trauma.

Gingivitis. In this disorder, reddened and edematous gums are characteristic. The gingivae between the teeth become bulbous and bleed easily with slight trauma. However, in *acute necrotizing ulcerative gingivitis,* bleeding is spontaneous. The gums also become so painful that the patient may be unable to eat.

Periodontal disease. Typically, chewing, toothbrushing, or gum probing initiates gum bleeding, or bleeding occurs spontaneously. As gingivae separate from the bone, pus-filled pockets develop around the teeth and, occasionally, pus can be expressed.

Pyogenic granuloma. Commonly affecting the gums, lips, tongue, and buccal mucosa, this granuloma may ulcerate and bleed spontaneously or with slight trauma.

Gastrointestinal
Cirrhosis. Gum bleeding is a late sign of cirrhosis that occurs with epistaxis and other bleeding tendencies.

Hematologic
Agranulocytosis. Spontaneous gum bleeding and other systemic hemorrhages may occur in this hematologic disorder. Typically, the disorder causes progressive fatigue and weakness followed by signs of infection, such as fever and chills.

Aplastic anemia. In this disorder, profuse or scant gum bleeding may follow trauma.

Familial thrombasthenia. This hereditary blood platelet disorder causes spontaneous bleeding from the oral cavity, especially the gums.

Hemophilia. Here, hemorrhage occurs from many sites in the oral cavity, especially the gums.

Hereditary hemorrhagic telangiectasia. This disorder is characterized by red to violet spiderlike hemorrhagic areas on the gums, which blanch on pressure and bleed spontaneously. These telangiectases may also occur on the lips, buccal mucosa, and palate as well as the face, ears, scalp, hands, arms, feet, and under the nails.

Hypofibrinogenemia. In this rare disorder, the patient has frequent, spontaneous episodes of severe gum bleeding.

Leukemia. Easy gum bleeding is an early sign of acute monocytic, lymphocytic, or myelocytic leukemia. It is accompanied by gum swelling, necrosis, and petechiae. The soft, tender gums appear glossy and bluish.

Polycythemia vera. In this disorder, engorged gums ooze blood after slight trauma. Usually, polycythemia vera turns the oral mucosa—especially the gums and tongue—a deep red-violet.

Thrombocytopenia. Blood usually oozes between the teeth and gums; however, severe bleeding may follow minor trauma.

Thrombocytopenic purpura (idiopathic). Profuse gum bleeding occurs in this disorder. Its classic feature, though, is spontaneous hemorrhagic skin lesions that range from pinpoint petechiae to massive hemorrhages.

Metabolic
Pernicious anemia. Gum bleeding and a sore tongue are characteristic in this disorder and often make eating painful.
Vitamin C deficiency. This deficiency causes swollen, spongy, tender gums that bleed easily. Between the teeth, the gums are red or purple. The teeth themselves become loose and may be surrounded by pockets filled with clotted blood.
Vitamin K deficiency. Usually, gums that bleed after toothbrushing are the first sign of vitamin K deficiency. Other signs of abnormal bleeding, such as ecchymosis, epistaxis, and hematuria, may occur.

Immunologic
Pemphigoid (benign mucosal). Most common in women between ages 40 and 50, this autoimmune disorder typically causes thick-walled gum lesions that rupture, desquamate, and then bleed easily. Extensive scars form with healing, and the gums remain red for months. Lesions may also develop on other parts of the oral mucosa, conjunctiva, and, less often, the skin.

Environmental
Chemical irritants. Occupational exposure to benzene may irritate the gums, resulting in bleeding.

Drugs
Coumadin and heparin interfere with blood clotting and may cause prolonged gum bleeding. Aspirin abuse may alter platelets, producing bleeding gums. Localized gum bleeding may also occur with mucosal "aspirin burn" caused by dissolving aspirin near an aching tooth.

Clinical considerations

If bleeding is profuse:
• Airway patency should be checked and maintained through suction and/or airway insertion.

Preventing Bleeding Gums

Follow these tips to improve oral hygiene and prevent bleeding gums:
• Eliminate between-meal snacks and reduce carbohydrate intake to help prevent plaque formation on teeth.
• Visit the dentist once every 6 months for thorough plaque removal.
• Avoid citrus fruits and juices, rough or spicy food, alcohol, and tobacco if they irritate mouth ulcers or sore gums and cause bleeding. Take vitamin C supplements if citrus fruits and juices cannot be consumed.
• If dentures make gums bleed, wear them *only* during meals.
• Avoid using toothpicks, which may cause gum injury and infection.
• Brush teeth gently after every meal, using a soft-bristle toothbrush held at a 45-degree angle to the gum line.
• If the doctor suggests not brushing, rinse with salt water or hydrogen peroxide and water. Avoid using commercial mouthwashes, which contain irritating alcohol.
• Floss teeth daily to remove plaque, unless flossing causes pain or bleeding.
• Use an oral irrigation device on the low pressure setting to massage gums.
• Use aspirin *sparingly* for toothaches or general pain relief.
• Control gum bleeding by applying direct pressure to the area with a gauze pad soaked in ice water.

• The physician should be notified and vital signs taken.
• Direct pressure should be applied to the bleeding site if it can be located.
If gum bleeding is not an emergency:
• A medical and dental history should be obtained and an oral examination performed.

• Diagnostic tests may include blood studies and facial X-rays.

• Meticulous mouth care should be provided. However, lemon-glycerin swabs should be avoided because they may irritate the gums; a soft toothbrush or one padded with sponge or gauze should be used instead.

• The patient should be taught how to perform mouth and gum care. (See *Preventing Bleeding Gums*, p. 179.)

Gums, swollen
(Gingival swelling)

Description
Gum swelling is an abnormal enlargement or overgrowth of the gingivae. This common sign may involve one or many papillae—the triangular-shaped bits of gum between adjacent teeth. Occasionally, the gums swell markedly, obscuring the teeth altogether. Usually, the swelling is most prominent on the labia and bucca.

Most commonly, gum swelling results from the effects of phenytoin. It may also result from nutritional deficiency and certain systemic disorders. Physiologic gum swelling and bleeding may occur during the first or second trimester of pregnancy when hormonal changes make the gums highly vascular; even slight irritation causes swelling and gives the papillae a characteristic raspberry hue (pregnancy epulis). Irritating dentures may also cause swelling associated with red, soft, moveable masses on the gums.

Mechanism
Gum swelling may result from one of two mechanisms: an increase in the size of existing gum cells (hypertrophy) or an increase in their number (hyperplasia).

Possible causes
Eyes, ears, nose, and throat
Fibrous hyperplasia (idiopathic). In this disorder, the gums become diffusely enlarged and may even cover the teeth. Large, firm, painless masses of fibrous tissue form on the gums and may prevent tooth eruption and cause lip protrusion and difficulty chewing.

Gastrointestinal
Crohn's disease. Granular or cobblestone gum swelling occurs in this disorder, which is characterized by cramping abdominal pain and diarrhea.

Hematologic
Leukemia. Gum swelling is commonly an early sign—especially in acute monocytic, lymphocytic, or myelocytic leukemia. Usually, the swelling is localized and accompanied by necrosis. The tender gums appear blue and glossy and bleed easily.

Metabolic
Vitamin C deficiency. The gums are spongy, tender, and edematous, and the papillae appear red or purple. The gums bleed easily, and inspection may reveal pockets filled with clotted blood around loose teeth.

Drugs
A common side effect of phenytoin is gum swelling. Cyclosporine, a drug used to prevent rejection of transplanted organs, also produces this sign in about 15% of patients.

Clinical considerations
• A medical and dental history should be obtained and an oral examination performed.

• Diagnostic tests may include blood studies.

• Meticulous mouth care should be provided. However, lemon-glycerin swabs should be avoided because they may irritate the gums; a soft toothbrush or one padded with sponge or gauze should be used instead.

• Because gum swelling may affect the patient's appearance, emotional support and reassurance that swelling usually resolves with treatment should be offered.

• To prevent further swelling, the patient should be taught the basics of good nutrition; encouraged to avoid gum irritants, such as commercial mouthwashes, alcohol, and tobacco; and advised to see a periodontist at least every 6 months.

Gynecomastia

Description

Occurring only in males, gynecomastia refers to excessive mammary gland development, resulting in increased breast size. This size change may be barely palpable or immediately obvious. Usually bilateral, gynecomastia may be associated with breast tenderness and milk secretion.

Gynecomastia commonly results from the effects of estrogens and other drugs. It may also result from hormone-secreting tumors and from endocrine, genetic, hepatic, and renal disorders. Physiologic gynecomastia may occur in neonatal, pubertal, and geriatric males due to normal fluctuations in hormone levels. In newborns, gynecomastia may be associated with galactorrhea ("witch's milk"). It usually disappears in a few weeks but may persist until age 2.

Mechanism

Normally, several hormones regulate breast development. Estrogens, growth hormone, and corticosteroids stimulate ductal growth, while progesterone and prolactin stimulate growth of the alveolar lobules. Although the pathophysiology of gynecomastia is not fully understood, hormonal imbalance—particularly a change in the estrogen-androgen ratio and an increase in prolactin—is a likely contributing factor.

Possible causes

Respiratory

Lung cancer. Bronchogenic carcinoma or metastasis to the lung from testicular choriocarcinoma may result in bilateral gynecomastia.

Endocrine

Adrenal carcinoma. Estrogen production by an adrenal tumor may produce a feminizing syndrome in males characterized by bilateral gynecomastia, loss of libido, impotence, testicular atrophy, and reduced facial hair growth. Cushingoid signs, like moon face and purple striae, may occur.

Hypothyroidism. Typically, this disorder produces bilateral gynecomastia along with bradycardia, cold intolerance, weight gain despite anorexia, and mental dullness.

Pituitary tumor. This hormone-secreting tumor causes bilateral gynecomastia accompanied by galactorrhea, impotence, and decreased libido. Other hormonal effects vary.

Testicular failure (secondary). Commonly associated with mumps or other infectious disorders, secondary testicular failure produces bilateral gynecomastia that appears after normal puberty.

Thyrotoxicosis. Bilateral gynecomastia may occur with loss of libido and impotence.

Gastrointestinal

Cirrhosis. A late sign of cirrhosis, bilateral gynecomastia results from failure of the liver to inactivate circulating estrogens. It is often accompanied by testicular atrophy, decreased libido, impotence, and loss of facial, chest, and axillary hair.

Hepatic carcinoma. This carcinoma may produce bilateral gynecomastia and other characteristics of feminization, such as testicular atrophy, impotence, and reduced facial hair growth.

Genitourinary

Renal failure (chronic). This disorder may produce bilateral gynecomastia accompanied by decreased libido and impotence. Among its more characteristic features, though, are ammonia breath odor, oliguria, fatigue, decreased mental acuity, convulsions, muscle cramps, and peripheral neuropathy.

Testicular tumor. Choriocarcinomas, Leydig's cell tumors, and other testicular tumors typically cause bilateral gynecomastia, nipple tenderness, and decreased libido.

Genetic
Hermaphroditism. In true hermaphroditism, ovarian and testicular tissues coexist, resulting in external genitalia with both feminine and masculine characteristics. At puberty, the patient typically develops marked bilateral gynecomastia. About half of these patients also display male menstruation in the form of cyclic hematuria.
Klinefelter's syndrome. Painless bilateral gynecomastia first appears during adolescence in this genetic disorder.
Reifenstein's syndrome. This genetic disorder produces painless bilateral gynecomastia that appears at puberty.
Obstetrics-Gynecology
Breast cancer. Painful unilateral gynecomastia develops rapidly in this disorder.
Drugs
Typically, drugs produce painful unilateral gynecomastia. Estrogens used to treat prostatic cancer, including diethylstilbestrol, estramustine, and chlorotrianisene, directly affect the estrogen-androgen ratio. Drugs that have an estrogen-like effect, such as digitalis and human chorionic gonadotropin, may do the same. Regular marijuana or heroin use reduces plasma testosterone levels, causing gynecomastia. Other drugs—such as spironolactone, cimetidine, and ketoconazole—produce this sign by interfering with androgen production or action. Some common drugs, including phenothiazines, tricyclic antidepressants, and antihypertensives, produce gynecomastia in an unknown way.
Treatments
Gynecomastia may develop within weeks of starting hemodialysis for chronic renal failure. It may also follow major surgery or testicular irradiation.

Clinical considerations
• A history should be obtained and a physical examination performed; the examination should focus on the breasts, testicles, and penis.

• Diagnostic tests may include chest and skull X-rays and blood hormone levels.
• To make the patient as comfortable as possible, cold compresses should be applied to his breasts and analgesics administered, as ordered.
• Because gynecomastia may alter the patient's body image, emotional support should be provided. The patient should be reassured that treatment can reduce the gynecomastia and that surgical removal of breast tissue can be done, if necessary.

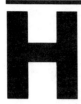

Halitosis

Description

Halitosis describes any breath odor that is unpleasant, disagreeable, or offensive. Usually it is easy to detect, but an embarrassed patient may take measures to hide it. Occasionally, the patient is not aware of halitosis, although he may complain of a bad taste in his mouth. Or he may believe he has halitosis, but no one else can detect it (psychogenic halitosis).

Certain types of halitosis characterize specific disorders; for example, a fruity breath odor typifies ketoacidosis. (See "Breath odor, ammonia;" "Breath odor, fecal;" "Breath odor, fruity;" and "Fetor hepaticus.") Other types of halitosis include putrid, foul, fetid, and musty breath odors.

This common sign may result from disorders of the oral cavity, nasal passages, sinuses, or respiratory tract. Halitosis may also stem from gastrointestinal disorders associated with belching, regurgitation, or vomiting. It may be a side effect of oral or inhalant drugs.

Usually, halitosis results from cigarette smoking and ingestion of alcohol and certain foods, such as garlic and onions. Poor oral hygiene—especially in the patient with an orthodontic device, dentures, or dental caries—commonly causes halitosis.

In children, halitosis commonly results from physiologic causes, such as continual mouth breathing and thumb or blanket sucking. However, phenylketonuria—a metabolic disorder that affects infants—may produce a musty or mousy breath odor.

Possible causes

Eyes, ears, nose, and throat

Gingivitis. Characterized by red, edematous gums, this disorder may also cause halitosis. The gingivae between the teeth become bulbous and bleed easily with slight trauma.

Acute necrotizing ulcerative gingivitis also causes fetid breath, a bad taste in the mouth, and ulcers—especially between the teeth—that may become covered with a gray exudate.

Necrotizing ulcerative mucositis (acute). A strong, putrid breath odor is characteristic here. Initially, this uncommon disorder causes slight cheek inflammation, which is rapidly followed by tooth loss and extensive bone sloughing in the mandible or maxilla.

Ozena. This severe, chronic form of rhinitis causes a musty or fetid breath odor. It also produces thick, green mucus and progressive anosmia.

Periodontal disease. In this disorder, halitosis is accompanied by an unpleasant taste. Typically, the patient's gums bleed spontaneously or with slight trauma and are marked by pus-filled pockets around the teeth.

Pharyngitis. Halitosis is a chief sign of this disorder.

Sinusitis. Acute sinusitis causes a purulent nasal discharge that leads to halitosis. *Chronic sinusitis* causes continuous mucopurulent discharge that leads to a musty breath odor.

Respiratory

Bronchiectasis. Usually, this disorder produces foul or putrid halitosis; however, some patients may have a sickeningly sweet breath odor. Typically, the patient also has a chronic productive cough with copious, foul-smelling, mucopurulent sputum.

Common cold. A musty breath odor may accompany the common cold.

Lung abscess. This disorder typically causes putrid halitosis. Its major sign, though, is a productive cough with copious, purulent, often bloody sputum.

Endocrine

Ketoacidosis. Both diabetic and starvation ketoacidosis produce a fruity breath odor.

Gastrointestinal

Bowel obstruction. Halitosis is a late sign of both small- and large-bowel obstruction. In *small-bowel obstruction*, vomiting of gastric, bilious, and then feculent material produces a related breath odor. In *large-bowel obstruction*, fecal vomiting produces fecal breath odor.

Esophageal cancer. In this disorder, halitosis may accompany classic findings of dysphagia, hoarseness, chest pain, and weight loss.

Gastric carcinoma. Halitosis is a late sign of this uncommon malignancy.

Gastrojejunocolic fistula. In this disorder, fecal vomiting is responsible for fecal breath odor. Typically, halitosis is preceded by intermittent diarrhea.

Hepatic encephalopathy. A characteristic late sign of this disorder is a musty, sweet, or mousy (new-mown hay) breath odor called fetor hepaticus.

Zenker's diverticulum. This esophageal disorder causes halitosis and a bad taste in the mouth associated with regurgitation.

Genitourinary

Renal failure (chronic). This disorder produces a urinous or ammonia breath odor.

Drugs

Triamterene and inhaled anesthetics can cause halitosis. So can paraldehyde, which is excreted through the lungs.

Clinical considerations

• A history should be obtained and an examination of the mouth, throat, and nose performed.

• If mouth and sinus examination does not reveal the cause of halitosis, upper GI and chest X-rays or endoscopy may be performed.

• To help control halitosis, good oral hygiene should be encouraged.

• If halitosis is drug-induced, the patient should be reassured that it will disappear as soon as his body eliminates the drug completely.

Hallucination

Description

A hallucination is sensory perception without corresponding external stimuli. Hallucinations may occur in depression, schizophrenia, bipolar disorder, organic brain disorders, and drug-induced and toxic conditions.

An *auditory hallucination* refers to the perception of nonexistent sounds—typically voices but occasionally music or other sounds. Occurring in schizophrenia, this is the most common type of hallucination.

An *olfactory hallucination*—a perception of nonexistent odors from the patient's own body or from some other person or object—is typically associated with somatic delusions. It occurs most often in temporal lobe lesions and may also occur in schizophrenia.

A *tactile hallucination* refers to the perception of nonexistent tactile stimuli, generally described as something crawling on or under the skin. It occurs mainly in toxic conditions and addiction to certain drugs. Formication—the sensation of insects crawling on the skin—most often occurs in alcohol withdrawal syndrome and cocaine abuse.

A *visual hallucination* is a perception of nonexistent images of people, flashes of light, or other scenes. It occurs most often in acute, reversible organic brain disorders but may also occur in drug and alcohol intoxication, schizophrenia, febrile illness, and encephalopathy.

A *gustatory hallucination* refers to the perception of nonexistent, usually unpleasant tastes. Head injury to the temporal area can cause this type of hallucination.

Halo vision
(Halos)

Description
Halo vision refers to seeing rainbow—like, colored rings around lights or bright objects. Occurring in ophthalmic disorders, halo vision usually develops suddenly; its duration depends on the causative disorder.

Nonpathologic causes of halos include poorly fitted or overworn contact lenses, emotional extremes, and exposure to intense light, as in snow blindness.

Mechanism
Halos may result from excessive tearing, corneal epithelial edema, or dispersion of light by abnormal opacities on the lens. The rainbowlike effect can be explained by this physical principle: as light passes through water (in the eye, through tears or the cells of various anteretinal media), it breaks up into spectral colors.

Possible causes
Eyes, ears, nose, and throat
Cataract. Halos may be an early symptom of painless, progressive cataract formation.
Corneal endothelial dystrophy. Typically, halos are a late symptom. Impaired visual acuity may also occur.
Glaucoma. Halos characterize all types of glaucoma. *Acute closed–angle glaucoma*—an ophthalmic emergency—also causes blurred vision followed by severe headache or

excruciating pain in and around the affected eye. Usually, *chronic closed–angle glaucoma* is asymptomatic until pain and blindness occur in advanced disease. Sometimes, halos and blurred vision develop slowly.

In *chronic open–angle glaucoma*, halos are a late symptom accompanied by mild eye ache, peripheral vision loss, and impaired visual acuity.

Clinical considerations
• A history should be obtained and visual acuity checked; an ophthalmoscopic examination should be performed.

• Tonometry should be performed to assess intraocular pressure.

• To help minimize halos, the patient should be reminded not to look directly at bright lights.

Hamman's sign

Description
Hammon's sign is a loud, crushing, crunching sound synchronous with the heart beat. Auscultated over the precordium, it reflects mediastinal emphysema, which occurs in such life–threatening conditions as pneumothorax and rupture of the trachea or bronchi. To detect this sign, the patient is placed in a left lateral recumbent position and gentle auscultation is performed over the precordium.

Harlequin sign

Description
Harlequin sign is a benign, erythematous color change occurring especially in low–birth–weight infants. This reddening of one longitudinal half of the body appears when the infant is placed on either side for a few minutes. When he is placed on his back, the sign usually disappears immediately but may persist up to 20 minutes.

Headache

Description

Headache refers to pain in the cranial vault, orbits, or nape of the neck (pain elsewhere in the face is not considered a headache). The most common neurologic symptom, a headache may be localized or generalized, producing mild–to–severe pain. About 90% of all headaches are benign (see *Comparing Benign Headaches*). Occasionally, though, this symptom indicates a severe neurologic disorder. A pathologic headache may result from disorders associated with intracranial inflammation, increased intracranial pressure, or meningeal irritation. In children over age 3, headache is the most common indicator of a brain tumor.

Headache may also result from ocular or sinus disorders and the effects of drugs, tests, and treatments. In certain metabolic disturbances—hypoxemia, hypercapnia, hyperglycemia, and hypoglycemia—headache may occur, but it is not a diagnostic or prominent symptom.

Among the many other causes of headache are fever, eyestrain, and dehydration. Some individuals get headaches from coughing, sneezing, heavy lifting, or stooping. Others experience headaches after seizures.

Mechanism

The basic mechanisms that result in headache are muscle contraction (tension headache), vascular (migraine or cluster headache), or a combination.

Possible causes

Central nervous system

Brain abscess. Here, headache is localized to the abscess site. Usually, it intensifies over a few days and is aggravated by straining. Accompanying the headache may be nausea, vomiting, and focal or generalized seizures. The patient's level of consciousness (LOC) will vary from drowsiness to deep stupor.

Brain tumor. Initially, this disorder causes a localized headache near the tumor site. The headache eventually becomes generalized as the tumor grows. Usually, it is intermittent, deep-seated and dull, and most intense in the morning. It is aggravated by coughing, stooping, Valsalva's maneuver, and changes in head position; it is relieved by sitting and rest.

Cerebral aneurysm (ruptured). Sudden, excruciating headache characterizes this life–threatening disorder. The headache may be unilateral and usually peaks within minutes of aneurysmal rupture. The patient may lose consciousness immediately or display a variably altered LOC.

Encephalitis. A severe, generalized headache is characteristic here. Typically, the patient's LOC then deteriorates within 48 hours—perhaps from lethargy to coma.

Epidural hemorrhage (acute). Usually, head trauma and immediate, brief loss of consciousness precede this hemorrhage, which causes a progressively severe headache. It is accompanied by nausea and vomiting, bladder distention, confusion, and then a rapid decrease in LOC.

Intracerebral hemorrhage. In some patients, this hemorrhage produces a severe generalized headache.

Meningitis. Sudden onset of a severe, constant, generalized headache that worsens with movement typifies this disorder.

Postconcussional syndrome. One to thirty days after head trauma, a generalized or localized headache may develop and last for 2 to 3 weeks. This characteristic symptom may be described as an aching, pounding, pressing, stabbing, or throbbing pain.

Subarachnoid hemorrhage. This hemorrhage commonly produces a sudden, violent headache.

Subdural hematoma. Typically associated with head trauma, both acute and chronic subdural hematomas may

Comparing Benign Headaches

Of the many patients who report headaches, only about 10% have an underlying medical disorder. The other 90% suffer from benign headaches, which may be muscle-contraction (tension), vascular (migraine and cluster), or a combination of both.

As the chart below shows, the two major types—muscle-contraction and vascular headaches—are quite different. In a combined headache, features of both appear. This headache may affect the patient with a severe muscle-contraction headache or a late-stage migraine. Treatment of a combined headache requires analgesics and sedatives.

Characteristics	Muscle-contraction headaches	Vascular headaches
Incidence	• Most common type, accounting for 80% of *all* headaches	• More common in women and those with a family history of migraines • Onset after puberty
Precipitating factors	• Stress, anxiety, or tension • Prolonged muscle contraction without structural damage • Eye, ear, and paranasal sinus disorders that produce reflex muscle contractions	• Hormone fluctuations • Alcohol • Emotional upset • Too little or too much sleep • Such foods as chocolate, cheese, monosodium glutamate, and cured meats • Weather changes, such as shifts in barometric pressure
Intensity and duration	• Produce an aching tightness or a band of pain around the head, especially in the neck, occipital, and temporal areas • Occur frequently and usually last for several hours	• May begin with an awareness of an impending migraine or a 5- to 15-minute prodrome of neurologic deficits such as visual disturbances; tingling of the face, lips, or hands; dizziness; or unsteady gait • Produce severe, constant, throbbing pain that's typically unilateral and may be incapacitating • Last for 4 to 6 hours
Associated signs and symptoms	• Tense neck and facial muscles	• Anorexia, nausea, and vomiting • Occasionally, photophobia, sensitivity to loud noises, weakness, and fatigue

(continued)

Comparing Benign Headaches (continued)

Characteristics	Muscle-contraction headaches	Vascular headaches
Associated signs and symptoms (continued)		• Depending on the type (classic, common, or hemiplegic migraine; or cluster headache), chills, depression, eye pain, ptosis, tearing, rhinorrhea, diaphoresis, and facial flushing may occur
Alleviating factors	• Mild analgesics, muscle relaxants, or other drugs during an attack • Measures to reduce stress, such as biofeedback, relaxation techniques and counseling, and posture correction to prevent attacks	• Methysergide and propranolol to prevent vascular headache • Ergot drugs at the first sign of a migraine • Rest in a quiet, darkened room • Elimination of irritating foods from diet

cause headache and decreased LOC. In *acute subdural hematoma*, head trauma produces immediate loss of consciousness followed by a latent period with headache, drowsiness, confusion, and agitation that may progress to coma.

Chronic subdural hematoma produces a dull, pounding headache that fluctuates in severity and is located over the hematoma.

Eyes, ears, nose, and throat

Glaucoma (acute closed–angle). This ophthalmic emergency may cause an excruciating headache.

Sinusitis (acute). Usually, a dull periorbital headache occurs in this disorder. The aching is typically aggravated by bending over or touching the face and is relieved by sinus drainage.

Cardiovascular

Hypertension. This disorder may cause a slightly throbbing occipital headache on awakening that decreases in severity during the day. However, if the patient's diastolic blood pressure exceeds 120 mm Hg, the headache remains constant.

Temporal arteritis. In this disorder, a throbbing unilateral headache in the temporal or frontotemporal region is typical.

Infectious diseases

Typhoid fever. Initially, this disorder causes a severe frontal headache, steadily increasing fever, abdominal discomfort, and constipation.

Infection

Influenza. A severe generalized or frontal headache usually begins suddenly with the flu. Accompanying signs and symptoms may last for 3 to 5 days and include stabbing retroorbital pain, weakness, diffuse myalgia, fever, chills, coughing, rhinorrhea, and occasionally hoarseness. However, cough and weakness may persist.

Psittacosis. Abrupt onset of an excruciating headache marks the beginning of this disorder. It is accompanied by fever, chills, malaise, and myalgia.

Drugs

Various drugs may cause headaches. For example, indomethacin produces headaches—usually in the morning—in about half of all patients. Vasodilators and drugs with a vasodilating effect, such as nitrates, typically cause a throbbing headache. This symptom may also follow withdrawal from vasopressors, such as caffeine, ergotamine, or sympathomimetic drugs.

Diagnostic tests
A pneumoencephalogram may produce a severe generalized headache, whereas a lumbar puncture or myelogram may produce a throbbing frontal headache.

Treatments
Cervical traction with pins commonly causes a headache, which may be generalized or localized to pin insertion sites.

Clinical considerations
• A history should be obtained and a neurologic assessment performed.

• Diagnostic tests may include skull X-rays, computed tomography, lumbar puncture, or cerebral arteriography.

• To help ease the headache, analgesics should be administered, as ordered. Also, the patient's room should be darkened and other stimuli minimized.

Hearing loss

Description
Affecting nearly 16 million Americans, hearing loss may be temporary or permanent and partial or complete. This common symptom may involve reception of low–, middle–, or high–frequency tones. If the hearing loss does not affect speech frequencies, the patient may be unaware of it.

Normally, sound waves enter the external auditory canal, then travel to the middle ear's tympanic membrane and ossicles (incus, malleus, and stapes) and into the inner ear's cochlea. The cochlear division of the eighth cranial (auditory) nerve carries the sound impulse to the brain. This type of sound transmission, called *air conduction*, is normally better than *bone conduction*—sound transmission through bone to the inner ear.

Hearing loss can be classified as conductive, sensorineural, mixed, and functional. *Conductive hearing loss* results from disorders of the external and middle ear that block sound transmission. *Sensorineural hearing loss*—also known as nerve deafness, perceptive deafness, or inner ear deafness—results from disorders of the inner ear, or the eighth cranial nerve. *Mixed hearing loss* combines aspects of both conductive and sensorineural hearing loss. *Functional hearing loss* results from psychological factors; no identifiable organic damage exists.

Hearing loss may result from trauma, infection, allergy, tumors, certain systemic and hereditary disorders, and the effects of ototoxic drugs and treatments. Most commonly, though, it results from presbycusis—a sensorineural hearing loss that usually affects those older than age 50. Other physiologic causes of hearing loss include cerumen (ear wax) impaction; barotitis media—unequal pressure on the eardrum—associated with descent in an airplane or elevator, diving, or close proximity to an explosion; and chronic exposure to noise over 90 decibels. This noise exposure can occur on the job, at a hobby, or from listening to live or recorded music.

Possible causes
Central nervous system
Head trauma. Sudden conductive or sensorineural hearing loss may result from ossicle disruption, ear canal fracture, or tympanic membrane perforation associated with head trauma. Typically, the patient will report a headache and have bleeding from his ear.

Multiple sclerosis. Rarely, this disorder causes sensorineural hearing loss associated with myelin destruction of the central auditory pathways. The hearing loss may be sudden and unilateral or intermittent and bilateral.

Differentiating Conductive and Sensorineural Hearing Loss

Conductive hearing loss produces:
- Abnormal Weber test
- Negative Rinne test
- Improved hearing in noisy areas
- Normal ability to discriminate sounds
- Difficulty hearing when chewing
- A quiet speaking voice

Sensorineural hearing loss produces:
- Abnormal Weber test
- Positive Rinne test
- Poor hearing in noisy areas
- Difficulty hearing high-frequency sounds
- Complaints that others mumble or shout
- Tinnitus

Eyes, ears, nose, and throat
Acoustic neuroma. This eighth cranial nerve tumor causes unilateral, progressive, sensorineural hearing loss.

Adenoid hypertrophy. Eustachian tube dysfunction gradually causes conductive hearing loss accompanied by intermittent ear discharge.

Allergies. Conductive hearing loss may result when an allergy produces eustachian tube and middle ear congestion.

Aural polyps. If a polyp occludes the external auditory canal, partial hearing loss may occur. Typically, the polyp bleeds easily and is covered by a purulent discharge.

Cholesteatoma. Gradual hearing loss characterizes this disorder. It is accompanied by vertigo and, occasionally, facial paralysis.

Cyst. Ear canal obstruction by a sebaceous or dermoid cyst causes progressive conductive hearing loss. On inspection, the cyst appears like a soft mass.

External ear canal tumor (malignant). Progressive conductive hearing loss is characteristic. It is accompanied by deep, boring ear pain, purulent discharge, and eventually facial paralysis.

Furuncle. A reversible conductive hearing loss may occur when one of these painful, hard nodules, or boils, forms in the ear.

Glomus jugulare tumor. Initially, this benign tumor causes a mild unilateral conductive hearing loss that becomes progressively more severe. The patient may report tinnitus that sounds like his heartbeat.

Glomus tympanium. This middle ear tumor causes slowly progressive hearing loss and throbbing or pulsating tinnitus.

Granuloma. A rare cause of conductive hearing loss, a granuloma may also produce fullness in the ear, deep-seated pain, and bloody discharge.

Ménière's disease. Initially, this inner ear disorder produces intermittent, unilateral sensorineural hearing loss that involves only low tones. Later, hearing loss becomes constant and affects other tones.

Myringitis. Rarely, *acute infectious myringitis* produces conductive hearing loss when fluid accumulates in the middle ear or a large bleb totally obstructs the ear canal.

Chronic granular myringitis produces a gradual hearing loss accompanied by pruritus and purulent discharge.

Nasopharyngeal cancer. This tumor causes mild, unilateral mixed hearing loss when it compresses the eustachian tube. Bone conduction is normal, and inspection reveals a retracted tympanic membrane backed by fluid.

Osteoma. Commonly affecting women and swimmers, osteoma may cause sudden or intermittent conductive hearing loss. Typically, bony projections are visible in the ear canal, but the tympanic membrane appears normal.

Otitis externa. Conductive hearing loss characterizes both acute and malignant otitis externa and results from debris in the ear canal.

Otitis media. Typically, this middle ear inflammation produces unilateral conductive hearing loss. In *acute suppurative otitis media*, the hearing loss develops gradually over a few hours. It is usually accompanied by an upper respiratory infection with sore throat, cough, nasal discharge, and headache. Hearing will return after the infection subsides. In *chronic otitis media*, hearing loss also develops gradually.

Often associated with an upper respiratory infection or nasopharyngeal carcinoma, *serous otitis media* commonly produces a stuffy feeling in the ear and pain that worsens at night.

Otosclerosis. In this hereditary disorder, unilateral conductive hearing loss usually begins in the early 20s and may gradually progress to bilateral mixed loss. The patient may report tinnitus and an ability to hear better in a noisy environment.

Ramsay Hunt syndrome. Associated with herpes infection, this syndrome causes sudden onset of severe unilateral mixed hearing loss. Vesicles appear in the external ear.

Tympanic membrane perforation. Often caused by trauma from sharp objects or rapid pressure changes, perforation of the tympanic membrane causes abrupt hearing loss.

Respiratory

Tuberculosis. This pulmonary infection may spread to the ear, resulting in eardrum perforation, mild conductive hearing loss, and cervical lymphadenopathy.

Cardiovascular

Temporal arteritis. This disorder may produce unilateral sensorineural hearing loss accompanied by throbbing unilateral facial pain, pain behind the eye, temporal or frontotemporal headache, and, occasionally, vision loss. Usually, the hearing loss is preceded by a prodrome of malaise, anorexia, weight loss, weakness, and myalgia that lasts for several days.

Endocrine

Hypothyroidism. This disorder may produce reversible sensorineural hearing loss.

Musculoskeletal

Skull fracture. Auditory nerve injury causes sudden unilateral sensorineural hearing loss.

Temporal bone fracture. This fracture causes sudden unilateral sensorineural hearing loss accompanied by hissing tinnitus. The tympanic membrane may be perforated, depending on the fracture's location.

Infectious diseases

Syphilis. In tertiary syphilis, sensorineural hearing loss may develop suddenly or gradually and usually affects one ear more than the other. It is usually accompanied by a gumma lesion—a chronic, superficial nodule or a deep, granulomatous lesion on the skin or mucous membranes.

Drugs

Typically, ototoxic drugs produce ringing or buzzing tinnitus and a feeling of fullness in the ear. Chloroquine, cisplatin, vancomycin, and aminoglycosides—especially neomycin, kanamycin, and amikacin—may cause irreversible hearing loss. Loop diuretics, such as furosemide, ethacrynic acid, and bumetanide, usually produce a brief, reversible hearing loss. Quinine, quinidine, or high doses of erythromycin or salicylates such as aspirin may also cause reversible hearing loss.

Treatments

Irradiation of the middle ear, thyroid, face, skull, or nasopharynx may cause eustachian tube dysfunction, resulting in hearing loss. Myringotomy, myringoplasty, simple or radical mastoidectomy, or fenestrations may cause scarring that interferes with hearing.

Clinical considerations

• A history should be obtained and an examination of the ear(s) performed.
• Hearing acuity should be evaluated.
• Audiometry and auditory evoked–response testing may be performed.

• After careful testing, the patient may require a hearing aid or cochlear implant to improve his hearing.
• The patient should be instructed to avoid exposure to loud noises to prevent further hearing loss.

Heat intolerance

Description
Heat intolerance refers to the inability to withstand high temperatures or to maintain a comfortable body temperature. It produces a continuous feeling of being overheated and, at times, profuse diaphoresis. Usually, this symptom develops gradually and is chronic.

Most often, heat intolerance results from thyrotoxicosis. In this disorder, excess thyroid hormone stimulates peripheral tissues, increasing basal metabolism and producing excess heat. Although rare, hypothalamic disease may also cause heat—and cold—intolerance by disrupting normal temperature control.

Possible causes
Endocrine
Hypothalamic disease. Among the common causes of this rare disease are pituitary adenoma and hypothalamic and pineal tumors. Here, body temperature fluctuates dramatically, causing alternating heat and cold intolerance.
Thyrotoxicosis. A classic symptom of thyrotoxicosis, heat intolerance may be accompanied by an enlarged thyroid, nervousness, weight loss despite increased appetite, diaphoresis, diarrhea, tremor, and palpitations. Although exophthalmos is characteristic, many patients do not display this sign. Associated findings may affect virtually every body system.
Drugs
Amphetamines and amphetamine–like appetite suppressants may increase basal metabolism, resulting in heat intolerance. Excessive doses of thyroid hormone may also cause heat intolerance.

Clinical considerations
• A history should be obtained and a physical examination performed.
• Diagnostic tests may include blood studies and skull X–rays.
• The patient's room temperature should be adjusted to a comfortable level.
• If the patient is diaphoretic, bed linens and clothing should be changed, as necessary; fluids should be encouraged.

Heberden's nodes

Description
Heberden's nodes are painless, irregular, bony enlargements of the distal finger joints. Approximately 2 to 3 mm in diameter, they develop on one or both sides of the dorsal midline. Usually, the dominant hand has larger nodes, which affect one or more fingers but not the thumb.

Repeated fingertip trauma may cause Heberden's nodes in only one joint ("baseball finger"). However, osteoarthritis is the most common

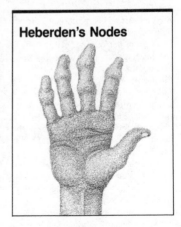

Heberden's Nodes

cause; in fact, Heberden's nodes occur in more than half of all osteoarthritic patients. Because the nodes are not associated with pain or loss of function, they are not a primary indicator of osteoarthritis but are a helpful adjunct to diagnosis.

Heberden's nodes reflect degeneration of articular cartilage, which irritates the bone and stimulates osteoblasts, causing bony enlargement.

Hematemesis

Description

Hematemesis is the vomiting of blood. It usually indicates gastrointestinal (GI) bleeding above the ligament of Treitz, which suspends the duodenum at its junction with the jejunum. Bright red or blood–streaked vomitus indicates fresh or recent bleeding. Dark red, brown, or black vomitus—about the color and consistency of coffee grounds—indicates that blood has been retained in the stomach and partially digested.

Most often, hematemesis results from GI disorders. It may also result from coagulation disorders and from treatments that irritate the GI tract. Swallowed blood from epistaxis or oropharyngeal erosions may also cause bloody vomitus.

Hematemesis is always an important sign, but its severity depends on the amount and source of the bleeding. Massive hematemesis (vomiting of 500 to 1,000 ml of blood) may rapidly be life–threatening. Hematemesis may be aggravated by straining, emotional stress, anti–inflammatory drugs, and alcohol ingestion.

Possible causes
Gastrointestinal
Achalasia. Rarely, this disorder produces hematemesis; passive regurgitation is much more common.

Esophageal carcinoma. A late sign of this disorder, hematemesis may be ac-

companied by steady chest pain that radiates to the back.

Esophageal injury. Ingestion of corrosive acids or alkalies produces esophageal injury associated with grossly bloody or "coffee ground" vomitus. This hematemesis is accompanied by epigastric and anterior or retrosternal chest pain that is intensified by swallowing. In 3 to 4 weeks, dysphagia, marked salivation, and fever may develop and worsen as strictures form.

Esophageal rupture. In this disorder, the severity of hematemesis depends on the cause of the rupture. When instrumentation damages the esophagus, hematemesis is usually slight. However, rupture from Boerhaave's syndrome—increased esophageal pressure from vomiting or retching—or other esophageal disorders typically causes more severe hematemesis.

Esophageal varices (ruptured). Life–threatening rupture of esophageal varices may produce "coffee ground" or massive, bright red vomitus. Signs of shock, such as hypotension or tachycardia, may follow or even precede hematemesis if the stomach fills with blood before vomiting occurs.

Gastric carcinoma. Painless bright red or dark brown hematemesis is a late sign of this uncommon cancer.

Gastritis (acute). Hematemesis and melena are the most common signs of this gastritis. In fact, they may be the only signs, although mild epigastric discomfort, nausea, fever, and malaise may also occur. Massive blood loss will precipitate signs of shock.

Gastroesophageal reflux disease. Although rare in this disorder, hematemesis may occur and even may lead to signs of shock, such as hypotension and tachycardia. It is accompanied by pyrosis, flatulence, dyspepsia, and postural regurgitation that is aggravated by laying down or stooping.

Gastrointestinal leiomyoma. Rarely, this benign tumor may involve the GI tract, eroding the mucosa or vascular

Managing Hematemesis with Intubation

If a patient has hematemesis, GI tube insertion should be anticipated to allow blood drainage, to aspirate gastric contents, or to perform gastric lavage. Here are some of the most common tubes and their uses.

Nasogastric tubes

The *Salem-Sump tube* (right), a double-lumen nasogastric tube, is used to remove stomach fluid and gas or to aspirate gastric contents. It may also be used for gastric lavage, drug administration, or feeding. Its main advantage over the *Levin tube*— a single-lumen nasogastric device—is that it allows atmospheric air to enter the patient's stomach so that the tube can float freely instead of risking adhesion and damage to the gastric mucosa.

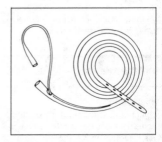

Wide-bore gastric tubes

The *Ewald tube,* a wide-bore tube that allows passage of a large amount of fluid and clots quickly, is especially useful for gastric lavage in patients with profuse GI bleeding or poison ingestion. Another wide-bore tube, the double-lumen *Levacuator,* has a large lumen for evacuation of gastric contents and a small one for lavage. The *Edlich tube* (right) has one wide-bore lumen with four openings near the closed distal tip. A funnel or syringe can be connected at the proximal end. Like the others, the Edlich can aspirate a large volume of gastric contents quickly.

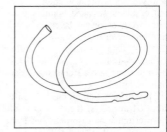

Esophageal tubes

The *Sengstaken-Blakemore tube* (right), a triple-lumen double-balloon esophageal tube, provides a gastric aspiration port that allows drainage from below the gastric balloon. It can also be used for instilling medication. A similar tube, the *Linton,* can aspirate esophageal and gastric contents without risking necrosis because it has no esophageal balloon. The *Minnesota esophagogastric tamponade tube,* which has four lumens and two balloons, provides pressure monitoring ports for both balloons without the need for Y connectors.

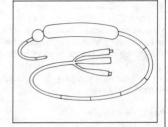

supply to produce hematemesis.

Mallory-Weiss syndrome. Characterized by a mucosal tear of the cardia or lower esophagus, this syndrome may produce hematemesis and melena. It is commonly triggered by severe vomiting, retching, or straining (as from coughing). Severe bleeding may precipitate signs of shock, such as tachycardia, hypotension, dyspnea, and cool, clammy skin.

Peptic ulcers. Hematemesis may occur here when a peptic ulcer penetrates an artery, vein, or highly vascular tissue. Massive—and possibly life–threatening—hematemesis is typical with penetration of an artery.

Hematologic

Coagulation disorders. Any disorder that disrupts normal clotting may cause GI bleeding and moderate–to–severe hematemesis. Bleeding may also occur in other body systems.

Treatments

Traumatic nasogastric or endotracheal intubation may cause hematemesis associated with swallowed blood. Nose or throat surgery may also cause this sign in the same way.

Clinical considerations

If the patient has massive hematemesis:
• Vital signs should be taken and the physician notified immediately.
• Emergency interventions should be anticipated to maintain an adequate airway and circulation, locate the bleeding site, and control the bleeding.
• The patient should be monitored closely and emergency equipment kept close by.

If the patient's hematemesis is not immediately life–threatening:
• A history should be obtained and a physical examination performed.
• Diagnostic tests may include serum electrolyte studies, endoscopy, and barium swallow.
• As the bleeding tapers off, hourly doses of antacids should be given by nasogastric tube, as ordered.

• Emotional support should be provided and frequent oral hygiene performed.

Hematochezia
(Rectal bleeding)

Description

Hematochezia is the passage of bloody stools. It usually indicates gastrointestinal (GI) bleeding below the ligament of Treitz. In fact, it may be the first sign of lower GI bleeding. However, hematochezia—usually preceded by hematemesis—may also accompany rapid hemorrhage of 1 liter or more from the upper GI tract.

Hematochezia ranges from formed, blood–streaked stools to liquid, bloody stools that may be bright red, dark mahogany, or maroon in color. Usually, hematochezia develops abruptly and is heralded by abdominal pain.

Although hematochezia commonly results from GI disorders, it may also result from coagulation disorders, the effects of toxins, and certain diagnostic tests. Always a significant sign, hematochezia may precipitate life–threatening hypovolemia.

Possible causes
Gastrointestinal

Anal fissure. Slight hematochezia characterizes this disorder; blood may streak the stool or appear on toilet tissue. Accompanying hematochezia is severe rectal pain that may make the patient reluctant to defecate, thereby causing constipation.

Angiodysplastic lesions. Most common in the elderly, these arteriovenous lesions of the ascending colon typically cause chronic, bright red rectal bleeding. Occasionally, this painless hematochezia may result in life–threatening blood loss and signs of shock, such as tachycardia and hypotension.

Anorectal fistula. Blood, pus, mucus, and occasionally stool may drain from this fistula.

Celiac disease. Rarely, this malabsorption syndrome causes bright red, liquid stools. More typically, it produces frothy, foul–smelling, fatty stools (steatorrhea) with diarrhea.

Colitis. *Ischemic colitis* often causes bloody diarrhea, especially in the elderly. The hematochezia may be slight or massive and is usually accompanied by severe cramping lower abdominal pain and hypotension. *Ulcerative colitis* typically causes bloody diarrhea that may also contain mucus. Occasionally, the hematochezia occurs at night. It is preceded by mild to severe abdominal cramps and may cause slight to massive blood loss.

Colon cancer. Although pain is the most common symptom here, bright red hematochezia is also a telling sign—especially in cancer of the left colon.

Colorectal polyps. These polyps are the most common cause of intermittent hematochezia in adults under age 60; however, they may cause no symptoms. When located high in the colon, polyps may cause blood–streaked stools; when closer to the rectum, they may bleed freely.

Crohn's disease. Although hematochezia is not a common sign of this disorder, it is usually associated with massive, life–threatening blood loss when it does occur.

Diverticulitis. Most common in the elderly, this disorder can suddenly cause mild–to–moderate rectal bleeding after the patient feels the urge to defecate. The bleeding may end abruptly or lead to life–threatening blood loss with signs of shock.

Esophageal varices (ruptured). In this life–threatening disorder, hematochezia may range from slight rectal oozing to grossly bloody stools. It may be accompanied by mild–to–severe hematemesis or melena. This painless—but massive—hemorrhage may precipitate signs of shock, such as tachycardia and hypotension. In fact, signs of shock occasionally precede overt signs of bleeding.

Hemorrhoids. Hematochezia may accompany external hemorrhoids, which typically cause painful defecation, resulting in constipation. Less painful internal hemorrhoids usually produce a constant oozing hematochezia that may eventually lead to signs of anemia, such as weakness and fatigue.

Peptic ulcers. GI bleeding is a frequent complication here. The patient may display hematochezia, hematemesis, or melena, depending on the rapidity and amount of bleeding.

Rectal melanoma (malignant). This rare rectal carcinoma typically causes recurrent rectal bleeding that arises from a painless, asymptomatic mass.

Small–intestine cancer. Rarely, this disorder produces slight hematochezia, or blood–streaked stools.

Ulcerative proctitis. Typically, this disorder causes an intense urge to defecate, but the patient passes only bright red blood, pus, or mucus.

Hematologic

Coagulation disorders. GI bleeding marked by moderate–to–severe hematochezia may occur. Bleeding may also occur in other body systems.

Infectious diseases

Typhoid fever. About 10% of patients with this disorder develop hematochezia, which is occasionally massive. However, melena is more common. Both signs of bleeding occur late and may be accompanied by mental dullness, marked abdominal distention, diarrhea, significant weight loss, and profound fatigue.

Infection

Dysentery. Bloody diarrhea is common in infection with *Shigella, Ameba,* and *Campylobacter*, but rare with *Salmonella*.

Leptospirosis. The severe form of this infection—Weil's syndrome—produces hematochezia or melena along with other signs of bleeding, such as epistaxis and hemoptysis. Typically, the bleeding is preceded by a sudden frontal headache and severe thigh and lumbar myalgia that may be accompanied by cutaneous hyperesthesia.

Environmental

Food poisoning (staphylococcal). One to six hours after ingesting food toxins, the patient may have bloody diarrhea. *Heavy metal poisoning.* Here, bloody diarrhea is accompanied by cramping abdominal pain, nausea, and vomiting.

Diagnostic tests

Certain procedures, such as colonoscopy and proctosigmoidoscopy, may cause bowel perforation and lead to rectal bleeding.

Clinical considerations

If the patient has severe hematochezia:
• Vital signs should be taken and the physician notified.
• If signs or symptoms of shock are present, emergency interventions should be anticipated to maintain circulation, locate the bleeding site, and control bleeding.
• The patient should be monitored closely for increased bleeding and signs and symptoms of shock.
If the patient's hematochezia is not immediately life–threatening:
• A history should be obtained and a physical examination performed.
• Diagnostic tests may include blood tests, endoscopy, and GI X–rays.
• The patient's stools should be visually examined and tested for occult blood. If necessary, a stool sample should be sent to the laboratory to check for parasites.
• Emotional support should be provided—hematochezia can be frightening for the patient.

Hematuria

Description

Hematuria is the presence of blood in the urine. By strict definition, it means three or more red blood cells per high–power microscopic field in the urine. Microscopic hematuria is confirmed by an occult blood indicator, whereas macroscopic hematuria is immediately visible. However, macroscopic hematuria must be distinguished from pseudohematuria (see *Confirming Hematuria,* p. 199). A cardinal indicator of renal and urinary tract disorders, this common sign may be continuous or intermittent, is often accompanied by pain, and may be aggravated by prolonged standing or walking.

Hematuria may be classified by the stage of urination it predominantly affects. Bleeding at the start of urination—*initial hematuria*—usually indicates urethral pathology; bleeding at the end of urination—*terminal hematuria*—usually indicates pathology of the bladder neck, posterior urethra, or prostate. Bleeding throughout urination—*total hematuria*—usually indicates pathology above the bladder neck. Another clue to the source of the bleeding is the color of hematuria. Usually, dark or brownish blood indicates renal or upper urinary tract bleeding, whereas bright red blood indicates lower urinary tract bleeding.

Although it usually results from renal and urinary tract disorders, hematuria may also result from certain gastrointestinal, prostate, vaginal, or coagulation disorders, or from the effects of drugs. Invasive therapy or diagnostic tests that involve manipulative instrumentation of the renal and urologic systems may also cause hematuria. Nonpathologic hematuria may result from fever and hypercatabolic states. Transient hematuria may also follow strenuous exercise.

Mechanism

Hematuria may result from one of two mechanisms: rupture or perforation of vessels in the renal system or urinary tract, or impaired glomerular filtration, which allows red blood cells to seep into the urine.

Possible causes

Cardiovascular

Endocarditis (subacute infective). Occasionally, this disorder produces embolization, resulting in renal infarction and microscopic or gross hematuria.

Renal vein thrombosis. Macroscopic, grossly bloody hematuria usually occurs with this thrombosis.

Vasculitis. Hematuria is usually microscopic in this disorder.

Gastrointestinal

Appendicitis. About 15% of appendicitis patients have either microscopic or macroscopic hematuria accompanied by bladder tenderness, dysuria, and urinary urgency.

Genitourinary

Bladder neoplasm. A primary cause of gross hematuria in men, this disorder may also produce pain in the bladder, rectum, pelvis, flank, back, or leg.

Bladder trauma. Gross hematuria is characteristic in traumatic rupture or perforation of the bladder. Typically, the hematuria is accompanied by lower abdominal pain and, occasionally, anuria despite a strong urge to void.

Calculi. Both bladder and renal calculi produce hematuria, which may be associated with signs of urinary tract infection, such as dysuria and urinary frequency and urgency. *Bladder calculi* usually cause gross hematuria, referred pain to the penile or vulvar area, and, in some patients, bladder distention. *Renal calculi* may produce microscopic or gross hematuria. The cardinal symptom, though, is colicky pain that travels from the costovertebral angle to the flank, the suprapubic region, and the external genitalia.

Cortical necrosis (acute). Accompanying gross hematuria in this renal disorder are intense flank pain, anuria, and fever.

Cystitis. Hematuria is a telling sign in all four types of cystitis. *Bacterial cystitis* usually produces macroscopic hematuria accompanied by urinary urgency and frequency, dysuria, nocturia, and tenesmus. More common in

women, *chronic interstitial cystitis* also causes grossly bloody hematuria. Both microscopic and macroscopic hematuria may occur in *tubercular cystitis*, which may also cause urinary urgency and frequency, dysuria, tenesmus, flank pain, fatigue, and anorexia. Usually, *viral cystitis* produces hematuria, urinary urgency and frequency, dysuria, nocturia, tenesmus, and fever.

Diverticulitis. When this disorder involves the bladder, it usually causes microscopic hematuria as well as urinary frequency and urgency, dysuria, and nocturia.

Glomerulonephritis. Usually, *acute glomerulonephritis* begins with gross hematuria that eventually tapers off to microscopic hematuria, which may persist for months.

Chronic glomerulonephritis usually causes microscopic hematuria accompanied by proteinuria, generalized edema, and increased blood pressure.

Nephritis (interstitial). Typically, this infection causes microscopic hematuria. However, some patients with *acute interstitial nephritis* may develop gross hematuria.

Obstructive nephropathy. This disorder may cause microscopic or macroscopic hematuria; however, it is rarely grossly bloody.

Polycystic kidney disease. This hereditary disorder may cause recurrent microscopic or gross hematuria.

Prostatic hypertrophy (benign). About 20% of these patients have macroscopic hematuria, usually when prostatic hypertrophy causes significant obstruction. Typically, the hematuria is preceded by diminished urinary stream, tenesmus, and a feeling of incomplete voiding.

Prostatitis. Whether it is acute or chronic, prostatitis may cause macroscopic hematuria, usually at the end of urination.

Pyelonephritis (acute). This infection typically produces microscopic or macroscopic hematuria that progresses to grossly bloody hematuria.

Confirming Hematuria

If the patient's urine appears blood-tinged, pseudohematuria—red- or pink-colored urine caused by urinary pigments—must be ruled out. First, the urine specimen should be carefully inspected. If it contains a red sediment, it is probably *true* hematuria.

  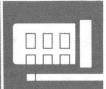

The patient's history should then be checked for use of drugs associated with pseudohematuria, including rifampin, chlorzoxazone, phenazopyridine, phenothiazines, doxorubicin, phensuximide, phenytoin, daunomycin, or laxatives with phenolphthalein.

The patient's diet should be assessed—intake of beets, berries, or foods with red dyes may color the urine red. Porphyrinuria or excess urate excretion may also cause pseudohematuria.

Finally, the urine should be tested using a chemical reagent strip, or "dip stick." This test can confirm hematuria—even if it's microscopic—and can also estimate the amount of blood present.

After the infection resolves, microscopic hematuria may persist for a few months.

Renal infarction. Typically, this disorder produces gross hematuria.

Renal neoplasm. The classic triad of signs and symptoms is macroscopic, grossly bloody hematuria; dull, aching flank pain; and a smooth, firm, palpable flank mass.

Renal papillary necrosis (acute). In this disorder, hematuria is usually macroscopic and grossly bloody.

Renal trauma. About 80% of patients with renal trauma will have microscopic or gross hematuria.

Renal tuberculosis. Gross hematuria is in many cases the first sign of this disorder.

Urethral trauma. Initial hematuria may occur here, possibly with blood at the urinary meatus, local pain, and penile or vulvar ecchymoses.

Musculoskeletal

Systemic lupus erythematosus. Gross hematuria and proteinuria may occur when this disorder involves the kidneys.

Hematologic

Coagulation disorders. Macroscopic hematuria is often the first sign of hemorrhage in coagulation disorders, such as thrombocytopenia or disseminated intravascular coagulation.

Sickle-cell anemia. In this hereditary disorder, gross hematuria may result from congestion of the renal papillae.

Obstetrics-Gynecology
Vaginitis. When this infection spreads to the urinary tract, it may produce macroscopic hematuria.
Infection
Schistosomiasis. This infection usually causes intermittent hematuria at the end of urination.
Drugs
Among common drugs that may cause hematuria are anticoagulants, cyclophosphamide (Cytoxan), metyrosine, phenylbutazone, oxyphenbutazone, and thiabendazole.
Treatments
Any therapy that involves manipulative instrumentation of the urinary tract, such as transurethral prostatectomy, may cause microscopic or macroscopic hematuria.
Diagnostic tests
Renal biopsy is the diagnostic test most commonly associated with hematuria. This sign may also result from biopsy or manipulative instrumentation of the urinary tract, as in cystoscopy.

Clinical considerations

• A history should be obtained and a physical examination performed.
• Diagnostic tests may include blood and urine studies, cystoscopy, and renal X-rays or biopsy.
• The patient should be taught how to collect serial urine specimens using the three–glass technique. This technique helps determine whether hematuria marks the beginning, end, or course of urination.
• Because hematuria may frighten and upset the patient, emotional support should be provided.
• Vital signs and fluid intake and output should be monitored at least every 4 hours.
• If appropriate, pain medications should be administered, as ordered.

Hemianopia

Description

Hemianopia is loss of vision in half the visual field (usually the vertical half) of one or both eyes. Its cause is a lesion affecting the optic chiasm, tract, or radiation. However, if the field defects are identical in both eyes but affect less than half the field of vision in each eye (incomplete homonymous hemianopia), the lesion may be in the occipital lobe; otherwise, it probably involves the parietal or temporal lobe. (See *Recognizing Types of Hemianopia*.)

Defects in visual perception due to cerebral lesions are usually associated with impaired color vision.

Possible causes
Central nervous system
Cerebrovascular accident (CVA). Hemianopia can result when a hemorrhagic, thrombotic, or embolic CVA affects any part of the optic pathway.
Occipital lobe lesion. The most common symptoms arising from a lesion of one occipital lobe include incomplete homonymous hemianopia, scotomas, and impaired color vision.
Parietal lobe lesion. This disorder produces homonymous hemianopia and sensory deficits, such as an inability to perceive body position or passive movement or to localize tactile, thermal, or vibratory stimuli. It may also cause apraxia and visual or tactile agnosia.
Cardiovascular
Carotid artery aneurysm. An aneurysm in the internal carotid artery can cause contralateral or bilateral defects in the visual fields.
Endocrine
Pituitary tumor. A tumor that compresses nerve fibers supplying the nasal half of both retinas causes complete

Recognizing Types of Hemianopia

Lesions of the optic pathways cause visual field defects. The lesion's site
determines the type of defect. For example, a lesion of the optic chiasm
involving only those fibers that cross over to the opposite side causes
bitemporal hemianopia—visual loss in the temporal half of each field. However, a lesion of the optic tract or a complete lesion of the optic radiation
produces visual loss in the same half of each field—either left or right
homonymous hemianopia.

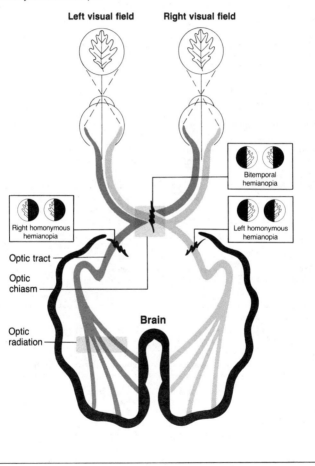

or partial bitemporal hemianopia that occurs first in the upper visual fields but later can progress to blindness.

Clinical considerations
• A history should be obtained and a complete neurologic and ophthalmologic examination performed.
• If the patient's visual field defect is significant, further visual field testing, such as perimetry or a tangent screen examination, may be done.
• The patient should be told the extent of his defect so that he learns to compensate for it. He should be advised to scan his surroundings frequently, turning his head in the direction of the defective visual field so he can directly view objects he would normally notice peripherally.
• The patient should be approached from the unaffected side. His bed should be positioned so his unaffected side faces the door; if he is ambulatory, objects that could cause falls should be removed and he should be alerted to other possible hazards.

Hemoptysis

Description
Hemoptysis is the expectoration of blood or bloody sputum from the lungs or tracheobronchial tree. It is sometimes confused with bleeding from the mouth, throat, nasopharynx, or gastrointestinal tract. (See *Identifying Hemoptysis*.) Expectoration of 200 ml of blood in a single episode suggests severe bleeding, whereas expectoration of 400 ml in 3 hours or more than 600 ml in 16 hours signals life–threatening crisis.

Hemoptysis most commonly results from chronic bronchitis, bronchogenic carcinoma, or bronchiectasis. However, it may also result from inflammatory, infectious, cardiovascular, or coagulation disorders—or, in up to 15% of patients, from unknown causes. Rarely, it stems from a ruptured aortic

aneurysm. The most common causes of *massive hemoptysis* are lung cancer, bronchiectasis, active tuberculosis, and cavitary pulmonary disease from necrotic infections or tuberculosis.

Mechanism
A number of pathophysiologic processes can cause hemoptysis. (See *What Happens in Hemoptysis*, p. 204.)

Possible causes
Eyes, ears, nose, and throat
Laryngeal cancer. Hemoptysis occurs with this disease, but hoarseness is the usual early sign.
Respiratory
Bronchial adenoma. This insidious disorder causes recurring hemoptysis in up to 30% of patients, along with a chronic cough and local wheezing.
Bronchiectasis. Inflamed bronchial surfaces and eroded bronchial blood vessels cause hemoptysis, which can vary from blood–tinged sputum to blood (in about 20% of patients). The patient's sputum may also be copious, foul–smelling, and purulent.
Bronchitis (chronic). The first sign of this disorder is typically a productive cough lasting at least 3 months. Eventually this leads to production of blood–streaked sputum; massive hemorrhage is unusual.
Lung abscess. In about 50% of patients, this disorder produces blood–streaked sputum resulting from bronchial ulceration, necrosis, and granulation tissue.
Lung cancer. Ulceration of the bronchus commonly causes recurring hemoptysis (an early sign), which can vary from blood–streaked sputum to blood.
Pneumonia. In up to 50% of patients, *Klebsiella pneumonia* produces dark brown or red (currant–jelly) sputum, which is so tenacious the patient has difficulty expelling it from his mouth. *Pneumococcal pneumonia* causes pinkish or rusty mucoid sputum.
Pulmonary arteriovenous fistula. Occurring in young adults, this genetic disor-

Identifying Hemoptysis

These guidelines can be used to help distinguish hemoptysis from epistaxis, hematemesis, and brown, red, or pink sputum.

Hemoptysis	Hematemesis	Brown, red, or pink sputum
Often frothy because it is mixed with air, hemoptysis is typically bright red with an alkaline pH (tested with nitrazine paper). It is strongly suggested by the presence of respiratory signs and symptoms—including a cough, a tickling sensation in the throat, and blood produced from repeated coughing episodes. (Epistaxis can be ruled out because the patient's nasal passages and posterior pharynx are usually clear.)	The usual site of hematemesis is the gastrointestinal tract; the patient vomits or regurgitates coffee-ground material that contains food particles, tests positive for occult blood, and has an acid pH. But he may vomit bright red blood or swallowed blood from the oral cavity and nasopharynx. After an episode of hematemesis, the patient may have stools with traces of blood. Many patients with hematemesis also complain of dyspepsia.	Brown, red, or pink sputum can result from oxidation of inhaled bronchodilators. Sputum that looks like old blood may result from rupture of an amebic abscess into the bronchus. Red or brown sputum may occur in a patient with pneumonia caused by the enterobacterium *Serratia marcescens*.

der causes intermittent hemoptysis.

Pulmonary contusion. Blunt chest trauma commonly causes a cough with hemoptysis.

Pulmonary edema. Severe cardiogenic or noncardiogenic pulmonary edema commonly causes frothy, blood–tinged pink sputum, which accompanies severe dyspnea, orthopnea, gasping, anxiety, cyanosis, diffuse crackles, a ventricular gallop, and cold, clammy skin.

Pulmonary embolism with infarction. Hemoptysis is a common finding in this life–threatening disorder, although massive hemoptysis is less common. Typical initial symptoms are dyspnea and anginal or pleuritic chest pain.

Pulmonary hypertension (primary). Features usually develop late. Hemoptysis, exertional dyspnea, and fatigue are common.

Pulmonary tuberculosis. Blood–streaked or –tinged sputum commonly occurs in this disorder; massive hemoptysis may occur in advanced cavitary tuberculosis.

Silicosis. Initially, this chronic disorder causes a productive cough with mucopurulent sputum. Subsequently, the sputum becomes blood–streaked and, occasionally, massive hemoptysis may occur.

Tracheal trauma. Torn tracheal mucosa may cause hemoptysis, hoarseness, dysphagia, neck pain, airway occlusion, and respiratory distress.

Cardiovascular

Aortic aneurysm (ruptured). Rarely, an aortic aneurysm ruptures into the tracheobronchial tree, causing hemoptysis and sudden death.

Wegener's granulomatosis. This multisystem disorder is characterized by necrotizing, granulomatous vasculitis. Pulmonary findings include hemoptysis, chest pain, cough, wheezing, dyspnea, epistaxis, severe sinusitis, and hemorrhagic skin lesions.

Musculoskeletal

Systemic lupus erythematosus. In 50% of patients with this disorder, pleuritis and pneumonitis cause hemoptysis, cough, dyspnea, pleuritic chest pain, and crackles.

Hematologic

Coagulation disorders. Such disorders as thrombocytopenia and disseminated intravascular coagulation can cause hemoptysis.

Diagnostic tests

Lung or airway injury from bronchoscopy, laryngoscopy, mediastinoscopy, or lung biopsy can cause bleeding and hemoptysis.

Clinical considerations

If hemoptysis is severe:

• Emergency interventions to maintain an adequate airway should be instituted and the physician notified immediately.

• Blood transfusion and fluid replacement should be anticipated.

• Emergency bronchoscopy should be anticipated to locate the bleeding site.

If hemoptysis is mild:

• A history should be obtained and a respiratory assessment performed.

• Diagnostic tests may include a complete blood count, a sputum culture and smear, chest X–rays, coagulation studies, bronchoscopy, lung biopsy, pulmonary arteriography, or a lung scan.

• The patient may react to this alarming sign with anxiety and apprehension. Consequently, he should be comforted and reassured and placed in a slight Trendelenburg position to promote drainage of blood from the lung. If necessary to protect the nonbleeding lung, he should be placed in the lateral decubitus position, with the suspected bleeding lung facing down.

• Cough suppression may or may not be desirable: cough suppressants can prevent blood from spreading throughout the lungs, but they can also lead to airway obstruction from accumulated blood.

• Although hemoptysis usually stops (but not abruptly) during treatment of

---

What Happens in Hemoptysis

Hemoptysis results from bleeding into the respiratory tract by bronchial or pulmonary vessels. Bleeding reflects alterations in the vascular walls and in blood-clotting mechanisms. It can reflect any of the following pathophysiologic processes.

Hemorrhage and diapedesis of red blood cells from the pulmonary microvasculature into the alveoli

Necrosis of lung tissue that causes inflammation and rupture of blood vessels or hemorrhage into the alveolar spaces

Rupture of an aortic aneurysm into the tracheobronchial tree

Rupture of distended endobronchial blood vessels from pulmonary hypertension caused by mitral stenosis

Rupture of a pulmonary arteriovenous fistula or of bronchial or pulmonary artery/pulmonary venous collateral channels

Sloughing of a caseous lesion into the tracheobronchial tree

Ulceration and erosion of the bronchial epithelium

the causative disorder, many chronic disorders cause recurrent hemoptysis. The patient should be instructed to report recurring episodes and to bring a sputum sample containing blood if he returns for treatment or reevaluation.

Hemorrhage, subungual

Description
Subungual hemorrhage refers to bleeding under the nail plate. Hemorrhagic lines, called splinter hemorrhages, run proximally from the distal edge and serve as an indicator of subacute bacterial endocarditis and trichinosis. Large hemorrhagic areas usually reflect nail bed injury.

Hepatomegaly

Description
Hepatomegaly means liver enlargement. This sign indicates potentially reversible primary or secondary liver disease. It is seldom a patient's major complaint. It usually comes to light during palpation and percussion of the GI system. Hepatomegaly may be confirmed by radiologic tests. It may be mistaken for displacement of the liver by the diaphragm in a respiratory disorder; by an abdominal tumor; by a spinal deformity such as kyphosis; by the gallbladder; or by fecal material or a neoplasm in the colon.

Mechanism
Hepatomegaly may stem from diverse pathophysiologic mechanisms: dilated hepatic sinusoids (in congestive heart failure), persistently high venous pressure leading to liver congestion (in chronic constrictive pericarditis), dysfunction and engorgement of hepatocytes (in hepatitis), fatty infiltration of parenchymal cells causing fibrous tissue (in cirrhosis), distention of liver cells with glycogen (in diabetes), and infiltration of amyloid (in amyloidosis).

Possible causes
Cardiovascular
Congestive heart failure. This disorder produces hepatomegaly due to visceral edema.

Pericarditis. In chronic constrictive pericarditis, an increase in systemic venous pressure produces marked congestive hepatomegaly.

Endocrine
Diabetes mellitus. Poorly controlled diabetes in overweight patients often produces fatty infiltration of the liver, hepatomegaly, and right upper quadrant tenderness along with polydipsia, polyphagia, and polyuria. These features are more common in Type II than in Type I diabetes. The chronically enlarged fatty liver is typically asymptomatic except for slight tenderness.

Gastrointestinal
Cirrhosis. Late in this disorder, the liver becomes enlarged, nodular, and hard. Other late signs and symptoms affect the entire body.

Hepatic abscess. Hepatomegaly may accompany fever (a primary sign), nausea, vomiting, chills, weakness, diarrhea, anorexia, and right upper quadrant pain and tenderness.

Hepatic neoplasms. Primary tumors commonly cause hepatomegaly, with pain or tenderness in the right upper quadrant and a friction rub or bruit over the liver.

Hepatitis. In viral hepatitis, early signs and symptoms include nausea, anorexia, vomiting, fatigue, malaise, photophobia, sore throat, cough, and headache. Hepatomegaly occurs in the icteric phase and continues during the recovery phase.

Pancreatic cancer. In this disorder, hepatomegaly accompanies such classic signs and symptoms as anorexia, weight loss, abdominal or back pain, and jaundice.

Hematologic
Leukemia and lymphomas. These proliferative blood cell disorders com-

monly cause moderate–to–massive hepatomegaly and splenomegaly as well as abdominal discomfort.

Metabolic

Amyloidosis. This rare disorder can cause hepatomegaly and mild jaundice.

Obesity. Hepatomegaly can result from fatty infiltration of the liver. Weight reduction reduces liver size.

Infection

Infectious mononucleosis. Occasionally, this disorder causes hepatomegaly.

Clinical considerations

• Diagnostic tests may include hepatic enzyme, alkaline phosphatase, bilirubin, albumin, and globulin studies to evaluate liver function and X–rays, liver scan, celiac arteriography, and ultrasonography to confirm hepatomegaly.

• Bed rest, relief from stress, and adequate nutrition should be provided to help protect liver cells from further damage and to allow the liver to regenerate functioning cells.

Hiccups
(Singultus)

A hiccup is a characteristic sound produced by involuntary diaphragm contraction followed by rapid closure of the glottis.

Usually benign and transient, hiccups are common and most often subside spontaneously or with simple treatment. However, in a patient with a neurologic disorder, they may indicate increasing intracranial pressure or extension of a brain stem lesion. They may also occur after ingestion of hot or cold liquids or other irritants, after exposure to cold, or with irritation from a drainage tube. Persistent hiccups cause considerable distress and may lead to vomiting.

Increased serum levels of carbon dioxide may inhibit hiccups; decreased levels may accentuate them.

Mechanism

Hiccups may result from irritations in the chest or abdomen that trigger transmission of impulses through the vagus (afferent) and the phrenic (efferent) nerves to the diaphragm. Hiccups occur as a two–stage process: an involuntary, spasmodic contraction of the diaphragm followed by sudden closure of the glottis. Their characteristic sound reflects the vibration of closed vocal cords as air suddenly rushes into the lungs.

Possible causes

Central nervous system

Brain stem lesion. Producing persistent hiccups, this lesion causes decreased level of consciousness, dysphagia, dysarthria, an absent corneal reflex on the side opposite the lesion, altered respiratory patterns, abnormal pupillary response, and ocular deviation.

Increased intracranial pressure. Early findings may include hiccups, drowsiness, and headache. Classic later signs include changes in pupillary reactions and respiratory pattern, increased systolic pressure, and bradycardia.

Respiratory

Pleural irritation. Besides hiccups, this condition may cause cough, dyspnea, or chest pain.

Gastrointestinal

Abdominal distention. The most common cause of hiccups, abdominal distention also causes a feeling of fullness and, depending on the cause, abdominal pain, nausea, and vomiting.

Gastric dilatation. Besides hiccups, possible clinical features include a sense of fullness, epigastric pain, and regurgitation or persistent vomiting.

Gastritis. This disorder can cause hiccups along with mild epigastric discomfort (sometimes the only symptom).

Pancreatitis. Hiccups, vomiting, and sudden and steady epigastric pain (often radiating to the back) may occur in this disorder.

Genitourinary

Chronic renal failure. Hiccups may occur in the late stages of this disorder.

Treatments

Occasionally, mild and transient attacks of hiccups may follow abdominal surgery.

Clinical considerations

• A history should be obtained and a physical examination performed.

• The patient should be taught simple methods of relieving hiccups, such as increasing his serum carbon dioxide level by holding his breath repeatedly or by rebreathing into a paper bag.

• Other treatments include gastric lavage or finger pressure on the eyeballs (applied through closed lids). If hiccups persist, a phenothiazine (especially chlorpromazine) or nasogastric intubation may provide relief. (*Caution*: The tube may cause vomiting.) If simpler methods fail, treatment may include a phrenic nerve block.

High birth weight

Description

High birth weight can be defined as neonatal weight that exceeds the 90th percentile for the gestational age of the infant. The high–birth–weight neonate is at increased risk for birth trauma, respiratory distress, hypocalcemia, hypoglycemia, and polycythemia.

Hill's sign

Description

Hill's sign is a femoral systolic pulse pressure 60 to 100 mm Hg higher in the right leg than in the right arm. Hill's sign may indicate severe aortic insufficiency. To detect this sign, the examiner places the patient in a supine position and takes blood pressure readings first in the right arm and then in the right leg, noting the difference.

Hirsutism

Description

Hirsutism is the excessive growth of dark, coarse body hair in females. Excessive androgen production stimulates hair growth on the pubic region, axilla, chin, upper lip, cheeks, anterior neck, sternum, linea alba, forearms, abdomen, back, and upper arms. In *mild hirsutism*, fine and pigmented hair appears on the sides of the face and the chin (but does not form a complete beard) and on the extremities, chest, abdomen, and perineum. In *moderate hirsutism*, coarse and pigmented hair appears on the same areas. In *severe hirsutism*, coarse hair also covers the whole beard area, the proximal interphalangeal joints, and the ears and nose.

Depending on the degree of excess androgen production, hirsutism may be associated with acne and increased skin oiliness, menstrual irregularity, and increased libido. Extremely high androgen levels cause further virilization, such as deepening of the voice, muscle hypertrophy, and temporal hair recession. Defeminization may also occur, producing signs such as amenorrhea, breast atrophy, and loss of female body contour.

Hirsutism may result from endocrine abnormalities and idiopathic causes. It may also occur in pregnancy due to transient androgen production by the placenta or corpus luteum, and in menopause due to increased androgen and decreased estrogen production.

Possible causes

Endocrine

Acromegaly. About 15% of patients with this chronic, progressive disorder display hirsutism.

Adrenocortical carcinoma. This disorder produces rapidly progressive hirsutism along with truncal obesity, buffalo hump, moon face, oligomenorrhea, amenorrhea, muscle wasting, and thin skin with purple striae.

Cushing's disease. Facial hirsutism is a common finding. This disorder also causes increased hair growth on the abdomen, breasts, chest, or upper thighs.

Hyperprolactinemia. This disorder produces hirsutism, hypogonadism, galactorrhea, amenorrhea, and acne.

Obstetrics-Gynecology

Ovarian overproduction of androgens. The most common cause of hirsutism, this condition is associated with anovulation progressing slowly over several years.

Ovarian tumor. Sometimes asymptomatic, this disorder can cause rapidly progressing hirsutism—but only if the tumor produces androgens. Amenorrhea and rapidly developing virilization are additional findings.

Polycystic ovary disease. Ovarian cysts—particularly chronic ones—can cause hirsutism. This usually occurs after the onset of menstrual irregularities, which may begin at puberty.

Drugs

Hirsutism can result from drugs containing androgens or progestins, aminoglutethimide, glucocorticoids, metoclopramide, cyclosporine, and minoxidil.

Clinical considerations

- A history should be obtained and a physical examination performed.
- Diagnostic tests may include tests to determine blood levels of luteinizing hormone, follicle–stimulating hormone, prolactin, and other hormones. Other studies may include computed tomography scan and ultrasonography.
- To relieve the patient's anxiety, the cause of excessive hair growth should be explained to her and she should be encouraged to talk about her self–image problems or fears. The family should be involved in discussions.
- At the patient's request, information should be provided on methods for eliminating excess hair—bleaching, tweezing, hot wax treatments, chemical depilatories, shaving, and electrolysis.

Hoarseness

Description

Hoarseness is a rough or harsh sound to the voice. It can result from infections or inflammatory lesions or exudates of the larynx, from laryngeal edema, and from compression or disruption of the vocal cords or recurrent laryngeal nerve. This common sign can also result from a thoracic aortic aneurysm, vocal cord paralysis, and systemic disorders, such as Sjögren's syndrome and rheumatoid arthritis. It is characteristically worsened by excessive alcohol intake, smoking, inhalation of noxious fumes, cheering, and shouting.

Hoarseness can be acute or chronic. For example, chronic hoarseness and laryngitis (an occupational hazard of clergymen and singers) result when irritating polyps form on the vocal cords. It may also result from progressive atrophy of the laryngeal muscles and mucosa due to aging, leading to diminished control of the vocal cords.

Possible causes

Eyes, ears, nose, and throat

Laryngeal cancer. Hoarseness is an early sign of vocal cord cancer, but may not occur until later in cancer of other laryngeal areas.

Laryngitis. Persistent hoarseness may be the only sign of *chronic laryngitis*. In *acute laryngitis*, hoarseness or a complete loss of voice develops suddenly.

Vocal cord paralysis. Unilateral vocal cord paralysis causes hoarseness and vocal weakness.

Vocal cord polyps. Raspy hoarseness, the chief complaint, accompanies a chronic cough and a crackling voice.

Respiratory

Inhalation injury. Inhalation injury from a fire or explosion produces hoarseness and coughing, singed nasal hairs, orofacial burns, and soot–stained sputum.

Pulmonary tuberculosis. In this disorder, hoarseness may be present if treatment has been delayed, but it is not an early finding.

Tracheal trauma. Torn tracheal mucosa may cause hoarseness, hemoptysis, dysphagia, neck pain, airway occlusion, and respiratory arrest.

Cardiovascular

Thoracic aortic aneurysm. Although typically asymptomatic, this aneurysm may cause hoarseness. Its most common symptom, however, is penetrating pain that is especially severe when the patient is supine.

Endocrine

Hypothyroidism. In this disorder, hoarseness may be an early sign.

Musculoskeletal

Rheumatoid arthritis. Hoarseness may signal laryngeal involvement.

Immunologic

Sjögren's syndrome. This immune disorder produces hoarseness, but its cardinal signs are dry eyes and mouth.

Treatments

Occasionally, surgical severing of the recurrent laryngeal nerve results in permanent unilateral vocal cord paralysis, leading to hoarseness. Prolonged intubation or a tracheostomy may cause temporary hoarseness.

Clinical considerations

• A history should be obtained and a physical examination performed.
• The patient should be carefully observed for stridor (which may indicate bilateral vocal cord paralysis), and other signs of respiratory distress.
• The doctor may perform indirect laryngoscopy, observing the larynx at rest and during phonation.
• The importance of resting the voice should be stressed: talking—even whispering—further traumatizes the vocal cords. Other ways to communicate (such as using pen and paper or body language) should be suggested, as needed.
• The patient should be urged to avoid alcohol, smoking, and smoke–filled environments.

• The patient should be told to report hoarseness lasting more than 2 weeks to the physician.

Hoehne's sign

Description

Hoehne's sign is the absence of uterine contractions during delivery, despite repeated doses of oxytocic drugs. This sign indicates a ruptured uterus.

Hoffmann's sign

Description

Hoffmann's sign is flexion of the terminal phalanx of the thumb and the second and third phalanx of another finger when the nail of the index, middle, or ring finger is snapped. A bilateral or strongly unilateral response suggests a pyramidal tract disorder, such as spastic hemiparesis. To elicit this sign, the examiner dorsiflexes the patient's wrist, has him flex his fingers, then snaps the nail of his index, middle, or ring finger.

Hoffman's sign also refers to increased sensitivity of sensory nerves to electrical stimulation, as in tetany.

Homans' sign

Description

Homans' sign is positive when deep calf pain results from strong and abrupt dorsiflexion of the ankle. This pain results from venous thrombosis or inflammation of the calf muscles. However, because a positive Homans' sign appears in only 35% of patients with these conditions, it is an unreliable indicator. Even when accurate, a positive Homans' sign does not indicate the extent of the venous disorder.

This elicited sign may be confused with continuous calf pain, which can

Eliciting Homans' Sign

To elicit this sign, the examiner first supports the patient's thigh with one hand and his foot with the other. He bends the patient's leg slightly at the knee, then firmly and abruptly dorsiflexes the ankle. Resulting deep calf pain indicates a positive Homans' sign. (The patient may also resist ankle dorsiflexion or flex the knee involuntarily if Homans' sign is positive.)

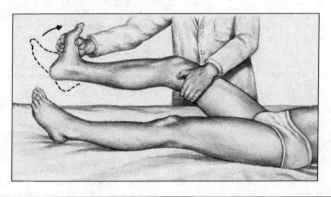

result from strains, contusions, cellulitis, or arterial occlusion; or with pain in the posterior ankle or Achilles' tendon (for example, in a woman with Achilles' tendons shortened from wearing high heels).

Possible causes
Cardiovascular
Deep vein thrombophlebitis. A positive Homans' sign and calf tenderness may be the only clinical features of this disorder.
Deep vein thrombosis (DVT). DVT causes a positive Homans' sign along with tenderness over the deep calf veins, slight edema of the calves and thighs, a low–grade fever, and tachycardia.

Clinical considerations
• A history should be obtained and the affected leg assessed.
• For further assessment, a blood pressure cuff that is wrapped around each calf should be inflated, as ordered, and the pressures at which the patient first reports pain compared. Pain occurring at a cuff pressure of less than 180 mm Hg indicates DVT or thrombophlebitis. However, because this test may dislodge a clot, the patient must be closely monitored for sudden onset of signs and symptoms of pulmonary embolism—dyspnea, cough, pleural pain, and tachycardia. If any of these occurs, the physician should be notified immediately.
• The patient should be placed on bed rest with the affected leg elevated above heart level and warm, moist compresses applied to the affected area.
• Mild oral analgesics should be administered, as ordered and needed.

Hoover's sign

Description
Hoover's sign is inward movement of one or both costal margins with inspiration. Bilateral movement occurs in

emphysema with acute respiratory distress. Unilateral movement occurs in intrathoracic disorders that cause flattening of one half of the diaphragm.

Hyperacusis

Description
Hyperacusis refers to abnormally acute hearing resulting from increased irritability of the auditory neural mechanism.

Hyperesthesia

Description
Hyperesthesia is increased cutaneous sensitivity to touch, temperature, or pain.

Hypernasality

Description
Hypernasality is a voice quality reflecting excessive expiration of air through the nose during speech. It is often associated with symptoms of dysarthria and possibly with swallowing defects. The sudden onset of hypernasality may indicate a neuromuscular disorder. This sign may also accompany cleft palate, a short soft and hard palate, abnormal nasopharyngeal size, and partial or complete velar paralysis. To detect this sign, the patient is asked to extend vowel sounds first with the nostrils open, then closed (pinched). A significant shift in tone may indicate hypernasality.

Hyperpigmentation
(Hypermelanosis)

Description
Hyperpigmentation is unusual darkening of the skin. It most commonly results from exposure to sunlight. However, it can also result from metabolic, endocrine, neoplastic, and inflammatory disorders; chemical poisoning; drugs; genetic defects; thermal burns; ionizing radiation; and localized activation by sunlight of certain photosensitizing chemicals on the skin.

Many types of benign hyperpigmented lesions occur normally. Some—such as acanthosis nigricans and carotenemia—may also accompany certain disorders, but their significance is unproven. Chronic nutritional insufficiency may lead to dyspigmentation—increased pigmentation in some areas and decreased pigmentation in others.

Typically asymptomatic and chronic, hyperpigmentation is a common problem that can have distressing psychological and social implications. It varies in location and intensity and may fade over time.

Mechanism
Hyperpigmentation usually reflects overproduction, abnormal location, or maldistribution of melanin—the dominant brown or black pigment found in skin, hair, mucous membranes, nails, brain tissue, cardiac muscle, and parts of the eye. This sign can also reflect abnormalities of other skin pigments: carotenoids (yellow), oxyhemoglobin (red), and hemoglobin (blue).

Possible causes
Endocrine
Acromegaly. This disorder results from a pituitary tumor that secretes excessive amounts of growth hormone after puberty. Hyperpigmentation (possibly acanthosis nigricans) may affect the face, neck, genitalia, axillae, palmar creases, and new scars.

Adrenocortical insufficiency. This disorder produces diffuse tan, brown, or bronze–to–black hyperpigmentation of both exposed and unexposed areas—the face, knees, knuckles, elbows, beltline, palmar creases, lips, gums, tongue, and buccal mucosa (where hyperpigmentation may be bluish black). Normally pigmented areas, moles, and scars become darker. Early in the disorder, hyperpigmentation occurs as persistent tanning after exposure to the sun.

Thyrotoxicosis. This disorder can cause hyperpigmentation on the face, neck, genitalia, axillae, and palmar creases as well as in new scars.

Gastrointestinal

Biliary cirrhosis. Hyperpigmentation is a classic feature of this disorder, which primarily affects women between the ages of 40 and 60. A widespread and accentuated brown hyperpigmentation appears on areas exposed to sunlight, but not on the mucosa.

Laennec's cirrhosis. After about 10 years of excessive alcohol ingestion, progressive liver dysfunction causes diffuse, generalized hyperpigmentation on sun–exposed areas.

Skin

Malignant melanoma. This form of cancer causes malignant lesions of pigmented skin, commonly moles. Common sites include the head and neck in men, the legs in women, and the backs in both men and women who are exposed to excessive sunlight; it rarely appears in the conjunctiva, choroid, pharynx, mouth, vagina, or anus. Up to 70% of lesions arise from a pre-existing nevus.

The cardinal sign of malignant melanoma is a skin lesion or nevus that enlarges, changes color, becomes inflamed, itches, ulcerates, bleeds, changes texture, or develops associated halo nevus or vitiligo. Coloring of lesions varies: brown or black around the edges and red, blue, black, or gray in the central raised area. Bleeding and ulceration may occur.

Porphyria cutanea tarda. Primarily affecting men between ages 40 and 60, this disorder produces generalized brownish hyperpigmentation on sun–exposed areas and extreme skin fragility (particularly on a bald scalp and on the face and hands).

Scleroderma. Localized and systemic scleroderma produce generalized dark brown hyperpigmentation that is related to sun exposure.

Hematologic

Hemochromatosis. In this inherited disorder (also called bronzed diabetes), most common in men between ages 40 and 60, early and progressive hyperpigmentation results from melanin (and possibly iron) deposits in the skin. Hyperpigmentation develops as generalized bronzing and metallic gray areas accentuated over sun–exposed areas, genitalia, and scars.

Environmental

Arsenic poisoning. Chronic arsenic poisoning can cause diffuse hyperpigmentation with scattered freckle–sized areas of normal or depigmented skin.

Drugs

Hyperpigmentation can stem from use of barbiturates, phenolphthalein, and salicylates; chemotherapeutic agents such as busulfan, cyclophosphamide, procarbazine, and nitrogen mustard; chlorpromazine; antimalarial drugs such as hydroxychloroquine; hydantoin; minocycline; metals such as silver (in argyria) and gold (in chrysiasis); adrenocorticotropic hormone; and phenothiazines.

Clinical considerations

• A history should be obtained and a physical examination performed, including a detailed assessment of the skin.
• Wood's lamp, a special ultraviolet light, may be used to help enhance the contrast between normal and hyperpigmented epidermis. A skin biopsy can help confirm the cause of hyperpigmentation.
• Emotional support should be provided because hyperpigmentation may persist even after treatment of the underlying disorder or withdrawal of the drug. Bleaching creams may not be effective either if most of the excess melanin lies in subepidermal skin layers. Over–the–counter bleaching creams tend to be in-

effective because they contain less then 2% hydroquinone.

• The patient should be advised to use corrective cosmetics, to avoid excessive sun exposure, and to apply a sunscreen or sunblocker, such as zinc oxide cream. The patient who stops using bleaching agents should be advised to continue using sunblockers, because rebound hyperpigmentation can occur.

• Every patient with a benign hyperpigmented area should be warned to consult the physician if the lesion's size, shape, or color changes; this may signal a developing malignancy.

Hyperpnea

Description
Hyperpnea indicates increased respiratory effort for a sustained period—a normal rate (at least 12 breaths/minute) with increased depth (a tidal volume greated that 500 ml), an increased rate (over 20 breaths/minute) with normal depth, or increased rate and depth. Hyperpnea differs from sighing (intermittent deep inspirations). However, it is also correctly called *tachypnea* (increased respiratory rate) when the depth of respirations remains normal, thereby increasing minute volume.

The typical patient with hyperpnea breathes at a normal or an increased rate and inhales deeply, displaying marked chest expansion. He may complain of shortness of breath if he has a respiratory disorder causing hypoxemia, or he may not be aware of his breathing if he has a metabolic or neurologic disorder causing involuntary hyperpnea. Other causes of hyperpnea include profuse diarrhea or dehydration, ureterosigmoidostomy, and loss of pancreatic juice or bile from gastrointestinal drainage. All these conditions cause a loss of bicarbonate ions, resulting in metabolic acidosis. Of course, hyperpnea may also accompany strenuous exercise, and voluntary

hyperpnea can aid relaxation in patients experiencing stress or pain—as in labor.

Hyperventilation, a form of hyperpnea associated with respiratory alkalosis, results in excessive exhalation of carbon dioxide (indicated by an arterial pH above 7.45 and a PCO_2 below 35). In central neurogenic hyperventilation, brain stem dysfunction (as in severe head injury) increases the rate and depth of respirations. In acute intermittent hyperventilation, the respiratory pattern may be a response to hypoxemia, anxiety, fear, pain, or excitement. It may also be a compensatory mechanism to metabolic acidosis.

Kussmaul's respirations, another form of hyperpnea, occur as a compensatory response to excessive carbon dioxide levels.

Possible causes
Central nervous system
Head injury. Hyperpnea that results from severe head injury is called central neurogenic hyperventilation. Whether its onset is acute or gradual, this type of hyperpnea indicates damage to the lower midbrain or upper pons. Accompanying signs of head injury reflect the site and extent of injury.
Respiratory
Hypoxemia. Many pulmonary disorders that cause hypoxemia—for example, pneumonia, pulmonary edema, chronic obstructive pulmonary disease, and pneumothorax—may cause hyperpnea and episodes of hyperventilation with chest pain, dizziness, and paresthesia.
Cardiovascular
Shock. Potentially life–threatening metabolic acidosis produces Kussmaul's respirations, hypotension, tachycardia, narrowed pulse pressure, weak pulse, dyspnea, oliguria, anxiety, restlessness, stupor that can progress to coma, and cool, clammy skin.
Metabolic
Ketoacidosis. Alcoholic ketoacidosis (occurring most often in females with a history of alcohol abuse) typically

follows cessation of drinking after a marked increase in alcohol consumption has caused severe vomiting. Kussmaul's respirations begin abruptly; they accompany vomiting for several days, slight dehydration, abdominal pain and distention, and absent bowel sounds. The patient is alert and has a normal blood glucose level, unlike the patient with diabetic ketoacidosis.

Diabetic ketoacidosis is potentially life–threatening and typically produces Kussmaul's respirations.

Starvation ketoacidosis is also potentially life–threatening and can cause Kussmaul's respirations. Its onset is gradual.
Genitourinary
Renal failure. Acute or chronic renal failure can cause life–threatening acidosis with Kussmaul's respirations.
Psychiatric
Hyperventilation syndrome. Acute anxiety triggers episodic hyperpnea, resulting in respiratory alkalosis.
Infection
Sepsis. A severe infection may cause lactic acidosis, resulting in Kussmaul's respirations.
Drugs
Toxic levels of salicylates, acetazolamide and other carbonic anhydrase inhibitors, and ammonium chloride cause Kussmaul's respirations. So can ingestion of methanol and ethylene glycol, found in antifreeze solutions.

Clinical considerations
If hyperpnea is detected in a patient with signs and symptoms of such life–threatening conditions as increased intracranial pressure, metabolic acidosis, diabetic ketoacidosis, or uremia:
• Rapid intervention should be carried out to provide ventilatory support and prevent cardiovascular collapse.
If the patient's condition is not serious:
• A history should be obtained and a physical examination performed.
• Vital signs should be monitored and the patient observed for signs of increasing respiratory distress or an irregular respiratory pattern signaling deterioration.
• Diagnostic tests include arterial blood gas analysis and blood chemistry studies.

Hypoesthesia

Description
Hypoesthesia is decreased cutaneous sensitivity to touch, temperature, or pain.

Hypopigmentation
(Hypomelanosis)

Description
Hypopigmentation is a decrease in normal skin, hair, mucous membrane, or nail color. This sign may be congenital or acquired, asymptomatic or associated with other findings. Its causes include genetic disorders, nutritional deficiency, chemicals and drugs, inflammation, infection, and physical trauma. Typically chronic, hypopigmentation can be difficult to identify if the patient is light–skinned or has only slightly decreased coloring.

Mechanism
Hypopigmentation results from deficiency, absence, or abnormal degradation of the pigment melanin.

Possible causes
Musculoskeletal
Discoid lupus erythematosus. This form of lupus erythematosus may produce hypopigmentation following inflammatory skin eruptions.
Skin
Idiopathic guttate hypomelanosis. Common in lightly pigmented people over age 30, this skin disorder produces sharply marginated, angular white spots on sun–exposed extremities. In blacks, hypopigmentation occurs mainly on the upper arms.

Leprosy. This chronic disorder affects the skin and peripheral nervous system. Erythematous or hypopigmented macules have decreased or absent sensation for light, touch, and warmth. The lesions do not sweat, so the skin feels dry and rough; it may be scaly.

Tinea versicolor. This benign fungal skin infection produces scaly, sharply defined hypopigmented lesions, usually on the upper trunk, neck, and arms.

Vitiligo. This common skin disorder produces sharply defined, flat white macules and patches ranging in diameter from 1 to over 20 cm. Usually bilaterally symmetrical, lesions appear on sun-exposed areas; in body folds; around the eyes, nose, mouth, and rectum; and over bony prominences. They are typically asymptomatic but may be pruritic. Hypopigmented patches (halo nevi) may surround pigmented moles.

Infectious diseases

Inflammatory and infectious disorders. Skin disorders, such as psoriasis, and infectious disorders, such as viral exanthems or syphilis, can cause transient or permanent hypopigmentation.

Environmental

Burns. Thermal and radiation burns can cause transient or permanent hypopigmentation.

Chemicals. Most phenolic compounds—for example, amylphenol and paratertiary butylphenol (PTBP), germicides used in many household and industrial products—can cause hypopigmentation. Monobenzyl ether of hydroquinone—contained in rubber products—produces permanent hypopigmented spots, resembling vitiligo, at the contact site (but they may spread).

Drugs

Topical or intralesional administration of corticosteroids causes hypopigmentation at the treatment site. Chloroquine, an antimalarial drug, may cause hair depigmentation (including eyebrows and lashes) and poor tanning. These effects occur 2 to 5 months after therapy begins.

Clinical considerations

• A history should be obtained and an examination of the skin performed.

• In fair-skinned patients, a special ultraviolet light (Wood's lamp) can help differentiate hypopigmented lesions, which appear pale, from depigmented lesions, which appear white.

• The patient should be advised to use corrective cosmetics to help hide skin lesions, and to use a sunblock because hypopigmented areas may sunburn easily.

• The patient should be encouraged to have regular examinations for early detection and treatment of lesions that may become premalignant or malignant.

• The doctor may prescribe repigmentation therapy, combining a photosensitizing drug (psoralen) and ultraviolet light, wavelength A.

• The patient should be referred for counseling, if appropriate, to reduce anxiety caused by skin lesions.

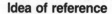

Idea of reference

Description
An idea of reference is a delusion that other people, statements, actions, or events have a meaning specific to oneself. This delusion occurs in schizophrenia and paranoid states.

Illusion

Description
An illusion is a misperception of external stimuli—usually visual or auditory (an example: the sound of the wind being perceived as a voice). Illusions occur normally as well as in schizophrenia and toxic states.

Impotence

Description
Impotence is the inability to achieve and maintain penile erection sufficient to complete satisfactory intercourse; ejaculation may or may not be affected. Impotence varies from occasional and minimal to permanent and complete. Occasional impotence occurs in about half of adult American men, whereas chronic impotence affects about 10 million American men.

Impotence can also be classified as primary or secondary. A man with *primary impotence* has never been potent with a partner but may achieve normal erections in other situations. This uncommon condition is difficult to treat. *Secondary impotence* carries a more favorable prognosis because, despite present erectile dysfunction, the patient has succeeded in completing intercourse in the past.

Organic causes of impotence may include vascular disease, diabetes mellitus, hypogonadism, a spinal cord lesion, alcohol and drug abuse, and surgical complications. (The incidence of organic impotence associated with other medical problems increases after age 50.) Psychogenic causes range from performance anxiety and marital discord to moral or religious conflicts.

Mechanism
Penile erection involves increased arterial blood flow secondary to psychological, tactile, or other sensory stimulation. Trapping of blood within the penis produces increased length, circumference, and rigidity. Impotence results when any component of this process—psychological, vascular, neurologic, or hormonal—malfunctions.

Possible causes
Central nervous system
Central nervous system disorders. Spinal cord lesions from trauma produce sudden impotence. A complete lesion above S2 (upper motor neuron lesion) disrupts descending motor tracts to the genital area, causing loss of voluntary erectile control but not the reflexive ability for erection and ejaculation. But a complete lesion in

the lumbosacral spinal cord (lower motor neuron lesions) causes loss of reflex ejaculation and reflex erection. Spinal cord tumors and degenerative diseases of the brain and spinal cord (such as multiple sclerosis and amyotrophic lateral sclerosis) cause progressive impotence.

Peripheral neuropathy. Systemic diseases, such as chronic renal failure and diabetes mellitus, can cause progressive impotence if they progress to peripheral neuropathy. This occurs in about 50% of male diabetics.

Cardiovascular

Vascular disorders. Various vascular disorders can cause impotence. These include advanced arteriosclerosis affecting both major and peripheral blood vessels; Leriche's syndrome—slowly developing occlusion of the terminal abdominal aorta; and arteriosclerosis, thrombosis, or embolization of smaller vessels supplying the penis.

Endocrine

Endocrine disorders. Hypogonadism from testicular or pituitary dysfunction may lead to impotence from deficient secretion of androgens (primarily testosterone). Adrenocortical and thyroid dysfunction and chronic hepatic disease may also cause impotence due to these organs' roles (although minor) in sex hormone regulation.

Genitourinary

Penile disorders. Peyronie's disease makes erection painful because the penis is bent, and may make penetration difficult and eventually impossible. Phimosis prevents erection until circumcision releases constricted foreskin. Other inflammatory, infectious, or destructive diseases of the penis may also cause impotence.

Trauma. Traumatic injury involving the penis, urethra, prostate, perineum, or pelvis may cause sudden impotence. This can result from structural alteration, nerve damage, or interrupted blood supply.

Psychiatric

Psychological distress. Impotence can result from diverse psychological

---

Impotence: An Unsought Effect

Many commonly used drugs—especially antihypertensives—can cause impotence that may be reversible if the drug is discontinued or the dosage reduced. Here are some examples.

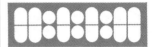

amitriptyline	methyldopa
atenolol	naproxen
cimetidine	nortriptyline
clonidine	perphenazine
desipramine	prazosin
digoxin	propranolol
hydralazine	thiazide diuretics
imipramine	thioridazine
methantheline bromide	tranylcypromine

---

causes, including depression, performance anxiety, memories of previous traumatic sexual experiences, moral or religious conflicts, and troubled emotional or sexual relationships.

Drugs

Alcohol and drug abuse are associated with impotence, as are many prescription drugs, especially antihypertensives. (See *Impotence: An Unsought Effect*.)

Treatments

Surgical injury to the penis, bladder neck, urinary sphincter, rectum, or perineum can cause impotence. So can injury to local nerves or blood vessels.

Clinical considerations

• A history should be obtained and a physical examination performed.

• Diagnostic tests may include screening tests for hormonal irregularities and for Doppler readings of penile blood pressure to rule out vascular insufficiency. Other possible tests include voiding studies, nerve conduction tests, evaluation of nocturnal penile tumescence, and psychological screening.

• Care should begin by establishing rapport with the patient. Probably no other medical condition in the male is as potentially frustrating, humiliating, even devastating to self–esteem and significant relationships as impotence.

• The patient should be made to feel comfortable about discussing his sexuality.

• Treatment for psychogenic impotence may include counseling of both the patient and his sexual partner; treatment for organic impotence focuses on reversing the cause, if possible. Other forms of treatment include surgical revascularization, drug–induction erection, surgical repair of venous leak, and penile prostheses.

• The patient should be encouraged to maintain follow–up appointments and treatment for underlying medical disorders.

Incontinence, fecal

Description

Fecal incontinence is the involuntary passage of feces. It follows any loss or impairment of external anal sphincter control and can result from various gastrointestinal, neurologic, and psychological disorders, the effects of drugs, and surgery. In some patients, it may even be a purposeful manipulative behavior.

Fecal incontinence may be temporary or permanent; its onset may be gradual, as in dementia, or sudden, as in spinal cord trauma. Although usually not a sign of severe illness, it can greatly affect the patient's physical and psychological well–being.

Possible causes

Central nervous system

Cerebrovascular accident. Temporary fecal incontinence occasionally occurs but usually disappears with the restoration of muscle tone and deep tendon reflexes. Persistent fecal incontinence may reflect extensive neurologic damage.

Dementias. Any of these chronic degenerative brain diseases can produce fecal incontinence.

Head trauma. Disruption of the neurologic pathways that control defecation can cause fecal incontinence.

Multiple sclerosis. Fecal incontinence occasionally appears as one of this disorder's extremely variable signs.

Spinal cord lesions. Any lesion that causes compression or transection of sensorimotor spinal tracts can lead to fecal incontinence. Incontinence may be permanent, especially with severe lesions of the sacral segments.

Gastrointestinal

Gastroenteritis. Severe gastroenteritis may result in temporary fecal incontinence manifested by explosive diarrhea.

Inflammatory bowel disease. Nocturnal fecal incontinence occurs occasionally with diarrhea.

Rectovaginal fistula. Fecal incontinence occurs in tandem with uninhibited passage of flatus.

Drugs

Chronic laxative abuse may cause insensitivity to a fecal mass or loss of the colonic defecation reflex.

Treatments

Pelvic, prostate, or rectal surgery occasionally produces temporary fecal incontinence. Colostomy or ileostomy causes permanent or temporary fecal incontinence.

Clinical considerations

• A history should be obtained and a physical examination performed.

• The pattern of incontinence should be determined and a stool sample obtained.

• Fecal impaction should be ruled out.

Bowel Retraining Tips

To help a patient control fecal incontinence, a bowel retraining program may be instituted, as described below.
● A specific time should be established for defecation. A typical schedule: once a day or once every other day after a meal, usually breakfast. However, the schedule should be kept flexible and consideration given to the patient's normal habits and preferences.
● If necessary, a suppository (either glycerin or bisacodyl) should be administered about 30 minutes before the time scheduled for defecation, to help ensure regularity. The routine use of enemas or laxatives should be avoided because they can cause dependence.
● To encourage regularity, privacy and a relaxed environment should be provided. If "accidents" occur, the patient should be assured that they are normal and do not represent a failure of the program.
● The patient's diet should be adjusted, if necessary, to provide adequate bulk and fiber; he should be encouraged to eat more raw fruits and vegetables and whole grains. A fluid intake of at least 1,000 ml/day should be ensured.
● If appropriate, the patient should be encouraged to exercise regularly to help stimulate peristalsis.
● Accurate intake and elimination records should be kept.

● Effective hygienic care should be maintained, including control of odors.
● Emotional support should be provided because the patient may feel deep embarrassment.
● For the patient with intermittent or temporary incontinence, Kegel exercises should be taught, as appropriate, to strengthen abdominal and perirectal muscles.

● For the neurologically capable patient with chronic incontinence, bowel retraining (see *Bowel Retraining Tips*) should be provided.

Incontinence, urinary

Description

Urinary incontinence is the uncontrollable passage of urine. It results from bladder abnormalities or neurologic disorders. A common urologic sign, incontinence may be transient or permanent, and may involve large volumes of urine or scant dribbling. It can be classified as stress, overflow, urge, or total incontinence. *Stress incontinence* refers to intermittent leakage resulting from a sudden physical strain, such as a cough, sneeze, or quick movement. *Overflow incontinence* is a dribble resulting from urine retention, which fills the bladder and prevents it from contracting with sufficient force to expel a urinary stream. *Urge incontinence* refers to the inability to suppress a sudden urge to urinate. *Total incontinence* is continuous leakage resulting from the bladder's inability to retain any urine.

Possible causes
Central nervous system

Cerebrovascular accident. Urinary incontinence may be transient or permanent.
Diabetic neuropathy. Autonomic neuropathy may cause painless bladder distention with overflow incontinence.
Guillain–Barré syndrome. Urinary incontinence may occur early in this disorder as a result of peripheral and autonomic nerve dysfunction.
Multiple sclerosis (MS). Urinary incontinence, urgency, and frequency are common urologic findings in MS.
Spinal cord injury. Complete cord transection above the sacral level causes flaccid paralysis of the bladder. Overflow incontinence follows rapid bladder distention.

Correcting Incontinence with Bladder Retraining

The incontinent patient typically feels frustrated, embarrassed, and sometimes hopeless. Fortunately, though, his problem can often be corrected by bladder retraining—a program that aims to establish a regular voiding pattern. Here are some guidelines for establishing such a program:

Before the program starts, the patient's intake pattern, voiding pattern, and behavior (for example, restlessness or talkativeness) should be assessed prior to each voiding episode.

The patient should be encouraged to use the toilet 30 minutes before he is usually incontinent. If this is not successful, the schedule should be readjusted. Once he is able to stay dry for 2 hours, the time between voidings should be increased by 30 minutes each day until he achieves a 3- to 4-hour voiding schedule.

When the patient voids, care should be taken to ensure that the sequence of conditioning stimuli is always the same.

The patient should have privacy while voiding—any inhibiting stimuli should be avoided.

To help reinforce the patient's efforts to remain continent, a record of continence and incontinence should be kept for 5 days.

Successful bladder retraining requires a positive attitude on the part of both patient and caregiver. Here are some additional tips that may help the patient succeed:

The patient should be kept close to a bathroom or portable toilet. A light should be kept on at night.

If the patient needs assistance getting out of his bed or chair, his call for help should be answered promptly.

To show the patient that the caregiver is confident he can remain continent, he should be encouraged to wear his accustomed clothing. Acceptable alternatives to diapers include condoms for the male patient and incontinence pads or panties for the female patient.

The patient should be encouraged to drink 2,000 to 2,500 ml of fluid each day. Less fluid does not prevent incontinence but does promote bladder infection. Limiting his intake after 5 p.m., however, will help him remain continent during the night.

The patient should be reassured that any episodes of incontinence do not signal a failure of the program. He should be encouraged to maintain a persistent, tolerant attitude.

Genitourinary

Benign prostatic hypertrophy. Overflow incontinence is common in this disorder as a result of urethral obstruction and urinary retention.

Bladder calculus. Overflow incontinence may occur if the stone lodges in the bladder neck.

Bladder cancer. Obstruction by a tumor may produce overflow incontinence.

Prostatic cancer. Urinary incontinence usually appears only in the advanced stages of this cancer.

Prostatitis (chronic). Urinary incontinence may occur as a result of urethral obstruction from an enlarged prostate.

Urethral stricture. Eventually, overflow incontinence may occur in this disorder.

Treatments

Urinary incontinence may occur after prostatectomy as a result of urethral sphincter damage.

Clinical considerations

• A history should be obtained and a physical examination performed.

• Diagnostic tests may include cystoscopy, cystometry, and a complete neurologic workup.

• Management of incontinence includes bladder retraining (see *Correcting Incontinence with Bladder Retraining*).

• Kegel exercises should be taught, as necessary, to strengthen pelvic floor muscles.

• If the patient's incontinence has a neurologic basis, he should be monitored for urinary retention, which may require periodic catheterizations. If appropriate, the patient should be taught self–catheterization techniques.

• A patient with permanent urinary incontinence may require surgical creation of a urinary diversion.

Insomnia

Description

Insomnia is the inability to fall asleep, remain asleep, or feel refreshed by sleep. Acute and transient during periods of stress, insomnia may become chronic and cause constant fatigue, extreme anxiety as the bedtime hour approaches, or even psychiatric disorders. A common complaint, it is experienced occasionally by about 25% of Americans and chronically by another 10%.

Physiologic causes of insomnia include jet lag, arguing, and lack of exercise. Its pathophysiologic causes range from medical and psychiatric disorders to pain, drug side effects, and idiopathic factors. Complaints of insomnia are subjective and require close investigation; the patient may mistakenly attribute to insomnia his fatigue from an organic cause, such as anemia.

Possible causes

Central nervous system

Nocturnal myoclonus. In this seizure disorder, involuntary and fleeting muscle jerks of the legs occur every 20 to 40 seconds, disturbing sleep.

Sleep apnea syndrome. Apneic periods begin with the onset of sleep, continue for 10 to 90 seconds, then end with a series of gasps and arousal. In *central sleep apnea*, respiratory movement ceases for the apneic period; in *obstructive sleep apnea*, upper airway obstruction blocks incoming air, although breathing movements continue. Some patients display both types of apnea. Repeated possibly hundreds of times during the night, this cycle alternates with bradycardia and tachycardia.

Endocrine

Pheochromocytoma. This rare disorder causes paroxysms of acute hypermetabolic activity, which can prevent or interrupt sleep.

Thyrotoxicosis. Chronic signs and symptoms of hypermetabolism include insomnia, in which the patient has difficulty falling asleep and sleeps for only a brief time.

Skin

Pruritic conditions. Localized skin infections and systemic disorders, such as liver failure, can cause pruritus with resultant insomnia.

Psychiatric

Affective disorders. Depression commonly causes chronic insomnia with difficulty falling asleep, waking and being unable to fall back to sleep, or waking early in the morning. Episodes of *mania* produce a decreased need for sleep with an elevated mood and irritability.

Generalized anxiety disorder. Hyperattentiveness from anxiety can cause chronic insomnia.

Drugs

Use or abuse of, or withdrawal from, sedatives or hypnotics may produce insomnia. Central nervous system stimulants—including amphetamines, theophylline derivatives, ephedrine, phenylpropanolamine, cocaine, and caffeine–containing beverages—may also produce insomnia. Abrupt cessation of alcohol after long–term use causes insomnia that may persist for up to 2 years.

Clinical considerations

• A history should be obtained and a physical examination performed.
• Diagnostic tests may include blood and urine studies for 17–hydroxycorticosteroids and catecholamines; sleep EEG; or polysomnography (including an EEG, electrooculography, and electrocardiography).
• As appropriate, the patient should be taught comfort and relaxation techniques to promote natural sleep.
• The patient should be advised to awaken and retire at the same time each day and to exercise regularly.
• The patient should be advised to get up but remain inactive when he cannot

sleep, and to use his bed only for sleeping, not relaxation.
• The patient should be advised to use tranquilizers or sedatives for acute insomnia only when relaxation techniques fail.
• If appropriate, the patient should be referred for counseling or to a sleep disorder clinic for biofeedback training or other interventions.

Intermittent claudication

Description

Most common in the legs, intermittent claudication is cramping limb pain brought on by exercise and relieved by 1 or 2 minutes of rest. It may be acute or chronic—when acute, it may signal acute arterial occlusion. Intermittent claudication occurs most often in men between the ages of 50 and 60; without treatment, it may progress to pain at rest. In chronic arterial occlusion, limb loss is uncommon because collateral circulation usually develops.

Mechanism

In occlusive artery disease, intermittent claudication results from an inadequate blood supply. Pain in the calf (the most common area) or foot indicates disease of the femoral or popliteal arteries; pain in the buttocks and upper thigh, disease of the aortoiliac arteries. During exercise, the pain typically results from the release of lactic acid due to anaerobic metabolism in the ischemic segment, secondary to atherosclerosis. When the patient stops exercising, the lactic acid clears and the pain subsides.

Intermittent claudication may also have a neurologic cause: narrowing of the vertebral column at the level of the cauda equina. This creates pressure on the nerve roots to the lower extremities. Walking stimulates circulation to the cauda equina, causing increased pressure on those nerves and pain.

Possible causes
Central nervous system
Neurogenic claudication. Neurospinal disease causes pain from intermittent claudication that requires a longer rest time than the 2 to 3 minutes needed in vascular claudication.
Cardiovascular
Acute arterial occlusion. This disorder produces intense intermittent claudication—sudden severe or aching leg pain aggravated by exercise.

Aortic arteriosclerotic occlusive disease. In this disorder, intermittent claudication occurs in the buttock, hip, thigh, and calf, along with absent or diminished femoral pulses.

Arteriosclerosis obliterans. This disorder usually affects the femoral and popliteal arteries, causing intermittent claudication (the most common symptom) in the calf.

Buerger's disease. Typically, this disorder produces intermittent claudication of the instep.

Clinical considerations
If the patient experiences *sudden intermittent claudication* along with severe or aching leg pain at rest:
• A rapid assessment of the affected leg should be performed and the physician notified immediately.
• The leg should be protected from pressure but not elevated.
• Surgery should be anticipated and the patient prepared acordingly.

If the patient has *chronic intermittent claudication*:
• A history should be obtained and a cardiovascular assessment performed.
• If intermittent claudication interferes with the patient's life–style, he may undergo diagnostic tests (Doppler flow studies, arteriography, and digital subtraction angiography) to determine the location and degree of occlusion.
• The patient with intermittent claudication should be counseled about risk factors. He should be encouraged to stop smoking, and be referred to a support group, if appropriate.

• Exercise should be promoted to improve collateral circulation and increase venous return, and the patient should be advised to avoid prolonged sitting or standing as well as crossing his legs at the knees.
• The patient should be taught to inspect his legs and feet for ulcers; to keep his extremities warm, clean, and dry; and to avoid injury.
• The patient should be instructed to immediately report skin breakdown that does not heal. He should also be urged to report any chest discomfort. (When circulation is restored to his legs, increased exercise tolerance may lead to angina if he has coronary artery disease that was previously asymptomatic as a result of exercise limitations.)

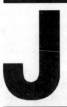

Janeway's spots

Description
Janeway's spots are small, erythematous lesions (1 to 4 mm in diameter) on the palms and soles. They are slightly raised, irregular, and nontender. Janeway's spots blanch with pressure and with elevation of the affected extremity; rarely, they form a diffuse rash over the trunk and extremities. They disappear spontaneously.

Janeway's spots are a common finding in infective acute and subacute endocarditis and may reflect an immunologic reaction to the infecting organism. They are a telltale sign of this disorder if other lesions (such as petechiae and Osler's nodes) and signs and symptoms of infection (such as fever) are present.

Jaundice
(Icterus)

Description
Jaundice is the yellow discoloration of the skin or mucous membranes. It indicates excessive levels of conjugated or unconjugated bilirubin in the blood. In fair-skinned patients, it is most noticeable on the face, trunk, and sclera. In dark-skinned patients, it is most noticeable on the hard palate, sclera, and conjunctiva.

Jaundice is most apparent in natural sunlight and may be undetectable in artificial or poor light. It is commonly accompanied by pruritus (because bile pigment damages sensory nerves), dark urine, and clay-colored stools. It may be the only warning sign of certain disorders, such as pancreatic carcinoma.

Mechanism
Jaundice occurs in three forms: prehepatic, hepatic, and posthepatic. In all three, bilirubin levels in the blood increase.

In *prehepatic jaundice,* certain conditions and disorders—such as transfusion reactions and sickle cell anemia—cause massive hemolysis. Red blood cells rupture faster than the liver can conjugate bilirubin, so large amounts of unconjugated bilirubin pass into the blood, causing increased intestinal conversion of this bilirubin to water-soluble urobilinogen for excretion in urine and stools. (Unconjugated bilirubin is insoluble in water, so it cannot be directly excreted in urine.)

Hepatic jaundice results from the liver's inability to conjugate or transport bilirubin, leading to increased blood levels of unconjugated bilirubin. This occurs in such disorders as hepatitis, cirrhosis, and metastatic cancer, and during prolonged use of drugs metabolized by the liver.

In *posthepatic jaundice,* occurring in biliary and pancreatic disorders, bilirubin forms at its normal rate; however, inflammation, scar tissue, a tumor, or gallstones block the flow of bile into the intestine. This causes an accumulation of conjugated bilirubin in the blood. Water soluble, the bilirubin is excreted in the urine.

Possible causes
Cardiovascular
Congestive heart failure. Jaundice caused by liver dysfunction occurs in severe right ventricular failure.
Gastrointestinal
Carcinoma. Carcinoma of the papilla of Vater initially produces fluctuating jaundice, mild abdominal pain, recurrent fever, and chills.

Hepatic carcinoma is usually metastatic; the resulting bile duct obstruction may cause jaundice.

In *pancreatic carcinoma*, progressive jaundice—possibly with pruritus—may be the only sign.

Cholangitis. Increased pressure and infection in the common bile duct cause Charcot's triad: jaundice, right upper quadrant pain, and high fever with chills.

Cholecystitis. This disorder produces jaundice (without pruritus) in about 25% of patients.

Cholelithiasis. This disorder commonly causes jaundice and biliary colic—the primary symptom.

Cholestasis. In benign recurrent intrahepatic cholestasis, attacks of severe, prolonged jaundice occur (sometimes several years apart) with pruritus.

Cirrhosis. In *Laennec's cirrhosis*, mild-to-moderate jaundice with pruritus usually signals hepatocellular necrosis.

In *primary biliary cirrhosis*, fluctuating jaundice may appear years after the onset of other signs and symptoms, such as pruritus that worsens at bedtime (often the first sign), weakness, fatigue, weight loss, and vague abdominal pain.

Dubin–Johnson syndrome. In this inherited syndrome, fluctuating jaundice—increasing with stress—is the major sign, appearing as late as age 40. Related findings include slight hepatic enlargement and tenderness, upper abdominal pain, nausea, and vomiting.

Hepatic abscess. Multiple abscesses may cause jaundice, but the primary effects are persistent fever with chills and sweating.

Hepatitis. Dark urine and clay–colored stools usually develop before jaundice in the late stages of acute viral hepatitis.

Pancreatitis (acute). Edema of the head of the pancreas and obstruction of the common bile duct can cause jaundice.
Hematologic
Glucose–6–phosphate dehydrogenase (G6PD) deficiency. Acute intravascular hemolysis after ingestion of such drugs as quinine or aspirin causes jaundice, pallor, dyspnea, tachycardia, and malaise.

Hemolytic anemia (acquired). This disorder may produce prominent jaundice along with dyspnea, fatigue, pallor, tachycardia, and palpitations.

Sickle cell anemia. Hemolysis produces jaundice in this disorder.
Drugs
Many drugs may cause hepatic injury and resultant jaundice. Some examples include phenylbutazone, I.V. tetracycline, isoniazid, oral contraceptives, sulfonamides, mercaptopurine, erythromycin estolate, niacin, troleandomycin, androgenic steroids, halothane, and phenothiazines.
Treatments
Upper abdominal surgery may cause postoperative jaundice. It occurs secondary to hepatocellular damage from manipulation of organs, leading to edema and obstructed bile flow; or from prolonged surgery with shock, blood loss, or blood transfusion.

A surgical shunt used to reduce portal hypertension (such as a portacaval shunt) may also produce jaundice.

Clinical considerations
• A history should be obtained and a physical examination performed.
• Diagnostic tests may include urine and fecal urobilinogen, serum bilirubin, hepatic enzymes and cholesterol, prothrombin time, complete blood count, ultrasonography, cholangiography, liver biopsy, and exploratory laparotomy.

• If the patient has pruritus, he should be bathed frequently and an antipruritic agent, such as calamine, applied to his skin.

• The patient may need to make dietary changes, such as a decreased protein intake and an increased carbohydrate intake.

• If the patient has obstructive jaundice, he should be encouraged to maintain a balanced, nutritious diet (avoiding high–fat foods) and frequent small meals.

Jellinek's sign

Description

Jellinek's sign is a brownish pigmentation on the eyelids, usually more prominent on the upper lid than on the lower one. This sign appears in Graves' disease.

Joffroy's sign

Description

Joffroy's sign is immobility of the facial muscles with upward rotation of the eyes, associated with exophthalmos in Graves' disease. To detect this sign, the patient's forehead is observed as he quickly rotates his eyes upward.

Joffroy's sign also refers to the inability to perform simple mathematics—a possible early sign of organic brain disorders.

Jugular vein distention

Description

Jugular vein distention is the abnormal fullness and height of the pulse waves in the internal or external jugular veins. When the supine patient's head is elevated 45°, a pulse wave height greater than 4 cm above the angle of Louis indicates distention. Engorged, distended veins reflect increased venous pressure in the right side of the heart. This sign characteristically occurs in congestive heart failure and other cardiovascular disorders, such as cardiac tamponade, hypervolemia, chronic constrictive pericarditis, and superior vena cava obstruction.

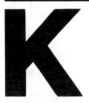

Kanavel's sign

Description
Kanavel's sign is an area of tenderness in the palm, caused by inflammation of the tendon sheath of the little finger. To detect this sign, pressure is applied to the palm proximal to the metacarpophalangeal joint of the little finger.

Kashida's sign

Description
Kashida's sign is hyperesthesia and muscle spasms produced by application of heat or cold. This sign occurs in tetany.

Keen's sign

Description
Keen's sign is an increased ankle circumference in Pott's fracture of the fibula. To detect this sign, the ankles are measured at the malleoli and their circumferences compared.

Kehr's sign

Description
A cardinal sign of hemorrhage within the peritoneal cavity, Kehr's sign is referred left shoulder pain from diaphragmatic irritation by intraperitoneal blood. Usually, the pain arises when the patient assumes the supine position or lowers his head. Such positioning increases the contact of free blood or clots with the left diaphragm, involving the phrenic nerve.

Kehr's sign usually develops right after the hemorrhage, although onset is sometimes delayed up to 48 hours. It is a classic sign of a ruptured spleen and also occurs with a ruptured ectopic pregnancy.

Kernig's sign

Description
Kernig's sign is combined resistance and hamstring muscle pain elicited when the examiner attempts to extend the supine patient's flexed leg. It may signal two life–threatening disorders: meningitis or subarachnoid hemorrhage.

Mechanism
In meningitis or subarachnoid hemorrhage, hamstring muscle pain results from stretching the blood– or exudate–irritated meninges surrounding spinal nerve roots.

Kernig's sign can also indicate a herniated disk or a spinal tumor. In these disorders, the pain results from disk or tumor pressure on spinal nerve roots.

Possible causes
Central nervous system
Lumbosacral herniated disk. A positive Kernig's sign may be elicited in this disorder, but the cardinal and ear-

liest feature is sciatic pain on the affected side or on both sides.

Meningitis. Usually, Kernig's sign is positive early in meningitis.

Spinal cord tumor. Kernig's sign can be elicited occasionally, but often the earliest symptom is pain felt locally or along the spinal nerve, commonly in the leg.

Subarachnoid hemorrhage. Kernig's sign and Brudzinski's sign can both be elicited within minutes after the initial bleed.

Clinical considerations

• If meningitis or subarachnoid hemorrhage is suspected, the physician should be notified immediately and emergency equipment kept readily available.

• Vital signs, neurologic status, and intracranial pressure should be monitored.

• Diagnostic tests include computed tomography, spinal X–ray, and myelography.

Kleist's sign

Description

Kleist's sign is flexion, or hooking, of the fingers when passively raised. It is associated with frontal lobe and thalamic lesions. To elicit this sign, the patient turns his palms down, and the examiner gently raises the fingers. If the patient's fingers hook onto the examiner's, the sign is present.

Koplik's spots

Description

Koplik's spots are small red spots with bluish white centers on the lingual and buccal mucosa. They are characteristic of measles. After this sign appears, the measles rash usually erupts in 1 to 2 days.

Kussmaul's respirations

Description

Kussmaul's respirations refer to an abnormal breathing pattern characterized by deep, rapid, sighing respirations. They are usually associated with metabolic acidosis.

Kussmaul's sign

Description

Kussmaul's sign is distention of the jugular veins on inspiration. It occurs in constrictive pericarditis and mediastinal tumor.

Kussmaul's sign also refers to a paradoxical pulse and to seizures and coma that result from absorption of toxins.

L

Langoria's sign

Description

Langoria's sign is relaxation of the extensor muscles of the thigh and hip joint, resulting from the intracapsular fracture of the femur. To elicit this sign, the examiner places the patient in a prone position, then presses firmly on the gluteus maximus and hamstring muscles on both sides, noting greater muscle relaxation on the affected sign. (The muscles are soft and spongy.)

Lasèque's sign

Description

Lasèque's sign is pain upon passive movement of the leg that distinguishes hip joint disease from sciatica. To elicit this sign, the examiner places the patient supine, raises one of his legs, and bends the knee to flex the hip joint. Pain with this movement indicates hip joint disease. With the hip still flexed, the examiner slowly extends the knee. Pain with this movement results from stretching an irritated sciatic nerve, indicating sciatica.

Laugier's sign

Description

Laugier's sign is an abnormal spatial relationship of the radial and ulnar styloid processes, resulting from fracture of the distal radius. To detect this sign, the patient's wrists are compared. Normally more distal than the ulnar process, the radial process may migrate proximally in fracture of the distal radius, so that it is level with the ulnar process.

Lead-pipe rigidity

Description

Lead-pipe rigidity is diffuse muscle stiffness occurring, for example, in Parkinson's disease.

Leichtenstern's sign

Description

Leichtenstern's sign is pain upon gentle tapping of the bones of an extremity. This sign occurs in cerebrospinal meningitis. The patient may wince, draw back suddenly, or cry out loudly.

Level of consciousness, decreased

Description

A decrease in level of consciousness (LOC)—from lethargy to stupor to coma—usually results from neurologic disorders and often signals life-threatening complications of hemorrhage, trauma, or cerebral edema.

However, this sign can also result from metabolic, gastrointestinal, musculoskeletal, urologic, and cardiopulmonary disorders; severe nutritional deficiency; the effects of toxins; and drug use. LOC can deteriorate suddenly or gradually and can remain altered temporarily or permanently.

Cerebral dysfunction characteristically produces the least dramatic decrease in a patient's LOC. In contrast, dysfunction of the reticular activating system (RAS) produces the most dramatic decrease in a patient's LOC—coma.

The most sensitive indicator of decreased LOC is a change in the patient's mental status. However, the Glasgow Coma Scale can also be used to quickly evaluate a patient's LOC, based on his ability to respond to verbal, sensory, and motor stimulation. (See *Glasow Coma Scale: Grading Level of Consciousness*.)

Mechanism

Consciousness is controlled by the RAS, an intricate network of neurons whose axons extend from the brain stem, thalamus, and hypothalamus to the cerebral cortex. Disturbance in any part of this integrated system prevents the intercommunication that makes consciousness possible.

Possible causes

Central nervous system

Brain abscess. Decreased LOC varies from drowsiness to deep stupor, depending on abscess size and site.

Brain tumor. LOC decreases slowly from lethargy to coma.

Cerebral aneurysm (ruptured). Somnolence, confusion, and, at times, stupor characterize a moderate bleed; deep coma occurs in severe bleeding, which is often fatal.

Cerebral contusion. Usually unconscious for a prolonged period, the patient may develop dilated, nonreactive pupils and decorticate or decerebrate posture. If he is conscious or recovers consciousness, he may be drowsy, confused, disoriented, agitated, or even violent.

Cerebrovascular accident (CVA). LOC changes vary in degree and onset but are not a CVA hallmark.

Encephalitis. Within 24 to 48 hours after onset, the patient may develop LOC changes ranging from lethargy to coma.

Encephalomyelitis (postvaccinal). This life-threatening disorder produces rapid LOC deterioration from drowsiness to coma.

Encephalopathy. In *hepatic encephalopathy,* signs and symptoms develop in four stages. *Prodromal stage:* slight personality changes (disorientation, forgetfulness, slurred speech) and slight tremor. *Impending stage:* tremor progressing to asterixis (the hallmark of hepatic encephalopathy), lethargy, aberrant behavior, and apraxia. *Stuporous stage:* stupor and hyperventilation, with the patient noisy and abusive when aroused. *Comatose stage:* coma with decerebrate posture, hyperactive reflexes, positive Babinski's reflex, and fetor hepaticus.

In life-threatening *hypertensive encephalopathy,* LOC progressively decreases from lethargy to stupor to coma.

In *hypoglycemia encephalopathy,* LOC rapidly deteriorates from lethargy to coma.

Depending on its severity, *hypoxic encephalopathy* produces a sudden or gradual decrease in LOC, leading to coma and brain death.

In *uremic encephalopathy,* LOC decreases gradually from lethargy to coma.

Epidural hemorrhage (acute). This life-threatening posttraumatic disorder produces momentary loss of consciousness followed by a lucid interval. While lucid, the patient has severe headache, nausea, vomiting, and bladder distention. Rapid deterioriation in consciousness follows, possibly leading to coma.

Intracerebral hemorrhage. This life-threatening disorder produces rapid, steady loss of consciousness within hours, often accompanied by severe headache, dizziness, nausea, and vomiting.

Meningitis. Confusion and irritability are expected, although stupor, coma, and seizures may occur in severe meningitis.

Pontine hemorrhage. A sudden, rapid decrease in LOC to the point of coma occurs within minutes, and death occurs within hours.

Seizure disorders. Complex partial seizure produces decreased LOC, manifested as a blank stare, purposeless behavior (picking at clothing, wandering, lip-smacking, or chewing motions), and unintelligible speech.

Absence seizure usually involves a brief change in LOC, indicated by blinking or eye rolling, blank stare, and slight mouth movements.

Glasgow Coma Scale: Grading Level of Consciousness

Terms such as *lethargic, obtunded,* or *stuporous* are sometimes used to describe progressive decrease in a patient's level of consciousness. However, the Glasgow Coma Scale provides a more accurate, less subjective method of recording such changes, grading consciousness in relation to eye opening and motor and verbal responses.

To use the Glasgow Coma Scale, the examiner tests the patient's ability to respond to verbal, motor, and sensory stimulation. The scoring system does not determine exact level of consciousness, but it does provide an easy way to describe the patient's basic status and helps to detect and interpret changes from baseline. A decreased reaction score in one or more categories may signal impending neurologic crisis. A patient scoring 7 or less is comatose and probably has severe neurologic damage.

Test		Reaction	Score
Eyes		Open spontaneously	4
		Open to verbal command	3
		Open to pain	2
		No response	1
Best motor response		Obeys verbal command	6
		Localizes painful stimulus	5
		Flexion—withdrawal	4
		Flexion—abnormal (decorticate rigidity)	3
		Extension (decerebrate rigidity)	2
		No response	1
Best verbal response		Oriented and converses	5
		Disoriented and converses	4
		Inappropriate words	3
		Incomprehensible sounds	2
		No response	1
Total			3 to 15

Generalized tonic-clonic seizure typically begins with a loud cry and sudden loss of consciousness. Consciousness returns after the seizure, but the patient remains confused and may have difficulty talking.

Atonic seizure produces sudden unconsciousness for a few seconds.

Status epilepticus, rapidly recurring seizures without intervening periods of physiologic recovery and return of consciousness, can be life-threatening.

Subdural hematoma (chronic). In this potentially life-threatening disorder, consciousness progressively decreases from somnolence to coma, preceded by agitation and confusion.

Transient ischemic attack. Abrupt decrease in LOC varies in severity and disappears gradually within 24 hours.

Respiratory

Hypercapnia with pulmonary disease. LOC decreases gradually from lethargy to coma, but prolonged coma is rare.

Hyperventilation syndrome. Brief episodes of unconsciousness follow stress-induced deep, rapid breathing associated with anxiety or agitation.

Cardiovascular

Shock. Decreased LOC—lethargy progressing to stupor and coma—occurs late in all forms of shock.

Endocrine

Adrenal crisis. Decreased LOC, ranging from lethargy to coma, may develop within 8 to 12 hours of onset.

Diabetic ketoacidosis. This potentially life-threatening disorder produces a fairly rapid decrease in LOC, ranging from lethargy to coma.

Hyperglycemic hyperosmolar nonketotic coma. LOC decreases rapidly from lethargy to coma.

Myxedema crisis. The patient may show swift LOC decrease to stupor or just slow mentation and confusion.

Thyroid storm. LOC decreases suddenly and can progress to coma.

Metabolic

Hypernatremia. This disorder, life-threatening if acute, causes LOC to deteriorate from lethargy to coma.

Hypokalemia. LOC gradually decreases to lethargy; coma is rare.

Hyponatremia. This disorder, life-threatening if acute, produces decreased LOC in late stages.

Environmental

Heatstroke. As body temperature increases, LOC gradually decreases from lethargy to coma.

Hypothermia. In severe hypothermia (temperature below 90° F. or 32.2 ° C.), LOC decreases rapidly from lethargy to coma.

Poisoning. Toxins such as lead, carbon monoxide, and snake and spider venoms can cause varying degrees of decreased LOC.

Drugs

Sedation and other degrees of decreased LOC can result from overdose of barbiturates, other central nervous system depressants, and aspirin.

Use of alcohol causes varying degrees of sedation, irritability, and incoordination; intoxication often causes stupor.

Clinical considerations

• A history should be obtained from the patient, if he is lucid, and from his family, and a physical examination performed.

• The patient's LOC and neurologic status should be assessed on a regular basis, as ordered.

• Precautions should be taken to ensure the patient's safety.

Lhermitte's sign

Description

Lhermitte's sign refers to sensations of sudden, transient, electriclike shocks spreading down the back and into the extremities, precipitated by forward flexion of the head. This sign occurs in multiple sclerosis, spinal cord degeneration, and cervical spinal cord injury.

Lichtheim's sign

Lichtheim's sign is an inability to speak associated with subcortical aphasia. However, the patient can indicate with his fingers the number of syllables in the word he wants to say.

Lid lag
(Graefe's sign)

Description

A cardinal sign of thyrotoxicosis, lid lag is the inability of the upper eyelid to follow the eye's downward move-

---

Differentiating Lid Lag and Bilateral Ptosis

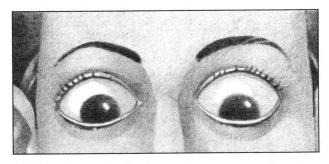

In lid lag (above), the upper eyelid is retracted—it *lags behind* the downward movement of the eye and exposes a rim of sclera above the iris.

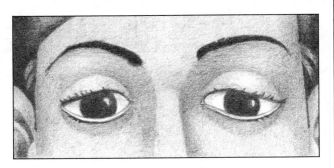

In bilateral ptosis (above), the upper eyelid *sags* and covers the sclera. Sometimes, ptosis is incorrectly called *lid lag*—a term that conveys an image of weakening and drooping.

ments. Testing for lid lag involves holding a finger, penlight, or other target above the patient's eye level, then moving it downward and observing eyelid movement as his eyes follow the target. This sign is demonstrated when a rim of sclera appears between the upper lid margin and the iris when the patient lowers his eyes, when one lid closes more slowly than the other, or when both lids close slowly and incompletely with jerky movements. (See *Differentiating Lid Lag and Bilateral Ptosis*, p. 233.) Lid lag results from chronic contraction of Müller's muscle in the upper eyelid.

Light flashes

Description

A cardinal symptom of vision-threatening retinal detachment, light flashes can occur locally or throughout the visual field. Usually, the patient reports seeing spots, stars, or lightning streaks. Light flashes can arise suddenly or gradually, and can indicate temporary or permanent vision impairment. Most often, light flashes signal the splitting of the posterior vitreous membrane into two layers; the inner layer detaches from the retina while the outer layer remains fixed to it.

Mechanism

The sensation of light flashes may result from vitreous traction on the retina, hemorrhage caused by a tear in the retinal capillary, or strands of solid vitreous floating in a local pool of liquid vitreous.

Possible causes

Central nervous system

Head trauma. A patient who has sustained minor head trauma may report "seeing stars" when the injury occurs.
Migraine headache. Light flashes—possibly accompanied by an aura—may herald a classic migraine headache.

Eyes, ears, nose, throat

Retinal detachment. Light flashes described as floaters or spots are localized in the portion of the visual field where the retina is detaching. With macular involvement, the patient may experience painless visual impairment resembling a curtain covering the visual field.
Vitreous detachment. Sudden onset of light flashes may be accompanied by visual floaters. Often both eyes are affected, but usually one at a time.

Clinical considerations

• A history should be obtained and an eye examination performed.
• If the patient has retinal detachment, he should be prepared for reattachment surgery.
• If the patient does not have retinal detachment, he should be reassured that the light flashes are temporary and do not indicate eye damage.

Linder's sign

Description

Linder's sign is pain upon neck flexion, indicating sciatica. To elicit this sign, the examiner places the patient in a supine or sitting position with his legs fully extended. Then she passively flexes his neck, noting if he experiences pain in the lower back or the affected leg resulting from stretching the irritated sciatic nerve.

Lloyd's sign

Description

Lloyd's sign is referred loin pain elicited by deep percussion over the kidney. This sign is associated with renal calculi.

Looseness of association

Description
Looseness of association is a cognitive disturbance marked by absence of a logical link between spoken statements. It occurs in schizophrenia, bipolar disorders, or other psychotic disorders.

Low birth weight

Description
Two groups of infants are born weighing less than the normal minimum birth weight of 5½ lb (2,500 g)—those who are born prematurely (before the 37th week of gestation) and those who are small for gestational age (SGA). The premature infant weighs an appropriate amount for his gestational age and probably would have matured normally if carried to term. Conversely, the SGA infant weighs less than the normal amount for his age, even if carried to term. Differentiating the two helps direct the search for a cause. In the premature infant, low birth weight usually results from a disorder that prevents the uterus from retaining the fetus, interferes with the normal course of pregnancy, causes premature separation of the placenta, or stimulates uterine contractions before term. In the SGA infant, intrauterine growth may be retarded by a disorder that interferes with the placental circulation, fetal development, or maternal health. Regardless of the cause, low birth weight is linked with higher infant morbidity and mortality and can signal a life-threatening emergency.

Possible causes
This section lists the fetal and placental causes of low birth weight as well as the associated signs and symptoms

---

Maternal Causes of Low Birth Weight

Various maternal factors can predispose an infant to low birth weight.
If the infant is small for his gestational age, these possible maternal causes should be considered:
- Alcohol and narcotics abuse
- Chronic maternal illness
- Cigarette smoking
- Hypertension
- Hypoxemia
- Malnutrition
- Toxemia
If the infant is born prematurely, these common maternal causes should be considered:
- Abruptio placentae
- Amnionitis
- Incompetent cervix
- Placenta previa
- Polyhydramnios
- Preeclampsia
- Premature rupture of membranes
- Severe maternal illness
- Urinary tract infection

---

present in the infant at birth. *(See Maternal Causes of Low Birth Weight* for other causes of low birth weight.)
Genetic
Chromosomal aberrations. Abnormalities in chromosomal number, size, or configuration cause low birth weight and possibly multiple congenital anomalies in a premature or SGA infant.
Obstetric-gynecologic
Placental dysfunction. Low birth weight and a wasted appearance occur in an infant who is SGA. The infant may be symmetrically short or may appear relatively long for his low weight. Additional findings reflect the underlying cause.
Infection
Cytomegalovirus infection. Although low birth weight in this disorder is

Ballard Scale: Calculating Gestational Age

The examiner tests the infant in each neuromuscular and physical category and assigns an appropriate score. At the end of the test, she totals the scores. Then, she checks the grading table at the bottom of p. 237 for the corresponding gestational age.

Neuromuscular maturity	0	1	2	3	4	5
Posture. Examiner places infant supine and observes degree of flexion in arms and legs.						
Square window. Examiner flexes infant's wrist against forearm, until she meets resistance, and measures angle.	90°	60°	45°	30°	0°	
Arm recoil. Examiner extends infant's forearm and releases; after arm recoils, she measures angle at elbow.	180°		100°-180°	90°-100°	<90°	
Popliteal angle. With infant's pelvis flat on a hard surface, examiner flexes his thigh at hip until knee is close to chest. Then, she extends his lower leg, until she meets resistance, and measures popliteal angle.	180°	160°	130°	110°	90°	<90°
Scarf sign. Examiner draws infant's hands across his chest as far over the opposite shoulder as it will go. She notes relationship of elbow to chest midline.						
Heel to ear. Examiner draws infant's foot toward his ear until she meets resistance. She notes distance between foot and ear.						

Ballard Scale: Calculating Gestational Age *(continued)*

Physical maturity	0	1	2	3	4	5
Skin. Examiner assesses skin over entire body, observing for cracking at wrist and ankle.	Gelatinous, red, transparent	Smooth, pink, visible veins	Superficial peeling and/or rash, few veins	Superficial cracking, pale area, rare veins	Parchment-like cracking, no vessels	Leathery, cracked, wrinkled
Lanugo. Examiner inspects infant's back for extent of body hair.	None	Abundant	Thinning	Bald areas	Mostly bald	
Plantar creases. Examiner inspects skin on soles of infant's feet and notes location of any creases.	No crease	Faint red marks	Anterior transverse crease	Creases over anterior two thirds	Creases over entire sole	
Breast. Examiner inspects, palpates, and measures breast tissue diameter to evaluate breast development and nipple formation.	Barely perceptible	Flat areola, no bud	Stippled areola, 1- to 2-mm bud	Raised areola, 3- to 4-mm bud	Full areola, 5- to 10-mm bud	
Ear. Examiner palpates infant's ear to determine extent of cartilage formation. She gently folds upper pinna toward infant's face, releases it, and observes response.	Pinna flat, stays folded	Slightly curved pinna, soft, with slow recoil	Well-curved pinna, soft with ready recoil	Formed and firm, with instant recoil	Thick cartilage, ear stiff	
Male genitalia. Examiner places infant in supine position and inspects and palpates scrotum.	Scrotum empty, no rugae		Testes descended, few rugae	Testes down, good rugae	Testes pendulous, deep rugae	
Female genitalia. Examiner places infant in supine position and inspects genitalia.	Prominent clitoris and labia minora		Labia majora and minora equally prominent	Labia majora large; minora small	Clitoris and labia minora completely covered	

Grading gestational age

Total score	5	10	15	20	25	30	35	40	45	50
Age (weeks)	26	28	30	32	34	36	38	40	42	44

usually associated with premature birth, some infants may be SGA.

Rubella (congenital). Usually, the low-birth-weight infant with this disease is born at term but is SGA.

Toxoplasmosis (congenital). The low-birth-weight infant may be either premature or SGA and may have hydrocephalus or microcephalus.

Varicella (congenital). Low birth weight is accompanied by cataracts and skin vesicles.

Clinical considerations

• A quick respiratory assessment should be performed, the physician notified of signs of respiratory distress, and emergency equipment kept readily available.

• When the infant's condition permits, neuromuscular and physical maturity should be assessed to determine gestational age. (See *Ballard Scale: Calculating Gestational Age*, pp. 236 and 237). A routine neonatal examination should then be performed.

Low-set ears

Description

Low-set ears are a position of the ears in which the superior helix lies lower than the eyes. This sign appears in several genetic syndromes, including Down's, Apert's, Turner's, Noonan's and Potter's, and may also appear in other congenital abnormalities.

Ludloff's sign

Description

Ludloff's sign is the inability to raise the thigh while sitting, along with edema and ecchymosis at the base of Scarpa's triangle (the depressed area just below the fold of the groin). Occurring in children, this sign indicates traumatic separation of the epiphyseal growth plate of the greater trochanter.

Lumbosacral hair tuft

Description

Lumbosacral hair tuft refers to an abnormal growth of hair over the lower spine, possibly accompanied by skin depression or discoloration. This may mark the site of spina bifida occulta or spina bifida cystica.

Lymphadenopathy

Description

Lymphadenopathy is the enlargement of one or more lymph nodes. This sign may be generalized (involving three or more node groups) or localized. Generalized lymphadenopathy may be caused by an inflammatory process, such as bacterial or viral infection; connective tissue disease; endocrine disorder; or neoplasm. Localized lymphadenopathy most commonly results from infection or trauma affecting the drained area.

Normally, lymph nodes range from 0.5 to 2.5 cm and are discrete, mobile, nontender, and nonpalpable. Nodes that exceed 3 cm are cause for concern. They may be tender and erythematous, suggesting a draining lesion. Or they may be hard and fixed, tender or nontender—suggesting malignant tissue.

Mechanism

Lymphadenopathy may result from increased production of lymphocytes or reticuloendothelial cells, or from infiltration of cells not normally present.

Possible causes

Various disorders can cause localized lymphadenopathy. (See *Reviewing Causes and Areas of Localized Lymphadenopathy*, pp. 240 and 241, for additional causes.)

Eyes, ears, nose, throat

Sjögren's syndrome. Lymphadenopathy of the parotid and submaxillary nodes may occur in this rare disorder.

Respiratory

Sarcoidosis. Generalized, bilateral hilar, and right paratracheal lymphadenopathy with splenomegaly are common.

Musculoskeletal

Rheumatoid arthritis. Lymphadenopathy is an early, nonspecific finding associated with fatigue, malaise, continuous low fever, weight loss, and vague arthralgias and myalgias.

Systemic lupus erythematosus. Generalized lymphadenopathy often accompanies the hallmark butterfly rash, photosensitivty, Raynaud's phenomenon, and joint pain and stiffness.

Hematologic

Leukemia (acute lymphocytic). Generalized lymphadenopathy is accompanied by fatigue, malaise, pallor, and low fever. The patient also experiences prolonged bleeding time, swollen gums, weight loss, bone or joint pain, and hepatosplenomegaly. Occasionally, dyspnea, tachycardia, palpitations, and abdominal pain may occur. Later findings may include confusion, headaches, vomiting, seizures, papilledema, and nuchal rigidity.

Leukemia (chronic lymphocytic). Generalized lymphadenopathy appears early, along with fatigue, malaise, and fever. As the disease progresses, hepatosplenomegaly, severe fatigue, and weight loss occur. Other late findings include bone tenderness, edema, pallor, dyspnea, tachycardia, palpitations, bleeding, and often macular or nodular lesions.

Waldenström's macroglobulinemia. Lymphadenopathy may occur with hepatosplenomegaly.

Neoplastic

Hodgkin's lymphoma. The extent of lymphadenopathy determines the stage of malignancy—from stage-one involvement of a single lymph node region to stage-four generalized lymphadenopathy. Usually, nodes in the neck enlarge first and become hard, swollen, movable, nontender, and discrete.

Mycosis fungoides. Lymphadenopathy occurs in stage three of this rare, chronic malignant lymphoma.

Non-Hodgkin's lymphoma. Painless enlargement of one or more peripheral lymph nodes is the most common sign of this cancer, with generalized lymphadenopathy characterizing stage four.

Infection

Brucellosis. Generalized lymphadenopathy most often affects cervical and axillary lymph nodes, making them tender.

Infectious diseases

Cytomegalovirus infection. Generalized lymphadenopathy occurs in the immunocompromised patient.

Infectious mononucleosis. Characteristic, painful lymphadenopathy involves cervical, axillary, and inguinal nodes. Typically, prodromal symptoms such as headache, malaise, and fatigue occur 3 to 5 days before the appearance of the classic triad of lymphadenopathy, sore throat, and temperature fluctuations with an evening peak of about 102° F. (38.9° C.). Hepatosplenomegaly may also develop, along with signs and symptoms of stomatitis, exudative tonsillitis, or pharyngitis.

Syphilis (secondary). Generalized lymphadenopathy occurs in stage two.

Tuberculous lymphadenitis. Lymphadenopathy may be restricted to superficial lymph nodes, or it may be generalized. Affected lymph nodes may become fluctuant and drain to surrounding tissue and may be accompanied by fever, chills, weakness, and fatigue.

Drugs

Phenytoin may cause generalized lymphadenopathy.

Treatments

Typhoid vaccination may also cause generalized lymphadenopathy.

Clinical considerations

• A history should be obtained and a physical examination performed, in-

Reviewing Causes and Areas of Localized Lymphadenopathy

When an enlarged lymph node is detected, the entire lymph node system should be palpated to determine the extent of lymphadenopathy. The lymph nodes indicated below should be included in the assessment.

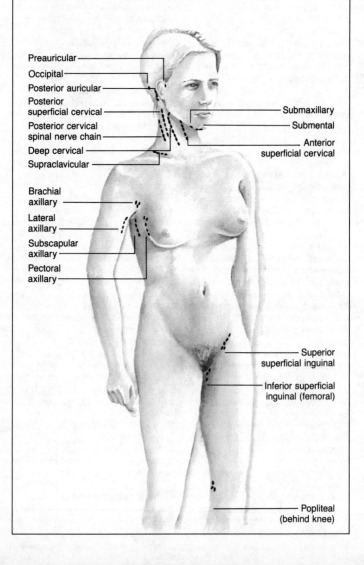

Preauricular

Occipital

Posterior auricular

Posterior superficial cervical

Posterior cervical spinal nerve chain

Deep cervical

Supraclavicular

Submaxillary

Submental

Anterior superficial cervical

Brachial axillary

Lateral axillary

Subscapular axillary

Pectoral axillary

Superior superficial inguinal

Inferior superficial inguinal (femoral)

Popliteal (behind knee)

Reviewing Causes and Areas of Localized Lymphadenopathy
(continued)

Various disorders can cause localized lymphadenopathy. Most often, this sign results from infection or trauma affecting the drained area. The list below matches some common causes of lymphadenopathy with the areas they affect.

Occipital

Roseola
Scalp infection
Seborrheic dermatitis
Tick bite
Tinea capitis

Auricular

Erysipelas
Herpes zoster ophthalmicus
Infection
Rubella
Squamous cell carcinoma
Styes or chalazion
Tularemia

Cervical

Cat-scratch fever
Facial or oral cancer
Infection
Mucocutaneous lymph node
  syndrome
Rubella
Rubeola
Thyrotoxicosis
Tonsillitis
Tuberculosis
Varicella

Submaxillary and Submental

Cystic fibrosis
Dental infection
Gingivitis
Glossitis

Supraclavicular

Neoplastic disease

Axillary

Breast cancer
Lymphoma

Inguinal and Femoral

Carcinoma
Chancroid
Lymphogranuloma venereum
Syphilis

Popliteal

Infection

cluding palpation of the entire lymph system (see *Reviewing Causes and Areas of Localized Lymphadenopathy*).
• Diagnostic tests include routine blood work, a platelet count, liver and renal function studies, chest X–ray, liver and spleen scan, lymph node biopsy, or lymphography to visualize the lymphatic system.

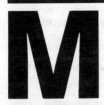

M

Macewen's sign

Description
Macewen's sign is a "cracked pot" sound heard on light percussion with one finger over an infant's or young child's anterior fontanelle. An early indicator of hydrocephalus, this sign may also occur in cerebral abscess.

Maisonneuve's sign

Description
Maisonneuve's sign is hyperextension of the wrist in Colles' fracture. Hyperextension results when a fracture of the lower radius causes posterior displacement of the distal fragment.

Malaise

Description
Malaise is listlessness, weariness, or absence of a sense of well–being. This nonspecific symptom may begin suddenly or gradually and may precede characteristic signs of an illness by several days or weeks. Malaise may reflect the metabolic alterations that precede or accompany infectious, endocrine, or neurologic disorders.

Malingering

Description
Malingering is exaggeration or simulation of symptoms to avoid an unpleasant situation or to gain attention or some other goal.

Mania

Description
Mania is an alteration in mood characterized by increased psychomotor activity, euphoria, flight of ideas, and pressured speech. It occurs most often in the manic phase of a bipolar disorder.

Mannkopf's sign

Description
Mannkopf's sign is an elevated pulse rate upon application of pressure over a painful area. It can help distinguish real pain from simulated pain.

Marcus Gunn phenomenon

Description
Marcus Gunn phenomenon is a unilateral reflexive elevation of an upper ptotic eyelid, associated with movement of the

lower jaw. This occurs in misdirectional syndrome, involving the oculomotor and trigeminal nerves (cranial nerves III and V). To elicit this sign, the patient is asked to open his mouth and move his lower jaw from side to side.

Marcus Gunn's pupillary sign

Description

Marcus Gunn's pupillary sign is a paradoxical dilatation of a pupil in response to afferent visual stimuli. This sign results from an optic nerve lesion or severe retinal dysfunction. However, visual loss in the affected eye is minimal. To detect this pupillary sign, the examiner darkens the room and instructs the patient to focus on a distant object. She shines a bright beam of light into the unaffected eye and observes for bilateral pupillary constriction. Then, she shines the light into the affected eye and observes for brief bilateral dilatation. Next, she returns the light beam to the unaffected eye, which she observes for prompt and persistent bilateral pupillary constriction.

Masklike facies

Description

Masklike facies is a total loss of facial expression. It results from bradykinesia—usually from extrapyramidal damage. Even the rate of eye blinking is reduced—to 1 to 4 blinks per minute—producing a characteristic "reptilian" stare. Although a neurologic disorder is the most common cause, masklike facies can also result from certain systemic diseases and the effects of drugs and toxins. The sign often develops insidiously, at first mistaken by the observer for depression or apathy.

Possible causes

Central nervous system
Parkinson's disease. Masklike facies occurs early but is often overlooked.

Musculoskeletal
Scleroderma. A late sign, masklike facies develops along with a smooth, wrinkle–free appearance, "pinching" of the mouth, and possible contractures, as facial skin becomes tight and inelastic.

Skin
Dermatomyositis. Masklike facies reflects muscle soreness and weakness extending from the face and neck to the shoulder and pelvic girdle.

Environmental
Carbon monoxide poisoning. Masklike facies usually develops several weeks after acute poisoning.

Manganese poisoning (chronic). Masklike facies develops gradually, along with a resting tremor and personality changes.

Drugs
Phenothiazines (particularly piperazine derivatives) and other antipsychotics frequently cause masklike facies and other extrapyramidal effects. Also, metoclopramide and metyrosine infrequently cause masklike facies. This sign usually improves when the drug is reduced or discontinued.

Clinical considerations
• A history should be obtained and a physical examination performed.
• If the patient's masklike facies results from Parkinson's disease, the family should be informed that the sign may hide facial clues to depression—a common symptom of Parkinson's disease.

Mayo's sign

Description
Mayo's sign is relaxation of the muscles controlling the lower jaw in deep anesthesia.

McBurney's sign

Description
McBurney's sign is tenderness elicited by palpating the right lower quadrant over McBurney's point (see *Eliciting McBurney's Sign*). It is a telltale indicator of localized peritoneal inflammation in appendicitis. Before McBurney's sign is elicited, the abdomen is inspected for distention and auscultated for hypoactive or absent bowel sounds.

McBurney's sign appears within the first 2 to 12 hours of appendicitis onset, after initial pain in the epigastric and periumbilical areas shifts to the right lower quadrant (McBurney's point). This persistent point pain increases with walking or coughing.

Rupture of the appendix causes a sudden cessation of pain. Signs of peritonitis, such as severe abdominal pain, pallor, hypoactive or absent bowel sounds, diaphoresis, and high fever then develop.

McMurray's sign

Description
McMurray's sign is a palpable, audible click or pop elicited by manipulating

Eliciting McBurney's Sign

To elicit McBurney's sign, the examiner positions the patient supine with his knees slightly flexed and his abdominal muscles relaxed. Then, the right lower quadrant is palpated deeply and slowly over McBurney's point—located one-third of the distance from the anterior superior iliac spine to the umbilicus. Point tenderness, a positive McBurney's sign, indicates appendicitis.

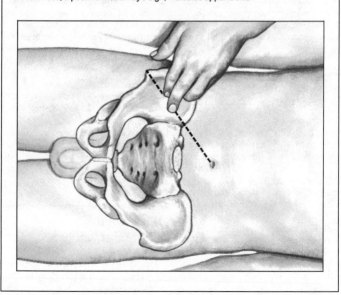

Eliciting McMurray's Sign

Eliciting this sign requires special training and gentle manipulation of the patient's leg to avoid extending a meniscal tear or locking the knee. To elicit McMurray's sign, the examiner places the patient in a supine position and flexes his affected knee until his heel nearly touches his buttock. She places her thumb and index finger on either side of the knee joint space and grasps his heel with her other hand. Then she rotates the foot and lower leg laterally to test the posterior meniscus. Keeping the patient's foot in a lateral position, she extends the knee to a 90° angle to test the anterior meniscus. A palpable or audible click—a positive McMurray's sign—indicates a meniscal tear.

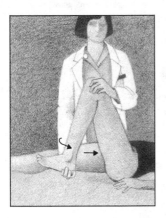 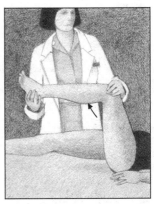

the leg (see *Eliciting McMurray's Sign*). It is frequently an indicator of meniscal injury and results when gentle manipulation of the leg traps torn cartilage and then lets it snap free. Because eliciting this sign forces the surface of the tibial plateau against the femoral condyles, it is contraindicated in patients with suspected fractures of the tibial plateau or femoral condyles.

A positive McMurray's sign augments other findings commonly associated with meniscal injury, such as severe knee pain and decreased range of motion.

Mean's sign

Description
Mean's sign is a lagging eye motion when the patient looks upward. In this sign of Graves' disease, the globe of the eye moves more slowly than the upper lid.

Meconium–stained amniotic fluid

Description
Meconium–stained amniotic fluid is greenish brown or yellow meconium

in the amniotic fluid during labor. Although not necessarily indicative of distress, this sign signals the need for close fetal monitoring to detect decreased variability or deceleration of heart rate. It may also signal the need for infant intubation and resuscitation at delivery to prevent meconium aspiration into the lungs.

Melena

Description
Melena is the passage of black, tarry stools. Characteristic color results from hydrochloric acid acting on the blood as it travels through the GI tract. At least 60 ml of blood is needed to produce this sign.

Severe melena can signal acute bleeding and life–threatening hypovolemic shock. Usually, melena indicates bleeding from the esophagus, stomach, or duodenum, although it can also indicate bleeding from the jejunum, ileum, or ascending colon. In addition, this sign can result from swallowing blood, as in epistaxis; from certain drugs; and from alcohol. Because false melena may occur from ingestion of lead, bismuth, or licorice (which produces black stools without the presence of blood), all black stools should be tested for the presence of occult blood.

Possible causes
Gastrointestinal
Colon cancer. On the *right* side of the colon, early tumor growth may cause melena accompanied by abdominal aching, pressure, or dull cramps.

On the *left* side, melena is a later sign. Early tumor growth commonly causes rectal bleeding accompanied by intermittent abdominal fullness or cramping and rectal pressure. As the disease progresses, the patient may develop obstipation, diarrhea, or pencil-shaped stools. At this stage, bleeding

from the colon becomes obvious, with melena or hematochezia and mucus in or on the stools.
Diverticulitis. Melena may occur as occult blood in the stool or as acute hemorrhage.
Esophageal carcinoma. Melena is a late sign.
Esophageal varices (ruptured). This life–threatening disorder can produce melena, possibly alternating with hematochezia, and hematemesis.
Gastric carcinoma. Melena and altered bowel habits may occur late in this uncommon cancer.
Gastritis. Melena and hematemesis are common.
Mallory–Weiss syndrome. Melena and hematemesis follow vomiting.
Mesenteric vascular occlusion. This life–threatening disorder produces slight melena with 2 to 3 days of persistent, mild abdominal pain.
Peptic ulcer. Melena may signal life–threatening hemorrhage from vascular penetration.
Hematologic
Thrombocytopenia. Melena or hematochezia may accompany other manifestations of bleeding tendency.
Infection
Malaria. Melena may accompany persistent high fever and orthostatic hypotension in severe malaria.
Infectious diseases
Typhoid fever. Melena or hematochezia occurs late in this disorder and may be accompanied by hypotension and hypothermia.
Yellow fever. Melena, hematochezia, and hematemesis are ominous signs of hemorrhage, a classic feature, along with jaundice.
Drugs
Aspirin, other nonsteroidal anti–inflammatories, and alcohol can cause melena as a result of gastric irritation.

Clinical considerations
If melena is severe:
• Vital signs should be taken and the physician notified of signs or symptoms of hypovolemic shock.

If the patient's condition permits:
• A history should be obtained and a physical examination performed.
• Diagnostic tests include blood studies, gastroscopy or other endoscopic studies, barium swallow, and upper GI series.
• Vital signs should be monitored and the patient observed closely for signs and symptoms of hypovolemic shock.

Menometrorrhagia

Description

Menometrorrhagia is an abnormal menstrual cycle marked by a prolonged flow (menorrhagia) with irregular, intermittent spotting between menses (metrorrhagia). Its causes include adenoacanthoma, endometriosis, follicular ovarian cysts, ovarian tumors, polycystic ovary disease, and submucosal leiomyoma.

Menorrhagia

Description

Menorrhagia is profuse or extended menstrual bleeding. It may occur as a single episode or a chronic sign. Normal menstrual flow lasts about 5 days and produces a total blood loss of 60 to 250 ml. In menorrhagia, the menstrual period may be extended and total blood loss can range from 80 ml to overt hemorrhage. Usually a result of gynecologic disorders, this relatively common sign can also result from endocrine and hematologic disorders, stress, certain drugs and procedures, and the use of intrauterine contraceptive devices.

Possible causes

Cardiovascular

Congestive heart failure. Chronic passive venous congestion occasionally produces persistent menorrhagia.

Endocrine

Hypothyroidism. Menorrhagia is a common early sign.
Blood dyscrasias. Menorrhagia is one of a number of possible signs of bleeding, such as epistaxis, bleeding gums, purpura, hematemesis, hematuria, or melena.

Obstetric-gynecologic

Dysfunctional uterine bleeding. Menorrhagia is a less common sign than metrorrhagia. The bleeding can be constant or intermittent.
Endometriosis. Menorrhagia is the most common sign of this disorder.
Uterine fibroids. Menorrhagia is the most common sign, but other forms of abnormal uterine bleeding, as well as dysmenorrhea or leukorrhea, can also occur.

Drugs

Use of oral contraceptives may cause sudden onset of profuse, prolonged menorrhagia. Anticoagulants can also produce menorrhagia.

Treatments

Cervical conization or cauterization can cause menorrhagia.

Clinical considerations

• Vital signs should be taken and the physician notified of any signs or symptoms of hypovolemic shock.
• When the patient's condition permits, a history should be obtained and a physical examination performed.
• Uterine blood loss should be estimated by recording the number of sanitary napkins or tampons used.
• To help decrease blood flow, the patient should be encouraged to rest and to avoid strenuous activities.

Metrorrhagia

Description

Metrorrhagia is uterine bleeding that occurs irregularly between menstrual periods. It is usually light, although it can range from staining to hemorrhage. Most often, this common sign reflects slight physiologic bleeding from the endometrium during ovulation. However, metrorrhagia may be the only indication of an underlying gynecologic disorder and can also result from stress, drugs, and treatments.

Possible causes
Obstetric-gynecologic
Cervicitis. This nonspecific infection may cause spontaneous bleeding, spotting, or posttraumatic bleeding.

Dysfunctional uterine bleeding. Abnormal uterine bleeding not caused by pregnancy or major gynecologic disorders usually occurs as metrorrhagia, although menorrhagia is possible. Bleeding may be profuse or scant, intermittent or constant.

Endometrial polyps. This disorder may produce metrorrhagia, but most patients are asymptomatic.

Endometriosis. Metrorrhagia may be the only indication of this disorder, or it may accompany pelvic discomfort and dyspareunia.

Endometritis. Infection of the endometrium results in metrorrhagia and purulent vaginal discharge.

Gynecologic carcinoma. Metrorrhagia often occurs as an early sign of these carcinomas.

Vaginal adenosis. This disorder commonly produces metrorrhagia.

Infectious diseases
Syphilis. Primary– or secondary–stage syphilis may cause metrorrhagia and postcoital bleeding.

Drugs
Anticoagulants and oral contraceptives may cause metrorrhagia.

Treatments
Cervical conization and cauterization may cause metrorrhagia.

Clinical considerations
• A thorough menstrual history should be obtained and a physical examination performed.

• Blood and urine specimens should be obtained, as ordered, for pregnancy testing.

• If bleeding is heavy, bed rest should be encouraged to reduce bleeding.

• The amount of bleeding should be monitored by recording the number of pads or tampons used.

Miosis

Description
Miosis is pupillary constriction caused by contraction of the sphincter muscle in the iris. It occurs normally as a response to fatigue, increased light, and administration of miotic drugs; as part of the eye's accommodation reflex; and as part of the aging process (pupil size steadily decreases from adolescence to about age 60). However, it can also stem from ocular and neurologic disorders, trauma, systemic drugs, and contact lens overuse. A rare form of miosis—Argyll Robertson pupils— can stem from tabes dorsalis and diverse neurologic disorders. Occurring bilaterally, these miotic (often pinpoint), unequal, and irregularly shaped pupils do not dilate properly with mydriatic drug use and fail to react to light, although they do constrict on accommodation.

Possible causes
Central nervous system
Cerebrovascular arteriosclerosis. Miosis is usually unilateral, depending upon the site and extent of vascular damage.

Cluster headache. Ipsilateral miosis, tearing, conjunctival injection, and ptosis often accompany a severe cluster headache.

Neuropathy. Diabetic and alcoholic neuropathy occasionally produce Argyll Robertson pupils.

Pontine hemorrhage. Bilateral miosis is characteristic in pontine hemorrhage.

Tabes dorsalis. Argyll Robertson pupils are present in this tertiary form of syphilis.

Eyes, ears, nose, throat
Corneal foreign body. Miosis in the affected eye occurs with pain, a foreign body sensation, slight vision loss,

conjunctival injection, photophobia, and profuse tearing.

Corneal ulcer. Miosis in the affected eye appears with moderate pain, visual blurring and possibly some vision loss, and diffuse conjunctival injection.

Horner's syndrome. Moderate miosis is common in this syndrome and occurs ipsilaterally to the lesion.

Hyphema. Usually the result of blunt trauma, hyphema can cause miosis.

Iritis (acute). Miosis typically occurs in the affected eye.

Parry–Romberg syndrome. This facial hemiatrophy typically produces miosis.

Uveitis. Anterior and posterior uveitis commonly produce miosis in the affected eye.

Environmental

Chemical burns. An opaque cornea may make miosis difficult to detect.

Drugs

Such topical drugs as acetylcholine, carbachol, demecarium bromide, echothiophate iodide, and pilocarpine are used to treat eye disorders specifically for their miotic effect. Such systemic drugs as barbiturates, cholinergics, cholinesterase inhibitors, clonidine (overdose), guanethidine, opiates, and reserpine also cause miosis, as does deep anesthesia.

Clinical considerations

• A history should be obtained and ophthalmologic and neurologic examinations performed.

Möbius' sign

Description

Möbius' sign is the inability to maintain convergence of the eyes. To detect this sign of Graves' disease, the examiner observes the patient's attempt to focus on any small object, such as a pencil, as she moves it toward him in line with his nose.

Moon face

Description

Moon face, a distinctive facial adiposity, usually indicates hypercortisolism resulting from ectopic or excessive pituitary production of adrenocorticotropic hormone (ACTH), adrenal adenoma or carcinoma, or long–term glucocorticoid therapy. Its typical characteristics include marked facial roundness, a double chin, prominent upper lip, and full supraclavicular fossae. Although the presence of moon face does not help differentiate causes of hypercortisolism, it indicates a need for diagnostic testing.

Moro's reflex

Description

Moro's reflex is a normal mass reflex in a young infant elicited by a sudden loud noise or by striking the table on which the infant lies, resulting in flexion of the legs, an embracing posture of the arms, and usually a brief cry. A bilaterally equal response is normal; an asymmetrical response may indicate a fractured clavicle or brachial nerve damage. The absence of a response may indicate hearing loss or severe central nervous system depression. Usually, this reflex disappears by about age 3 months. Its persistence after 6 months of age may indicate brain damage.

Mouth lesions

Description

Mouth lesions include ulcers (the most common type), cysts, firm nodules, hemorrhagic lesions, papules, vesicles, bullae, and erythematous lesions. They may occur anywhere on the lips, cheeks, hard and soft palate, salivary glands, tongue, gingivae, or mucous membranes. Many are painful and readily detected. Some, however, are asymptomatic; when these occur deep in the mouth, they may be discovered only through a complete oral examination.

Mouth lesions can result from trauma, infection, systemic diseases, drugs, and radiation therapy.

Possible causes

Eyes, ears, nose, throat

Actinomycosis (cervicofacial). This chronic fungal infection typically produces small, firm, flat, painful or painless swellings on the oral mucosa and under the skin of the jaw and neck. Swellings may indurate and abscess, producing fistulas with a characteristic purulent yellow discharge.

Behçet's syndrome. This chronic, progressive syndrome produces small, painful ulcers on the lips, gums, buccal mucosa, and tongue. In severe cases, the ulcers also develop on the palate, pharynx, and esophagus. Typically, the ulcers have a reddened border and are covered with a gray or yellow exudate.

Epulis (giant cell). This rare lesion occurs on the gingival or alveolar process, anterior to the molars. Dark red, pedunculated or sessile, and 0.5 to 1.5 cm in diameter, it commonly ulcerates to produce a concave defect in the underlying bone. Gingivae bleed easily with slight trauma.

Gingivitis (acute necrotizing ulcerative). This condition causes a sudden onset of gingival ulcers covered with a grayish white pseudomembrane.

Inflammatory fibrous hyperplasia. This painless nodular swelling of the buccal mucosa typically results from cheek trauma or irritation. It is characterized by pink, smooth, pedunculated areas of soft tissue.

Lichen planus. Oral lesions develop on the buccal mucosa or, less often, on the tongue as painless, white or gray, velvety, threadlike papules.

Mucous duct obstruction. Obstruction produces a ranula—a painless, slow-growing mucocele on the floor of the mouth near the ducts of the submandibular and sublingual glands.

Pyogenic granuloma. Often the result of trauma or irritation, this soft, painless nodule, papule, or polypoid mass most commonly appears on the gingivae but can also erupt on the lips, tongue, or buccal mucosa. The affected area may be smooth or have a warty surface; erythema develops in the surrounding mucosa. The lesions may ulcerate, producing a purulent exudate.

Squamous cell carcinoma. In this disease, a painless ulcer with an elevated, indurated border usually erupts in areas of leukoplakia. It is most common on the lower lip but may also occur on the lateral border of the tongue and on the floor of the mouth.

Stomatitis (aphthous). This common disease is characterized by recurrent, painful ulcerations of the oral mucosa, most often on the dorsum of the tongue, gingivae, and hard palate. In *recurrent aphthous stomatitis minor*, the ulcer begins as a single or multiple erosion covered by a gray membrane and surrounded by a red halo. It is commonly found on the buccal and lip mucosa and junction, tongue, soft palate, pharynx, gingivae, and all places not bound to the periosteum. In *recurrent aphthous stomatitis major*, large, painful ulcers are commonly found on the lips, cheek, tongue, and soft palate; they may last for up to 6 weeks and may leave a scar.

Musculoskeletal

Discoid lupus erythematosus. Oral lesions are common, typically appearing on the tongue, buccal mucosa, and palate as erythematous areas with white spots and radiating white striae.

Systemic lupus erythematosus. Oral lesions are common and appear as erythematous areas associated with edema, petechiae, a tendency to bleed, and a superficial ulcer with a red halo.

Skin
Erythema multiforme. This acute inflammatory skin disease produces sudden onset of vesicles and bullae on the lips and buccal mucosa.

Pemphigus. This chronic skin disease is characterized by vesicles and bullae that appear in cycles. On the oral mucosa, bullae rupture, leaving painful lesions that bleed easily.

Immunologic
Pemphigoid (benign mucosal). This autoimmune disease is characterized by vesicles on the oral mucous membranes, conjunctiva, and, less often, the skin. Mouth lesions typically develop months or even years before other manifestations and may occur as desquamative patchy gingivitis or as a vesicobullous eruption.

Infectious diseases
Candidiasis. This common fungal infection characteristically produces soft, elevated plaques on the buccal mucosa, tongue, and sometimes the palate, gingivae, and floor of the mouth; the plaques may be wiped away. The lesions of *acute atrophic candidiasis* are red and painful. In contrast, the lesions of *chronic hyperplastic candidiasis* are white and firm. Localized areas of redness, pruritus, and foul odor may be present.

Gonorrhea. Painful lip ulcerations may occur, along with rough, reddened, bleeding gingivae (possibly necrotic and covered by a yellowish pseudomembrane), and a swollen, ulcerated tongue.

Herpes simplex. In primary infection, a brief period of prodromal tingling and itching, accompanied by fever and pharyngitis, is followed by eruption of vesicles on any part of the oral mucosa, especially the tongue, gums, and cheeks. Vesicles form on an erythematous base, then rupture and leave a painful ulcer, followed by a yellowish crust.

Herpes zoster. This common viral infection may produce painful vesicles on the buccal mucosa, tongue, uvula, pharynx, and larynx.

Syphilis. *Primary* syphilis typically produces a solitary painful ulcer (chancre) on the lip, tongue, palate, tonsil, or gingiva. The ulcer appears as a crater with undulated, raised edges and a shiny center; lip chancres may develop a crust. During the *secondary* stage, multiple painless ulcers covered by a grayish white plaque may erupt on the tongue, gingivae, or buccal mucosa. At the *tertiary* stage, lesions (often gummas—chronic, painless, superficial nodules or deep granulomatous lesions) develop on the skin and mucous membranes, especially the tongue and palate.

Tuberculosis (oral mucosal). This rare disorder produces a painless ulcer (most often on the tongue) and, sometimes, caseation.

Environmental
Trauma. The most common cause of oral lesions, trauma can produce ulcers anywhere in the mouth.

Drugs
Various chemotherapeutic agents can directly produce stomatitis. In addition, allergic reactions to penicillin, sulfonamides, gold, quinine, streptomycin, phenytoin, aspirin, and barbiturates often cause lesions to erupt.

Treatments
Radiation therapy may produce mouth lesions.

Clinical considerations
• A history should be obtained and an oral examination performed.
• A topical anesthetic, such as lidocaine, may be used to relieve pain.
• The patient should be instructed to avoid highly seasoned foods, citrus fruits, alcohol, and tobacco.
• The use of lemon–glycerin swabs should be avoided because they can dry and irritate the lesions.
• If toothbrushing is contraindicated, the patient should be instructed to use a mouth rinse, such as normal saline solution or half–strength hydrogen peroxide, and to avoid commercial mouthwashes that contain alcohol.

Murmurs

Description

Murmurs are auscultatory sounds heard within the heart chambers or major arteries. They are classified by their timing and duration in the cardiac cycle, auscultatory location, loudness, configuration, pitch, and quality. *Timing* can be characterized as systolic, holosystolic (continuous throughout systole), diastolic, or continuous throughout systole and diastole; systolic and diastolic murmurs can be further characterized as early, middle, or late. *Location* refers to the area of maximum loudness, such as the apex, the lower left sternal border, or an intercostal space. *Loudness* is graded on a scale of I to VI, with I signifying the faintest audible murmur. *Configuration*, or shape, refers to the nature of loudness—crescendo, decrescendo, crescendo–decrescendo, decrescendo–crescendo, plateau (even), or variable (uneven). The murmur's *pitch* may be high or low. Its *quality* may be described as harsh, rumbling, blowing, scratching, buzzing, musical, or squeaking.

Murmurs can reflect accelerated blood flow through normal or abnormal valves; forward blood flow through a narrowed or irregular valve or into a dilated vessel; blood backflow through an incompetent valve, septal defect, or patent ductus arteriosus; or decreased blood viscosity. Often the result of organic heart disease, murmurs occasionally may signal an emergency situation—for example, a loud holosystolic murmur after acute myocardial infarction (MI) may signal papillary muscle rupture. Murmurs may also result from surgical implantation of a prosthetic valve.

Some murmurs are innocent or functional. An *innocent systolic murmur* is generally soft, medium–pitched, and loudest along the left sternal border at the second or third intercostal space. It is exacerbated by physical activity, excitement, fever, pregnancy, anemia, or thyrotoxicosis. Examples include *Still's murmur* in children and *mammary souffle*, often heard over either breast during late pregnancy and early postpartum.

Possible causes

Cardiovascular

Aortic regurgitation. Acute aortic regurgitation typically produces a soft, short diastolic murmur over the left sternal border that is best heard when the patient sits and leans forward. S_2 may be soft or absent. Sometimes, a soft, short midsystolic murmur may also be heard over the second right intercostal space.

Chronic aortic regurgitation causes a high–pitched, blowing, decrescendo diastolic murmur that is best heard over the second or third right intercostal space or the left sternal border with the patient sitting, leaning forward, and holding his breath after deep expiration. An Austin Flint murmur—a rumbling, mid– to late diastolic murmur best heard at the apex—may also occur.

Aortic stenosis. In this valvular disorder, the murmur is systolic, beginning after S_1 and ending at or before aortic valve closure. It is harsh and grating, medium–pitched, and crescendo–decrescendo. Loudest over the second right intercostal space, this murmur may also be heard at the apex, at the suprasternal notch (Erb's point), and over the carotid arteries. In advanced disease, S_2 may be heard as a single sound, with inaudible aortic closure. An early systolic ejection click at the apex is typical; it is absent when the valve is severely calcified.

Cardiomyopathy (hypertrophic obstructive). This disorder generates a harsh late systolic murmur, ending at S_2. Best heard over the left sternal border and at the apex, the murmur is often accompanied by an audible S_3 or S_4.

Complete heart block. This disorder commonly produces a short, crescendo–decrescendo diastolic murmur after atrial contraction, best heard at the apex. S_1 may be paradoxical.

Mitral prolapse. This disorder generates a mid– to late systolic click with a high–pitched late systolic crescendo murmur, best heard at the apex. Occasionally, multiple clicks may be heard, with or without a systolic murmur.

Mitral regurgitation. *Acute mitral regurgitation* is characterized by an early systolic or holosystolic decrescendo murmur at the apex, along with a widely split S_2 and often an S_4.

Chronic mitral regurgitation produces a high–pitched, blowing, holosystolic plateau murmur that is loudest at the apex and usually radiates to the axilla or back.

Mitral stenosis. In this valvular disorder, the murmur is soft, low–pitched, rumbling, decrescendo–crescendo, and diastolic, accompanied by a loud S_1 and an opening snap—a cardinal sign. It is best heard at the apex with the patient in the left lateral position. In severe stenosis, the murmur of mitral regurgitation may also be heard.

Myxomas. A *left atrial myxoma* (most common) usually produces a middiastolic murmur and a holosystolic murmur that is loudest at the apex, with an S_4, an early diastolic thudding sound (tumor plop), and a loud, widely split S_1.

A *right atrial myxoma* causes a late diastolic rumbling murmur, a holosystolic crescendo murmur, and tumor plop, best heard at the lower left sternal border.

A *left ventricular myxoma* (very rare) produces a systolic murmur best heard at the lower left sternal border.

A *right ventricular myxoma* commonly generates a systolic ejection murmur with delayed S_2 and a tumor plop, best heard at the left sternal border.

Papillary muscle rupture. In this life–threatening complication of acute MI, a loud holosystolic murmur can be auscultated at the apex.

Identifying Common Murmurs

The timing and configuration of a murmur can indicate its underlying cause. The characteristics of some common murmurs are shown below.

Aortic regurgitation (chronic)
Thickened valve leaflets fail to close correctly, permitting backflow of blood into the left ventricle.

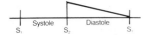

Aortic stenosis
Thickened, scarred, or calcified valve leaflets impede ventricular systolic ejection.

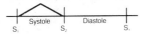

Mitral prolapse
Incompetent mitral valve bulges into the left atrium because of an enlarged posterior leaflet and elongated chordae tendineae.

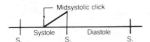

Mitral regurgitation (chronic)
Incomplete mitral valve closure permits backflow of blood into the left atrium.

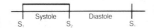

Mitral stenosis
Thickened or scarred valve leaflets cause valve stenosis and restrict blood flow.

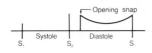

When Murmurs Mean Emergency

Although not normally a sign of an emergency, murmurs—especially newly developed ones—may signal a serious complication in patients with bacterial endocarditis or recent acute myocardial infarction (MI).

Care for a patient with known or suspected bacterial endocarditis should include careful auscultation for any new murmurs. Their development along with crackles, distended neck veins, orthopnea, and dyspnea may herald congestive heart failure.

Regular auscultation is also important in a patient who has experienced an acute MI. A loud decrescendo holosystolic murmur at the apex that radiates to the axilla and left sternal border or throughout the chest is significant, particularly in association with a widely split S_2 and an atrial gallop (S_4). This murmur, when accompanied by signs of acute pulmonary edema, usually indicates the development of acute mitral regurgitation from rupture of the chordae tendineae—a medical emergency.

Tricuspid regurgitation. This valvular abnormality is characterized by a soft, high–pitched, holosystolic blowing murmur that increases with inspiration (Carvallo's sign); it is best heard over the lower left sternal border and the xiphoid area.

Tricuspid stenosis. This valvular disorder produces a diastolic murmur similar to that of mitral stenosis, but louder with inspiration. S_1 may also be louder.

Treatments

Prosthetic valve replacement may cause variable murmurs, depending on the location, valve composition, and method of operation.

Clinical considerations

• If a murmur is discovered, the type must be determined through careful auscultation (see *Identifying Common Murmurs*, p. 253). Then a history should be obtained and a complete physical examination performed.

• Diagnostic tests include chest X-ray, EKG, and echocardiography.

• A newly developed murmur in a patient with bacterial endocarditis or recent acute MI may signal an emergency; the physician should be notified immediately (see *When Murmurs Mean Emergency*).

Murphy's sign

Description

Murphy's sign is the arrest of inspiratory effort when gentle finger pressure beneath the right subcostal arch and below the margin of the liver causes pain during deep inspiration. This classic (but not always present) sign of acute cholecystitis may also occur in hepatitis.

Muscle atrophy
(Muscle wasting)

Description

Muscle atrophy is a wasting or diminution of muscle size resulting from prolonged muscle immobility or disuse. Even slight atrophy usually causes some loss of motion or power.

Atrophy most commonly stems from neuromuscular disease or injury. However, it may also stem from certain metabolic and endocrine disorders and prolonged immobility. Some muscle atrophy also occurs with aging.

Mechanism

When deprived of regular exercise, muscle fibers lose both bulk and length, producing a visible loss of muscle size and contour and apparent emaciation or deformity in the affected area.

Possible causes

Central nervous system

Amyotrophic lateral sclerosis. Initial symptoms of this progressive disease include muscle weakness and atrophy that typically begin in one hand, spread to the arm, and then develop in the other hand and arm. Eventually, weakness and atrophy spread to the trunk, neck, tongue, larynx, pharynx, and legs; progressive respiratory muscle weakness leads to respiratory insufficiency.

Cerebrovascular accident (CVA). This disorder may produce contralateral or bilateral weakness, and eventually atrophy, of the arms, legs, face, and tongue.

Multiple sclerosis. This degenerative disease may produce arm and leg atrophy as a result of chronic progressive weakness; spasticity and contractures may also develop.

Parkinson's disease. In this disorder, muscle rigidity, weakness, and disuse may produce muscle atrophy.

Peripheral nerve trauma. Injury to or prolonged pressure on a peripheral nerve leads to muscle weakness and atrophy.

Peripheral neuropathy. In this disorder, muscle weakness progresses slowly to flaccid paralysis and eventually atrophy. Distal extremity muscles are usually affected first.

Spinal cord injury. Trauma to the spinal cord can produce severe muscle weakness and flaccid, then spastic, paralysis, eventually leading to atrophy.

Endocrine

Hypercortisolism. This disorder may cause limb weakness and eventually atrophy.

Hypothyroidism. Reversible weakness and atrophy of proximal limb muscles may occur in hypothyroidism.

Thyrotoxicosis. This disorder may produce insidious, generalized muscle weakness and atrophy.

Musculoskeletal

Compartment syndrome and Volkmann's ischemic contracture. In this acute disorder, muscle atrophy is a late sign of irreversible ischemia, along with contractures, paralysis, and loss of pulses.

Herniated disk. Here, pressure on nerve roots leads to muscle weakness, disuse, and ultimately atrophy.

Meniscal tear. Quadriceps muscle atrophy, resulting from prolonged knee immobility and muscle weakness, is a classic sign of this traumatic disorder.

Osteoarthritis. This chronic disorder eventually causes atrophy proximal to involved joints as a result of progressive weakness and disuse.

Rheumatoid arthritis. Muscle atrophy occurs in the late stages of this disorder, as joint pain and stiffness decrease range of motion and discourage muscle use.

Metabolic

Protein deficiency. Prolonged protein deficiency may lead to muscle weakness and atrophy.

Environmental

Burns. Fibrous scar tissue formation, pain, and loss of serum proteins from severe burns can limit muscle movement, resulting in atrophy.

Drugs

Prolonged steroid therapy interferes with muscle metabolism and leads to atrophy, most prominently in the limbs.

Treatments

Prolonged immobilization from bed rest, casts, splints or traction may cause muscle weakness and atrophy.

Clinical considerations

• A history should be obtained and a physical examination performed to determine the extent of atrophy. Limb circumference should be measured (see *Measuring Limb Circumference*, p. 256).

• Diagnostic tests include electromyography, nerve conduction studies, muscle biopsy, and X–rays or computed tomography scans.

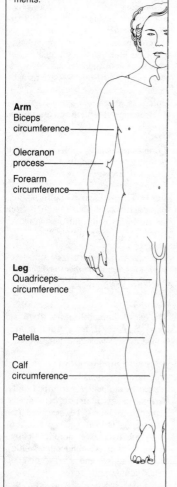

Measuring Limb Circumference

For accurate and consistent limb circumference measurements, a consistent reference point must be used each time and the limb must be fully extended. The diagram below shows the correct reference points for arm and leg measurements.

Arm
Biceps circumference

Olecranon process

Forearm circumference

Leg
Quadriceps circumference

Patella

Calf circumference

• Unless contraindicated, the patient should be instructed to perform active range–of–motion exercises.
• If the patient is unable to actively move a joint, active–assistive or passive exercises should be provided and splints or braces applied to maintain muscle length.
• Moist heat, a whirlpool bath, resistive exercises, ultrasound therapy, or surgery may be used to correct a contracture.

Muscle flaccidity
(Muscle hypotonicity)

Description
Flaccid muscles are profoundly weak and soft muscles, with decreased resistance to movement, increased mobility, and greater–than–normal range of motion. Flaccidity can be localized to a limb or muscle group or generalized over the entire body. Its onset may be acute, as in trauma, or chronic, as in neurologic disease. Muscle flaccidity may be life–threatening if it affects the respiratory system.

Mechanism
Muscle flaccidity is the result of disrupted muscle innervation.

Possible causes
Central nervous system
Amyotrophic lateral sclerosis. In this disorder, progressive muscle weakness and paralysis are accompanied by generalized flaccidity. Typically, these effects begin in one hand, spread to the arm, and then develop in the other hand and arm. Eventually, they spread to the trunk, neck, tongue, larynx, pharynx, and legs; progressive respiratory muscle weakness leads to respiratory insufficiency.
Brain lesions. Frontal and parietal lobe lesions may cause contralateral flaccidity, weakness or paralysis, and eventually spasticity.
Cerebellar disease. In this disease, generalized muscle flaccidity is ac-

companied by ataxia, dysmetria, intention tremor, slight muscle weakness, fatigue, and dysarthria.

Guillain–Barré syndrome. This disorder causes muscle flaccidity from rapidly progressive muscle deterioration. Progression is typically symmetrical and ascending, moving from the feet to the arms and facial nerves within 24 to 72 hours of onset.

Peripheral nerve trauma. Peripheral nerve damage can produce flaccidity, paralysis, and loss of sensation and reflexes in the innervated area.

Peripheral neuropathy. This disorder may produce muscle flaccidity, most commonly in the legs, as a result of chronic progressive muscle weakness and paralysis.

Poliomyelitis. Flaccidity develops late in this disorder from chronic muscle weakness that progresses to paralysis.

Seizure disorder. Brief periods of syncope and generalized flaccidity commonly follow a grand mal seizure. Muscle tone returns rapidly once the patient regains consciousness.

Spinal cord injury. Spinal shock can result in acute muscle flaccidity or spasticity below the level of injury.

Clinical considerations

If flaccidity results from trauma:
- The cervical spine should be stabilized and the physician notified.
- A quick respiratory assessment should be performed. If signs of respiratory insufficiency are present, oxygen should be administered and preparations made for intubation and mechanical ventilation.

If the patient is not experiencing respiratory distress:
- A history should be obtained and a physical examination performed.
- Diagnostic tests include cranial and spinal X-rays or computed tomography scans and electromyography.
- Regular, systematic, passive range–of–motion exercises should be provided to preserve joint mobility and to increase circulation.

- The patient with generalized flaccidity should be repositioned every 2 hours, as ordered, to prevent skin breakdown.
- Isolated flaccidity should be treated, as ordered, by supporting the affected limb in a sling or with a splint.
- Bony prominences and other pressure points should be padded.

Muscle rigidity

Description

Muscle rigidity is muscle tension, stiffness, and resistance to passive movement. This extrapyramidal symptom occurs in disorders affecting the basal ganglia and cerebellum, such as Parkinson's disease, Wilson's disease, Hallervorden–Spatz disease in adults, and kernicterus in infants.

Muscle spasms
(Muscle cramps)

Description

Muscle spasms are strong, painful contractions. They can occur in virtually any muscle but are most common in the calf and foot. Muscle spasms typically result from simple muscle fatigue, from exercise, and during pregnancy. However, they may also occur in electrolyte imbalances and neuromuscular disorders or as the result of certain drugs. They are often precipitated by movement and can usually be relieved by slow stretching.

Possible causes

Central nervous system

Amyotrophic lateral sclerosis. In this disorder, muscle spasms may accompany progressive muscle weakness and atrophy that typically begin in one hand, spread to the arm, and then spread to the other hand and arm. Eventually, muscle weakness and atrophy affect the trunk, neck, tongue, larynx, pharynx, and legs; progressive respiratory muscle weakness leads to respiratory insufficiency.

Spinal injury or disease. Muscle spasms can result from spinal injury, such as cervical extension injury or spinous process fracture, or from spinal disease, such as infection.

Arterial occlusive disease. Arterial occlusion typically produces spasms and intermittent claudication in the leg, with residual pain.

Endocrine

Hypothyroidism. Muscle involvement may produce spasms and stiffness, along with leg muscle hypertrophy or proximal limb weakness and atrophy.

Musculoskeletal

Fracture. Localized spasms and pain are mild if the fracture is nondisplaced, intense if it is severely displaced.

Muscle trauma. Excessive muscle strain may cause mild to severe spasms.

Metabolic

Dehydration. Sodium loss may produce limb and abdominal cramps.

Hypocalcemia. The classic feature is tetany—a syndrome of muscle cramps and twitching, carpopedal and facial muscle spasms, and convulsions, possibly with stridor.

Respiratory alkalosis. Acute onset of muscle spasms may be accompanied by twitching and weakness.

Drugs

Common spasm–producing drugs include diuretics, corticosteroids, and estrogens.

Clinical considerations

If hypocalcemia is suspected:

• A quick respiratory assessment should be performed and the patient observed for the development of laryngospasm.

• The physician should be notified of signs or symptoms of respiratory distress; oxygen should be administered, as ordered.

• Preparations should be made for intubation and mechanical ventilation.

If the patient has no signs of respiratory distress:

• A history should be obtained and a physical examination performed.

• Diagnostic studies include serum calcium and sodium levels, thyroid function tests, and blood flow studies or arteriography.

• Spasms may be alleviated by slowly stretching the affected muscle in the direction opposite the contraction.

• Analgesics should be administered, as needed and ordered, to relieve pain.

Muscle spasticity
(Muscle hypertonicity)

Description

Spasticity is a state of excessive muscle tone with increased resistance to stretching and heightened reflexes. It is detected by evaluating a muscle's response to passive movement; a spastic muscle offers an initial resistance that suddenly gives way—a phenomenon known as the clasp–knife reflex. Spasticity most commonly occurs in arm and leg muscles. Long-term spasticity results in muscle fibrosis and contractures.

Mechanism

Muscle spasticity is caused by an upper motor neuron lesion (see *How Spasticity Develops*).

Possible causes
Central nervous system

Amyotrophic lateral sclerosis. This disorder commonly produces spasticity.

Cerebrovascular accident (CVA). Spastic paralysis may develop on the affected side after the acute stage of CVA.

Epidural hemorrhage. In this disorder, bilateral limb spasticity is a late and ominous sign.

Multiple sclerosis. Muscle spasticity, hyperreflexia, and contractures may eventually develop in this disorder; earlier muscle changes include progressive weakness and atrophy.

How Spasticity Develops

Motor activity is controlled by pyramidal and extrapyramidal tracts that originate in the motor cortex and extend down the spinal cord. The pyramidal tract stimulates muscle action, whereas the extrapyramidal tract inhibits it. Nerve fibers from the two tracts converge and synapse at the anterior horn in the spinal cord. Together, they maintain segmental muscle tone through a mechanism known as the *stretch reflex arc*. This arc, shown in simplified form below, is basically a negative feedback loop in which muscle stretch (stimulation) causes reflexive contraction (inhibition), thus maintaining muscle length and tone.

Damage to the extrapyramidal tract (or to the originating area of the motor cortex) results in loss of inhibition and disruption of the stretch reflex arc. Uninhibited muscle stretch produces exaggerated, uncontrolled muscle activity, eventually resulting in spasticity.

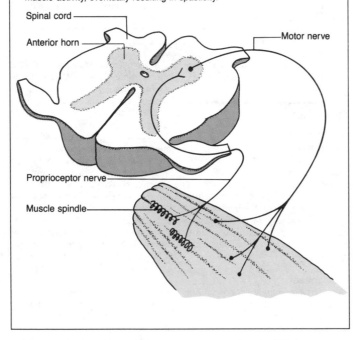

Spinal cord

Anterior horn

Motor nerve

Proprioceptor nerve

Muscle spindle

Spinal cord injury. Spasticity commonly results from cervical and high thoracic spinal cord injury, especially from incomplete lesions. Spastic paralysis in the affected limbs follows initial flaccid paralysis; typically, spasticity and muscle atrophy increase for 1½ to 2 years after the injury, then gradually regress to flaccidity.

Tetanus. This rare, life–threatening disease produces varying degrees of spasticity. As the disease progresses, painful involuntary spasms may spread and cause boardlike abdominal rigidity, opisthotonos, and a characteristic grotesque grin known as risus sardonicus. Reflex spasms may occur in any muscle group with the slightest stimulus. Glottal, pharyngeal, or respiratory muscle involvement can cause death by asphyxia or cardiac failure.

Clinical considerations

- A history should be obtained and a physical examination performed.
- Diagnostic tests include electromyography, muscle biopsy, or intracranial or spinal computed tomography scans.
- Passive range–of–motion exercises, splinting, traction, and application of heat may help relieve spasms and prevent contractures.
- Pain medications and antispasmodics should be administered, as ordered.
- A calm, quiet environment should be provided to help relieve spasms and prevent recurrence.
- Nerve blocks or surgical transection may be necessary for permanent relief.

Muscle weakness

Description

Muscle weakness is detected by measuring the strength of an individual muscle or a muscle group. It occurs in a variety of neurologic and musculoskeletal disorders; in certain metabolic, endocrine, and cardiovascular disorders; as a response to certain drugs; and as a result of prolonged immobilization.

Mechanism

Demonstrable muscle weakness can result from nerve degeneration or injury, or from altered chemical regulation at the neuromuscular junction or within the muscle itself.

Possible causes

Central nervous system

Amyotrophic lateral sclerosis. This progressive disease typically begins with muscle weakness and atrophy in one hand that rapidly spreads to the arm, and then to the other hand and arm. Eventually, these effects spread to the trunk, neck, tongue, larynx, pharynx, and legs; progressive respiratory muscle weakness leads to respiratory insufficiency.

Cerebrovascular accident (CVA). Depending on the site and extent of vascular damage, a CVA may produce contralateral or bilateral weakness of the arms, legs, face, and tongue, possibly progressing to hemiplegia and atrophy.

Guillain–Barré syndrome. In this disorder, rapidly progressive, symmetrical weakness ascends from the feet to the arms and facial nerves and may progress to total motor paralysis and respiratory failure.

Head trauma. Severe head injury can cause varying degrees of muscle weakness.

Multiple sclerosis. Muscle weakness in one or more limbs may progress to atrophy, spasticity, and contractures.

Myasthenia gravis. Gradually progressive skeletal muscle weakness and fatigue are the cardinal symptoms of this disorder. Typically, weakness is mild upon awakening but worsens during the day. Early signs may include weak eye closure, ptosis, and diplopia; a blank, masklike facies; difficulty chewing and swallowing; nasal regurgitation of fluid with hypernasality; and a hanging jaw and bobbing head. Respiratory muscle involvement may eventually lead to respiratory failure.

Parkinson's disease. Muscle weakness accompanies rigidity in this degenerative disorder.

Peripheral nerve trauma. Prolonged pressure on or injury to a peripheral nerve causes muscle weakness and atrophy.

Peripheral neuropathy. In this disorder, muscle weakness progresses slowly to flaccid paralysis, usually affecting distal extremities first.

Poliomyelitis. Rapidly developing asymmetrical muscle weakness, progressing to flaccid paralysis, occurs in *paralytic poliomyelitis. Bulbar paralytic poliomyelitis* produces symptoms of encephalitis along with facial weakness, dysphasia, dysphagia, and respiratory abnormalities.

Seizure disorder. Temporary generalized muscle weakness may occur after a grand mal seizure.

Spinal trauma and disease. Trauma can cause severe muscle weakness, leading to flaccidity or spasticity and, eventually, paralysis. Infection, tumor, and cervical spondylosis or stenosis can also cause muscle weakness.

Endocrine
Hypercortisolism. This disorder may cause limb weakness and, eventually, atrophy.

Hypothyroidism. Reversible weakness and atrophy of proximal limb muscles may occur in hypothyroidism.

Thyrotoxicosis. This disorder may produce insidious, generalized muscle weakness and atrophy.

Musculoskeletal
Herniated disk. In this disorder, pressure on nerve roots leads to muscle weakness, disuse, and ultimately atrophy.

Osteoarthritis. This chronic disorder causes progressive muscle disuse and weakness that leads to atrophy.

Paget's disease. As this disease progresses, muscle weakness or paralysis may develop, along with paresthesias and pain.

Polymyositis. This disorder produces insidious or acute onset of symmetrical limb and trunk muscle weakness and tenderness. Weakness may progress to facial, neck, pharyngeal, and laryngeal muscles.

Rheumatoid arthritis. In this disorder, muscle weakness may accompany increased warmth, swelling, and tenderness in involved joints; pain; and stiffness restricting motion.

Hematologic
Anemia. This disorder can cause varying degrees of muscle weakness and fatigue, exacerbated by exertion and temporarily relieved by rest.

Metabolic
Potassium imbalance. In *hypokalemia,* temporary generalized muscle weakness may be accompanied by nausea, vomiting, diarrhea, decreased mentation, leg cramps, diminished reflexes, malaise, polyuria, dizziness, hypotension, and dysrhythmias. In *hyperkalemia,* weakness may progress to flaccid paralysis accompanied by irritability and confusion, hyperreflexia, paresthesias or anesthesia, oliguria, anorexia, nausea, diarrhea, abdominal cramps, tachycardia or bradycardia, and dysrhythmias.

Protein deficiency. Prolonged protein deficiency may lead to muscle weakness and wasting.

Neoplastic
Hodgkin's lymphoma. Muscle weakness may accompany the classic sign of lymphadenopathy in this disease.

Drugs
Generalized muscle weakness can result from prolonged corticosteroid use, digitalis toxicity, and excessive doses of dantrolene. Aminoglycoside antibiotics may worsen weakness in patients with myasthenia gravis.

Treatments
Immobilization in a cast, a splint, or traction can lead to muscle weakness in the involved extremity; prolonged bed rest or inactivity results in generalized muscle weakness.

Clinical considerations
• A history should be obtained and a physical examination performed, focusing on evaluation of muscle strength (see *Testing Muscle Strength,* pp. 262 and 263).

• Diagnostic tests include muscle biopsy, electromyography, nerve conduction studies, and X-rays or computed tomography scans.

• Assistive devices should be provided, as necessary, and the patient protected from injury.

• If the patient has concomitant sensory loss, decubitus ulcer formation and thermal injury should be prevented.

• With chronic weakness, range-of-motion exercises should be provided or limbs splinted as necessary.

Testing Muscle Strength

To obtain an overall picture of the patient's motor function, the examiner tests strength in ten selected muscle groups. She asks the patient to attempt normal range-of-motion movements against her resistance. If the muscle group is weak, she varies the amount of resistance as necessary to permit accurate assessment. If necessary, she positions the patient so limbs do not have to resist gravity, and she repeats the test.

Arm Muscles

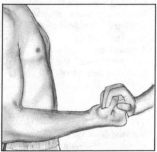

Biceps. With her hand on the patient's hand, the examiner has him flex his forearm against the examiner's resistance; she observes for biceps contraction.

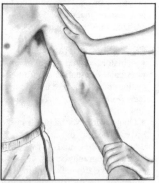

Deltoid muscle. With the patient's arm fully extended, the examiner places one hand over his deltoid muscle and the other on his wrist. She asks him to abduct his arm to a horizontal position against her resistance; as he does so, she palpates for deltoid contraction.

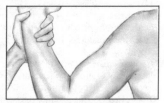

Triceps. The examiner has the patient abduct and hold his arm midway between flexion and extension. She holds and supports his arm at the wrist, and asks him to extend it against her resistance. She observes for triceps contraction.

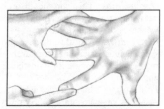

Dorsal interossei. The examiner has the patient extend and spread his fingers, and tells him to try resisting the examiner's attempt to squeeze them together.

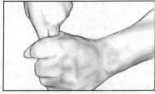

Forearm and hand (grip). The examiner has the patient grasp her middle and index fingers and squeeze as hard as he can.

Muscle strength is rated on a scale from 0 to 5:
0 = Total paralysis
1 = Visible or palpable contraction, but no movement
2 = Full muscle movement with force of gravity eliminated
3 = Full muscle movement against gravity, but no movement against resistance
4 = Full muscle movement against gravity; partial movement against resistance
5 = Full muscle movement against both gravity and resistance—normal strength

Leg Muscles

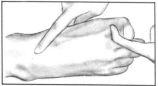

Extensor hallucis longus. With her finger on the patient's great toe, the examiner has him dorsiflex the toe against resistance. She palpates for extensor hallucis contraction.

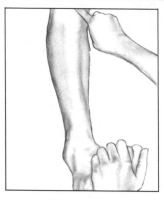

Anterior tibial. With the patient's leg extended, the examiner places her hand on his foot and asks him to dorsiflex his ankle against her resistance.

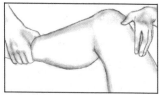

Quadriceps. The examiner has the patient bend his knee slightly while she supports his lower leg. Then she asks him to extend the knee against her resistance; as he is doing so, the examiner palpates for quadriceps contraction.

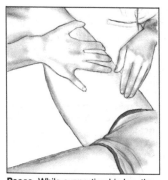

Psoas. While supporting his leg, the examiner has the patient raise his knee and then flex his hip against her resistance. She observes for psoas muscle contraction.

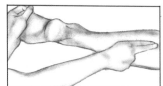

Gastrocnemius. With the patient on his side, the examiner supports his foot and asks him to plantar-flex his ankle against her resistance. She palpates for gastrocnemius contraction.

Mydriasis

Description

Mydriasis is pupillary dilation caused by contraction of the dilator of the iris. It is a normal response to decreased light, strong emotional stimuli, and topical administration of mydriatic and cycloplegic drugs. It can also result from ocular and neurologic disorders, eye trauma, and disorders that decrease level of consciousness. Mydriasis may be a side effect of antihistamines or other drugs.

Possible causes

Central nervous system

Brain stem infarction. This rare disorder may cause bilateral mydriatic, fixed pupils.

Eyes, ears, nose, throat

Adie's syndrome. This disorder is characterized by abrupt unilateral mydriasis, poor or absent pupillary reflexes, visual blurring, and cramplike eye pain.

Glaucoma (acute closed–angle). This ocular emergency is characterized by moderate mydriasis and loss of pupillary reflex in the affected eye, accompanied by abrupt onset of excruciating pain, decreased visual acuity, visual blurring, halo vision, conjunctival injection, and a cloudy cornea.

Oculomotor nerve palsy. Unilateral mydriasis is often the first sign of this disorder.

Cardiovascular

Aortic arch syndrome. Bilateral pupillary mydriasis commonly occurs late in this syndrome.

Carotid artery aneurysm. In this disorder, unilateral mydriasis may be accompanied by bitemporal hemianopia, decreased visual acuity, hemiplegia, decreased level of consciousness, headache, aphasia, behavioral changes, and hypoesthesia.

Environmental

Botulism. Botulinum toxin causes bilateral mydriasis, usually 12 to 36 hours after ingestion.

Traumatic iridoplegia. Eye trauma often paralyzes the sphincter of the iris, causing mydriasis and loss of pupillary reflex; usually, this is transient.

Drugs

Mydriasis can be caused by anticholinergics, antihistamines, sympathomimetics, barbiturates (in overdose), estrogens, and tricyclic antidepressants; it also occurs commonly early in anesthesia induction. Topical mydriatics and cycloplegics, such as phenylephrine, atropine, homatropine, scopolamine, cyclopentolate, and tropicamide, are administered specifically for their mydriatic effects.

Treatments

Traumatic mydriasis commonly results from ocular surgery.

Grading Pupil Size

For an accurate evaluation of pupillary size, the patient's pupils should be compared with the scale below. (However, maximum constriction may be less than 1 mm and maximum dilation greater than 9 mm.)

Clinical considerations

If the patient reports acute eye pain or trauma:

• The physician should be notified immediately because mydriasis may signal two ocular emergencies—acute closed–angle glaucoma or traumatic iridoplegia.

If the patient does not report acute eye pain or trauma:

• A history should be obtained and ophthalmologic and neurologic examinations performed. Pupil size should be evaluated (see *Grading Pupil Size*).

• If mydriasis is the result of mydriatic drugs received during an eye examination, the patient should be told he will likely experience some photophobia and loss of accommodation. He should also be advised to wear dark glasses and to avoid bright light and be reassured that the condition is temporary.

Myoclonus

Description

Myoclonus is a spasm of a muscle or a group of muscles. It occurs in various neurologic disorders and often heralds onset of a seizure. These contractions may be isolated or repetitive, rhythmic or arrhythmic, symmetrical or asymmetrical, synchronous or asynchronous, and generalized or focal. Often, they are precipitated by a sensory stimulus, such as bright flickering light or a loud sound. One type, *intention myoclonus*, is evoked by intentional muscle movement. Myoclonus occurs normally just before falling asleep and as a part of the natural startle reaction.

Possible causes
Central nervous system
Alzheimer's disease. Generalized myoclonus may occur in advanced stages. *Creutzfeldt–Jakob disease*. Diffuse myoclonic jerks appear early in this rapidly progressive dementia. Initially random, they gradually become more rhythmic and symmetrical.
Encephalitis (viral). In this disease, myoclonus is usually intermittent and either localized or generalized.

Encephalopathy. Hepatic encephalopathy occasionally produces myoclonic jerks in association with asterixis and focal or generalized seizures.

Hypoxic encephalopathy may produce generalized myoclonus or convulsions almost immediately after restoration of cardiopulmonary function.

Uremic encephalopathy often produces myoclonic jerks and seizures.
Epilepsy. In *idiopathic epilepsy*, localized myoclonus is usually confined to an arm or leg and occurs singly or in short bursts, often upon awakening. It is often more frequent and severe during the prodromal stage of a major generalized seizure.

Myoclonic jerks are usually the first signs of *myoclonic epilepsy*, the most common cause of progressive myoclonus. At first, myoclonus is infrequent and localized, but over a period of months it becomes more frequent and involves the entire body, disrupting voluntary movement (intention myoclonus).
Environmental
Poisoning. Acute intoxication with methyl bromide, bismuth, or strychnine may produce an acute onset of myoclonus and confusion.
Treatments
Facial or generalized myoclonus is an unusual complication of long–term hemodialysis.

Clinical considerations
• The physician should be notified immediately and the patient assessed for seizure activity.

If the patient is stable:

• A history should be obtained and a neurologic examination performed.

• An EEG may be ordered to evaluate myoclonus and related brain activity.

• Seizure precautions should be taken.

• As ordered, any of the following drugs should be administered to suppress myoclonus: ethosuximide, 5–hydroxytryptophan, phenobarbital, clonazepam, or carbidopa.

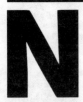

Nail dystrophy

Description
Nail dystrophy is a change in the nail plate, such as pitting, furrowing, splitting, or fraying. It most often results from injury, chronic nail infections, neurovascular disorders affecting the extremities, or collagen disorders.

Nail plate discoloration

Description
Nail plate discoloration is a change in the color of the nail plate. It results from infection or drugs. Blue–green discoloration may occur with *Pseudomonas* infection; brown or black, with fungal infection or fluorosis; and bluish gray, with excessive use of silver salts.

Nail plate hypertrophy

Description
Nail plate hypertrophy is a thickening of the nail plate resulting from the accumulation of irregular keratin layers. This condition is often associated with fungal infections of the nails, although it can be hereditary.

Nail separation

Description
Nail separation is the separation of the nail plate from the nail bed. This occurs primarily in injury or infection of the nail, and thyrotoxicosis.

Nasal flaring

Description
Nasal flaring is the abnormal dilatation of the nostrils. Usually occurring during inspiration, nasal flaring may occasionally occur during expiration or throughout the respiratory cycle. It indicates respiratory dysfunction, ranging from mild difficulty to potentially life–threatening respiratory distress.

Nasal flaring is an important sign of respiratory distress in infants and very young children, who cannot verbalize their discomfort. Common causes include airway obstruction, hyaline membrane disease, croup, and acute epiglottitis.

Possible causes
Respiratory
Adult respiratory distress syndrome (ARDS). ARDS causes increased respiratory difficulty, with nasal flaring, dyspnea, tachypnea, diaphoresis, cyanosis, scattered crackles, and rhonchi.
Airway obstruction. Complete obstruction above the tracheal bifurcation

causes sudden nasal flaring, absent breath sounds despite intercostal retractions and marked accessory muscle use, tachycardia, diaphoresis, cyanosis, decreasing level of consciousness, and eventually respiratory arrest.

Partial obstruction causes nasal flaring with inspiratory stridor, gagging, wheezing, violent cough, marked accessory muscle use, agitation, cyanosis, and hoarseness.

Anaphylaxis. Severe reactions can produce respiratory distress with nasal flaring, stridor, wheezing, accessory muscle use, intercostal retractions, and dyspnea.

Asthma (acute). An asthmatic attack can cause nasal flaring, dyspnea, tachypnea, prolonged expiratory wheezing, accessory muscle use, cyanosis, and a dry or productive cough.

Chronic obstructive pulmonary disease. Nasal flaring is accompanied by prolonged pursed–lip expiration; accessory muscle use; loose, rattling, productive cough; cyanosis; reduced chest expansion; crackles; rhonchi; wheezing; and dyspnea.

Pneumonia (bacterial). In this disease, nasal flaring occurs with dyspnea, tachypnea, high fever, and sudden shaking chills.

Pneumothorax. This acute disorder can result in respiratory distress with nasal flaring, dyspnea, tachypnea, shallow respirations, hyperresonance or tympany on percussion, agitation, distended neck veins, tracheal deviation, and cyanosis.

Pulmonary edema. This disorder typically produces nasal flaring, severe dyspnea, wheezing, and a cough that produces frothy, pink sputum.

Pulmonary embolus. Signs of this potentially life–threatening disorder may include nasal flaring, dyspnea, tachypnea, wheezing, cyanosis, pleural friction rub, and productive cough (possibly hemoptysis).

Diagnostic tests
Pulmonary function tests, such as vital capacity testing, can produce nasal flaring with forced inspiration or expiration.

Clinical considerations

• A quick respiratory assessment should be performed and the physician notified of signs or symptoms of acute respiratory distress.

• The Heimlich maneuver should be performed if airway obstruction is the suspected cause of nasal flaring and respiratory distress.

• Emergency equipment for intubation or tracheostomy and mechanical ventilation should be kept readily available.

• Oxygen should be administered, as ordered.

• The patient should be assisted to a high Fowler's position.

• Diagnostic tests include chest X–rays, lung scan, pulmonary arteriography, sputum culture, complete blood count, arterial blood gas analysis, and 12–lead EKG.

Nausea

Description
Nausea is a sensation of profound revulsion to food or of impending vomiting. Often accompanied by autonomic signs, such as hypersalivation, diaphoresis, tachycardia, pallor, and tachypnea, it is closely associated with anorexia and vomiting.

Nausea, a common symptom of GI disorders, also occurs with fluid andelectrolyte imbalances; infections; metabolic, endocrine, labyrinthine, and cardiac disorders; and as a result of drug therapy, surgery, and radiation. Often present during the first trimester of pregnancy, nausea may also arise from severe pain, anxiety, alcohol intoxication, overeating, or ingestion of distasteful food or liquids.

Possible causes

Central nervous system

Migraine headache. Nausea and vomiting may occur in the prodromal stage.

Eyes, ears, nose, throat

Labyrinthitis. Nausea and vomiting commonly occur with this acute inner ear inflammation.

Ménière's disease. This disease causes sudden, brief, recurrent attacks of nausea, vomiting, vertigo, tinnitus, diaphoresis, and nystagmus.

Cardiovascular

Congestive heart failure. This disorder may produce nausea and vomiting, particularly with right ventircular failure.

Myocardial infarction. Nausea and vomiting may occur, but the cardinal symptom is severe substernal chest pain that may radiate to the left arm, jaw, or neck.

Endocrine

Adrenal insufficiency. Common GI findings in this endocrine disorder include nausea, vomiting, anorexia, and diarrhea.

Thyrotoxicosis. In this disorder, nausea and vomiting may accompany the classic findings.

Gastrointestinal

Appendicitis. With acute appendicitis, a brief period of nausea may accompany onset of abdominal pain.

Cholecystitis (acute). Nausea often follows severe right upper quadrant pain that may radiate to the back or shoulders.

Cholelithiasis. In this disorder, nausea accompanies attacks of severe right upper quadrant or epigastric pain after ingestion of fatty foods.

Cirrhosis. Insidious early symptoms of cirrhosis typically include nausea and vomiting, anorexia, abdominal pain, and constipation or diarrhea.

Diverticulitis. Besides nausea, diverticulitis causes intermittent abdominal pain, constipation, low–grade fever, and commonly a palpable mass.

Gastric cancer. This rare cancer may produce vague GI symptoms—mild nausea, anorexia, upper abdominal discomfort, and chronic dyspepsia.

Gastritis. Nausea is common in this disorder, especially after ingestion of alcohol, aspirin, spicy foods, or caffeine.

Gastroenteritis. This disorder causes nausea, vomiting, diarrhea, and abdominal cramping.

Hepatitis. Nausea is an insidious early symptom of viral hepatitis.

Intestinal obstruction. Nausea occurs frequently, especially with high small intestinal obstruction. Vomiting may be bilious or fecal; abdominal pain is usually episodic and colicky but can become severe and steady with strangulation.

Irritable bowel syndrome. Nausea, dyspepsia, and abdominal distention may occur in this syndrome.

Pancreatitis (acute). Nausea, usually followed by vomiting, is an early symptom of pancreatitis.

Peptic ulcer. In this disorder, nausea and vomiting may follow attacks of sharp or burning epigastric pain.

Peritonitis. Nausea and vomiting usually accompany acute abdominal pain localized to the area of inflammation.

Mesenteric artery ischemia. In this disorder, nausea and vomiting may accompany severe cramping abdominal pain, especially after meals.

Mesenteric venous thrombosis. Insidious or acute onset of nausea, vomiting, and abdominal pain occur in this disorder.

Ulcerative colitis. Nausea, vomiting, and anorexia may occur in this disorder, but the most common symptom is recurrent diarrhea with blood, pus, and mucus.

Genitourinary

Renal and urologic disorders. Cystitis, pyelonephritis, calculi, uremia, and other disorders of this system can cause nausea.

Metabolic

Electrolyte imbalances. Such disturbances as hyponatremia or hypernatremia, hypokalemia, and hypercalcemia commonly cause nausea and vomiting.

Metabolic acidosis. This acid–base imbalance may produce nausea and vomiting, anorexia, and diarrhea.
Obstetric-gynecologic
Ectopic pregnancy. Nausea, vomiting, vaginal bleeding, and lower abdominal pain occur in this potentially life–threatening disorder.
Hyperemesis gravidarum. Unremitting nausea and vomiting that persist beyond the first trimester are characteristic of this disorder of pregnancy.
Preeclampsia. Nausea and vomiting commonly occur in this disorder of pregnancy.
Drugs
Common nausea–producing drugs include antineoplastic agents, opiates, ferrous sulfate, levodopa, oral potassium chloride replacements, estrogens, sulfasalazine, antibiotics, quinidine, anesthetic agents, and digitalis and theophylline (overdose).
Treatments
Radiation therapy may cause nausea and vomiting. Postoperative nausea and vomiting are common, especially after abdominal surgery.

Clinical considerations
• A history should be obtained and a physical examination performed; the history should focus on GI, endocrine, and metabolic disorders; recent infections; and cancer and its treatment.
• An antiemetic should be administered, as ordered.
• Room air should be kept fresh and clean–smelling by removing bedpans and emesis basins promptly after use and by providing adequate ventilation.
• The patient should be advised to breathe deeply to ease his nausea.
• The head of the bed should be elevated or the patient positioned on his side to prevent aspiration of vomitus.
• Because pain can precipitate or intensify nausea, pain medications should be administered promptly, as ordered.

Neologism

Description
Neologism is a new word or condensation of several words with special meaning for the patient but not readily understood by others. This coining occurs in schizophrenia and organic brain disorders.

Neuralgia

Description
Neuralgia is severe, paroxysmal pain over an area innervated by specific nerve fibers. The cause is often unknown, but it may be precipitated by pressure, cold, movement, or stimulation of a trigger zone. Usually brief, neuralgia may be accompanied by vasomotor symptoms, such as sweating or tearing.

Nicoladoni's sign

Description
Nicoladoni's sign is bradycardia resulting from finger pressure on an artery proximal to an arteriovenous fistula.

Night blindness
(*Nyctalopia*)

Description
Night blindness is impaired vision in the dark, especially after entering a darkened room or while driving at night. A symptom of choroidal and retinal degeneration, night blindness occurs in various ocular disorders and as an early indicator of vitamin A deficiency. In some patients, though, night blindness occurs without underlying pathology,

simply reflecting poor adaptation to the dark. In these patients, it is often accompanied by myopia.

Possible causes
Eyes, ears, nose, throat
Cataracts. Night blindness and halo vision occur early in senile–type cataract formation. As the cataract matures, it causes gradual, painless visual blurring and vision loss, sometimes with visible lens opacity.
Choroidal dystrophies. Night blindness and decreased peripheral vision may occur early in choroidal dystrophies.
Fundus albipunctatus. Night blindness is the chief complaint in this retinal and choroidal disease.
Fundus flavimaculatus. In this disease, night blindness may be pronounced or may be an incidental finding.
Glaucoma. Night blindness occurs late in chronic open–angle glaucoma, with halo vision, gradually impaired bilateral visual acuity, loss of peripheral vision, and possibly slight eye pain.
Goldman–Favre dystrophy. In this disorder, night blindness is usually the chief complaint.
Oguchi's disease. This rare, hereditary retinal and choroidal degeneration produces night blindness and a retina with a yellowish metallic sheen.
Optic nerve atrophy. This disorder may cause night blindness, visual field and color vision defects, and decreased visual acuity.
Retinitis pigmentosa. In this hereditary retinal degeneration, night blindness is characteristically the first symptom, usually arising in adolescence.
Vitamin A deficiency. Night blindness is typically the first symptom of vitamin A deficiency.

Clinical considerations
• A history should be obtained and an eye examination performed.
• The patient should be advised to take necessary safety precautions.

Nipple retraction

Description
Nipple retraction is the inward displacement of the nipple below the level of surrounding breast tissue. It may indicate an inflammatory breast lesion or cancer.

Mechanism
Nipple retraction results from scar tissue formation within a lesion or large mammary duct. As the scar tissue shortens, it pulls adjacent tissue in, causing nipple deviation, flattening, and finally retraction. Nipple retraction is sometimes confused with *inversion* (see *Differentiating Nipple Retraction and Inversion*).

Possible causes
Obstetric-gynecologic
Breast abscess. This disorder, most common in lactating women, occasionally produces unilateral nipple retraction.
Breast cancer. Unilateral nipple retraction is often accompanied by a hard, fixed nodule beneath the areola, as well as other breast nodules.
Mammary duct ectasia. Nipple retraction commonly occurs along with a poorly defined, rubbery nodule beneath the areola, with a blue–green skin discoloration.
Mastitis. Nipple retraction, deviation, cracking, or flattening may occur with this condition.

Clinical considerations
• A history should be obtained and a breast examination performed.
• Diagnostic tests include mammography, cytology of nipple discharge, and biopsy.

Differentiating Nipple Retraction and Inversion

Nipple retraction is often confused with nipple inversion, a common abnormality that is often congenital and does not usually signal underlying disease. A *retracted* nipple appears flat and broad, whereas an *inverted* nipple can be pulled out from the sulcus where it hides.

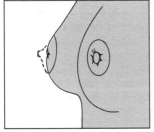

Nipple retraction

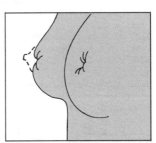

Nipple inversion

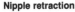

Nocturia

Description

Nocturia is excessive urination at night. It may result from disruption of the normal diurnal pattern of urine concentration or from overstimulation of the nerves and muscles that control urination. Normally, more urine is concentrated during the night than during the day. As a result, most persons excrete three to four times more urine during the day and can sleep for 6 to 8 hours during the night without being awakened. In nocturia, the patient may awaken one or more times during the night to empty his bladder and excrete 700 ml or more of urine.

Although nocturia usually results from renal and lower urinary tract disorders, it may result from certain cardiovascular, endocrine, and metabolic disorders. This common sign may also result from drugs that induce diuresis, particularly when they are taken at night, and from the ingestion of large quantities of fluids, especially caffeinated beverages or alcohol, at bedtime.

Possible causes

Cardiovascular

Congestive heart failure. Nocturia may develop early here—the result of increased glomerular filtration associated with movement of edematous fluid from dependent areas during recumbency.

Endocrine

Diabetes insipidus. The result of antidiuretic hormone deficiency, this disorder usually produces nocturia early in its course. It is characterized by periodic voiding of moderate to large amounts of urine.

Diabetes mellitus. An early sign of diabetes mellitus, nocturia involves frequent, large voidings.

Genitourinary

Benign prostatic hypertrophy. Common in men older than age 50, this disorder produces nocturia when significant urethral obstruction develops.

Bladder neoplasm. A late sign of this neoplasm, nocturia involves frequent voiding of small to moderate amounts of urine.

Cystitis. All three forms of cystitis (bacterial, chronic interstitial, and viral) may cause nocturia marked by frequent, small voidings and accompanied by dysuria and tenesmus.

Hypercalcemic nephropathy. In this disorder, nocturia involves the periodic voiding of moderate to large amounts of urine.

Hypokalemic nephropathy. In this disorder, nocturia involves the periodic voiding of moderate to large amounts of urine.

Prostatic neoplasm. The second leading cause of cancer deaths in men, this disorder is usually asymptomatic in early stages. Later, it produces nocturia characterized by infrequent voiding of moderate amounts of urine.

Pyelonephritis (acute). Nocturia occurs frequently in this inflammatory disorder; it is usually characterized by infrequent voiding of moderate amounts of urine. The urine may appear cloudy.

Renal failure (chronic). Nocturia occurs relatively early in this disorder and is usually characterized by infrequent voiding of moderate amounts of urine. As the disorder progresses, oliguria or even anuria develops.

Drugs

Any drug that mobilizes edematous fluid or produces diuresis (for example, diuretics and cardiac glycosides) may cause nocturia; obviously, this effect depends on when the drug is administered.

Clinical considerations

• A history should be obtained and a physical examination performed.

• Diagnostic tests include routine urinalysis, urine concentration and dilution studies, and serum blood urea nitrogen, creatinine, and electrolyte levels.

• Fluid and electrolyte status should be monitored.

• Diuretics should be administered during daytime hours.

Nodules

Description

Nodules are small, solid, circumscribed masses of differentiated tissue, detected on palpation.

Nuchal rigidity

Description

Nuchal rigidity refers to profound stiffness of the neck that prevents flexion. It is commonly an early sign of meningeal irritation. The patient may notice nuchal rigidity when he attempts to flex his neck during daily activities. To elicit this sign, the patient's neck is passively flexed so that his chin touches his chest. In nuchal rigidity, this maneuver triggers pain and muscle spasms.

This sign may herald life–threatening subarachnoid hemorrhage or meningitis. It may also be a late sign of cervical arthritis, in which joint mobility is gradually lost. Transient, mild neck stiffness may accompany muscle tension, muscle spasms, or myalgia and must be differentiated from true nuchal rigidity.

Possible causes

Central nervous system

Encephalitis. This viral infection may cause nuchal rigidity accompanied by other signs of meningeal irritation, such as positive Kernig's and Brudzinski's signs. Usually, nuchal rigidity appears abruptly and is preceded by headache, vomiting, and fever. The patient may display a rapidly decreasing level of consciousness, progressing from lethargy to coma within 24 to 48 hours of onset.

Meningitis. Nuchal rigidity is an early sign in this disorder. It is accompanied by other signs of meningeal irritation—positive Kernig's and Brudzinski's signs, hyperreflexia, and possibly opisthotonos.

Subarachnoid hemorrhage. In this acute disorder, nuchal rigidity develops immediately after bleeding into the subarachnoid space. Examination may detect positive Kernig's and Brudzinski's signs.

Musculoskeletal

Cervical arthritis. In this disorder, nuchal rigidity develops gradually. Initially, the patient may complain of neck stiffness in the early morning or after a period of inactivity. Stiffness then becomes increasingly severe and frequent. Pain on movement, especially with lateral motion or head turning, is common.

Clinical considerations

• A history should be obtained from the patient and/or a family member and a neurologic examination performed.

• Diagnostic tests include cultures of blood, cerebrospinal fluid, urine, and nose and throat secretions; lumbar puncture; computed tomography scans; and cervical spine X-rays.

• Vital signs and neurologic status should be monitored, as ordered.

Nystagmus

Description

Nystagmus refers to the involuntary oscillations of one or—more commonly—both eyeballs. These oscillations are usually rhythmic and may be horizontal, vertical, or rotary. They may be transient or sustained and may occur spontaneously or on deviation or fixation of the eyes. Although nystagmus is fairly easy to identify, the patient may be unaware of it unless it affects his vision.

Nystagmus may be classified as pendular or jerk. *Pendular nystagmus* consists of horizontal (pendular) or vertical (seesaw) oscillations that are equal in both directions and resemble the movements of a clock's pendulum. *Jerk nystagmus* (convergence–retraction, downbeat, and vestibular) has a fast component and then a slow—perhaps unequal—corrective component in the opposite direction (see *Classifying Nystagmus*, p. 274).

Nystagmus is considered a *supranuclear* ocular palsy; that is, it results from pathology in the visual perceptual area, vestibular system, cerebellum, or brain stem rather than in the extraocular muscles or cranial nerves III, IV, and VI. Its causes are varied and include brain stem or cerebellar lesions, multiple sclerosis, encephalitis, labyrinthine disease, and drug toxicity. Occasionally, nystagmus is entirely normal; it is also considered a normal response in the unconscious patient during the doll's eye test (oculocephalic stimulation) or the cold caloric water test (oculovestibular stimulation).

Possible causes

Central nervous system

Brain tumor. Insidious onset of jerk nystagmus may occur with tumors of the brain stem and cerebellum.

Cerebrovascular accident (CVA). A CVA involving the posterior inferior cerebellar artery may cause sudden horizontal or vertical jerk nystagmus that may be gaze-dependent.

Encephalitis. In this disorder, jerk nystagmus is typically accompanied by altered level of consciousness, ranging from lethargy to coma. Usually, it is preceded by sudden onset of fever, headache, and vomiting.

Head trauma. Brain stem injury may cause jerk nystagmus, which is usually horizontal.

Multiple sclerosis. In this disorder, jerk or pendular nystagmus may occur intermittently. Usually, it is preceded by diplopia, blurred vision, and paresthesias.

Classifying Nystagmus

Jerk Nystagmus

Convergence-retraction nystagmus refers to the irregular jerking of the eyes back into the orbit during upward gaze. It can indicate midbrain tegmental damage.

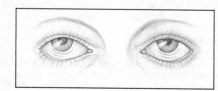

Downbeat nystagmus refers to the irregular downward jerking of the eyes during downward gaze. It can signal lower medullary damage.

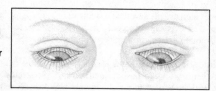

Vestibular nystagmus, the horizontal or rotary movements of the eyes, suggests vestibular disease or cochlear dysfunction.

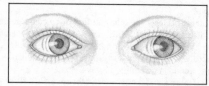

Pendular Nystagmus

Horizontal, or pendular, nystagmus refers to slow, steady oscillations of equal velocity around a center point. It can indicate congenital loss of visual acuity or multiple sclerosis.

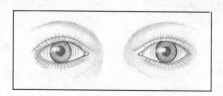

Vertical, or seesaw, nystagmus is the rapid, seesaw movement of the eyes: one eye appears to rise while the other appears to fall. It suggests an optic chiasm lesion.

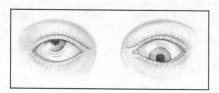

Eyes, ears, nose, throat

Labyrinthitis (acute). This inner ear inflammation causes sudden onset of jerk nystagmus, accompanied by dizziness, vertigo, tinnitus, nausea, and vomiting. The fast component of the nystagmus is toward the unaffected ear.

Ménière's disease. This inner ear disorder is characterized by acute attacks of jerk nystagmus, severe nausea and vomiting, dizziness, vertigo, progressive hearing loss, tinnitus, and diaphoresis. Typically, the direction of jerk nystagmus varies from one attack to the next. Attacks may last from 10 minutes to several hours.

Drugs

Jerk nystagmus may result from barbiturate, phenytoin, or carbamazepine toxicity or from alcohol intoxication.

Clinical considerations

• A history should be obtained and a neurologic examination performed.

• Diagnostic tests include electronystagmography and a cerebral computed tomography scan.

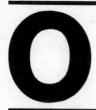

Obsession

Description
An obsession is a persistent, usually disturbing thought or image that cannot be eliminated by reason or logic. It is associated with an obsessive-compulsive personality disorder and occasionally schizophrenia.

Obturator sign

Description
The obturator sign is pain in the right hypogastric region, occurring with flexion of the right leg at the hip with the knee bent and internally rotated. It indicates irritation of the obturator muscle.

In children this sign may signal acute appendicitis because the appendix lies rectocecally over the obturator muscle.

Ocular deviation

Description
Ocular deviation refers to abnormal eye movement. It may be *conjugate* (both eyes move together) or *dysconjugate* (one eye moves differently from the other). This common sign may result from ocular, neurologic, endocrine, and systemic disorders that interfere with the muscles, nerves, or brain centers governing eye movement. Occasionally, it signals a life-threatening disorder, such as ruptured cerebral aneurysm (see *Ocular Deviation: Its Characteristics and Causes in Cranial Nerve Damage*).

Normally, eye movement is directly controlled by the extraocular muscles innervated by the oculomotor, trochlear, and abducens nerves (cranial nerves III, IV, and VI). Together, these muscles and nerves direct a visual stimulus to fall on corresponding parts of the retina. Dysconjugate ocular deviation may result from unequal muscle tone (nonparalytic strabismus) or from muscle paralysis associated with cranial nerve damage (paralytic strabismus). Conjugate ocular deviation may result from disorders that affect the centers in the cerebral cortex and brain stem responsible for conjugate eye movement. Typically, such disorders cause *gaze palsy*— difficulty moving the eyes in one or more directions.

Possible causes
Central nervous system
Brain tumor. Ocular deviation varies, depending on the site and extent of the tumor.
Cerebral aneurysm. When an aneurysm near the internal carotid artery compresses the oculomotor nerve, it may produce features that resemble third cranial nerve palsy. Typically, ocular deviation and diplopia are the presenting signs.
Cerebrovascular accident (CVA). This life-threatening disorder may cause ocular deviation, depending on the site and extent of the stroke.

Encephalitis. This infection causes ocular deviation and diplopia in some patients.

Head trauma. Ocular deviation varies with the site and extent of head trauma.

Multiple sclerosis. Ocular deviation may be an early sign of this disorder.

Myasthenia gravis. In this disorder, ocular deviation may accompany the more common presenting signs of diplopia and ptosis.

Ophthalmoplegic migraine. Most common in young adults, this disorder produces ocular deviation and diplopia, which persist for days after the pain subsides.

Eyes, ears, nose, throat

Cavernous sinus thrombosis. In this disorder, ocular deviation may be accompanied by diplopia, photophobia, exophthalmos, orbital and eyelid edema, corneal haziness, diminished or absent pupillary reflexes, and impaired visual acuity.

Orbital blow-out fracture. In this fracture, the inferior rectus muscle may become entrapped, resulting in limited extraocular movements and ocular deviation.

Orbital cellulitis. This disorder may cause sudden onset of ocular deviation and diplopia.

Orbital tumor. Ocular deviation occurs as the tumor gradually enlarges.

Endocrine

Diabetes mellitus. A leading cause of isolated third cranial nerve palsy, especially in the middle-aged patient with long-standing mild diabetes, this disorder may cause ocular deviation and ptosis.

Thyrotoxicosis. This disorder may produce exophthalmos—protruding eyes—which, in turn, causes limited extraocular movements and ocular deviation. Usually, the patient's upward gaze weakens first, followed by diplopia.

Clinical considerations

• A history should be obtained and a physical examination performed.

• Diagnostic tests include blood studies, orbital and skull X-rays, and computed tomography scan.

• If an acute neurologic disorder is suspected, the physician should be notified and vital signs and neurologic status monitored.

Ocular Deviation: Its Characteristics and Causes in Cranial Nerve Damage

Characteristics	Cranial Nerve and Extraocular Muscles Involved	Probable Causes
Inability to focus the eye upward, downward, inward, and outward; drooping eyelid; and, except in diabetes, a dilated pupil in the affected eye	Oculomotor nerve (III); medial rectus, superior rectus, inferior rectus, and inferior oblique muscles	Cerebral aneurysm, diabetes, temporal lobe herniation from increased intracranial pressure, brain tumor
Loss of downward and outward movement in the affected eye	Trochlear nerve (IV), superior oblique muscle	Head trauma
Loss of outward movement in the affected eye	Abducens nerve (VI), lateral rectus muscle	Brain tumor

Oculocardiac reflex

Description
The oculocardiac reflex is bradycardia in response to vagal stimulation, caused by application of pressure to the eyeball or carotid sinus. This reflex can help diagnose angina or relieve anginal pain. *Caution*: Repeated application of pressure to the eye to elicit this response may precipitate retinal detachment.

Oligomenorrhea

Description
Oligomenorrhea is abnormally infrequent menstrual bleeding characterized by three to six menstrual cycles per year. In most women, menstrual bleeding occurs every 28 days plus or minus 4 days. Although some variation is normal, menstrual bleeding at intervals of greater than 36 days may indicate oligomenorrhea. It may develop suddenly or after a period of gradually lengthening cycles. Although this sign may alternate with normal menstrual bleeding, it can progress to secondary amenorrhea.

Because oligomenorrhea is frequently associated with anovulation, it is common in infertile, early postmenarchal, and perimenopausal women. Usually, this sign reflects abnormalities of the hormones that govern normal proliferation and shedding of the endometrium. It may result from ovarian, pituitary, and other metabolic disorders and from the effects of certain drugs. It may also result from emotional or physical stress, such as sudden weight change, debilitating illness, or rigorous physical training.

Possible causes
Endocrine
Adrenal hyperplasia. In this disorder, oligomenorrhea may be accompanied by signs of androgen excess, such as clitoral enlargement and male distribution of hair, fat, and muscle mass. If this disorder is congenital, the patient may have never had normal menses.

Diabetes mellitus. Oligomenorrhea may be an early sign in this disorder. In juvenile–onset diabetes, the patient may have never had normal menses.

Prolactin–secreting pituitary tumor. Oligomenorrhea or amenorrhea may be the first sign of a prolactin–secreting pituitary tumor.

Sheehan's syndrome. This pituitary disorder usually follows severe obstetric hemorrhage. Oligomenorrhea or amenorrhea may be accompanied by failure to lactate, sparse pubic and axillary hair, decreased libido, and fatigue.

Thyrotoxicosis. This disorder may produce oligomenorrhea accompanied by reduced fertility.

Obstetric-gynecologic
Polycystic ovary disease. Nearly 25% of women with polycystic ovary disease have oligomenorrhea; however, some may have amenorrhea, menometrorrhagia, or irregular menses.

Psychiatric
Anorexia nervosa. Anorexia nervosa may cause sporadic oligomenorrhea or amenorrhea.

Drugs
Drugs that increase androgen levels—such as corticosteriods, ACTH, anabolic steroids, and danazol—may cause oligomenorrhea. Oral contraceptives may be associated with delayed resumption of normal menses when their use is discontinued; however, 95% of women resume normal menses within 3 months. Phenothiazine derivatives and amphetamines may also cause oligomenorrhea.

Clinical considerations
• A history should be obtained and a physical examination performed.
• Diagnostic tests include blood hormone levels, thyroid studies, and computed tomography scan.
• The patient should be requested to record basal body temperatures.

Oliguria

Description
Oliguria is clinically defined as urinary output of less than 400 ml per 24 hours. Typically, this sign occurs abruptly and may herald serious, possibly life-threatening, hemodynamic instability. Its causes can be classified as prerenal (decreased renal blood flow), intrarenal (intrinsic renal damage), or postrenal (urinary tract obstruction). Oliguria associated with a prerenal or postrenal cause is usually promptly reversible with treatment, although it may lead to intrarenal damage if untreated. However, oliguria associated with an intrarenal cause is usually more persistent and may be irreversible.

Mechanism
The pathophysiology of oliguria differs for each classification (see *How Oliguria Develops*, pp. 280 and 281).

Possible causes
Cardiovascular
Congestive heart failure. Oliguria may occur in left ventricular failure as a result of low cardiac output and decreased renal perfusion.

Hypovolemia. Any disorder that decreases circulating fluid volume can produce oliguria.

Gastrointestinal
Cirrhosis. In severe cirrhosis, hepatorenal syndrome may develop with oliguria.

Genitourinary
Acute tubular necrosis (ATN). An early sign of ATN, oliguria may occur abruptly (in shock) or gradually (in nephrotoxicity). Usually, it persists for about 2 weeks, followed by polyuria.

Benign prostatic hypertrophy. Common in men over age 50, this disorder often causes oliguria from urethral obstruction.

Bladder neoplasm. This disorder also produces oliguria from urethral obstruction.

Calculi. Oliguria or anuria may result from stones lodging in the kidneys, ureters, or the bladder outlet.

Glomerulonephritis (acute). This disorder produces oliguria or anuria.

Pyelonephritis (acute). Accompanying the sudden onset of oliguria in this disorder are high fever with chills, fatigue, flank pain, costovertebral angle (CVA) tenderness, weakness, nocturia, dysuria, hematuria, urinary frequency and urgency, and tenesmus. The urine may appear cloudy.

Renal artery occlusion (bilateral). This disorder may produce oliguria or, more commonly, anuria.

Renal failure (chronic). Oliguria is a major sign of end-stage chronic renal failure.

Renal vein occlusion (bilateral). This disorder occasionally causes oliguria accompanied by acute low back and flank pain; CVA tenderness; fever; pallor; hematuria; enlarged, palpable kidneys; and possibly signs of uremia.

Retroperitoneal fibrosis. Oliguria may result from bilateral ureteral obstruction by dense fibrous tissue.

Urethral stricture. This disorder produces oliguria accompanied by chronic urethral discharge, urinary frequency and urgency, dysuria, pyuria, and diminished urinary stream.

Obstetric-gynecologic
Toxemia of pregnancy. In severe preeclampsia, oliguria may be accompanied by elevated blood pressure, dizziness, diplopia, blurred vision, epigastric pain, nausea and vomiting, irritability, and severe frontal headache. Typically, the oliguria is preceded by generalized edema and sudden weight gain of more than 3 lb/week during the second trimester or more than 1 lb/week during the third trimester.

Infection
Sepsis. Any condition that results in sepsis may produce oliguria.

Drugs
Oliguria may result from drugs that cause decreased renal perfusion (diuretics), nephrotoxicity (most notably ami-

How Oliguria Develops

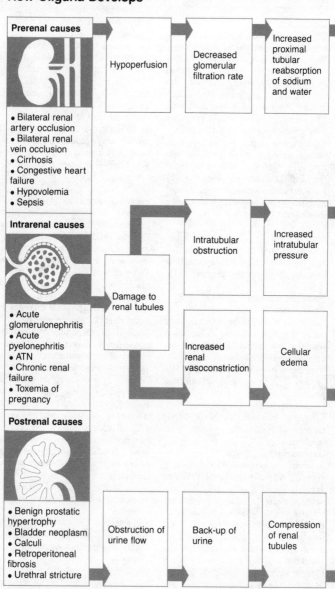

Prerenal causes

- Bilateral renal artery occlusion
- Bilateral renal vein occlusion
- Cirrhosis
- Congestive heart failure
- Hypovolemia
- Sepsis

Hypoperfusion → Decreased glomerular filtration rate → Increased proximal tubular reabsorption of sodium and water

Intrarenal causes

- Acute glomerulonephritis
- Acute pyelonephritis
- ATN
- Chronic renal failure
- Toxemia of pregnancy

Damage to renal tubules → Intratubular obstruction → Increased intratubular pressure

Increased renal vasoconstriction → Cellular edema

Postrenal causes

- Benign prostatic hypertrophy
- Bladder neoplasm
- Calculi
- Retroperitoneal fibrosis
- Urethral stricture

Obstruction of urine flow → Back-up of urine → Compression of renal tubules

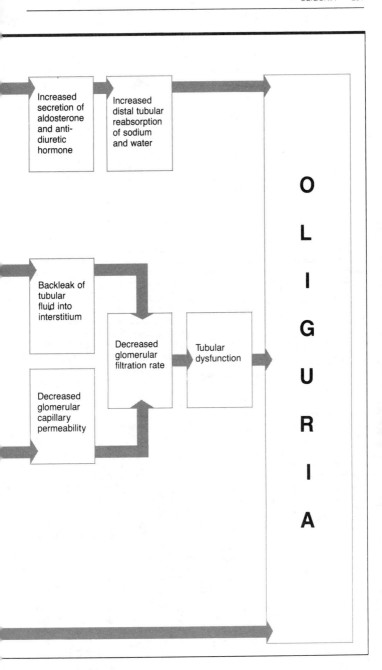

noglycosides and chemotherapeutic agents, such as cisplatin and methotrexate), urinary retention (adrenergic and anticholinergic agents) or urinary obstruction associated with precipitation of urinary crystals (sulfonamides).

Diagnostic tests

Radiographic studies that use contrast media may cause nephrotoxicity and oliguria.

Clinical considerations

• A history should be obtained and a physical examination performed.

• Diagnostic tests include serum blood urea nitrogen and creatinine levels, urea and creatinine clearance, urine sodium levels, urine osmolality, abdominal X-rays, ultrasonography, computed tomography scan, and a renal scan.

• Fluid and electrolyte levels should be monitored.

• The patient should be urged to adhere to fluid and dietary restrictions.

Opisthotonos

Description

Opisthotonos is a prolonged severe spasm of the muscles causing the back to arch acutely, the head to bend back on the neck, the heels to bend back on the legs, and the arms and hands to flex rigidly at the joints (see *Opisthotonos: A Sign of Meningeal Irritation*). Usually, this posture occurs spontaneously and continuously; however, it may be aggravated by movement.

Most commonly caused by meningitis, opisthotonos may also result from subarachnoid hemorrhage, Arnold–Chiari syndrome, and tetanus. Occasionally, it occurs in achondroplastic dwarfism, although not necessarily as an indicator of meningeal irritation.

Opisthotonos is far more common in children, especially infants, than in adults. It is also more exaggerated in children—the result of nervous system immaturity.

Mechanism

Presumably, opisthotonos represents a protective reflex because it immobilizes the spine, alleviating the pain associated with meningeal irritation.

Possible causes

Central nervous system

Arnold–Chiari syndrome. In this syndrome, opisthotonos is typically accompanied by hydrocephalus with its characteristic enlarged head; thin, shiny scalp with distended veins; and underdeveloped neck muscles.

Meningitis. In this infection, opisthotonos accompanies other signs of meningeal irritation, including nuchal rigidity, positive Brudzinski's and Kernig's signs, and hyperreflexia.

Subarachnoid hemorrhage. This disorder may also produce opisthotonos along with other signs of meningeal irritation, such as nuchal rigidity and positive Brudzinski's and Kernig's signs.

Tetanus. This life-threatening infection can cause opisthotonos. Initially, trismus occurs. Eventually, muscle spasms may affect the abdomen, producing boardlike rigidity; the back, resulting in opisthotonos; or the face, producing risus sardonicus.

Drugs

Phenothiazines and other antipsychotic drugs may cause opisthotonos, usually as part of an acute dystonic reaction.

Clinical considerations

• Opisthotonos should be reported to the physician at once.

• Vital signs and neurologic status should be assessed.

• If the patient is stuporous or comatose, resuscitative measures should be taken, as appropriate.

• The patient should be assisted to a side-lying position with pillows for support.

• When the patient's condition permits, a history should be obtained from the patient or a family member. A physical examination should be performed, focusing on neurologic status.

Opisthotonos: A Sign of Meningeal Irritation

In this characteristic posture, the back is severely arched with the neck hyperextended. The heels bend back on the legs, and the arms and hands flex rigidly at the joints, as shown.

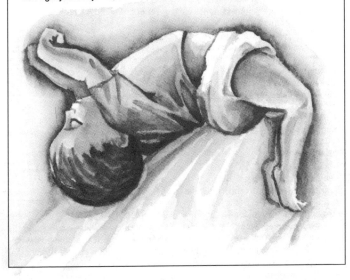

• Diagnostic tests include cerebrospinal fluid analysis and a computed tomography scan.

Orbicularis sign

Description

The orbicularis sign is the inability to close one eye at a time. It occurs in hemiplegia.

Orgasmic dysfunction

Description

Orgasmic dysfunction is a transient or persistent inhibition of the orgasmic phase of sexual excitement. In the female, orgasmic dysfunction is delayed or absent orgasm after a phase of sexual excitement. This results most commonly from psychological or interpersonal problems. It may also result from chronic disorders, congenital anomalies, and chronic vaginal or pelvic infections.

In the male, orgasmic dysfunction is delayed or absent ejaculation after a phase of sexual excitement. Its causes include psychological problems, neurologic disorders, and the effects of antihypertensive drugs (see "Impotence").

Orofacial dyskinesia

Description

Orofacial dyskinesia is abnormal movements involving muscles of the face, mouth, eyes, and occasionally neck. It may be unilateral or bilateral, and constant or intermittent. Sometimes described as a facial tic, this sign is more common in women than in men, especially after age 50.

Mechanism
The pathophysiology of orofacial dyskinesia is not clearly understood. Although the dyskinesia may result from hemifacial spasm disease and the effects of certain drugs, it is commonly idiopathic. Presumably, it results from pressure on the facial nerves associated with an extrapyramidal lesion or from a chemical imbalance. Psychogenic factors may also play a role—a theory supported by the fact that emotional upset aggravates the dyskinesia.

Possible causes
Musculoskeletal

Hemifacial spasm. This disorder is characterized by unilateral, intermittent spasms of muscles of the face, eye, and mouth. The patient may have some voluntary control over the spasms. Typically, the spasms are aggravated by emotional upset and disappear during sleep. Spasms may interfere with swallowing and speech.

Drugs

Phenothiazines and other antipsychotic drugs may cause orofacial dyskinesia and other extrapyramidal effects. Typically, the movements are sustained and involve the eyes, mouth, face, and neck. Lip retraction and difficulty swallowing are common. Among the *phenothiazines*, the piperazine derivatives—acetophenazine, perphenazine, prochlorperazine, fluphenazine, and trifluoperazine—most commonly cause this sign. The aliphatic phenothiazines—chlorpromazine, promazine, and triflupromazine—occasionally cause orofacial dyskinesia. The piperidine phenothiazines—thioridazine, piperacetazine, and mesoridazine—rarely cause orofacial dyskinesia. *Other antipsychotics*—haloperidol, thiothixene, and loxapine—commonly cause this sign.

Metoclopramide and metyrosine rarely cause orofacial dyskinesia.

Clinical considerations
• A history should be obtained and a neurologic examination performed.
• Diagnostic tests include a blood screening for drugs and computed tomography scan.
• If orofacial dyskinesia is drug–induced, the patient should be told that movements typically disappear 24 to 72 hours after stopping the drug.
• If orofacial dyskinesia is uncontrollable, the patient and his family should be advised that drug therapy—including phenobarbital, L–dopa, or carbamazepine—or psychotherapy may be beneficial.

Orthopnea

Description
Orthopnea is difficulty breathing in the supine position. It is a common symptom of cardiopulmonary disorders that produce dyspnea. It is often a subtle symptom; the patient may complain that he cannot catch his breath when lying down or mention that he sleeps comfortably in a reclining chair or propped up by pillows. Derived from this complaint is the common classification of two– or three–pillow orthopnea.

Orthopnea may be aggravated by obesity, which restricts diaphragmatic excursion. Assuming the upright position relieves orthopnea by impairing venous return, which reduces hydrostatic pressure, and by enhancing diaphragmatic excursion, which increases inspiratory volume.

Mechanism
Orthopnea presumably results from increased hydrostatic pressure in the pulmonary vasculature associated with increased venous return in the supine position.

Possible causes
Respiratory
Chronic obstructive pulmonary disease. This disorder typically produces orthopnea and other dyspneic complaints.

Mediastinal tumor. Orthopnea is an early sign of this disorder, resulting from pressure of the tumor against the trachea, bronchus, or lung when the patient lies down. However, many patients are asymptomatic until the tumor enlarges.

Cardiovascular
Left ventricular failure. Orthopnea occurs late in this disorder. If heart failure is acute, orthopnea may begin suddenly; if chronic, it may be constant. The earliest symptom of this disorder is progressively severe dyspnea.

Clinical considerations
• A history should be obtained and a respiratory assessment performed.
• Diagnostic tests include EKG, chest X–ray, and pulmonary function tests.
• Orthopnea may be relieved by a semi–Fowler's or high Fowler's position; if this does not help, the patient should be told to lean over a bedside table with his chest forward.
• Oxygen should be administered, as ordered.

Orthostatic hypotension
(Postural hypotension)

Description
In orthostatic hypotension, the patient's blood pressure drops 10 mm Hg or more when he rises from a supine to a sitting or standing position. It is typically associated with dizziness, syncope, or blurred vision and may occur in a hypotensive, normotensive, or hypertensive patient. Although commonly a nonpathologic sign in elderly patients, orthostatic hypotension may result from prolonged bed rest, fluid and electrolyte imbalance, endocrine or systemic disorders, and the effects of drugs.

Orthostatic hypotension is detected by comparing blood pressure readings with the patient supine, sitting, and then standing.

Mechanism
This common sign indicates failure of compensatory vasomotor responses to adjust to position changes.

Possible causes
Central nervous system
Diabetic autonomic neuropathy. Orthostatic hypotension may be accompanied by signs and symptoms of neuropathy in other areas of the body.

Cardiovascular
Hypovolemia. Mild to moderate hypovolemia may cause orthostatic hypotension.

Endocrine
Adrenal insufficiency. This disorder typically begins insidiously, with progressively severe signs and symptoms. Orthostatic hypotension may be accompanied by fatigue, muscle weakness, anorexia, nausea and vomiting, weight loss, abdominal pain, irritability, and a weak, irregular pulse.

Hyperaldosteronism. This disorder typically produces orthostatic hypotension with sustained elevated blood pressure.

Hematologic
Pheochromocytoma. Although this disorder may produce orthostatic hypotension, its cardinal sign is paroxysmal or sustained hypertension.

Metabolic
Hyponatremia. In this disorder, orthostatic hypotension is typically accompanied by other signs and symptoms of sodium deficit.

Drugs
Certain drugs may cause orthostatic hypotension by reducing circulating blood volume, causing blood vessel dilatation, or depressing the sympathetic nervous system. These drugs include antihypertensives (especially guanethidine and the initial dosage of prazosin), tricyclic antidepressants, phenothiazines, L–dopa, nitrates, mono-

Performing Preambulation Exercises

To help minimize the effects of orthostatic hypotension, such as dizziness and blurred vision when standing up, perform these leg exercises before getting out of bed.

Lie flat and flex one knee slightly, keeping heel on the bed.

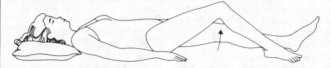

Lift the heel off the bed and try to straighten leg.

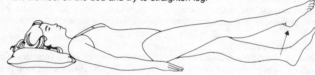

Flex knee again, and lower heel to the bed.

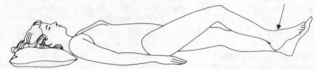

Straighten the leg.

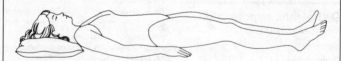

Repeat the procedure for the other leg. Alternating sides, perform the exercises six times for each leg.

amine oxidase inhibitors, morphine, bretylium, and spinal anesthesia. Large doses of diuretics can also cause orthostatic hypotension.

Treatments

Orthostatic hypotension is commonly associated with prolonged bed rest (24 hours or longer). It may also result from sympathectomy, which disrupts normal vasoconstrictive mechanisms.

Clinical considerations
• If orthostatic hypotension is detected, the patient should be assessed for other signs and symptoms of hypovolemic shock.

• A history should be obtained and a physical examination performed.

• Diagnostic tests include serum electrolyte and drug levels, urinalysis, 12–lead EKG, and chest X–ray.

• To help minimize orthostatic hypotension, the patient should be advised to change his position *gradually*. The head of the bed should be elevated and the patient assisted to a sitting position with his feet dangling over the side of the bed. If he can tolerate this position, he should be instructed to sit in a chair for brief periods. The patient should be returned immediately to bed if he becomes dizzy or pale or displays other signs of hypotension.

• Preambulation exercises may also be performed to minimize orthostatic hypotension (see *Performing Preambulation Exercises*).

• The patient should never be unattended while walking.

Orthotonos

Description
Orthotonos is a form of tetanic spasm producing a rigid, straight line of the neck, limbs, and body.

Ortolani's sign

Description
Ortolani's sign is a click or popping sensation that is felt and often heard on abduction of the newborn's thighs. It indicates congenital dislocation of the hip (congenital hip dysplasia). Screening for this sign is an important part of newborn care (see *Detecting Congenital Hip Dysplasia*, pp. 288 and 289). Early detection and treatment of congenital hip dysplasia improves the infant's chances of developing a healthy, functional joint. If treatment is delayed, congenital hip dysplasia may cause degenerative hip changes, lordosis, joint malformation,

and soft–tissue damage. Various methods of abduction are used to produce a stable joint, including double–diapering, soft splinting devices, and a plaster hip spica cast.

Ortolani's sign can be elicited only during the first 4 to 6 weeks of life. It is most common in females and in American Indians.

Osler's nodes

Description
Osler's nodes are tender, raised, pea-sized, red or purple lesions that erupt on the palms, soles, and especially the pads of the fingers and toes. They are a rare, but reliable, sign of infective endocarditis and are pathognomonic of the subacute form. However, the nodes usually develop after other telling signs and symptoms and disappear spontaneously within several days. How and why they develop is uncertain; they may result from emboli caught in peripheral capillaries or may reflect an immunologic reaction to the causative organism. Osler's nodes must be distinguished from the even less common Janeway's lesions—small, painless, erythematous lesions that erupt on the palms and soles.

Ostealgia

Description
Ostealgia is bone pain. It is associated with such disorders as osteomyelitis.

Otorrhagia

Description
Otorrhagia is bleeding from the ear. It occurs with a tumor, severe infection, or injury affecting the auricle, external canal, tympanic membrane, or temporal bone.

Detecting Congenital Hip Dysplasia

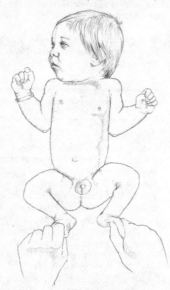

When assessing the newborn, the examiner attempts to elicit Ortolani's sign to detect congenital hip dsyplasia. With the infant in a supine position with his knees and hips flexed, the examiner observes for symmetry.

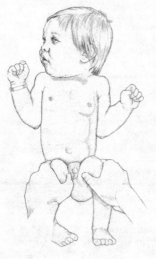

The examiner places her hands on the infant's knees, with the index fingers along his lateral thighs. Then she raises his knees at a 90° angle to his back.

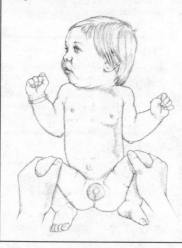

Next, the examiner abducts the infant's thighs, so that the lateral aspect of his knees lies almost flat on the table. If the infant has a dislocated hip, the examiner will feel and often hear a click or popping sensation (Ortolani's sign) as the head of the femur moves out of the acetabulum. The infant may also give a sudden cry of pain.

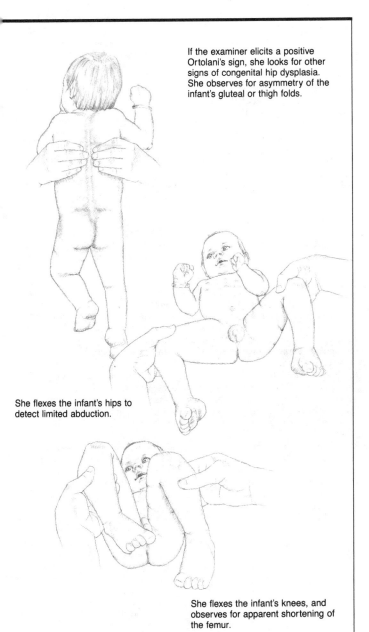

If the examiner elicits a positive Ortolani's sign, she looks for other signs of congenital hip dysplasia. She observes for asymmetry of the infant's gluteal or thigh folds.

She flexes the infant's hips to detect limited abduction.

She flexes the infant's knees, and observes for apparent shortening of the femur.

Otorrhea

Description

Otorrhea is drainage from the ear. It may be bloody (otorrhagia), purulent, clear, or serosanguineous. Its onset, duration, and severity provide clues to the underlying cause. This sign may result from disorders that affect the external ear canal or the middle ear, including allergy, infection, neoplasms, trauma, and collagen diseases. Otorrhea may occur alone or with other symptoms, such as ear pain. Otitis media is the most common cause of otorrhea in infants and young children.

Possible causes

Central nervous system

Basilar skull fracture. In this disorder, otorrhea may be clear and watery, representing cerebrospinal fluid leakage, or bloody, representing hemorrhage.

Epidural abscess. In this disorder, profuse, creamy otorrhea is accompanied by steady, throbbing ear pain; fever; and temporal or temporoparietal headache on the ipsilateral side.

Eyes, ears, nose, throat

Aural polyps. These polyps may produce foul, purulent, and perhaps blood–streaked discharge. If they occlude the external ear canal, the polyps may cause partial hearing loss.

Dermatitis of the external ear canal. In *contact dermatitis*, vesicles produce clear, watery otorrhea with edema and erythema of the external ear canal.

Infectious eczematoid dermatitis causes purulent otorrhea with erythema and crusting of the external ear canal.

In *seborrheic dermatitis*, otorrhea consists of greasy scales and flakes.

Mastoiditis. This disorder causes thick, purulent, yellow otorrhea that becomes increasingly profuse.

Myringitis (infectious). In *acute infectious myringitis*, small, reddened, blood–filled blebs erupt in the external ear canal, the tympanic membrane, and, occasionally, the middle ear. Spontaneous rupture of these blebs causes serosanguineous otorrhea.

Chronic infectious myringitis causes purulent otorrhea, pruritus, and gradual hearing loss.

Otitis externa. Acute otitis externa, commonly known as swimmer's ear, usually causes purulent, yellow, sticky, foul–smelling otorrhea. Inspection may reveal white–green debris in the external ear canal.

Chronic otitis externa usually causes scanty, intermittent otorrhea that may be serous or purulent and possibly foul-smelling. Its primary symptom is itching.

Life–threatening *malignant otitis externa* produces debris in the ear canal, which may build up against the tympanic membrane causing severe pain, which is especially acute during manipulation of the tragus or auricle.

Otitis media. In *acute otitis media*, rupture of the tympanic membrane produces bloody, purulent otorrhea and relieves continuous or intermittent ear pain.

In *acute suppurative otitis media*, the patient may also have signs and symptoms of upper respiratory infection—sore throat, cough, nasal discharge, headache. Other features may include dizziness, fever, nausea, and vomiting.

Chronic otitis media causes intermittent, purulent, foul–smelling otorrhea associated with frequent perforation of the tympanic membrane.

Perichondritis. In this disorder, multiple fistulas may open on the auricle or external ear canal, causing purulent otorrhea.

Tuberculosis. Pulmonary tuberculosis may spread through the upper airway to the middle ear, causing chronic ear infection. The tympanic membrane thickens, ruptures, and produces a watery otorrhea and mild hearing loss.

Tumor (benign). A benign tumor of the glomus jugulare (jugular bulb) may cause bloody otorrhea.

Tumor (malignant). Squamous cell carcinoma of the external ear causes purulent otorrhea with itching.

In *squamous cell carcinoma of the middle ear*, blood–tinged otorrhea occurs early, typically accompanied by hearing loss on the affected side.

Immunologic

Allergy. An allergy associated with tympanic membrane perforation may cause clear or cloudy otorrhea, rhinorrhea, and itchy, watery eyes.

Environmental

Trauma. Bloody otorrhea may result from trauma, such as a blow to the external ear, a foreign body in the ear, or barotrauma. Usually, the bleeding is minimal or moderate; it may be accompanied by partial hearing loss.

Clinical considerations

• A history should be obtained and an ear examination performed.

• An ear drainage specimen should be obtained, as ordered, for culture and sensitivity testing or cytology.

• Warm, moist compresses, heating pads, or hot water bottles should be applied, as needed and ordered, to the patient's ears to relieve inflammation and pain.

• To avoid channeling infected secretions into the middle ear, the patient with chronic ear problems should be advised to avoid forceful nose blowing when he has an upper respiratory infection. He should be instructed to blow his nose with his mouth open.

• A warm, wet washcloth may be used to remove drainage from the external ear canal.

• Until the tympanic membrane has healed, lubricated cotton balls should be inserted into the ear canal before the patient showers or shampoos.

P-Q

Pain, abdominal

Description

Usually, abdominal pain results from gastrointestinal disorders, but it can also result from reproductive, genitourinary, musculoskeletal, and vascular disorders (see *Abdominal Pain: Types and Location,* p. 294); drug use; and the effects of toxins. At times, it indicates life–threatening complications. In children, abdominal pain can signal a disorder with greater severity or different associated signs than in adults.

Abdominal pain arises from the abdominopelvic viscera, the parietal peritoneum, or the capsules of the liver, kidney, or spleen. It may be acute or chronic, diffuse or localized. Visceral pain develops slowly into a dull, aching pain that is poorly localized in the epigastric, periumbilical, or lower midabdominal region. In contrast, somatic pain produces a bright, sharp, more intense, and well–localized discomfort that rapidly follows the insult. Movement or coughing aggravates this pain.

Pain may also be referred to the abdomen from another site with the same or similar nerve supply. This sharp, well–localized, referred pain is felt in skin or deeper tissues and may coexist with skin hyperesthesia and muscle hyperalgesia.

Mechanism

Mechanisms that produce abdominal pain include stretching or tension of the gut wall, traction on the peritoneum or mesentery, vigorous intestinal contraction, inflammation, ischemia, or sensory nerve irritation.

Possible causes

Respiratory

Pleurisy. This disorder may produce upper abdominal or costal margin pain referred from the chest. Characteristic sharp, stabbing chest pain increases with inspiration and movement.

Pneumonia. Lower lobe pneumonia can cause pleuritic chest pain and referred, severe upper abdominal pain, tenderness, and rigidity that diminish with inspiration.

Pneumothorax. This potentially life–threatening disorder can cause pain across the upper abdomen and costal margin that is referred from the chest. Characteristic chest pain arises suddenly and worsens with deep inspiration or movement.

Cardiovascular

Abdominal aortic aneurysm (dissecting). Initially, this life–threatening disorder may produce dull abdominal, low back, or severe chest pain. More often, it produces constant upper abdominal pain, which may worsen when the patient lies down and abate when he leans forward or sits up.

Congestive heart failure. Right upper quadrant pain commonly accompanies this disorder's hallmarks: neck vein distention, dyspnea, tachycardia, and peripheral edema.

Mesenteric artery ischemia. Severe, constant, and diffuse abdominal pain is preceded by 2 to 3 days of colicky periumbilical pain and diarrhea.

Myocardial infarction. Substernal chest pain may radiate to the abdomen in this life–threatening disorder.

Endocrine

Adrenal crisis. Severe abdominal pain appears early, along with nausea, vomiting, weakness, anorexia, and fever.

Diabetic ketoacidosis. Rarely, severe, sharp, shooting, and girdling pain may persist for several days.

Gastrointestinal

Abdominal cancer. Abdominal pain usually occurs late in this disorder.

Abdominal trauma. Generalized or localized abdominal pain occurs with possible ecchymoses on the abdomen; abdominal tenderness; vomiting; and, with hemorrhage into the peritoneal cavity, abdominal rigidity.

Appendicitis. In this disorder, dull discomfort in the epigastric or umbilical region typically precedes anorexia, nausea, and vomiting. Pain localizes at McBurney's point in the right lower quadrant, accompanied by abdominal rigidity, increasing tenderness (especially over McBurney's point), rebound tenderness, and retractive respirations.

Cirrhosis. Dull abdominal aching occurs early, usually with anorexia, indigestion, nausea, vomiting, constipation, or diarrhea. Subsequent right upper quadrant pain worsens when the patient sits up or leans forward.

Cholecystitis. Severe pain in the right upper quadrant may arise suddenly or increase gradually over several hours and may radiate to the right shoulder, chest, or back.

Cholelithiasis. Sudden, severe, and paroxysmal pain in the right upper quadrant may last several minutes to several hours and may radiate to the epigastrium, back, or shoulder blades.

Crohn's disease. An *acute* attack causes severe, cramping pain in the lower abdomen, typically preceded by weeks or months of milder, cramping pain.

Milder *chronic* symptoms include right lower quadrant pain with diarrhea, steatorrhea, and weight loss.

Diverticulitis. Mild diverticulitis usually produces intermittent, diffuse abdominal pain, which is sometimes relieved by defecation or passage of flatus. Rupture causes left lower quadrant pain, abdominal rigidity, and posible signs of sepsis and shock (high fever, chills, and hypotension).

Duodenal ulcer. Localized abdominal pain—described as steady, gnawing, burning, aching, or hungerlike—may occur high in the midepigastrium or slightly off center, usually on the right. It usually does not radiate unless pancreatic penetration occurs. Usually, pain begins 2 to 4 hours after meals and may cause nocturnal awakening. Ingestion of food or antacids brings relief until the cycle starts again but also may produce weight gain.

Gastric ulcer. Diffuse, gnawing, burning pain in the left upper quadrant or epigastric area often occurs 1 to 2 hours after meals and may be relieved by food or antacids.

Gastritis. In gastritis, abdominal pain can range from mild epigastric discomfort to burning pain in the left upper quadrant.

Gastroenteritis. Cramping or colicky abdominal pain, which can be diffuse, originates in the left upper quadrant and radiates or migrates to the other quadrants.

Hepatic abscess. Abdominal pain that is steady, severe, and located in the right upper quadrant or midepigastrium commonly accompanies this rare disorder, although right upper quadrant tenderness is the most important finding.

Hepatic amebiasis. This disorder, rare in the United States, causes severe right upper quadrant pain and tenderness over the liver and possibly the right shoulder.

Hepatitis. Liver enlargement from any type of hepatitis causes discomfort or dull pain and tenderness in the right upper quadrant.

Intestinal obstruction. Short episodes of intense, colicky, cramping pain alternate with pain–free intervals in this life–threatening disorder.

Abdominal Pain: Types and Location

Affected Organ	Visceral Pain	Parietal Pain	Referred Pain
Stomach	Middle epigastrium	Middle epigastrium and left upper quadrant	Shoulders
Small intestine	Periumbilical area	Over affected site	Midback (rare)
Appendix	Periumbilical area	Right lower quadrant	Right lower quadrant
Proximal colon	Periumbilical area and right flank for ascending colon	Over affected site	Right lower quadrant and back (rare)
Distal colon	Hypogastrium and left flank for descending colon	Over affected site	Left lower quadrant and back (rare)
Gallbladder	Middle epigastrium	Right upper quadrant	Right subscapular area
Ureters	Costovertebral angle	Over affected site	Groin; scrotum in men, labia in women (rare)
Pancreas	Middle epigastrium and left upper quadrant	Middle epigastrium and left upper quadrant	Back and left shoulder
Ovaries, fallopian tubes, and uterus	Hypogastrium and groin	Over affected site	Inner thighs

Irritable bowel syndrome. Lower abdominal cramping or pain is aggravated by eating coarse or raw foods and may be alleviated by defecation or passage of flatus.

Pancreatitis. Life–threatening *acute pancreatitis* produces fulminating, continuous upper abdominal pain that may radiate to both flanks and to the back. To relieve this pain, the patient may bend forward, draw his knees to his chest, or move restlessly about.

Chronic pancreatitis produces severe left upper quadrant or epigastric pain that radiates to the back.

Perforated ulcer. In this life–threatening disorder, sudden, severe, and prostrating epigastric pain may radiate through the abdomen to the back.

Peritonitis. In this life–threatening disorder, sudden and severe pain can be diffuse or localized in the area of the underlying disorder; movement worsens pain.

Splenic infarction. Fulminating pain in the left upper quadrant occurs along with chest pain that may worsen on inspiration. Pain often radiates to the left shoulder with splinting of the left diaphragm, abdominal guarding, and occasionally a splenic friction rub.

Ulcerative colitis. This disorder may begin with vague abdominal discomfort that leads to cramping lower abdominal pain. As the disorder progresses, pain can become steady and diffuse, increasing with movement and coughing. The most common symptom—recurrent and possibly severe diarrhea with blood, pus, and mucus—may relieve the pain.

Genitourinary

Cystitis. Abdominal pain and tenderness are usually suprapubic.

Prostatitis. Vague abdominal pain or discomfort in the lower abdomen, groin, perineum, or rectum may develop.

Pyelonephritis (acute). Progressive lower quadrant pain in one or both sides, flank pain, and costovertebral angle (CVA) tenderness characterize this disorder. Pain may radiate to the lower midabdomen or to the groin.

Renal calculi. Depending on the location of calculi, severe abdominal or back pain may occur. However, the classic symptom is severe, colicky pain that travels from the CVA to the flank, the suprapubic region, and the external genitalia. The pain may be excruciating or dull and constant.

Uremia. This disorder is characterized by generalized or periumbilical pain that shifts and varies in intensity.

Musculoskeletal

Systemic lupus erythematosus. Generalized abdominal pain is unusual but may occur after meals.

Hematologic

Sickle cell crisis. Sudden, severe abdominal pain may accompany chest, back, hand, or foot pain.

Obstetric-gynecologic

Ectopic pregnancy. Lower abdominal pain may be sharp, dull, or cramping, and constant or intermittent in this potentially life–threatening disorder. Rupture of the fallopian tube produces sharp lower abdominal pain, which may radiate to the shoulders and neck and become extreme with cervical or adnexal palpation.

Endometriosis. Constant, severe pain in the lower abdomen usually begins 5 to 7 days before menstruation begins and may be aggravated by defecation.

Ovarian cyst. Torsion or hemorrhage causes pain and tenderness in the right or left lower abdominal quadrant. Sharp and severe if the patient suddenly stands or stoops, the pain becomes brief and intermittent if the torsion self-corrects, or dull and diffuse after several hours if it does not.

Pelvic inflammatory disease. Pain in the right or left lower quadrant ranges from vague discomfort worsened by movement to deep, severe, and progressive pain. Sometimes metrorrhagia precedes or accompanies the onset of pain. Extreme pain accompanies cervical or adnexal palpation.

Infection

Herpes zoster. Herpes zoster of the thoracic, lumbar, or sacral nerves can cause localized abdominal and chest pain in the area these nerves serve.

Environmental

Insect toxins. Generalized, cramping abdominal pain usually occurs with low–grade fever, nausea, vomiting, abdominal rigidity, tremors, and burning sensations in the hands or feet.

Drugs

Salicylates and nonsteroidal anti–inflammatory drugs commonly cause burning, gnawing pain in the left upper quadrant or epigastric area, along with nausea and vomiting.

Clinical considerations

If the patient is experiencing sudden and severe abdominal pain:

• Vital signs should be taken quickly and a rapid assessment performed.

- The physician should be notified immediately.
- Emergency intervention, including surgery, should be anticipated and the patient prepared accordingly.

If the patient has no life–threatening signs or symptoms:

- A history should be taken and an abdominal assessment performed.
- Diagnostic tests may include pelvic or rectal examination; blood, urine, and stool tests; X–rays; barium studies; ultrasonography; endoscopy; or biopsy.
- If ordered, vasogastric or intestinal intubation should be performed.
- Preparations should be made to assist with peritoneal lavage or abdominal paracentesis, if ordered.
- The patient should be closely monitored—abdominal pain can signal a life–threatening disorder.
- The patient should be assisted to a comfortable position, if possible, to ease his distress.
- Analgesics should be administered, as ordered, only *after* a diagnosis has been made, as these drugs mask symptoms.

Pain, arm

Description

Usually, arm pain results from musculoskeletal disorders, but it can also result from neurovascular or cardiovascular disorders. Its location, onset, and character provide clues to its cause. The pain may affect the entire arm or only the upper arm or forearm. It may arise suddenly or gradually and be constant or intermittent. Arm pain can be described as sharp or dull, burning or numbing, shooting or penetrating. Diffuse arm pain may be difficult to describe, especially if it is not associated with injury.

Possible causes

Central nervous system
Cervical nerve root compression. Compression of the cervical nerves supplying the upper arm produces chronic arm and neck pain that may worsen with movement or prolonged sitting.

Cardiovascular
Angina. This disorder may cause inner arm pain, as well as chest and jaw pain. Typically, the pain follows exertion and persists for a few minutes.

Myocardial infarction. In this life–threatening disorder, the patient may complain of left arm pain as well as the characteristic deep and crushing chest pain.

Musculoskeletal
Biceps rupture. Rupture of the biceps after excessive weight lifting or osteoarthritic degeneration of bicipital tendon insertion at the shoulder can cause pain in the upper arm. Forearm flexion and supination aggravate the pain.

Compartment syndrome. Severe pain with passive muscle stretching is the cardinal sign of this syndrome.

Fractures. In fractures of the cervical vertebrae, humerus, scapula, clavicle, radius, or ulna, pain can occur at the injury site and radiate throughout the entire arm. Pain at a fresh fracture site is intense and worsens with movement.

Muscle contusion. This disorder may cause generalized pain in the area of injury.

Muscle strain. Acute or chronic muscle strain causes mild to severe pain with movement.

Osteomyelitis. This disorder typically begins with the sudden onset of localized arm pain and fever.

Skin
Cellulitis. Typically, this disorder affects the legs, but it can also affect the arms. It produces pain as well as redness, tenderness, edema, and, at times, fever, chills, tachycardia, headache, and hypotension.

Neoplastic
Neoplasms of the arm. This disorder produces continuous, deep, and penetrating arm pain that worsens at night. Occasionally, redness and swelling accompany arm pain; later, skin breakdown, impaired circulation, and paresthesia may occur.

Causes of Local Pain

Various disorders cause hand, wrist, elbow, or shoulder pain. In some disorders, pain may radiate from the injury site to other areas.

Hand pain
Arthritis
Buerger's disease
Carpal tunnel syndrome
Dupuytren's contracture
Elbow tunnel syndrome
Fracture
Ganglion
Infection
Occlusive vascular disease
Radiculopathy
Raynaud's disease
Shoulder-hand syndrome (reflex
  sympathetic dystrophy)
Sprain or strain
Thoracic outlet syndromes
Trigger finger

Wrist pain
Arthritis
Carpal tunnel syndrome
Fracture
Ganglion
Sprain or strain
Tenosynovitis (de Quervain's disease)

Elbow pain
Arthritis
Bursitis

Dislocation
Fracture
Lateral epicondylitis (tennis elbow)
Tendonitis

Shoulder pain
Acromioclavicular separation
Acute pancreatitis
Adhesive capsulitis (frozen shoulder)
Angina pectoris
Arthritis
Bursitis
Cholecystitis/cholelithiasis
Clavicle fracture
Diaphragmatic pleurisy
Dislocation
Dissecting aortic aneurysm
Gastritis
Humeral neck fracture
Infection
Pancoast's syndrome
Perforated ulcer
Pneumothorax
Ruptured spleen (left shoulder)
Shoulder-hand syndrome
Subphrenic abscess
Tendonitis

Clinical considerations
• If the patient reports arm pain after an injury, a brief history should be taken and a quick assessment of the arm performed; the arm should be immobilized to prevent further injury.
• If a patient has a cast, splint, or restrictive dressing, a neurovascular assessment should be performed distal to the site.
• If the patient reports generalized or intermittent arm pain, a detailed history should be obtained and a thorough examination performed.
• Diagnostic tests include X–rays of the affected arm.
• The patient's comfort should be promoted by elevating the arm, applying ice, and administering analgesics, as ordered.

Pain, back

Description
Back pain affects an estimated 80% of the population; it is second only to the common cold for lost time from work. Although this symptom may herald a spondylogenic disorder, it may also result from genitourinary, gastrointestinal, cardiovascular, or neoplastic disorders. Postural imbalance associated with pregnancy may also cause back pain.

Back pain most commonly occurs in the lower back, or lumbosacral area. Back pain may also be referred from the abdomen or flank, possibly signaling life–threatening perforated ulcer, acute pancreatitis, or dissecting abdominal aortic aneurysm.

The onset, location, and distribution of pain and its response to activity and rest provide important clues about the causative disorder. Pain may be acute or chronic, constant or intermittent. It may remain localized in the back or radiate along the spine or down one or both legs. Pain may be exacerbated by activity—most commonly, bending, stooping, or lifting—and alleviated by rest, or it may be unaffected by both.

Mechanism
Intrinsic back pain results from muscle spasm, nerve root irritation, fracture, or a combination of these mechanisms.

Possible causes
Central nervous system
Chordoma. A slow–developing malignant tumor, chordoma causes persistent pain in the lower back, sacrum, and coccyx.

Spinal neoplasm (benign). Typically, this disorder causes severe, localized back pain and scoliosis.

Cardiovascular
Abdominal aortic aneurysm (dissecting). Life–threatening dissection of this aneurysm may initially cause low back pain or dull abdominal pain. More often, it produces constant upper abdominal pain.

Gastrointestinal
Appendicitis. In this life–threatening disorder, a vague and dull discomfort in the epigastric or umbilical region migrates to McBurney's point in the right lower quadrant. In retrocecal appendicitis, pain may also radiate to the back. The shift in pain is preceded by anorexia and nausea.

Cholecystitis. This disorder produces severe pain in the right upper quadrant that may radiate to the right shoulder, chest, or back. The pain may arise suddenly or may increase gradually over several hours.

Pancreatitis (acute). This life–threatening disorder usually produces fulminating, continuous upper abdominal pain that may radiate to both flanks and to the back. To relieve this pain, the patient may bend forward, draw his knees to his chest, or move restlessly about.

Perforated ulcer. In some patients, perforation of a duodenal or gastric ulcer causes sudden, prostrating epigastric pain that may radiate throughout the abdomen and to the back.

Genitourinary
Prostatic carcinoma. Chronic, aching back pain may be the only symptom of prostatic carcinoma. This disorder may also produce cloudy urine or hematuria.

Pyelonephritis (acute). This disorder produces progressive flank and lower abdominal pain accompanied by back pain or tenderness (especially over the costovertebral angle [CVA]).

Renal calculi. The colicky pain of this disorder usually results from irritation of the ureteral lining, which increases the frequency and force of peristaltic contractions. This pain travels from the CVA to the flank, the suprapubic region, and the external genitalia. Its intensity varies but may become excruciating if calculi travel down a ureter.

Musculoskeletal
Ankylosing spondylitis. This chronic, progressive disorder causes sacroiliac pain, which radiates up the spine and is aggravated by lateral pressure on the pelvis. The pain is usually most severe in the morning or after a period of inactivity and is not relieved by rest.

Intervertebral disk rupture. This disorder produces gradual or sudden low back pain with or without leg pain (sciatica). Rarely, it produces leg pain alone. More often, pain begins in the back and radiates to the buttocks and leg. The pain is exacerbated by activity, coughing, and sneezing and is eased by rest.

Exercises for Chronic Low Back Pain

The exercises illustrated here may help relieve discomfort and prevent further lumbar deterioration. Keep in mind the following points:
• Breathe slowly, inhaling through the nose and exhaling completely through pursed lips.
• Begin gradually, performing each exercise only once per day and progressing to 10 repetitions.
• Exercise moderately; expect mild discomfort, but stop if you experience severe pain.

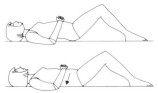

Back press
Lie flat, with arms on chest and knees bent. Press the small (lower portion) of back to the floor while tightening the abdominal muscles and buttocks. Count to 10, then slowly relax.

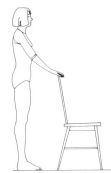

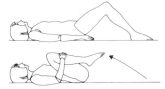

Knee grasp
Lie flat, with knees bent. Bring one knee to chest, grasping it firmly with both hands; lower the knee. Repeat with the other knee—then with *both* knees, as shown here.

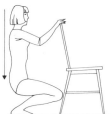

Knee bend
Stand with hands on the back of a chair for support. Keeping back straight, slowly bend knees to a squatting position. Return to starting position.

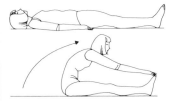

Sit-up
Lie flat, with arms at sides. Using the abdominal muscles, slowly sit up and reach for toes, touching them if possible.

Lumbosacral sprain. This disorder causes aching, localized pain and tenderness associated with muscle spasm on lateral motion. The recumbent patient will typically flex his knees and hips to help ease pain. Flexion of the spine intensifies pain, whereas rest helps relieve it.

Myeloma. Back pain caused by this primary malignant tumor commonly begins abruptly and worsens with exercise.

Reiter's syndrome. In some patients, sacroiliac pain is the first sign of this disorder. It is accompanied by the classic triad of conjunctivitis, urethritis, and arthritis.

Sacroiliac strain. This disorder causes sacroiliac pain that may radiate to the buttock, hip, and lateral aspect of the thigh. The pain is aggravated by weight bearing on the affected extremity and by abduction with resistance of the leg.

Spinal stenosis. Resembling a ruptured intervertebral disk, this disorder produces back pain with or without sciatica.

Spondylolisthesis. A major structural disorder characterized by forward slippage of one vertebra onto another, spondylolisthesis may be asymptomatic or cause low back pain with or without nerve root involvement.

Transverse process fracture. This fracture causes severe localized back pain with muscle spasm and hematoma.

Vertebral compression fracture. Initially, this fracture may be painless. Several weeks later, it causes back pain aggravated by weight bearing and local tenderness. Fracture of a thoracic vertebra may cause referred pain in the lumbar area.

Vertebral osteomyelitis. Initially, this disorder causes insidious back pain. As it progresses, the pain may become constant, more pronounced at night, and aggravated by spinal movement.

Vertebral osteoporosis. This disorder causes chronic, aching back pain that is aggravated by activity and somewhat relieved by rest.

Obstetric-gynecologic

Endometriosis. This disorder causes deep sacral pain and severe, cramping pain in the lower abdomen. The pain worsens just before or during menstruation and may be aggravated by defecation.

Neoplastic

Metastatic tumors. These tumors commonly spread to the spine, causing low back pain in at least 25% of patients. Typically, the pain begins abruptly, is accompanied by cramping muscular pain, and is not relieved by rest.

Diagnostic tests

Lumbar puncture and myelography can produce transient back pain.

Clinical considerations

If back pain suggests a life–threatening cause:

• Vital signs should be taken quickly and a rapid, well–focused assessment performed.

• The physician should be notified.

• Emergency intervention, including surgery, should be anticipated and the patient prepared accordingly.

If life–threatening causes of back pain are ruled out:

• A complete history should be obtained and a physical examination performed.

• Diagnostic tests may include a rectal or pelvic examination; routine blood tests; urinalysis; X–rays of the chest, abdomen, and spine; computed tomography scan of the spine; and appropriate biopsies.

• Until a diagnosis is made, analgesics should be withheld, as ordered, because they may mask symptoms.

• The patient should be positioned as comfortably as possible.

• If the patient has chronic back pain, instructions regarding bed rest, therapeutic warm baths, analgesics, anti–inflammatory drugs, and exercise should be reinforced (see *Exercises for Chronic Low Back Pain*, p. 299).

• The patient may be fitted for a corset or lumbosacral support device.

• The patient should be helped to make necessary life–style changes; for example, he should be advised to lose weight or correct poor posture.

- The patient should be taught about alternatives to analgesic drugs, such as biofeedback and transcutaneous electrical nerve stimulation.
- Heat or cold therapy, a backboard, an egg–crate mattress, or pelvic traction may also be used to relieve pain.
- Back pain is notoriously associated with malingering. The patient should be referred to other professionals, such as a physical therapist, occupational therapist, or psychologist, when indicated.

Pain, breast
(Mastalgia)

Description
An unreliable indicator of cancer, this symptom commonly results from benign breast disease. It may occur during rest or movement and may be aggravated by manipulation or palpation. (Breast *tenderness* refers to pain *elicited* by physical contact.) Breast pain may be unilateral or bilateral; cyclic, intermittent, or constant; and dull or sharp. It may result from surface cuts, furuncles, contusions, and similar lesions (superficial pain); nipple fissures and inflammation in the papillary ducts and areolae (severe, localized pain); stromal distention in the breast parenchyma; a tumor that affects nerve endings (severe, constant pain); or inflammatory lesions that not only distend the stroma but also irritate sensory nerve endings (severe pain). Breast pain may radiate to the back, the arms, and sometimes the neck.

Breast tenderness in women may occur before menstruation and during pregnancy. Before menstruation, breast pain or tenderness stems from increased mammary blood flow resulting from hormonal changes. During pregnancy, breast tenderness and throbbing, tingling, or pricking sensations may occur, also influenced by hormonal changes.

In men, breast pain may stem from gynecomastia (especially during puberty and senescence), reproductive tract anomalies, and organic disease of the pituitary, adrenal cortex, and thyroid glands.

Possible causes
Obstetric-gynecologic
Areolar gland abscess. Tender, palpable abscesses on the periphery of the areola follow inflammation of the sebaceous glands of Montgomery.

Breast abscess (acute). In the affected breast, local pain, tenderness, erythema, peau d'orange, and warmth are associated with a nodule.

Breast cancer. Breast pain is an infrequent symptom. However, when reported, the pain may be described as momentary and snatching, a pricking sensation, or infrequent but bothersome twinges.

Breast cyst. A breast cyst that enlarges rapidly may cause acute, localized, and usually unilateral pain.

Fat necrosis. Local pain and tenderness may develop in this benign disorder. A history of trauma may be present.

Intraductal papilloma. Unilateral breast pain or tenderness may accompany this condition, although the primary sign is a serous or bloody nipple discharge.

Mammary duct ectasia. Burning pain and itching around the areola may occur, although ectasia is commonly asymptomatic at first. The history may include one or more episodes of inflammation with pain, tenderness, erythema, and acute fever, or with pain and tenderness alone, which develop and then subside spontaneously within 7 to 10 days.

Mastitis. Unilateral pain may be severe, particularly when the inflammation occurs near the skin surface.

Proliferative (fibrocystic) breast disease. In this common cause of breast pain, cysts develop and may cause pain before menstruation and be asymptomatic after it. Later in the disease's course, pain and tenderness may persist throughout the cycle.

Sebaceous cyst (infected). Breast pain may be reported with this cutaneous cyst.

Clinical considerations

• A history should be obtained and a breast examination performed.

• Diagnostic tests may include mammography, thermography, cytology of nipple discharge, biopsy, or culture of any aspirate.

• Analgesics should be administered, as ordered.

• The patient should be advised to wear a well–fitting brassiere for support, especially if her breasts are large or pendulous.

• Emotional support should be provided for the patient and, when appropriate, the importance of monthly breast self–examination emphasized. The patient should be taught how to perform this examination and instructed to call the physician immediately if she detects any breast changes.

Pain, eye
(Ophthalmalgia)

Description

Eye pain may be described as a burning, throbbing, aching, or stabbing sensation in or around the eye. It may also be characterized as a foreign–body sensation. This sign varies from mild to severe; its duration and exact location provide clues to the causative disorder.

Most commonly, eye pain results from corneal abrasion. It may also result from glaucoma and other eye disorders, trauma, and neurologic and systemic disorders. Any of these may stimulate nerve endings in the cornea or external eye, producing pain.

Possible causes

Central nervous system

Migraine headache. Pain may be so severe in this disorder that the eyes also ache.

Subdural hematoma. Following head trauma, a subdural hematoma commonly causes severe eye ache and headache.

Eyes, ears, nose, throat

Acute closed–angle glaucoma. Blurred vision and sudden, excruciating pain in and around the eye characterize this disorder; the pain may be so severe that it causes nausea and vomiting.

Astigmatism. Uncorrected astigmatism commonly causes headache and eye fatigue, aching, and redness.

Blepharitis. Burning pain in both eyelids is accompanied by itching, sticky discharge, and conjunctival injection.

Chalazion. A chalazion causes localized tenderness and swelling on the upper or lower eyelid.

Conjunctivitis. Some degree of eye pain and excessive tearing occurs with four types of conjunctivitis. *Allergic conjunctivitis* causes mild, burning, bilateral pain accompanied by itching, conjunctival injection, and a characteristic ropy discharge. *Bacterial conjunctivitis* causes pain only when it affects the cornea. Otherwise, it produces burning and a foreign–body sensation. If it affects the cornea, *fungal conjunctivitis* may cause pain and photophobia. *Viral conjunctivitis* produces itching, red eyes accompanied by a foreign–body sensation, visible conjunctival follicles, and eyelid edema.

Corneal abrasions. In this type of injury, eye pain is characterized by a foreign–body sensation.

Corneal erosion (recurrent). Severe pain occurs on waking and continues throughout the day. Accompanying the pain are conjunctival injection and photophobia.

Corneal ulcers. Both bacterial and fungal corneal ulcers cause severe eye pain.

Dacryoadenitis. Temporal pain may affect both eyes in this disorder.

Dacryocystitis. Pain and tenderness near the tear sac characterize acute dacryocystitis.

Episcleritis. Deep eye pain occurs as tissues over sclera become inflamed.

Erythema multiforme major. This disorder commonly produces severe eye pain, entropion, trichiasis, purulent conjunctivitis, photophobia, and decreased tear formation.

Foreign bodies in the cornea and conjunctiva. Sudden severe pain is common but vision usually remains intact.

Herpes zoster ophthalmicus. Eye pain occurs with severe unilateral facial pain, usually several days before vesicles erupt.

Hordeolum (stye). Usually, this lesion produces localized eye pain that increases as the stye grows.

Hyphema. Occurring after eye injury or surgery, hyphema accompanies sudden pain in and around the eye.

Interstitial keratitis. Associated with congenital syphilis, this corneal inflammation produces eye pain with photophobia, blurred vision, prominent conjunctival injection, and grayish pink corneas.

Iritis (acute). Moderate to severe eye pain occurs with severe photophobia, dramatic conjunctival injection, and blurred vision.

Keratoconjunctivitis sicca. This condition—known as dry eye syndrome—causes chronic burning pain in both eyes, itching, a foreign–body sensation, photophobia, dramatic conjunctival injection, and difficulty moving the eyelids.

Lacrimal gland tumor. This neoplastic lesion usually produces unilateral eye pain, impaired visual acuity, and some degree of exophthalmos.

Ocular laceration and intraocular foreign bodies. Penetrating eye injuries usually cause mild to severe unilateral eye pain and impaired visual acuity.

Optic neuritis. Pain in and around the eye occurs with eye movement in this disorder.

Orbital cellulitis. This disorder causes dull, aching pain in the affected eye, some degree of exophthalmos, eyelid edema and erythema, purulent discharge, impaired extraocular movement, and, occasionally, decreased visual acuity and fever.

Orbital floor fracture. Sometimes called a blow–out fracture, this injury causes eye pain, dramatic eyelid edema, and, possibly, enophthalmos and diplopia.

Orbital pseudotumor. This disorder causes deep, boring eye pain and diplopia in about 50% of patients. However, prominent exophthalmos and lateral ocular deviation are more characteristic.

Scleritis. This inflammation produces severe eye pain and tenderness, along with conjunctival injection, bluish purple sclera, and, possibly, photophobia and excessive tearing.

Sclerokeratitis. Inflammation of the sclera and cornea causes pain, burning, irritation, and photophobia.

Trachoma. Along with pain in the affected eye, trachoma causes excessive tearing, photophobia, eye discharge, eyelid edema and redness, and visible conjunctival follicles.

Uveitis. Anterior *uveitis* causes sudden onset of severe pain, dramatic conjunctival injection, photophobia, and a small, nonreactive pupil. *Posterior uveitis* causes insidious onset of similar features, plus gradual blurring of vision and distorted pupil shape. *Lens–induced uveitis* causes moderate eye pain, conjunctival injection, pupil constriction, and severely impaired visual acuity.

Skin
Pemphigus. In this disorder, bilateral eye pain and irritation may be accompanied by blurred vision and a thick discharge.

Environmental
Burns. In *chemical burns*, sudden and severe eye pain may occur with erythema and blistering of the face and eyelids, photophobia, miosis, conjunctival injection, blurring, and inability to keep the eyelids open. In *ultraviolet radiation burns*, moderate to severe pain occurs about 12 hours after exposure along with photophobia and vision changes.

Treatments

Contact lenses may cause eye pain and a foreign–body sensation. Ocular surgery may also produce eye pain, ranging from a mild ache to a severe pounding or stabbing sensation.

Clinical considerations

If the patient's eye pain results from a chemical burn:

• The physician should be notified immediately.

• The eye should be irrigated with at least 1 liter of normal saline solution over 10 minutes.

If the patient's eye pain does not result from a chemical burn:

• A complete history should be obtained and an ocular assessment performed.

• Visual acuity should be checked.

• Diagnostic tests may include tonometry and orbital X–rays.

• To help ease eye pain, the patient should be instructed to lie down in a darkened, quiet environment and close his eyes.

Pain, facial

Description

This symptom may result from various neurologic, vascular, or infectious disorders. It can also be referred to the face in disorders of the ear, nose, paranasal sinuses, teeth, neck, and jaw. Its most common cause is trigeminal neuralgia, or tic douloureux.

Typically paroxysmal and intense, facial pain may occur along the pathway of a specific facial nerve or nerve branch, usually cranial nerve V (trigeminal nerve) or cranial nerve VII (facial nerve). Differentiating facial pain from the more diffuse pain of headache is sometimes difficult, since many patients refer to all head and facial pain as headache.

Possible causes

Central nervous system

Multiple sclerosis. Facial pain may resemble that of trigeminal neuralgia accompanied by jaw and facial weakness.

Postherpetic neuralgia. Burning, itching, prickly pain persists along any of the three trigeminal nerve divisions and worsens with contact or movement. Mild hypoesthesia or paresthesia and vesicles (with possible scarring) affect the area before the onset of pain.

Sphenopalatine neuralgia. Unilateral, deep, boring pain occurs below the ear and may radiate to the eye, ear, cheek, nose, palate, maxillary teeth, temple, back of the head, neck, or shoulder.

Trigeminal neuralgia. Paroxysms of intense pain, lasting up to 15 minutes, shoot along the superior maxillary or mandibular division of the trigeminal nerve. The pain can be triggered by touching the nose, cheek, or mouth; by hot or cold weather; by consuming hot or cold foods and beverages; or even by smiling or talking. Between attacks, the pain may diminish to a dull ache or may disappear.

Eyes, ears, nose, throat

Dental caries. Caries in the mandibular molars can produce ear, preauricular, and temporal pain. In contrast, caries in the maxillary teeth can produce orbital, retroorbital, and parietal pain.

Herpes zoster oticus. Severe pain localizes around the ear, followed by the appearance of vesicles in the ear and on the oral mucosa, tonsils, and posterior tongue.

Sinus carcinoma. In *ethmoid sinus carcinoma*, facial pain is a late symptom, preceded by exophthalmos. In rare *frontal sinus carcinoma*, late–stage forehead pain may be accompanied by local erythema, unilateral epistaxis or purulent discharge, exophthalmos, and swelling and hypoesthesia in the cheek. In *maxillary sinus carcinoma*, persistent pain along the second division of cranial nerve V is a late symptom.

Sinusitis. Acute maxillary sinusitis produces unilateral or bilateral pressure, fullness, or burning pain behind the eyes and over the cheek, nose, and upper teeth. Bending or stooping increases the pain.

Frontal sinusitis commonly produces dull, aching pain above or around the eyes, which worsens with bending or stooping.

In *sphenoid sinusitis*, dull pain persists behind the eyes and nose.

Cardiovascular

Temporal arteritis. Unilateral pain occurs behind the eye or in the scalp, jaw, tongue, or neck. A typical episode consists of a severe throbbing or boring temporal headache with redness, swelling, and nodulation of the temporal artery.

Musculoskeletal

Temporomandibular joint syndrome. Intermittent pain, usually unilateral, is described as a severe, dull ache or intense spasm that radiates to the cheek, temple, lower jaw, ear, or mastoid area.

Clinical considerations

• A history should be obtained and a neurologic assessment performed.

• Diagnostic tests may include sinus, skull, or dental X–rays; sinus transillumination; and intracranial computed tomography.

• Analgesics and muscle relaxants should be administered, as ordered.

• Direct heat should be applied, if ordered, to help relieve pain.

Pain, flank

Description

Flank pain refers to pain in the area extending from the ribs to the ilium. It is a leading indicator of renal and upper urinary tract disease or trauma. Depending on the cause, this symptom may vary from a dull ache to severe stabbing or throbbing pain and may be unilateral or bilateral and constant or

Major Nerve Pathways of the Face

Cranial nerve V has three branches. The *ophthalmic branch* supplies sensation to the anterior scalp, forehead, upper nose, and cornea. The *maxillary branch* supplies sensation to the midportion of the face, lower nose, upper lip, and mucous membrane of the anterior palate. The *mandibular branch* supplies the lower face, lower jaw, mucous membrane of the cheek, and base of the tongue.

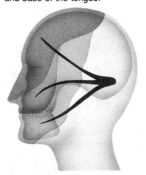

Cranial nerve V

Cranial nerve VII innervates the facial muscles. Its motor branch controls the muscles of the forehead, eye orbit, and mouth.

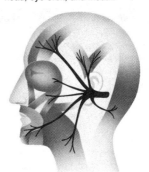

Cranial nerve VII

intermittent. It is aggravated by costovertebral angle (CVA) percussion and, in patients with renal or urinary tract obstruction, by increased fluid intake or ingestion of alcohol, caffeine, and diuretic drugs. Unaffected by position changes, flank pain typically responds only to analgesics or to treatment of the underlying disorder.

Possible causes
Cardiovascular
Renal vein thrombosis. Severe unilateral flank and low back pain with CVA and epigastric tenderness typify the rapid onset of venous obstruction. Bilateral flank pain, oliguria, and other uremic signs (nausea, vomiting, and uremic fetor) typify bilateral obstruction.

Gastrointestinal
Pancreatitis (acute). Bilateral flank pain may develop as severe epigastric or left upper quandrant pain radiates to the back.

Genitourinary
Bladder neoplasm. Dull, constant flank pain may be unilateral or bilateral and may radiate to the leg, back, and perineum. Commonly, the first sign of this neoplasm is gross, painless, intermittent hematuria, often with clots.

Calculi. Renal and ureteral calculi produce intense unilateral, colicky flank pain. Typically, initial CVA pain radiates to the flank, suprapubic region, and perhaps the genitalia, with abdominal and low back pain also possible. Nausea and vomiting often accompany severe pain.

Cortical necrosis (acute). Unilateral flank pain is usually severe.

Cystitis (bacterial). Unilateral or bilateral flank pain occurs secondary to an ascending urinary tract infection.

Glomerulonephritis (acute). Flank pain is bilateral, constant, and moderately intense.

Obstructive uropathy. In acute obstruction, flank pain may be excruciating; in gradual obstruction, it is typically a dull ache. In both, the pain may also localize in the upper abdo-

men and may radiate to the groin.

Papillary necrosis (acute). Intense bilateral flank pain occurs along with renal colic, CVA tenderness, and abdominal pain and rigidity.

Perirenal abscess. Intense unilateral flank pain and CVA tenderness accompany dysuria, persistent high fever, chills, and, in some patients, a palpable abdominal mass.

Polycystic kidney disease. Dull, aching, bilateral flank pain is often the earliest symptom. The pain can become severe and colicky if cysts rupture and clots migrate or cause obstruction.

Pyelonephritis (acute). Intense, constant, unilateral or bilateral flank pain develops over a few hours or days along with typical urinary features: dysuria, nocturia, hematuria, urgency, frequency, and tenesmus.

Renal infarction. Unilateral, constant, severe flank pain and tenderness typically accompany persistent, severe upper abdominal pain.

Renal neoplasm. Unilateral flank pain, gross hematuria, and a palpable flank mass form the classic clinical triad. Flank pain is usually dull and vague, although severe colicky pain can occur during bleeding or passage of clots.

Renal trauma. Variable bilateral or unilateral flank pain is a common symptom. A visible or palpable flank mass may also exist, along with CVA or abdominal pain—possibly severe and radiating to the groin.

Clinical considerations
If the patient suffered trauma:
• A rapid assessment should be performed and the physician notified.
• An indwelling (Foley) catheter should be inserted, as ordered.
• Emergency intervention should be anticipated.
If the patient's condition is not serious:
• A complete history should be obtained and a physical examination performed.
• Diagnostic tests may include serial urine and serum analysis, I.V. pyelog-

raphy, flank ultrasonography, computed tomography scan, voiding cystourethrography, cytoscopy, and retrograde ureteropyelography, urethrography, and cystography.

• Analgesics should be administered, as ordered.

• Fluid intake and output should be monitored and recorded precisely.

Pain, jaw

Description

Jaw pain may arise from either or both of the bones that hold the teeth in the jaw—the maxilla, or upper jaw, and the mandible, or lower jaw. Jaw pain also includes pain in the temporomandibular joint (TMJ), where the mandible meets the temporal bone.

Jaw pain may develop gradually or abruptly and may range from barely noticeable to excruciating, depending on its cause. It usually results from disorders of the teeth, soft tissue, or glands of the mouth or throat, or from local trauma or infections. Systemic causes include musculoskeletal, neurologic, cardiovascular, endocrine, immunologic, metabolic, or infectious disorders. Such life-threatening disorders as myocardial infarction (MI) or tetany also produce jaw pain, as do drugs (especially phenothiazines) and dental or surgical procedures.

Jaw pain is seldom a primary indicator of any one disorder, but some of its causes represent medical emergencies.

Possible causes

Central nervous system

Trigeminal neuralgia. This disorder causes paroxysmal attacks of intense unilateral jaw pain (stopping at the facial midline) or rapid-fire shooting sensations in one of the divisions of the trigeminal nerve (usually the superior mandibular or maxillary division). This superficial pain, felt mainly over the lips and chin and in the teeth, lasts from 1 to 15 minutes.

Eyes, ears, nose, throat

Head and neck cancer. Many types of head and neck cancer, especially of the oral cavity and nasopharynx, produce aching jaw pain of insidious onset.

Ludwig's angina. Infection of the sublingual and submandibular spaces produces severe jaw pain in the mandibular area with tongue elevation, sublingual edema, and drooling.

Sialolithiasis. In this disorder, stones form in the salivary glands and cause painful swelling that makes chewing uncomfortable. Jaw pain occurs in the lower jaw, the floor of the mouth, and the TMJ. It may also radiate to the ear or neck.

Sinusitis. Maxillary sinusitis produces intense boring pain in the maxilla and cheek that may radiate to the eye. *Sphenoid sinusitis* causes chronic pain at the mandibular ramus, vertex of the head, and temporal area, and a scanty nasal discharge.

Suppurative parotitis. Bacterial infection of the parotid gland by *Staphylococcus aureus* tends to develop in debilitated patients with dry mouth or poor oral hygiene. Besides abrupt onset of jaw pain, high fever, and chills, findings include redness and edema of the overlying skin; a tender, swollen gland; and pus at the second top molar (Stensen's ducts).

Trauma. Injury to the face, head, or neck, and particularly fracture of the maxilla or mandible, may produce jaw pain and swelling and decreased jaw mobility.

Cardiovascular

Angina pectoris. Angina pectoris may produce jaw pain (usually radiating from the substernal area) and left arm pain.

Myocardial infarction. Initially this life-threatening disorder causes intense, crushing, substernal pain unrelieved by rest or nitroglycerin. It may radiate to the lower jaw, left arm, neck, back, or shoulder blades. (Rarely, jaw pain occurs without chest pain.)

Temporal arteritis. Common in patients over age 60, this disorder produces sharp jaw pain after chewing or talking.

Musculoskeletal

Arthritis. In *osteoarthritis*, which usually affects the small hand joints, aching jaw pain increases with activity (talking, eating) and subsides with rest. *Rheumatoid arthritis* causes symmetrical pain in all the joints, including the jaw (commonly affecting proximal finger joints first).

Osteomyelitis. Bone infection after trauma, sinus infection, or dental injury may produce diffuse, aching jaw pain along with warmth, swelling, tenderness, erythema, and restricted jaw movement.

TMJ syndrome. This common syndrome produces jaw pain at the TMJ; spasm and pain of the masticating muscle; clicking, popping, or crepitus of the TMJ; and restricted jaw movement. Unilateral, localized pain may radiate to other head and neck areas.

Metabolic

Hypocalcemic tetany. Besides painful muscle contractions of the jaw and mouth, this life-threatening disorder produces paresthesias and carpopedal spasm.

Environmental

Tetanus. A rare life-threatening disorder caused by a bacterial toxin, tetanus produces stiffness and pain in the jaw and difficulty opening the mouth.

Drugs

Some drugs, such as phenothiazines, affect the extrapyramidal tract, causing dyskinesias; others cause tetany of the jaw secondary to hypocalcemia.

Clinical considerations

• A history should be obtained and an examination of the jaw performed.

• Diagnostic tests may include jaw X-rays.

• Analgesics should be administered, as ordered, and ice packs applied to relieve pain and swelling.

• The patient should be advised to avoid talking or moving his jaws excessively.

Pain, leg

Description

Although leg pain often signifies a musculoskeletal disorder, this symptom can also result from more serious vascular or neurologic disorders. The pain may arise suddenly or gradually and may be localized or affect the entire leg. Constant or intermittent, it may feel dull, burning, sharp, shooting or tingling. Leg pain often affects locomotion, limiting weight bearing. Severe leg pain that follows cast application for a fracture may signal limb-threatening compartment syndrome. Sudden onset of severe leg pain in a patient with underlying vascular insufficiency may signal acute deterioration, possibly requiring an arterial graft or amputation.

Possible causes

Cardiovascular

Occlusive vascular disease. Continuous cramping pain in the legs and feet may worsen with walking, inducing claudication. The patient may report increased pain at night and complain of cold feet and cold intolerance.

Thrombophlebitis. Discomfort may range from calf tenderness to severe pain accompanied by swelling, warmth, and a feeling of heaviness in the affected leg.

Varicose veins. Mild to severe leg symptoms may develop, including nocturnal cramping; a feeling of heaviness; diffuse, dull aching after prolonged standing or walking; and aching during menses.

Venous stasis ulcers. Localized pain and bleeding arise from infected ulcerations on the calves.

Musculoskeletal

Bone neoplasm. Continuous deep or boring pain, often worse at night, may be the first symptom.

Compartment syndrome. Progressive, intense, lower leg pain that increases with passive muscle stretching is a cardinal sign of this limb-threatening disorder. Restrictive dressings or traction may aggravate the pain, which typically worsens despite analgesia.

Fracture. Severe, acute pain accompanies swelling and ecchymosis in the affected leg. Movement produces extreme pain, and the leg may be unable to bear weight.

Infection. Local leg pain, erythema, swelling, and warmth characterize both soft tissue and bone infections.

Sciatica. Pain radiates down the back of the leg along the sciatic nerve. Pain may be described as shooting, aching, or tingling. Typically, activity exacerbates the pain and rest relieves it. The patient may limp to avoid aggravating the leg pain and may have difficulty moving from a sitting to a standing position.

Strain or sprain. Acute strain causes sharp, transient pain and rapid swelling, followed by leg tenderness and ecchymosis. Chronic strain produces stiffness, soreness, and generalized leg tenderness several hours after the injury; active and passive motion may be painful or impossible. A sprain causes local pain, especially during joint movement; ecchymosis and possibly local swelling and loss of mobility develop.

Clinical considerations

If the patient has acute leg pain:

• Vital signs should be taken and a brief history obtained quickly. An assessment of the leg should be performed, including its neurovascular status.

• The physician should be notified if the affected leg is cool, pale, and pulseless; these findings may indicate impaired circulation, which could necessitate emergency surgery.

• If a fracture is suspected, the leg should be immobilized.

If the patient's condition does not suggest an emergency:

• A history should be obtained and a physical examination performed.

Highlighting Causes of Local Leg Pain

Various disorders cause hip, knee, ankle, or foot pain, which may radiate to surrounding tissues and be reported as leg pain.

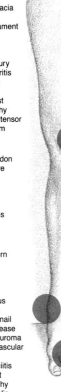

Hip pain
Arthritis
Avascular necrosis
Bursitis
Dislocation
Fracture
Sepsis
Tumor

Knee pain
Arthritis
Bursitis
Chondromalacia
Contusion
Cruciate ligament
  injury
Dislocation
Fracture
Meniscal injury
Osteochondritis
  dissecans
Phlebitis
Popliteal cyst
Radiculopathy
Ruptured extensor
  mechanism
Sprain

Ankle pain
Achilles' tendon
  contracture
Arthritis
Dislocation
Fracture
Sprain
Tenosynovitis

Foot pain
Arthritis
Bunion
Callus or corn
Dislocation
Flat foot
Fracture
Gout
Hallux rigidus
Hammertoe
Ingrown toenail
Köhler's disease
Morton's neuroma
Occlusive vascular
  disease
Plantar fasciitis
Plantar wart
Radiculopathy
Tabes dorsalis
Tarsal tunnel syndrome

• Diagnostic tests may include X-rays, venography, Doppler ultrasonography, and plethysmography.

• Analgesics should be administered, as ordered, once a preliminary diagnosis has been made.

• If the patient has chronic leg pain, he should be instructed in using anti-inflammatory drugs and performing range-of-motion exercises.

• If necessary, the patient should be taught how to use a cane, walker, or other assistive device.

• Any life-style changes that may be necessary until leg pain resolves should be explored with the patient and his family.

• If physical therapy is ordered, the importance of establishing a daily exercise regimen should be stressed.

Pain, neck

Description

Neck pain may originate from any neck structure, ranging from the meninges and cervical vertebrae to its blood vessels, muscles, and lympathic tissue. This symptom can also be referred from other areas of the body. Its location, onset, and pattern help determine its origin and underlying causes. Neck pain most commonly results from trauma and degenerative, congenital, inflammatory, metabolic, and neoplastic disorders.

Possible causes

Central nervous system

Hemorrhage (subarachnoid). This life-threatening condition may cause moderate to severe neck pain and rigidity, headache, and a decreased level of consciousness.

Meningitis. Neck pain may accompany characteristic nuchal rigidity.

Eyes, ears, nose, throat

Laryngeal cancer. Neck pain that radiates to the ear develops late in this disorder.

Respiratory

Tracheal trauma. *Fracture of the tracheal cartilage*, a life-threatening condition, produces moderate to severe neck pain and respiratory difficulty.

Torn tracheal mucosa produces mild to moderate pain and may result in airway occlusion, hemoptysis, hoarseness, and dysphagia.

Endocrine

Thyroid trauma. Besides mild to moderate neck pain, thyroid trauma may cause local swelling and ecchymosis.

Gastrointestinal

Esophageal trauma. An esophageal mucosal tear or a pulsion diverticulum may produce mild neck pain, chest pain, edema, hemoptysis, and dysphagia.

Musculoskeletal

Ankylosing spondylitis. Intermittent moderate to severe neck pain and stiffness with severely restricted range of motion is a classic finding in this disorder.

Cervical extension injury. Anterior or posterior neck pain may develop within hours or days after a whiplash injury. Anterior pain usually diminishes within several days, but posterior pain persists and may even intensify.

Cervical fibrositis. This disorder may produce anterior neck pain that radiates to one or both shoulders. Pain is intermittent and variable, often changing with weather patterns.

Cervical spine fracture. Fracture at C1 to C4 often results in sudden death; survivors may experience severe neck pain that restricts all movement, intense occipital headache, quadriplegia, and respiratory paralysis.

Cervical spine infection. Acute infection can cause moderate neck pain that restricts motion.

Cervical spine tumor. Metastatic tumors typically produce persistent neck pain that increases with movement and is not relieved by rest; *primary tumors* cause mild to severe pain along a specific nerve root.

Cervical spondylosis. This degenerative process produces posterior neck pain that restricts movement and is aggravated by it. Pain may radiate down either arm and may accompany paresthesias and weakness.

Cervical stenosis. This slowly progressive disorder, commonly asymptomatic, may produce nonspecific neck pain, paresthesias, and muscle weakness or paralysis.

Herniated cervical disk. This disorder characteristically causes variable neck pain that restricts movement and is aggravated by it.

Neck sprain. Minor sprains typically produce pain, slight swelling, stiffness, and restricted range of motion. *Ligament rupture* causes pain, marked swelling, ecchymosis, muscle spasms, and nuchal rigidity with head tilt.

Osteoporosis. Neck pain occurs rarely in this disorder, which usually affects the thoracic or lumbar vertebrae. Cervical vertebrae involvement produces tenderness and deformity.

Paget's disease. This slowly developing disease is often asymptomatic in its early stages. As it progresses, cervical vertebrae deformity may produce severe, persistent neck pain, along with paresthesias and arm weakness or paralysis.

Rheumatoid arthritis. This disorder most often affects peripheral joints, but it can also involve the cervical vertebrae. Acute inflammation may cause moderate to severe pain that radiates along a specific nerve root; increased warmth, swelling, and tenderness in involved joints; stiffness restricting range of motion; paresthesias and muscle weakness; low-grade fever; anorexia; malaise; and fatigue. Some pain and stiffness remain after the acute phase.

Spinous process fracture. Fracture near the cervicothoracic junction produces acute pain radiating to the shoulders.

Torticollis. In this neck deformity, severe neck pain accompanies recurrent unilateral stiffness and muscle spasms that produce a characteristic head tilt.

Neoplastic
Hodgkin's lymphoma. This disorder eventually may result in generalized pain that may affect the neck.

Infection
Lymphadenitis. In this disorder, enlarged and inflamed cervical lymph nodes cause acute pain and tenderness.

Clinical considerations

If the patient's neck pain is from trauma:
- Cervical spine immobilization must be ensured and an adequate airway maintained.
- Vital signs should be taken and a brief history obtained.
- The neck should be examined and a quick neurologic assessment performed.

If neck pain is not associated with trauma:
- A complete history should be obtained and a physical examination performed.
- Diagnostic tests may include X-rays, computed tomography scan, blood tests, and cerebrospinal fluid analysis.
- Analgesics should be administered, as ordered.

Pain, rectal

Description

Rectal pain is discomfort that arises in the anal-rectal area. It is a common symptom of anorectal disorders. Although the anal canal is separated from the rest of the rectum by the internal sphincter, the patient may refer to all local pain as rectal pain.

Because the mucocutaneous border of the anal canal and the perianal skin contains somatic nerve fibers, lesions in this area are especially painful. This pain may result from or be aggravated by diarrhea, constipation, or passage of hardened stools. It may also be aggravated by intense pruritus and continued scratching associated with drainage of mucus, blood, or fecal matter that irritates the skin and nerve endings.

Possible causes
Gastrointestinal
Anal carcinoma. Rectal pain, bleeding, and tenesmus are typical findings in this rare disorder.

Anal fissure. This longitudinal crack in the anal lining causes sharp rectal pain on defecation. Typically, the patient experiences a burning sensation and gnawing pain that can continue up to 4 hours after defecation. Fear of provoking this pain may lead to acute constipation.

Anorectal abscess. This abscess can occur in various locations in the rectum and anus, causing pain in the perianal area. Typically, a superficial abscess produces constant, throbbing local pain that is exacerbated by sitting or walking. The local pain associated with a deeper abscess may begin insidiously, often occurring high in the rectum or even in the lower abdomen, and is accompanied by an indurated anal mass.

Anorectal fistula. Pain develops when a tract formed between the anal canal and skin temporarily seals. It persists until drainage resumes.

Cryptitis. This disorder results when particles of stool that are lodged in the anal folds decay and cause infection, which may produce dull anal pain or discomfort and anal pruritus.

Hemorrhoids. Thrombosed or prolapsed hemorrhoids cause rectal pain that may worsen during defecation and abate after it. The patient's fear of provoking the pain may lead to constipation. Usually, rectal pain is accompanied by severe itching.

Proctalgia fugax. In this disorder, muscle spasms of the rectum and pelvic floor produce sudden, severe episodes of rectal pain that last up to several minutes and then disappear. The patient may report being awakened by the pain.

Genitourinary
Prostatic abscess. This disorder occasionally produces rectal pain.

Clinical considerations
• A history should be obtained and a rectal examination performed.

• Diagnostic tests may include anoscopic examination and proctosigmoidoscopy to determine the cause of the rectal pain.

• Analgesic ointments should be applied or suppositories administered, as ordered; stool softeners should be administered, if needed and ordered.

• The patient should be taught how to apply hot or cool moist compresses, as appropriate, to relieve pain.

• Sitz baths may be given to help relieve the sphincter spasm associated with most anorectal disorders.

• Proper dietary instructions should be given to maintain a soft stool and thus avoid aggravating rectal pain during defecation.

• Because the patient may feel embarrassed by treatments and diagnostic tests involving the rectum, emotional support and as much privacy as possible should be provided.

Pain, testicular

Description
Testicular pain is unilateral or bilateral pain localized in or around the testicle and possibly radiating along the spermatic cord and into the lower abdomen. It usually results from trauma, infection, or torsion. Typically its onset is sudden and severe; however, its intensity can vary from sharp pain accompanied by nausea and vomiting to a chronic, dull ache. In a child, sudden onset of severe testicular pain is a urologic emergency. Torsion should be assumed as the cause until disproven. If a young male complains of abdominal pain, the scrotum should always be carefully examined because abdomi-

nal pain often precedes testicular pain in testicular torsion.

Pain, throat
(Sore throat)

Description

Throat pain refers to discomfort in any part of the pharynx—the nasopharynx, the oropharynx, or the hypopharynx. This common symptom ranges from a sensation of scratchiness to severe pain.

It is often accompanied by ear pain because cranial nerves IX and X innervate the pharynx as well as the middle and external ear.

Throat pain may result from infection, trauma, allergy, neoplasms, and certain systemic disorders. It may also follow surgery and endotracheal intubation. Nonpathologic causes include dry mucous membranes associated with mouth breathing and laryngeal irritation associated with alcohol consumption, inhaling smoke or chemicals such as ammonia, and vocal strain.

Possible causes

Eyes, ears, nose, throat

Allergic rhinitis. Occurring seasonally or year-round, this disorder may produce sore throat.

Contact ulcers. Common in men with stressful jobs, contact ulcers appear symmetrically on the vocal cords, resulting in sore throat. The pain is aggravated by talking and may be accompanied by referred ear pain and, occasionally, hemoptysis. Typically the patient also has a history of chronic throat clearing.

Eagle's syndrome. This syndrome results when an unusually long styloid process becomes trapped in a tonsillectomy scar. Palpation of this area will cause throat pain.

Foreign body. A foreign body lodged in the palatine or lingual tonsil and pyriform sinus may produce localized throat pain. The pain may persist after the foreign body is dislodged until mucosal irritation resolves.

Glossopharyngeal neuralgia. Triggered by a specific pharyngeal movement, such as yawning or swallowing, this condition causes unilateral, knifelike throat pain in the tonsillar fossa that may radiate to the ear.

Laryngeal cancer. In extrinsic laryngeal cancer, the chief symptom is pain or burning in the throat when drinking citrus juice or hot liquids, or a lump in the throat.

Laryngitis (acute). This disorder produces sore throat. Its cardinal sign, though, is mild to severe hoarseness—perhaps with temporary loss of voice.

Lymph follicular hypertrophy. In this disorder, mild sore throat is accompanied by diffuse edema of the oropharynx.

Necrotizing ulcerative gingivitis (acute). Also known as trench mouth, this disorder usually begins abruptly with sore throat and tender gums that ulcerate and bleed.

Peritonsillar abscess. A complication of bacterial tonsillitis, this abcess typically causes severe throat pain that radiates to the ear.

Pharyngeal burns. First- or second-degree burns of the posterior pharynx may cause throat pain and dysphagia.

Pharyngitis. Whether bacterial, fungal, or viral, pharyngitis may cause sore throat and localized erythema and edema. *Bacterial pharyngitis* begins abruptly with unilateral sore throat. Also known as thrush, *fungal pharyngitis* causes diffuse sore throat—often described as a burning sensation—accompanied by pharyngeal erythema and edema. In *viral pharyngitis*, findings include diffuse sore throat, malaise, fever, and mild erythema and edema of the posterior oropharyngeal wall.

Pharyngomaxillary space abscess. A complication of untreated pharyngeal or tonsillar infection or tooth extraction, this abscess causes mild throat pain.

Posterior tongue carcinoma. In this disease, localized throat pain may occur around a raised white lesion or ulcer. The pain may radiate to the ear and be accompanied by dysphagia.

Reflux laryngopharyngitis. In this disorder, an incompetent gastroesophageal sphincter allows gastric juices to enter the hypopharynx and irrritate the larynx, resulting in chronic sore throat and hoarseness.

Sinusitis (acute). This disorder may cause sore throat accompanied by purulent nasal discharge and postnasal drip, resulting in halitosis.

Supraglottic cancer. Early features include throat pain that radiates to the ear, dsyphagia, and a muffled voice.

Tonsillar carcinoma. Sore throat is the presenting symptom of this disease. Unfortunately, the carcinoma is usually quite advanced before this symptom occurs. The pain radiates to the ear and is accompanied by a superficial ulcer on the tonsil or one that extends to the base of the tongue.

Tonsillitis. In *acute tonsillitis*, mild to severe sore throat is usually the first symptom. The pain may radiate to the ears and be accompanied by dysphagia and headache. *Chronic tonsillitis* causes mild sore throat, malaise, and tender cervical lymph nodes. Unilateral throat pain just above the hyoid bone occurs in *lingual tonsillitis*.

Uvulitis. This inflammation may cause throat pain or a sensation of something in the throat.

Respiratory

Bronchitis (acute). This disorder may produce lower throat pain.

Hematologic

Agranulocytosis. In this disorder, sore throat may accompany other signs of infection, such as fever, chills, and headache. Typically it follows progressive fatigue and weakness.

Infection

Common cold. Sore throat may accompany cough, sneezing, nasal congestion, rhinorrhea, fatigue, headache, myalgia, and arthralgia.

Herpes simplex virus. Sore throat may result from lesions on the oral mucosa, especially the tongue, gingivae, and cheeks. After causing brief prodromal discomfort (tingling and itching), lesions erupt into erythematous vesicles that eventually rupture and leave a painful ulcer, followed by a yellowish crust.

Infectious mononucleosis. Sore throat, lymphadenopathy, and fluctuating temperature are the three classic findings in this infection.

Influenza. Patients with the flu commonly complain of sore throat, fever with chills, headache, weakness, malaise, muscle aches, cough, and occasionally hoarseness and rhinorrhea.

Treatments

Endotracheal intubation and local surgery, such as tonsillectomy and adenoidectomy, commonly cause sore throat.

Clinical considerations

• A history should be obtained and a throat examination performed.

• Diagnostic tests may include throat culture, complete blood count, and a Monospot test.

• Analgesic sprays and lozenges should be administered, as ordered.

Pallor

Description

Pallor is abnormal paleness or loss of skin color, which may develop suddenly or gradually. Although generalized pallor affects the entire body, it is most apparent on the face, conjunctiva, oral mucosa, and nail beds. Localized pallor commonly affects a single limb.

How easily pallor is detected varies with skin color and the thickness and vascularity of underlying subcutaneous tissue. At times, it is merely a subtle lightening of skin color. It may be difficult to detect in dark-skinned persons; sometimes it is evident only on the conjunctiva and oral mucosa.

Mechanism

Pallor may result from decreased peripheral oxyhemoglobin *or* decreased total oxyhemoglobin. The former reflects diminished peripheral blood flow associated with peripheral vasoconstriction or arterial occlusion or with low cardiac output. (Transient peripheral vasoconstriction may occur with exposure to cold, causing nonpathologic pallor.) The latter most commonly results from anemia, the chief cause of pallor.

Possible causes

Cardiovascular

Arterial occlusion (acute). Pallor develops abruptly in the extremity with the occlusion, which usually results from an embolus. A line of demarcation develops, separating the cool, pale, cyanotic, and mottled skin below the occlusion from the normal skin above it.

Arterial occlusive disease (chronic). Pallor is specific to an extremity—usually one leg—but occasionally both legs or an arm. It develops gradually from obstructive arteriosclerosis or thrombus formation and is aggravated by elevating the extremity.

Cardiac dysrhythmias. Cardiac dysrhythmias that seriously reduce cardiac output, such as complete heart block and attacks of tachyarrhythmia, may cause acute onset of pallor.

Orthostatic hypotension. In this condition, pallor occurs abruptly on rising from a recumbent position to a sitting or standing position. A precipitous drop in blood pressure and dizziness are also characteristic.

Raynaud's disease. Pallor of the fingers upon exposure to cold or stress is a hallmark of this disease. Typically, the fingers abruptly turn pale, then cyanotic; with rewarming, they become red and paresthetic.

Shock. Hypovolemic and cardiogenic shock initially cause acute onset of pallor and cool, clammy skin, along with other typical signs and symptoms.

Vasopressor syncope. Sudden onset of pallor immediately precedes or accompanies loss of consciousness during syncopal attacks.

Hematologic

Anemia. Typically, pallor develops gradually in this disorder. The patient's skin color may also appear sallow or grayish.

Environmental

Frostbite. Pallor is localized to the frostbitten area, such as the feet, hands, or ears. Typically, the area feels cold, waxy, and perhaps hard in deep frostbite. As the area thaws, the skin turns purplish blue.

Clinical considerations

If the patient suddenly develops generalized pallor:
• Vital signs should be taken, a rapid assessment performed, and the physician notified.
• Emergency interventions should be taken, if necessary, to maintain adequate circulation.

If the patient's condition does not suggest an emergency:
• A history should be obtained and a complete cardiovascular assessment performed.
• If the patient has chronic generalized pallor, diagnostic tests may include blood studies and, possibly, bone marrow biopsy. If the patient has localized pallor, arteriography may be required to accurately determine the cause.
• The patient's vital signs, fluid intake and output, EKG, and hemodynamic status should be monitored frequently.

Palmar crease, abnormal

Description

An abnormal palmar crease is an abnormal line pattern on the palms, resulting from faulty embryonic development during the 2nd and 4th months of gestation. This pattern may occur normally but most commonly appears in Down's syndrome (called the *simian crease*) as a single transverse crease formed by fusion of the proximal and distal palmar creases. It also appears in Turner's syndrome and congenital rubella syndrome.

Palpitations

Description
Palpitations are defined as a conscious awareness of one's heartbeat. They are usually felt over the precordium or in the throat or neck. The patient may describe them as pounding, jumping, turning, fluttering, flopping, or as missing or skipping beats. They may be regular or irregular, fast or slow, paroxysmal or sustained.

Although frequently insignificant, this common symptom may result from cardiac and metabolic disorders and from the effects of certain drugs. Nonpathologic palpitations may occur with a newly implanted prosthetic valve because its clicking sound heightens the patient's awareness of his heartbeat. Transient palpitations may accompany emotional stress, such as fright, anger, and anxiety; or physical stress, such as exercise and fever. They can also accompany use of stimulants, such as tobacco and caffeine.

To help characterize the palpitations, the patient should be asked to simulate their rhythm by tapping his finger on a hard surface. An irregular "skipped beat" rhythm points to premature ventricular contractions, whereas an episodic racing rhythm that ends abruptly suggests paroxysmal atrial tachycardia.

Possible causes
Cardiovascular
Aortic insufficiency. This disorder may produce sustained or paroxysmal palpitations accompanied by anginal pain, pallor, or dyspnea.

Cardiac dysrhythmias. Paroxysmal or sustained palpitations may occur with this disorder, with dizziness, weakness, and fatigue.

Hypertension. In this disorder, the patient may be asymptomatic or may complain of sustained palpitations alone or with headache, dizziness, tinnitus, and fatigue. Typically, his blood pressure exceeds 140/90 mm Hg.

Mitral prolapse. This valvular disorder may cause paroxysmal palpitations accompanied by sharp, stabbing, or aching precordial pain. Its hallmark is a midsystolic click followed by an apical systolic murmur.

Mitral stenosis. Early features of this disorder typically include sustained palpitations with dyspnea and fatigue on exertion.

Endocrine
Pheochromocytoma. This rare adrenal medulla tumor causes episodic hypermetabolism, commonly associated with paroxysmal palpitations. Its cardinal sign is dramatically elevated blood pressure, which may be sustained or paroxysmal.

Thyrotoxicosis. Sustained palpitations, a characteristic symptom in this disorder, may be accompanied by tachycardia, dyspnea, weight loss despite increased appetite, diarrhea, tremors, nervousness, diaphoresis, heat intolerance, and, possibly, exophthalmos and an enlarged thyroid.

Hematologic
Anemia. Palpitations may occur in anemia, especially on exertion.

Metabolic
Hypocalcemia. Typically, this disorder produces palpitations, weakness, and fatigue.

Hypoglycemia. When blood glucose levels drop significantly, the sympathetic nervous system triggers adrenalin production, which may cause sustained palpitations accompanied by fatigue, irritability, hunger, cold sweats, tremors, tachycardia, anxiety, and headache.

Psychiatric
Acute anxiety attack. In this disorder, palpitations may be accompanied by diaphoresis, facial flushing, and trembling.

Drugs
Palpitations may result from drugs that precipitate cardiac dysrhythmias or increase cardiac output, such as cardiac glycosides, sympathomimetics, ganglionic blockers, and atropine.

Clinical considerations
If the patient is in distress:
- Vital signs should be taken and cardiac monitoring initiated.
- The physician should be notified.
- Emergency intervention should be performed, if necessary, to restore normal cardiac rhythm.

If the patient is not in distress:
- A history should be obtained and a complete physical examination performed.
- Diagnostic tests may include EKG and chest X-ray.
- Emotional support should be provided—even mild palpitations may cause the patient much concern.
- A quiet, comfortable environment should be maintained to minimize anxiety and perhaps decrease palpitations.

Paradoxical respirations

Description
Paradoxical respirations refer to an abnormal breathing pattern marked by paradoxical movement of an injured portion of the chest wall—it contracts on inspiration and bulges on expiration. This ominous sign is characteristic of flail chest, a thoracic injury involving multiple free-floating, fractured ribs.

Paralysis

Description
Paralysis is the total loss of voluntary motor function. It results from severe cortical or pyramidal tract damage. It occurs in cerebrovascular disorders and degenerative neuromuscular dis-

ease or as a result of trauma, tumors, or central nervous system infection. Acute paralysis may be an early indicator of a life-threatening disorder, such as Guillain-Barré syndrome. Paralysis can be local or widespread, symmetrical or asymmetrical, transient or permanent, and spastic or flaccid. It is often classified according to location and severity as paraplegia (sometimes transient paralysis of the legs), quadriplegia (permanent paralysis of the arms, legs, and body below the level of the spinal lesion), or hemiplegia (unilateral paralysis of varying severity and permanence). Incomplete paralysis with profound weakness (paresis) may precede total paralysis in some patients.

Possible causes
Central nervous system
Amyotrophic lateral sclerosis. This invariably fatal disorder produces spastic or flaccid paralysis in the body's major muscle groups, eventually progressing to total paralysis.

Bell's palsy. Bell's palsy, a disease of cranial nerve VII, causes transient, unilateral facial muscle paralysis. The affected muscles sag and eyelid closure is impossible.

Brain abscess. Advanced abscess in the frontal or temporal lobe can cause hemiplegia accompanied by other late findings, such as ocular disturbances, unequal pupils, decreased level of consciousness, ataxia, tremors, and signs of infection.

Brain tumor. A tumor affecting the motor cortex of the frontal lobe may cause contralateral hemiparesis that progresses to hemiplegia. Onset is gradual, but paralysis is permanent without treatment.

Cerebrovascular accident (CVA). A CVA involving the motor cortex can produce contralateral paresis or paralysis. Onset may be sudden or gradual, and paralysis may be transient or permanent.

Encephalitis. Variable paralysis develops in the late stages of this disorder.

Understanding Spinal Cord Syndromes

When the patient's spinal cord is incompletely severed, he will have partial motor and sensory loss. Most incomplete cord lesions fit into one of the syndromes described below.

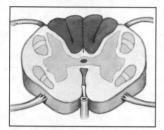

Anterior cord syndrome, most commonly resulting from a flexion injury, causes motor paralysis and loss of pain and temperature sensation below the level of injury. Touch, proprioception, and vibration sensation are usually preserved.

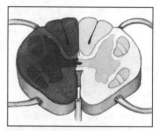

Brown-Séquard syndrome can result from flexion, rotation, or penetration injuries. It is characterized by unilateral motor paralysis ipsilateral to the injury and loss of pain and temperature sensation contralateral to the injury.

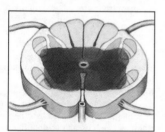

Central cord syndrome is caused by hyperextension or flexion injuries. Motor loss is variable and greater in the arms than in the legs; sensory loss is usually slight.

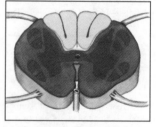

Posterior cord syndrome, produced by a cervical hyperextension injury, causes only a loss of proprioception and loss of light touch sensation. Motor function remains intact.

Guillain-Barré syndrome. This syndrome is characterized by a rapidly developing, but reversible, ascending paralysis. It commonly begins as leg muscle weakness and progresses symmetrically, sometimes affecting even the cranial nerves, producing dysphagia, nasal speech, and dysarthria. Respiratory muscle paralysis may be life threatening.

Head trauma. Cerebral injury can cause paralysis resulting from cerebral edema and increased intracranial pressure. Onset is usually sudden. Location and extent vary depending on the injury.

Migraine headache. Hemiparesis, scotomas, paresthesias, confusion, dizziness, photophobia, or other transient symptoms may precede the onset of a throbbing unilateral headache and may persist after it subsides.

Multiple sclerosis. In this disorder, paralysis commonly waxes and wanes until the later stages, when it may become permanent. Its extent can range from monoplegia to quadriplegia. In most patients, visual and sensory disturbances (paresthesias) are the earliest symptoms.

Myasthenia gravis. In this neuromuscular disease, profound muscle weakness and abnormal fatigability may produce paralysis of certain muscle groups. Paralysis is usually transient in the early stages but becomes more persistent as the disease progresses.

Neurosyphilis. Irreversible hemiplegia may occur in the late stages of neurosyphilis.

Parkinson's disease. Tremor, bradykinesia, and lead-pipe or cogwheel rigidity are the classic signs of Parkinson's disease. Extreme rigidity can progress to paralysis, particularly in the extremities. In most cases, paralysis resolves with prompt treatment of the disease.

Peripheral nerve trauma. Severe injury to a peripheral nerve or group of nerves results in the loss of motor and sensory function in the innervated area. Muscles become flaccid and atrophied, and reflexes are lost. If transection is not complete, paralysis may be temporary.

Peripheral neuropathy. Typically, this syndrome produces muscle weakness that may lead to flaccid paralysis and atrophy.

Poliomyelitis. This disorder can produce insidious, permanent flaccid paralysis and hyporeflexia. Sensory function remains intact, but the patient loses voluntary muscle control.

Seizure disorders. Seizures, particularly focal seizures, can cause transient local paralysis (Todd's paralysis). Any part of the body may be affected, although paralysis tends to occur contralateral to the side of the irritable focus.

Spinal cord injury. Complete spinal cord transection results in permanent spastic paralysis below the level of injury. Reflexes may return after resolution of spinal shock. Partial transection causes variable paralysis and paresthesias, depending on the location and extent of the injury (see *Understanding Spinal Cord Syndromes*).

Spinal cord tumors. Paresis, pain, paresthesias, and variable sensory loss may occur along the nerve distribution pathway served by the affected cord segment. Eventually, this may progress to spastic paralysis with hyperactive deep tendon reflexes (unless the tumor is in the cauda equina, which produces hyporeflexia) and, perhaps, bladder and bowel incontinence. Paralysis is permanent without treatment.

Subarachnoid hemorrhage. This potentially life-threatening disorder can produce sudden paralysis. Duration may be temporary, resolving with decreased edema, or permanent, if tissue destruction has occurred.

Syringomyelia. This degenerative spinal cord disease produces segmental paresis, leading to flaccid paralysis of the hands and arms.

Thoracic aortic aneurysm. Occlusion of spinal arteries by a ruptured thoracic aortic aneurysm may cause sudden onset of transient bilateral paralysis.

Transient ischemic attack (TIA). Episodic TIAs may cause transient unilateral paresis or paralysis accompanied by paresthesias, blurred or double vision, dizziness, aphasia, dysarthria, decreased level of consciousness, and other site-dependent effects.

Psychiatric

Conversion disorder. Hysterical paralysis, a classic conversion symptom, is characterized by the loss of voluntary movement with no obvious physical cause. It can affect any muscle group, appears and disappears unpredictably, and may occur with histrionic behavior (manipulative, dramatic, vain, irrational) or a strange indifference.

Environmental

Botulism. This bacterial toxin infection can cause rapidly descending muscle weakness that progresses to paralysis within 2 to 4 days after the ingestion of contaminated food. Respiratory muscle paralysis leads to dyspnea and respiratory arrest.

Rabies. This acute disorder produces progressive flaccid paralysis, vascular collapse, coma, and death within 2 weeks of contact with an infected animal.

Drugs

Therapeutic use of neuromuscular blocking agents, such as pancuronium or curare, produces paralysis.

Treatments

Electroconvulsive therapy can produce acute, but transient, paralysis.

Clinical considerations

If the patient's paralysis has developed suddenly:

• Trauma or an acute vascular incident should be suspected.

• The patient's spine should be immobilized and the physician notified immediately.

• A rapid assessment should be performed and emergency intervention performed, if necessary, to maintain adequate respiration.

• To help determine the nature of the injury, an account of the precipitating events should be obtained. If the patient is unable to respond, an attempt should be made to find an eyewitness.

If the patient is not in immediate danger:

• A history should be obtained and a complete neurologic assessment performed.

• Diagnostic tests may include X-rays, myelography, electromyography, computed tomography, and blood studies.

• Because a paralyzed patient is particularly susceptible to the complications of prolonged immobility, frequent position changes, meticulous skin care, and frequent chest physiotherapy should be provided.

• The patient may benefit from passive range-of-motion exercises to maintain muscle tone, application of splints to prevent contractures, and the use of footboards or other devices to prevent footdrop.

• If his cranial nerves are affected, the patient will have difficulty chewing and swallowing; therefore, a liquid or soft diet should be provided and suction equipment kept on hand in case aspiration occurs.

• Feeding tubes or I.V. hyperalimentation may be necessary in severe paralysis.

• Paralysis and accompanying visual disturbances may make ambulation hazardous; a call light should be placed close by and the patient shown how to call for help.

• As appropriate, arrangements should be made for physical, speech, or occupational therapy.

Paranoia

Description

Paranoia is an extreme suspiciousness related to delusion of persecution by another person, group, or institution. This may occur in schizophrenia, drug-induced or toxic states, or paranoid disorders.

Paresthesias

Description

Paresthesias are abnormal sensations—often described as numbness, prickling, or tingling—felt along peripheral nerve pathways. These sensations usually are not painful; unpleasant or painful sensations are termed *dysesthesias.* Paresthesias may develop suddenly or gradually and may be transient or permanent.

A common symptom of many neurologic disorders, paresthesias may also result from certain systemic disorders and the effects of drugs.

Mechanism

Paresthesias reflect damage to or irritation of the parietal lobe, thalamus, spinothalamic tract, or spinal or peripheral nerves—the circuit responsible for transmission and interpretation of sensory stimuli.

Possible causes

Central nervous system

Brain tumor. Tumors affecting the sensory cortex in the parietal lobe may cause progressive contralateral paresthesias accompanied by agnosia, apraxia, agraphia, homonymous hemianopia, and loss of proprioception.

Cerebrovascular accident (CVA). Although contralateral paresthesias may occur in CVA, sensory loss is more common.

Guillain-Barré syndrome. In this syndrome, transient paresthesias may precede muscle weakness, which usually begins in the legs and ascends to the arms and facial nerves.

Head trauma. Unilateral or bilateral paresthesias may occur when head trauma causes concussion or contusion; however, sensory loss is more common.

Herpes zoster. An early symptom of this disorder, paresthesias occur in the dermatome supplied by the affected spinal nerve. Within several days this dermatome is marked by a pruritic, erythematous, vesicular rash associated with sharp, shooting, or burning pain.

Migraine headache. Paresthesias in the hands, face, and perioral area may herald an impending migraine headache.

Multiple sclerosis (MS). In this disorder, demyelination of the sensory cortex or spinothalamic tract may produce paresthesias—often one of the earliest symptoms of MS. Like other effects of MS, paresthesias commonly wax and wane until the later stages, when they may become permanent.

Peripheral nerve trauma. Injury to any of the major peripheral nerves may cause paresthesias—often dysesthesias—in the area supplied by that nerve. Paresthesias begin shortly after trauma and may be permanent.

Peripheral neuropathy. This syndrome may cause progessive paresthesias in all extremities.

Seizure disorders. Seizures originating in the parietal lobe usually cause paresthesias of the lips, fingers, and toes. Paresthesias may also be an aura that warns of tonic-clonic seizures.

Spinal cord injury. Paresthesias may occur in partial spinal cord transection, after spinal shock resolves. They may be unilateral or bilateral, occurring at or below the level of the lesion. Associated sensory and motor loss is variable (see *Understanding Spinal Cord Syndromes*, p. 318).

Spinal cord tumors. Typically, these tumors produce paresthesias, paresis, pain, and variable sensory loss along the nerve distribution pathway served by the affected cord segment.

Tabes dorsalis. In this form of neurosyphilis, paresthesias—especially of the legs—are a common, but late, symptom.

Transient ischemic attack (TIA). Typically, paresthesias occur abruptly in an attack and are limited to one arm or another isolated part of the body. They usually last about 10 minutes and are accompanied by paralysis or paresis.

Cardiovascular

Arterial occlusion (acute). In this disorder, sudden paresthesias and coldness may develop in one or both legs with a saddle embolus. Paresis, intermittent claudication, and aching pain at rest are also characteristic.

Arteriosclerosis obliterans. This disorder produces paresthesias, intermittent claudication (most common symptom), diminished or absent popliteal and pedal pulses, pallor, paresis, and coldness in the affected leg.

Buerger's disease. In this inflammatory occlusive disorder, exposure to cold makes the feet cold, cyanotic, and numb; later, they redden, become hot, and tingle.

Raynaud's disease. Exposure to cold or stress makes the fingers turn pale, cold, and cyanotic; with rewarming, they become red and paresthetic.

Thoracic outlet syndrome. Paresthesias occur suddenly in this syndrome when the affected arm is raised and abducted.

Musculoskeletal

Arthritis. Rheumatoid or osteoarthritic changes in the cervical spine may cause paresthesias in the neck, shoulders, and arms. Less commonly, the lumbar spine is affected, causing paresthesias in one or both legs and feet.

Herniated disk. Herniation of a lumbar or cervical disk may cause acute or gradual onset of paresthesias along the distribution pathways of affected spinal nerves.

Systemic lupus eythematosus. This disorder seldom causes paresthesias.

Metabolic

Hypocalcemia. An early symptom of hypocalcemia, asymmetrical paresthesias usually occur in the fingers, toes, and circumoral area.

Vitamin B deficiency. Chronic thiamine or vitamin B_{12} deficiency may cause paresthesias and weakness in the arms and legs.

Psychiatric

Hyperventilation syndrome. Usually triggered by acute anxiety, this syndrome may produce transient paresthesias in the hands, feet, and perioral area, accompanied by agitation, vertigo, syncope, pallor, muscle twitching and weakness, carpopedal spasm, and cardiac dysrhythmias.

Environmental

Heavy metal or solvent poisoning. Exposure to industrial or household products containing lead, mercury, thallium, or organophosphates may cause paresthesias of acute or gradual onset.

Rabies. Paresthesias, coldness, and itching at the site of an animal bite herald the prodromal stage of rabies.

Drugs

Phenytoin, chemotherapeutic agents (such as vincristine, vinblastine, and procarbazine), D-penicillamine, isoniazid, nitrofurantoin, chloroquine, and parenteral gold therapy may produce transient paresthesias that disappear when the drug is discontinued.

Treatments

Long-term radiation therapy may eventually cause peripheral nerve damage, producing paresthesias.

Clinical considerations

• A history should be obtained and a neurologic assessment performed.

• Diagnostic tests may include X-rays, myelography, computed tomography, electromyography, and blood studies.

• Since paresthesias are often accompanied by patchy sensory loss, the patient should be taught safety measures.

Paroxysmal nocturnal dyspnea

Description

Typically dramatic and terrifying to the patient, this sign refers to an attack of dyspnea that abruptly awakens the patient. An attack often causes diaphoresis, coughing, and wheezing. It abates after the patient sits up or stands for several minutes, but may recur every 2 to 3 hours.

Paroxysmal nocturnal dyspnea is an early sign of left ventricular failure. It can reflect decreased respiratory drive, impaired left ventricular function, enhanced reabsorption of interstitial fluid, and increased thoracic blood volume. All these pathophysiologic mechanisms cause dyspnea to worsen when the patient lies down.

Pastia's sign

Description

Pastia's sign is petechiae appearing along skin creases in such areas as the antecubital fossa, the groin, and the wrists. They accompany the rash of scarlet fever as a response to the erythrogenic toxin produced by scarlatinal strains of group A streptococci.

Peau d'Orange

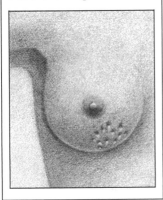

Peau d'orange
("Orange-peel" skin)

Description
Peau d'orange is the edematous thickening and pitting of breast skin. Usually developing slowly and appearing as a late sign of breast cancer, peau d'orange can also occur with breast or axillary lymph node infection. Its striking orange-peel appearance stems from lymphatic edema around deepened hair follicles.

Pel-Ebstein fever

Description
Pel-Ebstein fever is a recurrent pattern characterized by several days of high fever alternating with afebrile periods that last for days or weeks. Typically, the fever becomes progressively higher and continuous. Pel-Ebstein fever occasionally occurs in Hodgkin's disease.

Perez's sign

Description
Perez's sign is crackles auscultated over the lungs when a seated patient raises and lowers his arms. This sign commonly occurs in fibrous mediastinitis and may also occur in aortic arch aneurysm.

Pericardial friction rub

Description
Often transient, a pericardial friction rub is a scratching, grating, or crunching sound that occurs when two inflamed layers of the pericardium slide over one another. Ranging from faint to loud, this abnormal sound is best heard along the lower left sternal border during deep inspiration. It is the hallmark of acute pericarditis, which can result from acute infection, cardiac and renal disorders, postpericardiotomy syndrome, and certain drugs, such as procainamide and antineoplastic agents.

Occasionally, a pericardial friction rub can resemble a murmur or a pleural friction rub (see *Comparing Auscultation Findings,* p. 327). However, the classic pericardial friction rub has three components (see *Understanding Pericardial Friction Rubs,* p. 324).

Peristaltic waves, visible

Description
Visible peristaltic waves occur in gastrointestinal (GI) obstruction. Typically, these waves appear suddenly and vanish quickly because increased peristalsis overcomes the obstruction or the GI tract becomes atonic. Peristal-

Understanding Pericardial Friction Rubs

The complete, or classic, rub is triphasic. Its three sound components are linked to phases of the cardiac cycle: the *presystolic* component (A) reflects atrial systole and precedes the first heart sound (S_1). The *systolic* component (B)—usually the loudest—reflects ventricular systole and occurs between the first and second heart sounds (S_2). The *early diastolic* component (C) reflects ventricular diastole and follows the second heart sound.

Sometimes, the early diastolic component merges with the presystolic component, producing a diphasic to-and-fro sound on auscultation. In other patients, auscultation may detect only one component—a monophasic rub, typically during ventricular systole.

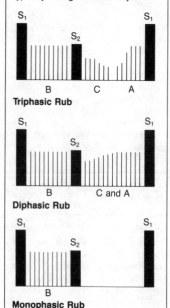

Triphasic Rub

Diphasic Rub

Monophasic Rub

tic waves are best detected by stooping at the supine patient's side and inspecting the abdominal contour.

Mechanism

In intestinal obstruction, peristalsis temporarily increases in strength and frequency as the intestine tries to force its contents past the obstruction. As a result, visible peristaltic waves may roll across the abdomen.

Visible peristaltic waves may also reflect normal stomach and intestinal contractions in thin patients or in malnourished patients with abdominal muscle atrophy.

Possible causes
Gastrointestinal

Large-bowel obstruction. Visible peristaltic waves in the upper abdomen are an early sign of this obstruction. Obstipation, however, may be the earliest finding.

Pyloric obstruction. Peristaltic waves may be detected in a swollen epigastrium or in the left upper quadrant, usually beginning near the left rib margin and rolling from left to right.

Small-bowel obstruction. Early signs of mechanical obstruction of the small bowel include peristaltic waves rolling across the upper abdomen and intermittent, cramping periumbilical pain.

Clinical considerations
• A thorough abdominal examination should be performed.
• Diagnostic tests may include abdominal X-rays and barium studies.
• Because visible peristaltic waves are often an early sign of intestinal obstruction, the patient's status should be monitored closely.

Peroneal sign

Description
The peroneal sign is dorsiflexion and abduction of the foot upon tapping over the common peroneal nerve. To elicit

this sign of latent tetany, the examiner taps over the lateral neck of the fibula with the patient's knee relaxed and slightly flexed.

Phobia

Description
A phobia is an irrational and persistent fear of an object, situation, or activity. Occurring in phobic disorders, it may interfere with normal functioning. Typical manifestations include faintness, fatigue, palpitations, diaphoresis, nausea, tremor, and panic.

Photophobia

Description
A common symptom, photophobia is an abnormal sensitivity to light. In many patients, photophobia simply indicates increased eye sensitivity without an underlying pathology. In some patients, it can indicate excessive wearing of contact lenses or poorly fitted lenses. But, in others, this symptom can indicate systemic disorders, ocular disorders or trauma, or use of certain drugs.

Possible causes
Central nervous system
Meningitis (acute bacterial). A common symptom of this disorder, photophobia may occur with other signs of meningeal irritation, such as nuchal rigidity, hyperreflexia, and opisthotonos. Brudzinski's and Kernig's signs can be elicited.

Migraine headache. Photophobia and noise sensitivity are prominent features of a common migraine.

Eyes, ears, nose, throat
Conjunctivitis. When conjunctivitis affects the cornea, it causes photophobia.

Corneal abrasion. A common finding with corneal abrasion, photophobia is usually accompanied by excessive tearing, conjunctival injection, visible corneal damage, and a foreign body sensation in the eye.

Corneal foreign body. Photophobia may occur with miosis, intense eye pain, a foreign body sensation, slightly impaired vision, conjunctival injection, and profuse tearing.

Corneal ulcer. This vision-threatening disorder causes severe photophobia and eye pain that is aggravated by blinking.

Dry eye syndrome. This disorder may produce photophobia but more characteristically causes eye pain, conjunctival injection, a foreign–body sensation, itching, excessive mucus secretion, and possibly decreased tearing and difficulty moving the eyelids.

Iritis (acute). Severe photophobia may result from this disorder, along with marked conjunctival injection, moderate to severe eye pain, and blurred vision.

Keratitis (interstitial). This corneal inflammation causes photophobia, eye pain, blurred vision, dramatic conjunctival injection, and grayish pink corneas.

Scleritis. This disorder may cause photophobia, severe eye pain, conjunctival injection, and a bluish purple sclera. The eye may tear profusely.

Sclerokeratitis. Inflammation of the sclera and cornea causes photophobia, eye pain, burning, and irritation.

Trachoma. In its early stages, trachoma resembles bacterial conjunctivitis, producing photophobia, visible conjunctival follicles, red and edematous eyelids, pain, increased tearing, and discharge.

Uveitis. Both anterior and posterior uveitis can cause photophobia.

Environmental
Burns. In *chemical burns,* photophobia and eye pain may be accompanied by erythema and blistering on the face and lids, miosis, diffuse conjunctival injection, and corneal changes.

In *ultraviolet radiation burns,* photophobia occurs with moderate to severe eye pain. These symptoms develop about 12 hours after exposure to the rays of a welding arc or sun lamp.

Drugs
Mydriatics—such as phenylephrine, atropine, scopolamine, cyclopentolate, and tropicamide—can cause photophobia from ocular dilation. Amphetamines, cocaine, and ophthalmic antifungal drugs—such as trifluridine, vidarabine, and idoxuridine—can also cause photophobia.

Clinical considerations
• A history should be obtained and careful neurologic and eye examinations performed.
• Diagnostic tests may include corneal scraping and slit-lamp examination.
• The patient's comfort can be ensured by darkening the room and telling him to close both eyes.
• If photophobia persists at home, the patient should be advised to wear dark glasses.

Pica

Description
Pica refers to the craving and ingestion of normally inedible substances, such as plaster, charcoal, clay, wool, ashes, paint, or dirt. In children, the most commonly affected group, pica typically results from nutritional deficiencies, such as iron-deficiency anemia and malnutrition. However, in adults, pica may reflect a psychological disturbance.

Depending on the substance eaten, pica can lead to poisoning and gastrointestinal disorders.

Piotrowski's sign

Description
Piotrowski's sign is dorsiflexion and supination of the foot on percussion of the anterior tibial muscle. Excessive flexion may indicate a central nervous system disorder.

Pitres' sign

Description
Pitres' sign is hyperesthesia of the scrotum in tabes dorsalis. This sign also refers to the anterior deviation of the sternum in pleural effusion.

Pleural friction rub

Description
A pleural friction rub is a loud, coarse, grating, creaking, or squeaking sound that may be auscultated over one or both lungs during late inspiration or early expiration. Usually resulting from pulmonary disorders or trauma, it is heard best over the low axilla or the anterior, lateral, or posterior bases of the lung fields with the patient upright. Sometimes intermittent, it may resemble crackles or a pericardial friction rub (see *Comparing Auscultation Findings*).

Mechanism
A pleural friction rub indicates inflammation of the visceral and parietal pleural lining, which causes congestion and edema. The resultant fibrinous exudate covers both pleural surfaces, displacing the fluid that is normally between them and causing the surfaces to rub together.

Possible causes
Respiratory
Asbestosis. Besides a pleural friction rub, this disorder may cause dyspnea on exertion, a cough, chest pain, and crackles.
Lung cancer. A pleural friction rub may be heard in the affected area of the lung.
Pleurisy. A pleural friction rub occurs early in this disorder. However, the

Comparing Auscultation Findings

A pleural friction rub, a pericardial friction rub, or crackles—three abnormal sounds that are often confused—may be detected during auscultation. This chart can be used to help identify auscultation findings.

Abnormal Sound	Pleural Friction Rub	Pericardial Friction Rub	Crackles
Cause	Caused by inflamed visceral and parietal pleural surfaces rubbing against each other	Caused by inflamed layers of the pericardium rubbing against each other	Caused by air suddenly entering fluid-filled airways
Quality	Loud and grating, creaking, or squeaking	Hard and grating, scratching, or crunching	Nonmusical clicking or rattling
Location	Best heard over the low axilla or the anterior, lateral, or posterior bases of the lung	Best heard along the lower left sternal border	Best heard at less distended and more dependent areas of the lungs, usually at the bases
Timing	Occurs in late inspiration and early expiration but ceases when the patient holds his breath; persists during coughing	Occurs in relation to heart-beat. Most noticeable during deep inspiration and continues even when the patient holds his breath	Occurs chiefly during inspiration

cardinal symptom is sudden, intense chest pain that is usually unilateral and located in the lower and lateral parts of the chest.

Pneumonia (bacterial). A pleural friction rub occurs in this disorder, which usually starts with a dry, painful, hacking cough that rapidly becomes productive.

Pulmonary embolism. An embolism can cause a pleural friction rub over the affected area of the lung. Usually, the first symptom is sudden dyspnea that may be accompanied by anginal or pleuritic chest pain.

Tuberculosis (pulmonary). In this disorder, a pleural friction rub may occur over the affected part of the lung.

Musculoskeletal

Rheumatoid arthritis. This disorder seldom causes a unilateral pleural friction rub.

Systemic lupus erythematosus. Pulmonary involvement can cause a pleural friction rub, hemoptysis, dyspnea, pleuritic chest pain, and crackles.

Treatments

Thoracic surgery and radiation therapy can cause a pleural friction rub.

Clinical considerations

• An attempt should be made to characterize the pleural friction rub by auscultating the lungs as the patient sits upright and breathes deeply and slowly through his mouth.

• If signs of respiratory distress are detected, emergency intervention should be performed, if necessary.
• Diagnostic tests include chest X-rays.
• The patient's respiratory status and vital signs should be monitored closely.

Plummer's sign

Description
Plummer's sign is the inability to ascend stairs or step up onto a chair. This sign can be demonstrated in Graves' disease.

Pneumaturia

Description
Pneumaturia is the passage of gas in the urine while voiding. Causes include a fistula between the bowel and bladder, sigmoid diverticulitis, rectosigmoid cancer, and gas-forming urinary tract infections.

Polydipsia

Description
Polydipsia refers to excessive thirst. It is a common symptom associated with endocrine disorders and certain drugs. It may reflect reduced fluid intake, increased urinary output (as in diabetes mellitus), or excessive loss of water and salt (as in profuse sweating).

Possible causes
Endocrine
Diabetes insipidus. This disorder characteristically produces polydipsia.
Diabetes mellitus. Polydipsia is a classic finding in this disorder.
Sheehan's syndrome. Polydipsia, polyuria, and nocturia occur in this syndrome of postpartum pituitary necrosis.
Thyrotoxicosis. This disorder seldom causes polydipsia.

Genitourinary
Renal disorders (chronic). Chronic renal disorders, such as glomerulonephritis and pyelonephritis, damage the kidneys, causing polydipsia and polyuria.
Hematologic
Sickle cell anemia. As nephropathy develops, polydipsia and polyuria occur.
Metabolic
Hypercalcemia. As this disorder progresses, the patient develops polydipsia, polyuria, nocturia, constipation, paresthesias, and, occasionally, hematuria and pyuria.
Hypokalemia. This electrolyte imbalance can cause nephropathy, resulting in polydipsia, polyuria, and nocturia.
Psychiatric
Psychogenic polydipsia. This uncommon disorder causes polydipsia and polyuria, usually without nocturnal awakening. Signs of psychiatric disturbances, such as anxiety or depression, typically occur.
Drugs
Diuretics and demeclocycline may produce polydipsia. Phenothiazines and anticholinergics can cause dry mouth, making the patient so thirsty that he drinks compulsively.

Clinical considerations
• A history should be obtained and a physical examination performed.
• Diagnostic tests include urine and blood studies.
• Because thirst is usually the body's way of compensating for water loss, the patient should be given ample liquids (orally or intravenously).
• Fluid intake and output should be monitored closely.

Polyphagia
(Hyperphagia)

Description
Polyphagia refers to voracious or excessive eating before satiety. This common symptom can be persistent or intermittent, resulting primarily from

endocrine and psychological disorders, as well as from certain drugs. Depending on the underlying cause, polyphagia may or may not cause weight gain.

Possible causes
Central nervous system
Migraine headache. Polyphagia sometimes precedes a migraine headache.
Endocrine
Diabetes mellitus. In this disorder, polyphagia occurs with weight loss, polydipsia, and polyuria.
Thyrotoxicosis. This disorder can produce weight loss despite constant polyphagia.
Obstetric-gynecologic
Premenstrual syndrome. Appetite changes, typified by food cravings and binges, are common in this syndrome.
Psychiatric
Anxiety. Polyphagia may result from mild to moderate anxiety or emotional stress.
Bulimia. Most common in women ages 18 to 29, bulimia causes polyphagia that alternates with self-induced vomiting, fasting, or diarrhea.
Drugs
Corticosteroids and cyproheptadine may increase appetite, causing weight gain.

Clinical considerations
• A history should be obtained, focusing on dietary habits, and a physical examination performed.
• Emotional support should be provided and, if necessary, the patient and his family referred for psychological counseling.

Polyuria

Description
Polyuria is the daily production and excretion of more than 2,500 ml (2.5 liters) of urine. A relatively common sign, it is usually reported by the patient as increased voidings, especially when it occurs at night. Polyuria is aggravated by overhydration, consumption of caffeine or alcohol, and excessive ingestion of salt, glucose, or other hyperosmolar substances.

Polyuria most commonly results from drugs, such as diuretics, and from psychological, neurologic, and renal disorders.

Mechanism
Polyuria can reflect central nervous system dysfunction that diminishes or suppresses secretion of antidiuretic hormone (ADH), which regulates fluid balance. Or, when ADH levels are normal, it can reflect renal impairment. In both of these pathophysiologic mechanisms, the renal tubules fail to reabsorb sufficient water, causing polyuria.

Possible causes
Endocrine
Diabetes insipidus. Extreme polyuria—up to 30 liters/day—can occur in this disorder. However, polyuria of about 5 liters/day with a specific gravity of 1.005 or less is a more common finding.
Diabetes mellitus. In this disorder, polyuria seldom exceeds 5 liters/day, whereas urine specific gravity typically exceeds 1.020.
Sheehan's syndrome. This syndrome of postpartum pituitary necrosis may cause polyuria of over 5 liters/day with a specific gravity of 1.001 to 1.005.
Genitourinary
Acute tubular necrosis. During the diuretic phase of this disorder, polyuria of less than 8 liters/day gradually subsides after 8 to 10 days. Urine specific gravity (1.010 or less) increases as the polyuria subsides.
Glomerulonephritis (chronic). Polyuria gradually progresses to oliguria in this disorder. Urine output is usually less than 4 liters/day; specific gravity is about 1.010.
Postobstructive uropathy. After resolution of a urinary tract obstruction, polyuria—usually more than 5 liters/day with a specific gravity of less than

1.010—occurs for several days before gradually subsiding.

Pyelonephritis. Acute pyelonephritis usually results in polyuria of less than 5 liters/day with a low but variable specific gravity. *Chronic pyelonephritis* produces polyuria of less than 5 liters/day that declines as renal function worsens. Usually, urine specific gravity is about 1.010, but it may be higher if proteinuria is present.

Hematologic
Sickle cell anemia. This disorder may cause nephropathy, typically producing polyuria that amounts to less than 5 liters/day with a specific gravity of about 1.020.

Metabolic
Hypercalcemia. Elevated plasma calcium levels may lead to nephropathy, usually producing polyuria of less than 5 liters/day with a specific gravity of about 1.010.

Hypokalemia. Prolonged potassium depletion may lead to nephropathy, producing polyuria—usually less than 5 liters/day with a specific gravity of about 1.010.

Psychiatric
Psychogenic polydipsia. Most common in women over age 30, this disorder usually produces dilute polyuria of 3 to 15 liters/day, depending on fluid intake.

Drugs
Diuretics characteristically produce polyuria. Cardiotonics, vitamin D, demeclocycline, phenytoin, lithium, methoxyflurane, and propoxyphene can also produce polyuria.

Diagnostic tests
Transient polyuria can result from radiographic tests that use contrast media.

Clinical considerations

• A history should be obtained and the patient assessed for hypovolemia.
• Diagnostic tests may include serum electrolyte, osmolality, blood urea nitrogen, and creatinine studies and a fluid deprivation test.
• Fluid balance should be maintained and intake and output monitored.
• The patient should be weighed daily.

Pool-Schlesinger sign

Description
Pool-Schlesinger sign is muscle spasm of the forearm, hand, and fingers or of the leg and foot in tetany. To detect this sign, the patient's arm is forcefully abducted and elevated with his forearm extended, or the patient's extended leg is flexed forcefully at the hip. Spasm results from tension on the brachial plexus or the sciatic nerve.

Postnasal drip

Description
Postnasal drip is a sinus or nasal discharge that flows behind the nose and into the throat. This symptom typically results from infection or allergies—a thick, tenacious, and purulent discharge suggests infection, whereas a watery discharge usually suggests an allergy. Postnasal drip may also result from environmental irritants.

Possible causes
Eyes, ears, nose, throat
Rhinitis. Two types of rhinitis—allergic and vasomotor—can produce postnasal drip. In *allergic rhinitis*, symptoms can occur seasonally, as with hay fever, or year-round, as with chronic rhinitis. A recurrent postnasal drip occurs with *vasomotor rhinitis*, which can be aggravated by dry air.
Sinusitis. This disorder commonly produces postnasal drip.

Environmental
Environmental irritants. Exposure to environmental irritants, such as fumes, smoke, or dust, may cause postnasal drip.

Clinical considerations
• A history should be obtained and the nose, oropharynx, nasopharynx, and sinuses examined.

- Diagnostic tests may include sinus X-rays and culture and sensitivity studies.
- If sinus pain accompanies postnasal drip, wet hot packs should be applied, as needed, to the sinuses.
- The patient should be instructed to avoid nasal irritants, such as tobacco smoke.
- The patient should be taught how to use medications safely. For example, he should be reminded not to use decongestants for more than a month at a time and to avoid overuse of nose drops, which can produce rebound rhinitis.
- If the patient has hypertension, he should be instructed to avoid systemic decongestants.

Potain's sign

Description

Potain's sign is dullness on percussion over the aortic arch, extending from the manubrium to the third costal cartilage on the right. This occurs in aortic dilatation.

Prehn's sign

Description

Prehn's sign is the relief of pain with elevation and support of the scrotum, occurring in epididymitis. This sign differentiates epididymitis from testicular torsion. Both disorders produce severe pain, tenderness, and scrotal swelling.

Pressured speech

Description

Pressured speech is verbal expression that is accelerated, difficult to interrupt, and at times unintelligible. This may accompany flight of ideas in the manic phase of a bipolar disorder.

Prévost's sign

Description

Prévost's sign is the conjugate deviation of the head and eyes in hemiplegia. Typically, the eyes gaze toward the affected hemisphere.

Priapism

Description

Priapism is a persistent, painful erection that is unrelated to sexual excitation. Indicating a urologic emergency, this relatively rare sign may begin during sleep and appear to be a normal erection, but it may last for several hours or days. It is usually accompanied by a severe, constant, dull aching in the penis. Despite this, the patient may be too embarrassed to seek medical help and may try to achieve detumescence through continued sexual activity.

Without prompt treatment, penile ischemia and thrombosis occur. In about half of all cases, priapism is idiopathic and develops without apparent predisposing factors. Secondary priapism results from blood disorders, neoplasms, trauma, and certain drugs.

Mechanism

Priapism occurs when the veins of the corpora cavernosa fail to drain correctly, resulting in persistent engorgement of the tissues.

Possible causes

Central nervous system
Cerebrovascular accident (CVA). A CVA may cause priapism, but sensory loss and aphasia may prevent the patient from noticing or describing it.
Spinal cord injury. In this condition, the patient may be unaware of the onset of priapism.

Genitourinary
Genitourinary infection. Priapism occurs rarely with infection.
Penile carcinoma. Carcinoma that exerts pressure on the corpora cavernosa can cause priapism.
Penile trauma. Priapism can occur with bruising, abrasions, swelling, pain, and hematuria.
Hematologic
Granulocytic leukemia (chronic). Priapism is an uncommon sign of this disorder.
Sickle cell anemia. In this disorder, painful priapism can occur without warning, usually on awakening. A history of priapism, impaired growth and development, and increased susceptibility to infection may be present.
Thrombocytopenia. This disorder uncommonly produces priapism.
Drugs
Priapism can result from phenothiazines, thioridazine, trazodone, androgenic steroids, and some antihypertensives.

Clinical considerations
• The physician should be notified immediately.
• As ordered, ice packs should be applied to the penis and analgesics administered.
• An indwelling (Foley) catheter may be inserted to relieve urinary retention.
• If surgery is required, the patient should be prepared accordingly.

Prognathism

Description
Prognathism is an enlarged, protuberant jaw associated with normal mandible condyles and temporomandibular joints. This sign most commonly appears in acromegaly.

Pruritus
(Itching)

Description
Often provoking scratching in an attempt to gain relief, this unpleasant sensation affects the skin, certain mucous membranes, and the eyes. Most severe at night, pruritus may also worsen with increased skin temperature, poor skin turgor, local vasodilation, dermatoses, and stress.

The most common symptom of dermatologic disease, pruritus may also result from local and systemic disorders and from drug use. Physiologic pruritus, such as pruritic urticarial papules and plaques of pregnancy, may occur in primigravidas late in the third trimester. It can also stem from emotional upsets or contact with skin irritants.

Possible causes
Eyes, ears, nose, throat
Conjunctivitis. Regardless of the type, conjunctivitis causes eye itching, burning, and pain along with photophobia, conjunctival injection, a foreign–body sensation, excessive tearing, and a feeling of fullness around the eye.
Myringitis (chronic). This disorder produces pruritus in the affected ear, along with a purulent discharge and gradual hearing loss.
Endocrine
Thyrotoxicosis. Generalized pruritus may precede or accompany this disorder's characteristic effects.
Gastrointestinal
Hemorrhoids. Anal pruritus may occur, along with rectal pain and constipation.
Hepatobiliary disease. An important diagnostic clue to liver and gallbladder disease, pruritus is often accompanied by jaundice and may be generalized or localized to the palms and soles.

Genitourinary

Renal failure (chronic). Pruritus may develop gradually or suddenly in this disorder.

Skin

Dermatitis. Several types of dermatitis can cause pruritus accompanied by a skin lesion. *Atopic dermatitis* begins with intense, severe pruritus and an erythematous rash on dry skin at flexion points (anticubital fossa, popliteal area, and neck).

Mild irritants and allergies can cause *contact dermatitis,* with itchy small vesicles that may ooze and scale and are surrounded by redness. Severe reaction can produce marked localized edema.

Dermatitis herpetiformis, most common in men between ages 20 and 50, initially causes intense pruritus and stinging. Eight to twelve hours later, symmetrically distributed lesions form on the buttocks, shoulders, elbows, and knees. Sometimes they also form on the neck, face, and scalp.

Herpes zoster. In this disorder, pruritus may precede eruption of lesions and may be accompanied by malaise, fever, erythema, and sharp, shooting, or burning pain.

Lichen planus. This common skin disease can cause moderate to severe pruritus that is aggravated by stress.

Lichen simplex chronicus. Persistent rubbing and scratching cause localized pruritus and a circumscribed scaling patch with sharp margins.

Pityriasis rosea. Typically, this disorder produces mild to severe pruritus that is aggravated by a hot bath or shower.

Psoriasis. Pruritus and pain are common in this disorder.

Tinea pedis. This fungal infection causes severe foot pruritus, pain with walking, scales and blisters between the toes, and a dry, scaly squamous inflammation on the entire sole.

Hematologic

Anemia (iron deficiency). This disorder occasionally produces pruritus.

Controlling Itching

To reduce itching and increase comfort, follow these simple steps:
• Avoid scratching or rubbing the itchy areas. Ask your family to let you know if you're scratching, because you may be unaware of it. Keep fingernails short to avoid skin damage from any unconscious scratching.
• Wear cool, light, loose bedclothes. Avoid wearing rough clothing—particularly wool—over the itchy area.
• Take tepid baths, using little soap and rinsing thoroughly. Try a skin-soothing oatmeal or cornstarch bath for a change.
• Apply an emollient lotion after bathing to soften and cool the skin.
• Apply cold compresses to the itchy area.
• Use topical ointments and take prescribed medications, as directed.
• Avoid prolonged exposure to excessive heat and humidity. For maximum comfort, keep room temperatures at 68° to 70° F. (20° to 21.1° C.) and humidity at 30% to 40%.
• Take up an enjoyable hobby that distracts from the itching during the day and leaves you tired enough to sleep at night.

Leukemia (chronic lymphocytic). Pruritus occurs uncommonly in this disorder.

Polycythemia vera. This hematologic disorder can produce pruritus that is generalized or localized to the head, neck, face, and extremities. Typically, the pruritus is aggravated by a hot bath or shower and can last from a few minutes to an hour.

Immunologic

Urticaria. Extreme pruritus and stinging occur as transient erythematous or whitish wheals form on the skin or mucous membranes.

Psychiatric

Psychogenic pruritus. Localized or generalized pruritus occurs without symptoms of dermatologic or systemic disease. Anxiety or emotional lability may be evident.

Obstetric-gynecologic

Vaginitis. This disorder seldom causes localized pruritus and a foul-smelling vaginal discharge that may be purulent, white or gray, and curdlike.

Neoplastic

Hodgkin's lymphoma. This disorder, which is most common in young adults, initially causes mild pruritus on the lower part of the body. As the disorder progresses, the pruritus may become severe and unresponsive to treatment.

Mycosis fungoides. Pruritus may precede other symptoms of this neoplastic disease by 10 years. It may persist into the first, or premycotic, stage, accompanied by erythematous lesions.

Environmental

Cimex lectularius (bedbugs). Typically, bedbug bites produce itching and burning over the ankles and lower legs, along with clusters of purpuric spots.

Pediculosis (lice). A prominent symptom, pruritus occurs in the area of infestation.

Scabies. Typically, scabies causes localized pruritus that intensifies at night. The pruritus may become generalized and persist up to 2 weeks after treatment.

Drugs

When mild and localized, an allergic reaction to such drugs as penicillin and sulfonamides can cause pruritus, erythema, an urticarial rash, and edema. However, in a severe drug reaction, anaphylaxis may occur.

Clinical considerations

• A history should be obtained and an examination of the affected area performed.

• If a localized infection or skin lesion is not present, diagnostic studies will focus on finding a systemic cause. Tests may include a complete blood count and differential, erythrocyte sedimentation rate, protein electrophoresis, and radiologic studies.

• As ordered, topical corticosteroids should be applied and antihistamines and tranquilizers administered.

• Methods to control pruritus at home should be suggested (see *Controlling Itching*, p. 333).

Psoas sign

Description

A positive psoas sign is increased abdominal pain when the patient moves his leg against resistance. It indicates direct or reflexive irritation of the psoas muscles. This sign, which can be elicited on the right or left side, usually indicates appendicitis but may also occur with localized abscesses. It is elicited in a patient with abdominal or lower back pain *after* completion of the abdominal examination to prevent spurious assessment findings (see *Eliciting Psoas Sign*).

Psychotic behavior

Description

Psychotic behavior reflects an inability or unwillingness to recognize and acknowledge reality and to relate with others. It may begin suddenly or insidiously, progressing from vague complaints of fatigue, insomnia, or headache to withdrawal, social isolation, and preoccupation with certain issues.

Various behaviors together or separately can constitute psychotic behavior. These include delusions, illusions, hallucinations, bizarre language, and perseveration. *Delusions* are persistent beliefs that have no basis in reality or in the patient's knowledge or experience, such as delusions of grandeur. *Illusions* are misinterpretations of external sensory stimuli, such as a mirage in the desert. In contrast,

Eliciting Psoas Sign

The two techniques described below can be used to elicit a psoas sign in an adult with abdominal pain. With either technique, increased abdominal pain is a positive result, indicating psoas muscle irritation from an inflamed appendix or a localized abscess.

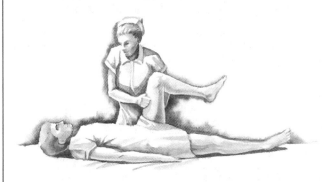

With the patient in a supine position, the examiner instructs him to move his flexed left leg against her hand to test for a left psoas sign. Then she performs this maneuver on the right leg to test for a right psoas sign.

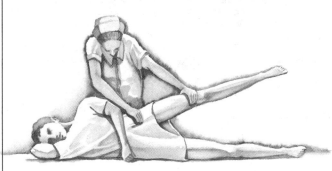

To test for a left psoas sign, the examiner turns the patient on his right side. Then she instructs him to push his left leg upward from the hip against her hand. Next, she turns the patient onto his left side and repeats this maneuver to test for a right psoas sign.

hallucinations are sensory perceptions that do not result from external stimuli. *Bizarre language* reflects a communication disruption. It can range from echolalia (purposeless repetition of a word or phrase) and clang association (repetition of words or phrases that sound similar) to neologisms (creation and use of words whose meaning only the patient knows). *Perseveration,* a persistent verbal or motor response, may indicate organic brain disease. Motor changes include inactivity, excessive activity, and repetitive movements. In children, psychotic behavior may result from early infantile autism, symbiotic infantile psychosis, and childhood schizophrenia—all of which can retard development of language, abstract thinking, and socialization.

The adolescent patient with psychotic behavior may have a history of several days' drug use or lack of sleep or food, which must be corrected before therapy can begin.

Mechanism
Psychotic behavior may stem from a primary biologic defect or vulnerability, learned maladaptive defenses, or a combination of these causes.

Possible causes
Organic disorders
Various disorders may produce psychotic behavior. These include alcohol withdrawal syndrome, cerebral hypoxia, and nutritional disorders. Endocrine disorders, such as adrenal dysfunction, and severe infections, such as encephalitis, can also cause psychotic behavior. Neurologic causes include Alzheimer's disease and other dementias.
Psychiatric disorders
Psychotic behavior usually occurs with bipolar disorders, personality disorders, schizophrenia, and traumatic stress disorders.
Drugs
Certain drugs can cause psychotic behavior (see *Psychotic Behavior: An Untoward Drug Effect*). However, al-

most any drug can provoke psychotic behavior as a rare, severe adverse or idiosyncratic reaction.
Treatments
After surgery, postoperative delirium and depression may produce psychotic behavior.

Clinical considerations
• A history should be obtained and a psychiatric assessment performed.
• Because the patient's behavior can make it difficult—or potentially dangerous—to obtain pertinent information, the interview should be conducted in a calm, safe, and well-lit room. Enough personal space should be provided to avoid threatening or agitating the patient.
• These specific guidelines for controlling psychotic behavior should be followed:
—Potentially dangerous objects, such as belts or metal utensils, should be removed from the patient's environment.
—The caregiver should help the patient discern what is real and unreal in an honest and genuine way.
—The caregiver should be straightforward, concise, and nonthreatening when speaking to the patient. Simple, concrete subjects should be discussed and theories or philosophical issues avoided.
—The patient's perceptions of reality should be positively reinforced and his misperceptions of reality corrected in a matter-of-fact way.
—The caregiver should *never* argue with the patient. However, she should not support his misperceptions.
—If the patient is frightened, the caregiver should stay with him.
—The patient should be touched to provide reassurance only if this has been tested before and proven safe.
—The patient should be moved to a safer, less stimulating environment.
—One-on-one nursing care should be provided if the patient's behavior is extremely bizarre, disturbing to other patients, or dangerous to himself.
• Antipsychotic drugs should be administered, as ordered.

Psychotic Behavior: An Untoward Drug Effect

Certain drugs can cause psychotic behavior and other psychiatric signs and symptoms, ranging from depression to violent behavior. Usually, these effects occur during therapy and resolve when the drug is discontinued. If a patient is receiving one of these common drugs and exhibits the behavior described below, the physician should be notified immediately. He may want to change the dosage or substitute another drug.

Drug	Psychiatric Signs and Symptoms
albuterol	Hallucinations, paranoia
alprazolam	Anger, hostility
amantadine	Visual hallucinations, nightmares
asparaginase	Confusion, depression, paranoia
atropine and anticholinergics	Auditory, visual, and tactile hallucinations; memory loss; delirium; fear; paranoia
bromocriptine	Mania, delusions, sudden relapse of schizophrenia, paranoia, aggressive behavior
cardiac glycosides	Paranoia, euphoria, amnesia, visual hallucinations
cimetidine	Hallucinations, paranoia, confusion, depression, delirium
clonidine	Delirium, hallucinations, depression
corticosteroids (prednisone, ACTH, cortisone)	Mania, catatonia, depression, confusion, paranoia, hallucinations
cycloserine	Anxiety, depression, confusion, paranoia, hallucinations
dapsone	Insomnia, agitation, hallucinations
diazepam	Suicidal thoughts, rage, hallucinations, depression
disopyramide	Agitation, paranoia, auditory and visual hallucinations, panic
disulfiram	Delirium, auditory hallucinations, paranoia, depression
indomethacin	Hostility, depression, paranoia, hallucinations
lidocaine	Disorientation, hallucinations, paranoia

(continued)

Psychotic Behavior: An Untoward Drug Effect (continued)

Drug	Psychiatric Signs and Symptoms
methyldopa	Severe depression, amnesia, paranoia, hallucinations
methysergide	Depersonalization, hallucinations
propranolol	Severe depression, hallucinations, paranoia, confusion
thyroid hormones	Mania, hallucinations, paranoia
vincristine	Hallucinations

Ptosis

Description
Ptosis is the excessive drooping of the upper eyelid. In severe ptosis, the patient may not be able to raise his eyelids voluntarily.

This sign can be constant, progressive, or intermittent, and unilateral or bilateral. When it is unilateral, it is easy to detect by comparing the eyelids' relative positions. When it is bilateral or mild, it is difficult to detect— the eyelids may be abnormally low, covering the upper part of the iris or even part of the pupil instead of overlapping the iris slightly. Other clues include a furrowed forehead or a tipped-back head—both of these help the patient see under his drooping lids. However, because ptosis can resemble enophthalmos, exophthalmometry may be required.

Ptosis can be classified as congenital or acquired. Congenital ptosis results from levator muscle underdevelopment or disorders of the third cranial (oculomotor) nerve. Acquired ptosis may result from trauma to or inflammation of these muscles and nerves, or from certain drugs, systemic diseases, intracranial lesions, and life-threatening aneurysms. The most common cause, however, is age, which reduces muscle elasticity and produces senile ptosis.

Possible causes
Central nervous system
Cerebral aneurysm. An aneurysm that compresses the oculomotor nerve can cause sudden ptosis, along with diplopia, a dilated pupil, and inability to rotate the eye. These may be the first signs of this life-threatening disorder.
Myasthenia gravis. Gradual bilateral ptosis is often the first sign of this disorder. It may be mild to severe and accompanied by weak eye closure and diplopia.
Myotonic dystrophy. This disorder may cause mild to severe bilateral ptosis.
Subdural hematoma (chronic). Ptosis may be a late sign, along with unilateral pupillary dilation and sluggishness.
Eyes, ears, nose, throat
Dacryoadenitis. Ptosis may accompany unilateral exophthalmos, limited extraocular movements, eyelid edema and erythema, conjunctival injection, eye pain, and diplopia.
Hemangioma. This orbital tumor can produce ptosis, exophthalmos, limited extraocular movements, and blurred vision.

Horner's syndrome. This disorder causes moderate unilateral ptosis that almost disappears when the patient opens his eye widely.

Lacrimal gland tumor. This disorder commonly produces mild to severe ptosis, depending on the tumor's size and location.

Ocular muscle dystrophy. In this disorder, bilateral ptosis progresses slowly to complete eyelid closure.

Ocular trauma. Trauma to the nerve or muscles that control the eyelids can cause mild to severe ptosis.

Parinaud's syndrome. This form of ophthalmoplegia can cause ptosis, enophthalmos, nystagmus, lid retraction, dilated pupils with absent or poor light response, and papilledema.

Psychiatric

Alcoholism. Long-term alcohol abuse can cause ptosis and such complications as severe weight loss, jaundice, ascites, and mental disturbances.

Environmental

Botulism. Acute cranial nerve dysfunction causes hallmark signs of ptosis, dysarthria, dysphagia, and diplopia.

Lead poisoning. Usually, ptosis develops over 3 to 6 months.

Drugs

Vinca alkaloids can produce ptosis.

Clinical considerations

• A history should be obtained and a neurologic assessment performed.

• Diagnostic tests may include the Tensilon test and a slit-lamp examination.

• Surgery may be necessary to correct levator muscle dysfunction.

• Special spectacle frames that suspend the eyelid by traction with a wire crutch may be provided, as ordered. Most often, these frames are used to help patients with temporary paresis or those who are not good candidates for surgery.

Pulse, absent or weak

Description

An absent or weak pulse may be generalized or affect only one extremity. When generalized, this sign is an important indicator of such life-threatening conditions as shock. Localized loss or weakness of a pulse that is normally present and strong may indicate arterial occlusion, which could require emergency surgery. However, the pressure of palpation may temporarily diminish or obliterate superficial pulses, such as the posterior tibial or the dorsal pedal. Thus, bilateral weakness or absence of these pulses does not necessarily indicate underlying pathology.

Possible causes

Respiratory

Pulmonary embolism. This disorder causes generalized weak, rapid pulse.

Cardiovascular

Aortic aneurysm (dissecting). When the dissecting aneurysm affects circulation to the innominate, left common carotid, subclavian, or femoral arteries, it causes weak or absent arterial pulses distal to the affected area. However, 25% of patients with this life-threatening condition may have normal peripheral pulses.

Aortic arch syndrome. This syndrome produces weak or abruptly absent carotid pulses and unequal or absent radial pulses. Usually, this is preceded by night sweats, pallor, nausea, anorexia, weight loss, arthralgia, and Raynaud's phenomenon.

Aortic bifurcation occlusion (acute). This rare disorder produces abrupt absence of all leg pulses.

Aortic stenosis. In this disorder, the carotid pulse is sustained, but weak. Dyspnea, chest pain, and syncope dominate the clinical picture.

Arterial occlusion. In *acute occlusion*, arterial pulses distal to the obstruction are unilaterally weak and then absent. In *chronic occlusion,* occurring in disorders such as arteriosclerosis or Buerger's disease, pulses in the affected limb weaken gradually.

Cardiac tamponade. Life-threatening cardiac tamponade causes a weak, rapid pulse accompanied by these classic findings: pulsus paradoxus, jugular vein distention, hypotension, and muffled heart sounds.

Dysrhythmias. Cardiac dysrhythmias may produce generalized weak pulses accompanied by cool, clammy skin.

Peripheral vascular disease. This disorder causes a gradual weakening and loss of peripheral pulses.

Shock. In *anaphylactic shock,* pulses become rapid and weak and then uniformly absent within seconds or minutes after exposure to an allergen. Before this, the patient experiences hypotension, anxiety, restlessness, feelings of doom, intense itching, a pounding headache, and possibly urticaria.

In *cardiogenic shock,* peripheral pulses are absent and central pulses are weak, depending on the degree of vascular collapse.

In *hypovolemic shock,* all pulses in the extremities become weak and then uniformly absent, depending on the severity of hypovolemia. As shock progresses, remaining pulses become thready and more rapid.

In *septic shock,* all pulses in the extremities first become weak. Depending on the degree of vascular collapse, pulses may then become uniformly absent.

Thoracic outlet syndrome. A patient with this syndrome may have a gradual or abrupt weakness or loss of the pulses in the arms, depending on how quickly vessels in the neck compress. These pulse changes commonly occur after the patient works with his hands above his shoulders, lifts a weight, or abducts his arm.

Treatments

Localized pulse absence may occur distal to arteriovenous fistulas or shunts for dialysis.

Clinical considerations

- All other arterial pulses should be palpated quickly to distinguish localized from generalized pulse loss or weakness.
- Vital signs should be taken, a brief history obtained, and a rapid cardiopulmonary assessment performed.
- The physician should be notified.
- Depending on assessment findings, emergency interventions may need to be performed to maintain adequate oxygenation and circulation.
- Diagnostic tests may include arteriography, aortography, and Doppler ultrasonography.
- The patient should be monitored closely.

Pulse, bounding

Description

A bounding pulse is a strong and easily palpable pulse that may be visible over superficial peripheral arteries. It is characterized by regular, recurrent expansion and contraction of the arterial walls and is not obliterated by the pressure of palpation. A healthy person develops a bounding pulse during exercise, pregnancy, or periods of anxiety. However, this sign also results from fever and certain endocrine, hematologic, and cardiovascular disorders that increase the basal metabolic rate. Bounding pulse can be normal in infants or children because arteries lie close to the skin surface. It can also result from patent ductus arteriosus if the left-to-right shunt is large.

Mechanism

A bounding pulse is produced by large waves of pressure as blood ejects from the left ventricle with each contraction.

Possible causes

Cardiovascular

Aortic insufficiency. Sometimes called a water-hammer pulse, the bounding pulse associated with this condition is characterized by a rapid, forceful expansion of the arterial pulse followed by rapid contraction.

Endocrine

Thyrotoxicosis. This disorder produces a rapid, full, bounding pulse.

Hematologic

Anemia. In this disorder, bounding pulse may be accompanied by capillary pulsations, a systolic ejection murmur, tachycardia, an atrial gallop (S_4), and a systolic bruit over the carotid artery.

Psychiatric

Alcoholism (acute). Vasodilation of acute alcoholism produces a rapid, bounding pulse and flushed face.

Clinical considerations

• Vital signs should be taken and the physical examination completed.
• Cardiac monitoring should be initiated, if appropriate.
• Diagnostic tests may include EKG, echocardiography, chest X-ray, and blood studies.

Pulse pressure, narrowed

Description

Narrowed pulse pressure is a difference of less than 30 mm Hg between systolic and diastolic blood pressures. (Normally, systolic pressure is about 40 mm Hg higher than diastolic.) In conditions that cause mechanical obstruction, such as aortic stenosis, pulse pressure is directly related to the severity of the underlying condition. Usually a late sign, narrowed pulse pressure alone does not signal an emergency, even though it commonly occurs in shock and other life-threatening disorders.

Mechanism

Narrowed pulse pressure occurs when peripheral vascular resistance increases, cardiac output declines, or intravascular volume markedly decreases (see *Understanding Pulse Pressure Changes*, p. 342).

Possible causes

Cardiovascular

Aortic stenosis. Narrowed pulse pressure occurs late in significant stenosis.

Cardiac tamponade. In this life-threatening disorder, pulse pressure narrows approximately 10 to 20 mm Hg.

Congestive heart failure. Narrowed pulse pressure occurs relatively late.

Shock. Narrowed pulse pressure occurs as a late sign in all types of shock.

Clinical considerations

• The physical examination should be completed and the physician notified.
• Diagnostic tests may include echocardiography and chest X-rays.
• The patient should be monitored closely for changes in pulse rate or quality of pulse rate and for hypotension.

Pulse pressure, widened

Description

Widened pulse pressure is a difference greater than 50 mm Hg. It commonly occurs as a physiologic response to fever, hot weather, or exercise. However, it can also result from certain neurologic and cardiovascular disorders that reduce arterial compliance or cause backflow of blood into the heart with each contraction; chief among these is a life-threatening increase in intracranial pressure (ICP). Widened pulse pressure can easily be identified by monitoring arterial blood pressure and is commonly detected during routine sphygmomanometric recordings.

Mechanism

(See *Understanding Pulse Pressure Changes*, p. 342.)

Possible causes

Central nervous system

Increased ICP. Widening pulse pressure is an intermediate to late sign of increased ICP. Although decreased level of consciousness is the earliest and most

Understanding Pulse Pressure Changes

Two major factors affect pulse pressure—the amount of blood, or *stroke volume,* that the ventricles eject into the arteries with each beat, and the arteries' *peripheral resistance* to blood flow. These two factors affect systolic and diastolic blood pressures and, as a result, pulse pressure. For example, pulse pressure narrows when systolic pressure falls (lower right), diastolic pressure rises (upper left), or both. These changes reflect decreased stroke volume, increased peripheral resistance, or both.

Pulse pressure widens when systolic pressure rises (upper right), diastolic pressure falls (lower left), or both. These changes reflect increased stroke volume, decreased peripheral resistance, or both.

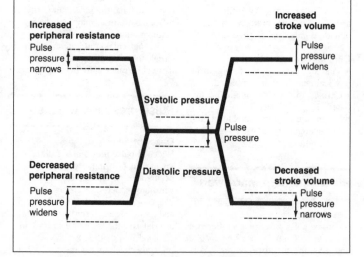

sensitive indicator of this life-threatening condition, the onset and progression of widening pulse pressure also parallel rising ICP. (Even a gap of only 50 mm Hg can signal a rapid deterioration in the patient's condition.)

Cardiovascular

Aortic insufficiency. In acute aortic insufficiency, pulse pressure widens progressively as the valve deteriorates, and a bounding pulse and an atrial gallop (S_4) develop.

Arteriosclerosis. In this disorder, reduced arterial compliance causes progressive widening of pulse pressure, which becomes permanent without treatment of the underlying disorder. It is preceded by moderate hypertension and accompanied by signs of vascular insufficiency, such as claudication and speech disturbances.

Clinical considerations

If the patient's level of consciousness is decreased and if increased ICP is the suspected cause of his widened pulse pressure:

• The physician should be notified immediately.

• Emergency intervention should be performed, as needed, to maintain a patent airway and reduce ICP.

• A neurologic assessment should be performed.

• The patient should be monitored closely for signs of increasing ICP.

If increased ICP is not suspected:

• A history should be obtained and a cardiovascular assessment performed.

• Diagnostic tests may include X-rays of the skull and chest, computed tomography, echocardiography, and blood tests.

Pulse rhythm, abnormal

Description

An abnormal pulse rhythm is an irregular expansion and contraction of the peripheral arterial walls. It may be persistent or sporadic, and rhythmic or arrhythmic. Detected by palpating the radial or carotid pulse, an abnormal rhythm is typically reported first by the patient, who complains instead of palpitations. This important finding reflects an underlying cardiac dysrhythmia, which may range from benign to life threatening. Dysrhythmias are commonly associated with cardiovascular, renal, respiratory, metabolic, and neurologic disorders, as well as the effects of drugs, diagnostic tests, and treatments.

Possible causes
Cardiovascular

Dysrhythmias. An abnormal pulse rhythm may be the only sign of a cardiac dysrhythmia (see *Abnormal Pulse Rhythm: Clue to Cardiac Dysrhythmias,* pp. 344 to 347). The patient may complain of palpitations, a fluttering heartbeat, or weak and skipped beats. Pulses may be weak and rapid or slow.

Clinical considerations

If the patient has signs of reduced cardiac output:

• The physician should be notified immediately.

• Cardiac monitoring should be initiated.

• Emergency intervention, including cardiopulmonary resuscitation, should be anticipated.

If the patient's condition permits:

• A history should be obtained and a cardiovascular assessment performed.

• Diagnostic tests may include chest X-ray; EKG; blood samples for serum electrolyte, cardiac enzyme, and drug level studies; and 24-hour Holter monitoring.

• The patient should be monitored closely.

• The patient should be instructed to avoid smoking and caffeine, which increase dysrhythmias.

• Medication compliance should be stressed.

Pulsus alternans

Description

Pulsus alternans is a beat-to-beat change in the size and intensity of a peripheral pulse. It is a sign of severe left ventricular failure. Although pulse rhythm remains regular, strong and weak contractions alternate (see *Comparing Arterial Pressure Waves,* pp. 348 and 349). An alternation in the intensity of heart sounds and of existing heart murmurs may accompany this sign.

Pulsus alternans is thought to result from the change in stroke volume that occurs with beat-to-beat alteration in the left ventricle's contractility. Recumbency or exercise increases venous return and reduces the abnormal pulse, which often disappears with treatment for heart failure. Rarely, a patient with normal left ventricular function has pulsus alternans, but the abnormal pulse seldom persists for more than 12 beats.

Although most easily detected by sphygmomanometry, pulsus alternans can be detected by palpating the brachial, radial, or femoral artery when systolic pressure varies from beat to beat by more than 20 mm Hg. Because the

Abnormal Pulse Rhythm:
Clue to Cardiac Dysrhythmias

An abnormal pulse rhythm may be the only clue that the patient has a cardiac dysrhythmia. But this sign does not help pinpoint the specific type of dysrhythmia. For that, a cardiac monitor or an electrocardiogram (EKG) machine is needed. These devices record the electrical current generated by the heart's conduction system and display this information on an

Dysrhythmia

Sinus arrhythmia

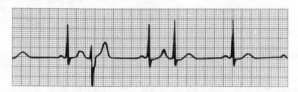

Premature atrial contractions (PACs)

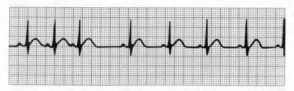

Paroxysmal atrial tachycardia

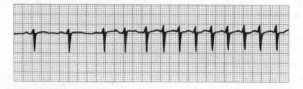

Atrial fibrillation

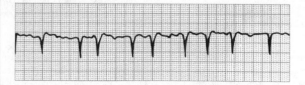

oscilloscope screen or a strip-chart recorder. Besides rhythm disturbances, they can identify conduction defects and electrolyte imbalances.

The EKG strips below show some common cardiac dysrhythmias that can cause abnormal pulse rhythms.

Pulse Rhythm and Rate	Clinical Implications
Irregular rhythm; fast, slow, or normal rate.	• Vagal effect of respiration on heart rate increases with inspiration and decreases with expiration. • May result from drugs, as in digitalis toxicity. • Occurs most often in children and young adults.
Irregular rhythm during PACs; fast, slow, or normal rate.	• Occasional PAC may be normal. • Isolated PACs indicate atrial irritation—for example, from anxiety or excessive caffeine intake. Increasing PACs may herald other atrial dysrhythmias. • May result from congestive heart failure, ischemic heart disease, acute respiratory failure, chronic obstructive pulmonary disease (COPD), or use of digitalis, aminophylline, or adrenergic drugs.
Irregular rhythm at abrupt onset or end of dysrhythmia; heart rate exceeds 140 beats/minute.	• May occur in otherwise normal, healthy persons with physical or psychological stress, hypoxia, or hypokalemia; may be associated with excessive use of caffeine or other stimulants, with use of marijuana, and with digitalis toxicity. • Indicates intrinsic abnormality of atrioventricular (AV) conduction system; may herald more serious ventricular dysrhythmia or precipitate angina or CHF.
Irregular rhythm; atrial rate exceeds 400 beats/minute; fast, slow, or normal ventricular rate.	• May result from congestive heart failure, COPD, hyperthyroidism, sepsis, pulmonary embolus, mitral valve disease, digitalis toxicity (rarely), atrial irritation, postcoronary bypass, or valve replacement surgery. • Because atria do not contract, preload is not consistent, so cardiac output changes with each beat. Emboli may also result.

(continued)

Abnormal Pulse Rhythm:
Clue to Cardiac Dysrhythmias *(continued)*

Dysrhythmia

Premature junctional contractions (PJCs)

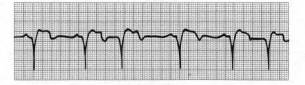

Second-degree AV heart block, Mobitz Type I (Wenckebach)

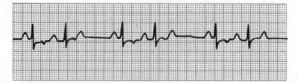

Second-degree AV heart block, Mobitz Type II

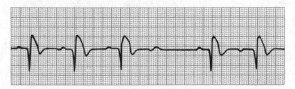

Premature ventricular contractions (multifocal)

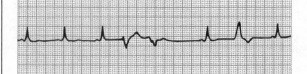

Pulse Rhythm and Rate	Clinical Implications
Irregular rhythm during PJCs; fast, slow, or normal rate.	• May result from myocardial infarction (MI) or ischemia, excessive caffeine intake, and most commonly digitalis toxicity (from enhanced automaticity). • Increasing PJCs may herald other dysrhythmias.
Irregular rhythm; fast, slow, or normal rate.	• Often transient; may progress to complete heart block. • May result from inferior wall MI, digitalis or quinidine toxicity, vagal stimulation, and arteriosclerotic heart disease.
Irregular rhythm; slow or normal rate.	• May progress to complete heart block. • May result from degenerative disease of conduction system, ischemia of AV node in anterior MI, anteroseptal infarction, or digitalis or quinidine toxicity.
Usually irregular rhythm with a long pause after the premature beat; fast, slow, or normal rate.	• Indicates ventricular irritability; may initiate ventricular tachycardia or ventricular fibrillation. • May result from heart failure, old or acute MI, contusion with trauma, myocardial irritation by a ventricular catheter, hypoxia, drug toxicity, electrolyte imbalance, or stress.

small changes in arterial pressure that occur during normal respirations may obscure this abnormal pulse, the patient is told to hold his breath during palpation. *Light* pressure should be applied to avoid obliterating the weaker pulse.

When using a sphygmomanometer to detect pulsus alternans, the cuff is inflated 10 to 20 mm Hg above the systolic pressure as determined by palpation, then slowly deflated. At first, only the strong beats will be heard. With further deflation, all beats will become audible and palpable, and then equally intense. (The difference between this point and the peak systolic level is often used to determine the degree of pulsus alternans.) When the cuff is removed, pulsus alternans returns.

Occasionally, the weak beat is so small that no palpable pulse is detected at the periphery. This produces total pulsus alternans, an apparent halving of the pulse rate.

Pulsus bisferiens

Description
Pulsus bisferiens is a hyperdynamic, double-beating pulse characterized by two systolic peaks separated by a mid-systolic dip. Both peaks may be equal or either may be larger; most often, though, the first peak is taller or more forceful than the second. The first peak (percussion wave) is believed to be the pulse pressure and the second (tidal wave), reverberation from the periphery (see *Comparing Arterial Pressure Waves*).

Pulsus bisferiens can be palpated in peripheral arteries or observed on an arterial pressure wave recording.

To detect pulsus bisferiens, the carotid, brachial, radial, or femoral artery is lightly palpated. (The pulse is easiest to palpate in the carotid artery.) At the same time, the patient's heart sounds are auscultated to determine

Comparing Arterial Pressure Waves

The percussion wave in the **normal arterial pulse** reflects ejection of blood into the aorta (early systole). The tidal wave is the peak of the pulse wave (later systole). And the dicrotic notch marks the beginning of diastole.

Pulsus alternans is a beat-to-beat alternation in pulse size and intensity. Although the rhythm of pulsus alternans is regular, the volume varies. During blood pressure measurement in a patient with this abnormality, a loud Korotkoff sound then a soft sound is heard; the sounds continually alternate. Pulsus alternans commonly accompanies states of poor contractility that occur with left ventricular failure.

Pulsus bisferiens is a double-beating pulse with two systolic peaks. The first beat reflects pulse pressure and the second beat reflects reverberation from the periphery. Pulsus bisferiens commonly occurs in aortic insufficiency or high cardiac output states.

Pulsus paradoxus is an exaggerated decline in blood pressure during inspiration, resulting from an increase in negative intrathoracic pressure. A pulsus paradoxus that exceeds 10 mm Hg is considered abnormal and may result from cardiac tamponade, constrictive pericarditis, or severe lung disease.

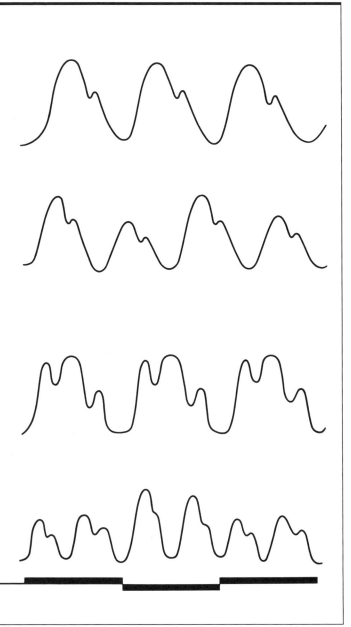

whether the two palpable peaks occur during systole. If they do, the double pulse will be felt between the first and second heart sounds.

Mechanism
Pulsus bisferiens occurs in conditions such as aortic insufficiency in which a large volume of blood is rapidly ejected from the left ventricle.

Possible causes
Cardiovascular
Aortic insufficiency. This heart defect is the most common organic cause of bisferiens pulse.

Aortic stenosis with aortic insufficiency. A bisferiens pulse is commonly seen in aortic stenosis when moderately severe aortic insufficiency also occurs. In aortic stenosis, the pulse rises slowly and the second wave of the double beat is the more forceful one. Frequently, this is accompanied by dyspnea and fatigue.

High cardiac output states. Pulsus bisferiens commonly occurs in high-output states, such as anemia, thyrotoxicosis, fever, or exercise.

Hypertrophic obstructive cardiomyopathy. About 40% of patients with this disorder have pulsus bisferiens because of a pressure gradient in the left ventricular outflow tract. Recorded more often than it is palpated, the pulse rises rapidly, and the first wave is the more forceful one.

Clinical considerations
• A history should be obtained and the cardiac assessment completed.

• Diagnostic tests may include EKG, chest X-ray, cardiac catheterization, or angiography.

Pulsus paradoxus
(Paradoxical pulse)

Description
Paradoxical pulse is an exaggerated decline in blood pressure during inspira-

tion. Normally, systolic pressure falls less than 10 mm Hg during inspiration. In pulsus paradoxus, however, it falls more than 10 mm Hg (see *Comparing Arterial Pressure Waves,* pp. 348 and 349). When systolic pressure falls more than 20 mm Hg, the peripheral pulses may be barely palpable or may disappear during inspiration.

To accurately detect and measure paradoxical pulse, a sphygmomanometer or intraarterial monitoring device is used. The blood pressure cuff is inflated 10 to 20 mm Hg beyond the peak systolic pressure. Then the cuff is deflated at a rate of 2 mm Hg/second until the first Korotkoff sound is heard during expiration. The systolic pressure should be noted. As the cuff is slowly deflated, the patient's respiratory pattern is observed. If a paradoxical pulse is present, the Korotkoff sounds will disappear with inspiration and return with expiration. Cuff deflation should continue until Korotkoff sounds are heard during both inspiration and expiration, and, again, the systolic pressure is noted. This reading is then subtracted from the first one to determine the degree of paradoxical pulse. A difference of more than 10 mm Hg is abnormal.

Paradoxical pulse can also be detected by palpating the radial pulse over several cycles of slow inspiration and expiration. Marked pulse diminution during inspiration indicates paradoxical pulse. When checking for paradoxical pulse, the examiner should remember that irregular heart rhythms and tachycardia cause variations in pulse amplitude and must be ruled out before a true paradoxical pulse can be identified.

Mechanism
Pulsus paradoxus is thought to result from an inspirational increase in negative intrathoracic pressure. Normally, systolic pressure drops during inspiration because of blood pooling in the pulmonary system. This, in turn, reduces left ventricular filling and stroke

volume and transmits negative intrathoracic pressure to the aorta. Such conditions as chronic obstructive pulmonary disease or cardiac tamponade further impede blood flow from the left ventricle during inspiration and produce paradoxical pulse.

Possible causes
Respiratory
Chronic obstructive pulmonary disease. The wide fluctuations in intrathoracic pressure characteristic of this disorder produce pulsus paradoxus and possibly tachycardia.

Pulmonary embolism (massive). Decreased left ventricular filling and stroke volume in massive pulmonary embolism produces pulsus paradoxus.

Cardiovascular
Cardiac tamponade. Pulsus paradoxus commonly occurs in this disorder. However, if intrapericardial pressure rises abruptly and profound hypotension occurs, paradoxical pulse may be difficult to detect. In severe tamponade, assessment also reveals these classic findings: hypotension, diminished or muffled heart sounds, and jugular vein distention. If cardiac tamponade develops gradually, paradoxical pulse may be accompanied by weakness, anorexia, and weight loss.

Pericarditis (chronic constrictive). Paradoxical pulse can occur in up to 50% of patients with this disorder.

Right ventricular infarction. This infarction may produce pulsus paradoxus and elevated jugular venous or central venous pressure.

Clinical considerations
• The patient's other vital signs should be taken quickly and the physician notified.

• Emergency intervention may be necessary to aspirate blood or fluid from the pericardial sac (pericardiocentesis).

• When appropriate, a history should be obtained and a complete cardiopulmonary assessment performed.

• Diagnostic tests may include chest X-rays and echocardiography.

• The patient should be monitored closely.

Pupils, nonreactive

Description
Nonreactive (fixed) pupils fail to constrict in response to light or dilate when the light is removed. The development of a unilateral or bilateral nonreactive response indicates an important change in the patient's condition and could signal a life-threatening emergency and possibly brain death. It also occurs with use of certain optic drugs.

To assess pupillary reaction to light, the patient's *direct light reflex* is tested first. The room is darkened, and one of the patient's eyes is covered while the opposite eyelid is held open. Using a bright penlight, the light is brought toward the patient from the side and is shone directly into his opened eye. If normal, the pupil will promptly constrict. The *consensual light reflex* is tested next. The patient's eyelids are held open and the light is shone into one eye while the pupil of the opposite eye is observed. If normal, both pupils will promptly constrict. Both procedures are repeated in the opposite eye. A unilateral or bilateral nonreactive response indicates dysfunction of cranial nerves II and III, which mediate the pupillary light reflex (see *Innervation of Direct and Consensual Light Reflexes,* p. 352).

Possible causes
Central nervous system
Adie's syndrome. This syndrome produces abrupt onset of unilateral mydriasis, along with sluggish or nonreactive pupillary response. It also may produce blurred vision and cramplike eye pain. Eventually, both eyes may be affected.

Innervation of Direct and Consensual Light Reflexes

Two reactions—direct and consensual—constitute the pupillary light reflex. Normally, when a light is shined directly onto the retina of one eye, the parasympathetic nerves are stimulated to cause brisk constriction of that pupil—the *direct light reflex.* The pupil of the opposite eye also constricts—the *consensual light reflex.* The optic nerve (CN II) mediates the afferent arc of this reflex from each eye, while the oculomotor nerve (CN III) mediates the efferent arc to both eyes. A nonreactive or sluggish response in one or both pupils indicates dysfunction of these cranial nerves—usually due to degenerative disease of the central nervous system.

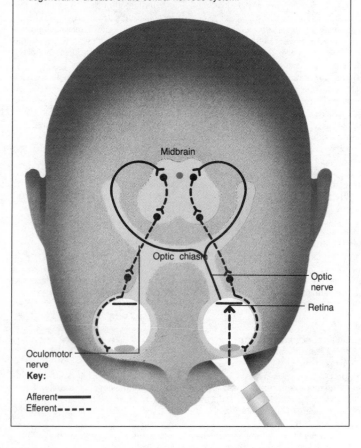

Midbrain

Optic chiasm

Optic nerve

Retina

Oculomotor nerve

Key:

Afferent ━━━━
Efferent ━ ━ ━ ━

Encephalitis. As this disease progresses, initally sluggish pupils become dilated and nonreactive.

Midbrain lesions. Although rare, these lesions produce bilateral midposition nonreactive pupils.

Wernicke's disease. Nonreactive pupils are a late sign in this disease, which initially produces intention tremor accompanied by sluggish pupillary reaction.

Eyes, ears, nose, throat
Glaucoma (acute closed-angle). In this ophthalmic emergency, examination reveals a moderately dilated, nonreactive pupil in the affected eye.

Iris disease (degenerative or inflammatory). This disease causes pupillary nonreactivity in the affected eye(s).

Ocular trauma. Severe damage to the iris or optic nerve may produce a nonreactive, dilated pupil in the affected eye (traumatic iridoplegia). It is usually transitory but can be permanent.

Oculomotor nerve palsy. Often, the first signs of this oculomotor ophthalmoplegia are a dilated, nonreactive pupil and loss of the accommodation reaction. These findings may occur in one eye or both, depending on whether the palsy is unilateral or bilateral. Among the causes of total third cranial nerve paralysis is life-threatening brain herniation. *Central herniation* causes bilateral midposition nonreactive pupils, whereas *uncal herniation* initially causes a unilateral dilated, nonreactive pupil.

Uveitis. A small, nonreactive pupil typifies *anterior uveitis,* appearing suddenly with severe eye pain, conjunctival injection, and photophobia. In *posterior uveitis,* similar features develop insidiously.

Environmental
Botulism. Bilateral mydriasis and nonreactive pupils usually appear 12 to 36 hours after ingestion of tainted food.

Drugs
Instillation of topical mydriatics and cycloplegics may induce a temporarily nonreactive pupil in the affected eye.

Use of glutethimide and deep ether anesthesia produces medium-sized or slightly enlarged pupils, which remain nonreactive for several hours. Opiates, such as heroin and morphine, cause pinpoint pupils with a minimal light response that can be seen only with a magnifying glass. Atropine poisoning produces widely dilated, nonreactive pupils.

Clinical considerations
If the patient is unconscious:
- The physician should be notified.
- Vital signs should be taken and a rapid neurologic assessment performed.
- Emergency intervention, including surgery, should be anticipated to decrease ICP and to maintain a patent airway and adequate oxygenation.
- The patient's eyes should be closed to prevent corneal exposure. (Tape may be used to secure the eyelids, if needed.)

If the patient is conscious:
- A brief history should be obtained and a complete neurologic assessment performed.
- Diagnostic tests may include X-rays and computed tomography of the skull, tonometry, and slit-lamp and ophthalmoscopic examination.
- The patient's pupillary light reflex should be monitored to detect changes.

Pupils, sluggish

Description
Sluggish pupillary reaction is an abnormally slow pupil response to light. It can occur in one pupil or both, unlike the normal reaction, which is always bilateral. A sluggish reaction accompanies degenerative disease of the central nervous system and diabetic neuropathy. It can occur normally in the elderly, whose pupils become smaller and less responsive with age. Sluggish pupillary reaction is not diagnostically significant, although it occurs in a variety of disorders.

To assess pupillary reaction to light, the examiner first tests the patient's *direct light reflex*. She darkens the room and covers one of the patient's eyes while holding open the opposite eyelid. Using a bright penlight, she brings the light toward the patient from the side and shines it directly into his open eye. If normal, the pupil will promptly constrict. She then tests the *consensual light reflex*. She holds both of the patient's eyelids open and shines the light into one eye while watching the pupil of the opposite eye. If normal, both pupils will promptly constrict. She repeats both procedures to test light reflexes in the opposite eye. A sluggish reaction in one or both pupils indicates dysfunction of cranial nerves II and III, which mediate the pupillary light reflex (see *Innervation of Direct and Consensual Light Reflexes*, p. 352).

Possible causes
Central nervous system
Adie's syndrome. This syndrome produces abrupt onset of unilateral mydriasis and sluggish pupillary response, possibly progressing to a nonreactive response.

Diabetic neuropathy. A patient with long-standing diabetes mellitus may have a sluggish pupillary response.

Encephalitis. This disorder initially produces a bilateral sluggish pupillary response. Later, pupils become dilated and nonreactive, and decreased accommodation may occur, along with other cranial nerve palsies, such as dysphagia and facial weakness.

Herpes zoster. The patient with herpes zoster affecting the nasociliary nerve may have a sluggish pupillary response.

Multiple sclerosis. This disorder may produce small, irregularly shaped pupils that react better to accommodation than to light.

Myotonic dystrophy. In this disorder, sluggish pupillary reaction may be accompanied by lid lag, ptosis, miosis, and possibly diplopia.

Tertiary syphilis. Sluggish pupillary reaction (especially in Argyll Robertson pupils) occurs in the late stage of neurosyphilis, along with marked weakness of the extraocular muscles, visual field defects, and possibly cataractous changes in the lens.

Wernicke's disease. Initially, this disorder produces intention tremor accompanied by sluggish pupillary reaction. Later, pupils may become nonreactive.

Eyes, ears, nose, throat
Iritis (acute). In this disorder, the affected eye exhibits a sluggish pupillary response and conjunctival injection. The pupil may remain constricted; if posterior synechiae have formed, the pupil will also be irregularly shaped.

Clinical considerations
• Visual acuity should be tested in both eyes and pupillary reaction to accommodation assessed.

• Ophthalmoscopic and slit-lamp examinations will be performed.

• Intraocular pressure may be measured.

Purple striae

Description
Purple striae are thin, purple streaks on the skin. They characteristically occur in hypercortisolism along with other cushingoid signs, such as a buffalo hump and moon face. Although hypercortisolism can result from adrenocortical carcinoma, adrenal adenoma, and pituitary adenoma, it most commonly results from excessive use of glucocorticoid drugs.

The catabolic action of excess glucocorticoids on skin, fat, and muscle produces purple striae by inhibiting fibroblast activity, resulting in loss of collagen and connective tissue. This causes extreme thinning of the skin, which, along with erythrocytosis, is responsible for the striae's purple color. Although purple striae are most common over the abdominal area, they may also occur over the breasts, hips, buttocks, thighs, and axillae. They develop gradually and, with treatment, may gradually fade or decrease in size.

Purpura

Description

Purpura is the extravasation of red blood cells from the blood vessels into the skin, subcutaneous tissue, or mucous membranes. It is characterized by discoloration—usually purplish or brownish red—that is easily visible through the epidermis. Purpuric lesions include petechiae, ecchymoses, and hematomas (see *Identifying Purpuric Lesions*, p. 356). Purpura differs from erythema in that it does not blanch with pressure because it involves blood in the tissues, not just dilated vessels.

Purpura results from damage to the endothelium of small blood vessels, coagulation defects, ineffective perivascular support, capillary fragility and permeability, or a combination of these factors. In turn, these faulty hemostatic factors can result from thrombocytopenia or other hematologic disorders, invasive procedures, and, of course, anticoagulant drugs.

Additional causes are nonpathologic. Purpura can be a consequence of aging, when loss of collagen decreases connective tissue support of upper skin blood vessels. In the elderly or cachectic person, skin atrophy and inelasticity and loss of subcutaneous fat increase susceptibility to minor trauma, causing purpura to appear along the veins of the forearms, hands, legs, and feet. Prolonged coughing or vomiting can produce crops of petechiae in loose face and neck tissue. Violent muscle contraction, as occurs in seizures or weight lifting, sometimes results in localized ecchymoses from increased in-

traluminal pressure and rupture. High fever, which increases capillary fragility, can also produce purpura.

Possible causes

Cardiovascular

Stasis. Chronic stasis usually affects the elderly, producing dusky reddish purpura on the legs after prolonged standing.

Gastrointestinal

Liver disease. Hepatic disease may cause purpura, particularly ecchymoses and other bleeding tendencies.

Musculoskeletal

Systemic lupus erythematosus. This chronic inflammatory disorder may produce purpura accompanied by other cutaneous findings, such as scaly patches on the scalp, face, neck, and arms; diffuse alopecia; telangiectasis; urticaria; and ulceration.

Hematologic

Disseminated intravascular coagulation. This syndrome can cause varying degrees of purpura, depending on its severity and underlying cause. Rarely, the patient develops life-threatening purpura fulminans, with symmetrical cutaneous and subcutaneous lesions on the arms and legs.

Dysproteinemias. In *multiple myeloma,* petechiae and ecchymoses accompany other bleeding tendencies: hematemesis, epistaxis, gum bleeding, and excessive bleeding after surgery. Similar findings occur in *cryoglobulinemia,* whch may also produce a malignant maculopapular purpura. *Hyperglobulinemia* typically begins insidiously with occasional attacks of purpura over the lower legs and feet. Attacks eventually become more frequent and extensive, involving the entire lower leg and possibly the trunk. The purpura usually occurs after prolonged standing or exercise and may be heralded by skin burning or stinging. Leg edema, knee or ankle pain, and low-grade fever may precede or accompany the purpura, which gradually fades over 1 or 2 weeks.

Identifying Purpuric Lesions

Petechiae are painless, round, pinpoint lesions, 1 to 3 mm in diameter. Caused by extravasation of red blood cells into cutaneous tissue, these red or brown lesions usually arise on dependent portions of the body. They appear and fade in crops and can group to form ecchymoses.

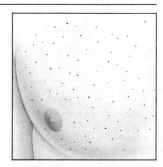

Ecchymoses, another form of blood extravasation, are larger than petechiae. These purple, blue, or yellow-green bruises vary in size and shape and can arise anywhere on the body as a result of trauma. Ecchymoses usually appear on the arms and legs of patients with bleeding disorders.

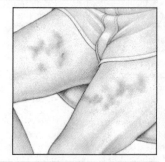

Hematomas are palpable ecchymoses that are painful and swollen. Usually the result of trauma, superficial hematomas are red, whereas deep hematomas are blue. Hematomas often exceed 1 cm in diameter, but their size varies widely.

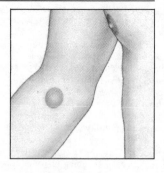

Idiopathic thrombocytopenic purpura (ITP). Chronic ITP typically begins insidiously, with scattered petechiae that are most common on the distal arms and legs. Deep-lying ecchymoses may also occur.

Leukemia. This disorder produces widespread petechiae on the skin, mucous membranes, retina, and serosal surfaces that persist throughout the course of the disease. Confluent ecchymoses are uncommon but may occur.

Myeloproliferative disorders. These disorders paradoxically can cause hemorrhage accompanied by ecchymoses and ruddy cyanosis.

Septicemia. Thrombocytopenia or the effects of toxins in acute infection can lead to purpura, especially in the form of petechiae.

Thrombotic thrombocytopenic purpura. Generalized purpura is usually a presenting sign in this disorder.

Metabolic

Nutritional deficiencies. In *vitamin C deficiency,* the characteristic pattern of purpura is perifollicular petechiae, which coalesce to form ecchymoses, in the "saddle area" of the thighs and buttocks. *Vitamin K deficiency* produces abnormal bleeding tendencies, such as ecchymosis, gum bleeding, epistaxis, and hematuria. It also causes GI and intracranial bleeding. *Vitamin B_{12} deficiency* can cause varying degrees of purpura. *Folic acid deficiency* also can cause varying degrees of purpura.

Immunologic

Autoerythrocyte sensitivity. In this syndrome, painful ecchymoses appear either singly or in groups, usually preceded by local itching, burning, or pain.

Drugs

The anticoagulants heparin and coumadin can produce purpura.

Treatments

Any procedures that disrupt circulation, coagulation, or platelet activity or production may cause purpura. These include pulmonary and cardiac surgery, radiation therapy, chemotherapy, hemodialysis, multiple blood transfusions with platelet-poor blood, and use of plasma expanders, such as dextran.

Diagnostic tests

Invasive procedures, such as venipuncture and arterial catheterization, may produce local ecchymoses and hematomas due to extravasated blood.

Clinical considerations

• Diagnostic tests may include a peripheral blood smear, bone marrow examination, and blood tests to determine platelet count, bleeding and coagulation times, capillary fragility, clot retraction, one-stage thromboplastin time, and fibrinogen levels.

• Purpuric lesions are not permanent and will fade if the underlying cause can be treated successfully.

• The patient should not use fade creams or other products in an attempt to reduce pigmentation.

• If the patient has a hematoma, pressure and cold compresses should be applied initially to help reduce bleeding and swelling. After the first 24 hours, hot compresses should be applied to help speed absorption of blood.

Pyrosis
(Heartburn)

Description

Pyrosis is a substernal burning sensation that rises in the chest and may radiate to the neck or throat. Caused by reflux of gastric contents into the esophagus, it is commonly accompanied by regurgitation. Because increased intraabdominal pressure contributes to reflux, pyrosis often occurs with pregnancy, ascites, or obesity. It also accompanies various GI disorders, connective tissue disease, and use of numerous drugs. Usually, pyrosis develops after meals or when the patient lies down (especially on his right side), bends over, lifts heavy objects, or exercises vigorously. Typically, pyrosis worsens with swallowing and improves when the patient sits upright or takes antacids.

Other signs and symptoms—such as dyspnea, tachycardia, palpitations, nausea, and vomiting—will help distinguish MI from pyrosis.

Mechanism

A barrier to reflux, the lower esophageal sphincter (LES) normally relaxes only to allow food to pass from the esophagus into the stomach. But hormonal fluctuations, mechanical stress, and the effects of certain foods and drugs can lower LES pressure. When LES pressure falls and intraabdominal or intragastric pressure rises, the normally contracted LES relaxes inappropriately and allows reflux of gastric acid or bile secretions into the lower esophagus. There, the reflux irritates and inflames the esophageal mucosa, producing pyrosis.

Possible causes

Gastrointestinal

Esophageal cancer. Pyrosis may be a sign of this cancer, depending on tumor size and location. The first and most common symptom is painless dysphagia that progressively worsens.

Esophageal diverticula. Although usually asymptomatic, this disorder may cause pyrosis, regurgitation, and dysphagia.

Gastroesophageal reflux disease. Pyrosis, frequently severe, is the most common symptom of this disorder. The pyrosis tends to be chronic, usually occurs 30 to 60 minutes after eating, and may be triggered by certain foods or beverages. It worsens when the patient lies down or bends and abates when he sits or stands upright or takes antacids.

Peptic ulcer disease. Pyrosis and indigestion usually signal the start of a peptic ulcer attack.

Musculoskeletal

Scleroderma. This connective tissue disease may cause esophageal dysfunction resulting in reflux with pyrosis, the sensation of food sticking behind the breastbone, odynophagia, bloating after meals, and weight loss.

Metabolic

Obesity. Increased intraabdominal pressure can contribute to reflux and resulting pyrosis.

Drugs

Various drugs may cause or aggravate pyrosis. Among these offenders are acetohexamide, tolbutamide, lypressin, aspirin, anticholinergic agents, and drugs that have anticholinergic effects.

Clinical considerations

• Diagnostic tests may include barium swallow, upper GI series, esophagoscopy, and laboratory studies to test esophageal motility and acidity.

• After the causative disorder is determined, the patient should be taught how to avoid a recurrence of pyrosis. He should be advised to eat frequent small meals, to sit upright (especially after a meal), and to avoid lying down for at least 2 hours after a meal. He should be instructed to avoid highly seasoned foods, caffeine, acidic juices, alcohol, bedtime snacks, and foods high in fat or carbohydrates, which reduce LES pressure. He should avoid bending, coughing, engaging in vigorous exercise, wearing tight clothing, or gaining weight, thereby preventing increased intraabdominal pressure. He should be advised to refrain from smoking and using drugs that reduce sphincter control.

• If the patient's pyrosis is severe, he should be advised to sleep with extra pillows or with 6″ wooden blocks under the head of the bed to reduce reflux.

• The patient should be instructed to take antacids, as ordered (usually 1 hour after meals and at bedtime).

• The physician may order medications that increase LES contraction, such as bethanechol.

Quinquaud's sign

Description

Quinquaud's sign is trembling of the fingers in alcoholism. To detect this sign, the examiner has the patient spread his hand, flex his fingers at the metacarpophalangeal joints, and touch her palm with his fingers at a 90° angle to her hand.

Raccoon's Eyes

Description

Raccoon's eyes refer to bilateral periorbital ecchymoses that do not result from facial trauma. Usually an indicator of basilar skull fracture, this sign develops when damage at the time of fracture tears the meninges and causes the venous sinuses to bleed into the arachnoid villi and the cranial sinuses. Raccoon's eyes may be the only indicator of basilar skull fracture, which is not always visible on skull X-rays. Their appearance signals the need for careful assessment to detect any underlying trauma, since a basilar skull fracture can injure cranial nerves, blood vessels, and the brain stem. Raccoon's eyes can also occur after a craniotomy if the surgery causes a meningeal tear.

Rash, butterfly

Description

A butterfly rash is a characteristic rash that appears in a malar distribution across the nose and cheeks. When present, butterfly rash is a cardinal sign of systemic lupus erythematosus. However, it can also signal dermatologic disorders.

Similar rashes may appear on the neck, scalp, and other areas. Butterfly rash is sometimes mistaken for sunburn, since it can be provoked or aggravated by ultraviolet rays.

Possible causes
Musculoskeletal

Discoid lupus erythematosus. This benign form of lupus erythematosus may present with a unilateral or butterfly rash that consists of mildly scaling, erythematous, raised, sharply demarcated plaques with follicular plugging and central atrophy. The rash may also involve the scalp, ears, chest, or any part of the body exposed to sun.

Systemic lupus erythematosus (SLE). Occurring in about 40% of patients with this connective tissue disorder, butterfly rash appears as a red, scaly, sharply demarcated macular eruption. The rash may be transient in acute SLE or may progress slowly to include the forehead, chin, the area around the ears, and other exposed areas.

Skin

Erysipelas. In this streptococcal infection, butterfly rash appears as warm, indurated, tender, pruritic, edematous, and erythematous plaques, enlarging peripherally with sharply elevated margins; vesicles and bullae may form. Commonly, the rash appears abruptly and covers the bridge of the nose and one or both cheeks, halting at the hairline of the scalp or beard. However, the rash may also appear on the hands and genitals.

Polymorphous light eruption. Butterfly rash appears as erythema, vesicles, plaques, and multiple small papules that may later become eczematized, lichenized, and excoriated. Provoked by ultraviolet rays, the rash appears on the cheeks and bridge of the nose, the hands and arms, and other areas, beginning a few hours to several days after exposure. The rash may be accompanied by pruritus.

Rosacea. Initially, the butterfly rash may appear as a prominent, nonscaling, intermittent erythema limited to the lower half of the nose or including the chin, cheeks, and central forehead. As rosacea develops, the duration of the rash increases; instead of disappearing after each episode, the rash varies in intensity and is often accompanied by telangiectasia.

Seborrheic dermatitis. The butterfly rash appears as greasy, scaling, slightly yellow macules and papules of varying size; the scalp, beard, eyebrows, portions of the forehead above the bridge of the nose, nasolabial fold, or trunk may also be involved.

Drugs

Hydralazine and procainamide can cause an SLE–like syndrome.

Clinical considerations

• A history should be obtained and an examination of the affected area performed.

• Diagnostic tests may include immunologic studies, complete blood count, and liver studies.

• The patient should be told to avoid exposure to the sun or to use a sunscreen.

• The patient should be advised to wear hypoallergenic makeup to help conceal facial lesions, if appropriate.

Rash, papular

Description

A papular rash consists of small, raised, circumscribed—and perhaps discolored—lesions known as papules. It may erupt anywhere on the body in various configurations and may be acute or chronic. Papular rashes characterize many cutaneous disorders; they may also result from allergy and from infectious, neoplastic, and systemic disorders.

Possible causes

Respiratory

Sarcoidosis. This multisystem granulomatous disorder may produce crops of small, erythematous or yellow-brown papules around the eyes and mouth and on the nose, nasal mucosa, and upper back.

Cardiovascular

Necrotizing vasculitis. In this systemic disorder, crops of purpuric, but otherwise asymptomatic, papules are typical.

Musculoskeletal

Systemic lupus erythematosus (SLE). This disorder is characterized by a butterfly rash of erythematous maculopapules or discoid plaques that appears in a malar distribution across the nose and cheeks. Similar rashes may appear elsewhere, especially on exposed body areas.

Skin

Acne vulgaris. In this disorder, rupture of enlarged comedones produces inflamed—and perhaps painful and pruritic—papules, pustules, nodules, or cysts on the face and sometimes the shoulders, chest, and back.

Dermatomyositis. Grotton's papules—flat, violet lesions on the dorsum of the finger joints—are pathognomonic of this disorder, as is the dusky lilac discoloration of periorbital tissue and lid margins.

Follicular mucinosis. In this cutaneous disorder, perifollicular papules or plaques are accompanied by prominent alopecia.

Fox–Fordyce disease. This chronic disorder is marked by pruritic papules on the axillae, pubic area, and areolae associated with apocrine sweat gland inflammation.

Granuloma annulare. This benign, chronic disorder produces papules that usually coalesce to form plaques. The papules spread peripherally to form a ring with a normal or slightly depressed center. They usually appear on the feet, legs, hands, or fingers, and may be pruritic or asymptomatic.

Lichen amyloidosus. This idiopathic cutaneous disorder produces discrete, firm, hemispherical, pruritic papules on the anterior tibiae. Papules may be brown or yellow, smooth or scaly.

Lichen planus. Characteristic lesions of this disorder are discrete, flat, angular or polygonal, violet papules, often marked with white lines or spots. They may be linear or may coalesce into plaques and most commonly appear on the lumbar region, genitalia, ankles, anterior tibiae, and the wrists. Lesions usually develop first on the buccal mucosa as a lacy network of white or gray threadlike papules or plaques.

Parapsoriasis (chronic). This disorder mimics psoriasis, producing small–to–moderate-sized, asymptomatic papules with a thin, adherent scale, primarily on the trunk, hands, and feet.

Perioral dermatitis. This inflammatory disorder causes an erythematous eruption of discrete, tiny papules and pustules on the nasolabial fold, chin, and upper lip area. This eruption may be pruritic and painful.

Pityriasis rosea. This disorder begins with an erythematous "herald patch"— a slightly raised, oval lesion about 2 to 6 cm in diameter that may appear anywhere on the body. A few days to weeks later, yellow–to–tan or erythematous patches with scaly edges appear on the trunk, arms, and legs, often erupting along body cleavage lines in a characteristic "pine tree" pattern. These pruritic patches are 0.5 to 1 cm in diameter.

Pityriasis rubra pilaris. This rare chronic disorder initially produces scaling seborrhea on the scalp that spreads to the face and ears. Scaly red patches then develop on the palms and soles; these patches thicken, become keratotic, and may develop painful fissures. Later, follicular papules erupt on the hands and forearms, then spread over wide areas of the trunk, neck, and extremities. These papules coalesce into large, scaly, erythematous plaques. Striated fingernails may appear.

Polymorphic light eruption. Abnormal reactions to light may produce papular, vesicular, or nodular rashes on sun–exposed areas. Other symptoms may include pruritus, headache, and malaise.

Psoriasis. Typically, this disorder begins with small, erythematous papules on the scalp, chest, elbows, knees, back, buttocks, and genitalia. These papules are pruritic and sometimes painful. Eventually they enlarge and coalesce, forming elevated, red, scaly plaques covered by characteristic silver scales, except in moist areas such as the genitalia. These scales may flake off easily or thicken, covering the plaque.

Rosacea. This hyperemic disorder is characterized by persistent erythema, telangiectasia, and recurrent eruption of papules and pustules on the forehead, malar areas, nose, and chin. Eventually, eruptions recur more frequently and erythema deepens.

Seborrheic keratosis. In this cutaneous disorder, benign skin tumors begin as small, yellow–brown papules on the chest, back, or abdomen; they eventually enlarge and become deeply pigmented. However, in blacks, these papules may remain small and affect only the malar part of the face (dermatosis papulosa nigra).

Neoplastic

Kaposi's sarcoma. This neoplastic disorder is characterized by purple or blue papules or macules on the extremities, ears, and nose. These lesions decrease in size upon firm pressure and then return to their original size within 10 to 15 seconds. They may become scaly and ulcerate with bleeding. Two variants—classic and acute generalized—affect the elderly and acquired immune deficiency syndrome patients.

Mycosis fungoides. Stage I (premycotic stage) of this rare malignant lymphoma is marked by the eruption of erythematous, pruritic macules on the trunk and extremities. In Stage II, these lesions coalesce into papules and plaques, and nodes become irregular. Stage III is characterized by large, irregular, brown–to–red tumors that ulcerate and are painful and itchy.

Syringoma. In this disorder, adenoma of the sweat glands produces a yellow-

Recognizing Common Skin Lesions

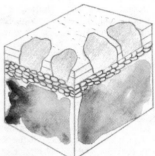

Macule
A small (usually less than 1 cm in diameter), flat blemish or discoloration that can be brown, tan, red, or white; texture is the same as surrounding skin

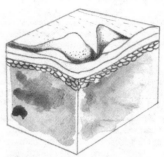

Vesicle
A small (less than 0.5 cm in diameter), thin-walled, raised blister containing clear, serous, purulent, or bloody fluid

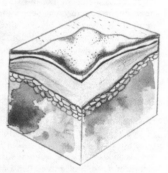

Bulla
A raised, thin-walled blister greater than 0.5 cm in diameter, containing clear or serous fluid

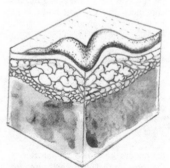

Pustule
A circumscribed, pus- or lymph-filled elevation that varies in diameter and may be firm or soft and white or yellow

ish or erythematous papular rash on the face (especially the eyelids), neck, and upper chest.
Infection
Gonococcemia. In this chronic infection, sporadic eruption of an erythematous macular rash is characteristic, although fistulas and petechiae may appear. Typically, the rash affects the distal extremities and rapidly becomes maculopapular, vesiculopustular, and frequently hemorrhagic. Bullae may form. The mature lesion is raised, has a

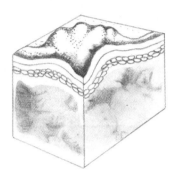

Wheal
A slightly raised, firm lesion of variable size and shape, surrounded by edema; skin may be red or pale

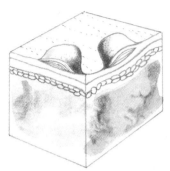

Papule
A small, solid, raised lesion less than 1 cm in diameter, with red-to-purple skin discoloration

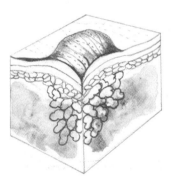

Nodule
A small, firm, circumscribed elevation approximately 1 to 2 cm in diameter; skin discoloration may be present

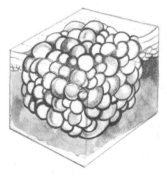

Tumor
A solid, raised mass, usually larger than 2 cm in diameter; skin discoloration may be present

gray, necrotic center, and is surrounded by erythema; it heals in 3 to 4 days.

Infectious mononucleosis. A maculo-papular rash that resembles rubella is an early sign of this infection in 10% of patients. Typically, it is preceded by headache, malaise, and fatigue.

Leprosy. This chronic infectious disorder produces a variety of skin lesions. Early papular or macular lesions are symmetrical, erythematous, or hypopigmented and may spread over the entire skin surface. Later, plaques and

nodules form, especially on the ear lobes, nose, eyebrows, and forehead.
Syphilis. A discrete, reddish brown, mucocutaneous rash and general lymphadenopathy herald the onset of secondary syphilis. The rash may be papular, macular, pustular, or nodular. Typically, it erupts between rolls of fat on the trunk and proximally on the arms, palms, soles, face, and scalp. Lesions in warm, moist areas enlarge and erode, producing highly contagious, pink or grayish white condylomata lata.

Environmental
Erythema chronicum migrans. Transmitted through a tick bite, this rare systemic disorder is characterized by a papular or macular rash that starts from a single lesion (usually on the leg) that spreads at the margins while clearing centrally. The rash commonly appears on the thighs, trunk, or upper arms, and may exceed 50 cm in diameter.
Insect bites. Venom from insect bites—especially ticks, lice, flies, and mosquitoes—may produce an allergic reaction associated with a papular, macular, or petechial rash.
Rat–bite fever. A maculopapular or petechial rash develops on the palms and soles several weeks after a bite from an infected rodent.

Drugs
Transient maculopapular rashes, usually on the trunk, may accompany reactions to many drugs, including antibiotics, such as tetracycline, ampicillin, cephalosporins, and sulfonamides; benzodiazepines, such as diazepam; lithium; phenylbutazone; gold salts; allopurinol; isoniazid; and salicylates.

Clinical considerations
• A history should be obtained and a complete examination of the affected areas performed.
• Diagnostic tests may include biopsies and blood studies.
• Cool compresses or antipruritic lotions should be applied, as ordered and needed.

• The patient should be advised to keep his skin clean and dry, to wear loose–fitting, nonirritating clothing, and to avoid scratching his rash.
• The patient should be instructed to promptly report any change in the rash's color, size, or configuration, and the onset of itching or bleeding.
• The patient should be told to avoid excessive exposure to direct sunlight and to apply a protective sunscreen before going outdoors.

Rash, pustular

Description
A pustular rash is made up of crops of pustules—vesicles and bullae that fill with purulent exudate. These lesions vary greatly in size and shape and can be generalized or localized. Pustules appear in skin and systemic disorders, with use of certain drugs, and with exposure to skin irritants. For example, people who have been swimming in salt water commonly develop a papulopustular rash under the bathing suit or elsewhere on the body from irritation by sea organisms (see *Recognizing Common Skin Lesions*, pp. 362 and 363). Although many pustular lesions are sterile, pustular rash usually indicates infection. Any vesicular eruption, or acute contact dermatitis, can become pustular if secondary infection occurs.

Possible causes
Skin
Acne vulgaris. Pustules typify inflammatory lesions of this disorder, which is accompanied by papules, nodules, cysts, and open comedones (blackheads). Lesions commonly appear on the face, shoulders, back, and chest.
Folliculitis. This bacterial infection of hair follicles produces individual pustules, each pierced by a hair and possibly attended by pruritus. *Hot–tub folliculitis* produces pustules on areas covered by a bathing suit.

Furunculosis. Crops of furuncles (purulent skin lesions involving hair follicles and sebaceous glands) typify this disorder. Furuncles usually begin as small, tender red pustules at the base of hair follicles. They are likely to occur on the face, neck, forearm, groin, axillae, buttocks, and legs, and to produce local pain, swelling, and redness. The pustules usually remain tense for 2 to 4 days and then become fluctuant. Rupture discharges pus and necrotic material. Then pain subsides, but erythema and edema may persist.

Nummular or annular dermatitis. In this disorder, coinlike (nummular) or ringed (annular) pustular lesions appear. Often, they ooze a purulent exudate, itch severely, and rapidly become crusted and scaly. There may be two or three lesions on the hands, but most often numerous lesions appear on the extensor surfaces of the extremities, posterior trunk, buttocks, and lower legs. A few small, scaling patches may remain for some time.

Pompholyx. This common recurrent disorder characteristically produces symmetrical vesicular lesions that can become pustular. The lesions appear on the palms and, less often, on the soles and may be accompanied by minimal erythema and recurrent pruritus.

Pustular miliaria. This anhidrotic disorder causes pustular lesions that begin as tiny erythematous papulovesicles located at sweat pores. Diffuse erythema may radiate from the lesion. The rash and associated burning and pruritus worsen with sweating.

Pustular psoriasis. Small vesicles form and eventually become pustules in this disorder. The patient may report pruritus, burning, and pain. Localized pustular psoriasis usually affects the hands and feet. Generalized pustular psoriasis erupts suddenly in patients with psoriasis, psoriatic arthritis, or exfoliative psoriasis. Although generalized pustular psoriasis rarely occurs, it can occasionally be fatal.

Rosacea. This chronic hyperemic disorder often produces telangiectasia with acute episodes of pustules, papules, and edema.

Infection

Blastomycosis. This fungal infection produces small, painless, nonpruritic macules or papules that can enlarge to well–circumscribed, verrucous, crusted, or ulcerated lesions edged by pustules. Localized infection may cause only one lesion; systemic infection, many lesions on the hands, feet, face, and wrists.

Gonococcemia. This disorder produces a rash of scanty, pinpoint erythematous macules that rapidly become vesiculopustular, maculopapular, and, frequently, hemorrhagic. Bullae may form. Mature lesions are elevated, with dirty gray necrotic centers and surrounding erythema. The rash appears on the distal part of the arms and legs, usually during the first day that other findings, such as fever and joint pain, occur. The rash disappears after 3 or 4 days but may recur with each episode of fever.

Environmental

Scabies. Threadlike channels or burrows under the skin characterize this disorder, which can also produce pustules, vesicles, and excoriations. The lesions are 1 to 10 cm long, with a swollen nodule or red papule that contains the itch mite. In men, crusted lesions often develop on the glans, shaft, and scrotum. In women, lesions may form on the nipples. Lesions also develop on wrists, elbows, axillae, and waist. Related pruritus worsens with inactivity and warmth.

Drugs

Bromides and iodides commonly cause pustular rash. Other drug causes include adrenocorticotropic hormone, corticosteroids, dactinomycin, trimethadione, lithium, phenytoin, phenobarbital, isoniazid, oral contraceptives, androgens, and anabolic steroids.

Clinical considerations

• A history should be obtained and an examination of the skin performed.

- Wound and skin isolation procedures should be observed until infection is ruled out by a Gram stain or culture and sensitivity test of the pustule's contents.
- If the organism is infectious, drainage should not be allowed to touch unaffected skin.
- The patient should be instructed to keep toilet articles and linen separate from those of other family members.
- Associated pain and itching, altered body image, or stress of isolation may result in loss of sleep, anxiety, and depression. Medications should be given, as ordered, to relieve pain and itching, and the patient should be encouraged to express his feelings.

Rash, vesicular

Description
A vesicular rash is a scattered or linear distribution of vesicles—sharply circumscribed lesions filled with clear, cloudy, or bloody fluid. The lesions, which are usually less than 0.5 cm in diameter, may occur singly or in groups. (See *Recognizing Common Skin Lesions*, pp. 362 and 363.) They sometimes occur with bullae—fluid–filled lesions larger than 0.5 cm in diameter.

A vesicular rash may be mild, or severe and temporary, or permanent. It can result from infection, inflammation, or allergic reactions.

Possible causes
Skin
Dermatitis. In *contact dermatitis*, a severe hypersensitivity reaction produces an eruption of small vesicles surrounded by redness and marked edema. The vesicles may ooze, scale, and cause severe pruritus.

Dermatitis herpetiformis, occurring most often in men between the ages of 20 and 50, produces a chronic inflammatory eruption marked by vesicular, papular, bullous, pustular, or erythematous lesions. Usually, the rash is symmetrically distributed on the buttocks, shoulders, extensor surfaces of the elbows and knees, and sometimes the face, scalp, and neck. Other symptoms include severe pruritus, burning, and stinging.

In *nummular dermatitis*, groups of pinpoint vesicles and papules appear on erythematous or pustular lesions that are nummular (coinlike) or annular (ringlike). Often, the pustular lesions ooze a purulent exudate, itch severely, and rapidly become crusted and scaly. Two or three lesions may develop on the hands, but the lesions most commonly develop on the extensor surfaces of the limbs and on the buttocks and posterior trunk.

Dermatophytid. This allergic reaction to fungal infection produces vesicular lesions on the hands, usually in response to tinea pedis. The lesions are extremely pruritic and tender and may be accompanied by fever, anorexia, generalized adenopathy, and splenomegaly.

Erythema multiforme. This acute inflammatory skin disease is heralded by a sudden eruption of erythematous macules, papules, and, occasionally, vesicles and bullae. The characteristic rash appears symmetrically over the hands, arms, feet, legs, face, and neck and tends to reappear. Vesicles and bullae may also erupt on the eyes and genitalia. Most often, though, vesiculobullous lesions appear on the mucous membranes—especially the lips and buccal mucosa—where they rupture and ulcerate, producing a thick, yellow or white exudate.

Herpes zoster. A vesicular rash is preceded by erythema and, occasionally, by a nodular skin eruption and unilateral sharp, shooting chest pain that mimics a myocardial infarction. About 5 days later, the lesions erupt and commonly spread unilaterally over the thorax or vertically over the arms and legs. The pain becomes burning. Vesicles dry and scab about 10 days after eruption.

Pemphigoid (bullous). Generalized pruritus or an urticarial or eczematous eruption may precede the classic bullous rash. Bullae are large, tense, and irregular, and most often form on an erythematous base. They usually appear on the lower abdomen, groin, inner thighs, and forearms.

Pemphigus. In *chronic familial pemphigus*, groups of tiny vesicles erupt on erythematous or normal skin. The vesicles are flaccid and easily broken, producing small denuded areas that become covered with crust; itching and burning are common. The eruption remits spontaneously but recurs.

Pemphigus foliaceus usually develops slowly and may begin with bullous lesions, commonly on the head and trunk. As these lesions spread to other areas, they become moist, scaly, and foul-smelling. Nikolsky's sign is present, and denudation of lesions results in extensive erythema, with large, loose scales and crusts. Pruritus and burning are common.

Pemphigus vulgaris may be acute and rapidly progressive, or chronic. The bullae may be tender or painful and large or small, and are usually flaccid. When they rupture, denuded skin exudes a clear, bloody, or purulent discharge. Commonly, the bullae first erupt in a specific location, such as the mouth or scalp, and eventually become widespread. Nikolsky's sign and pruritus may be present.

Pompholyx. This common, recurrent disorder produces symmetrical vesicular lesions that can become pustular. The pruritic lesions appear on the palms more frequently than on the soles and may be accompanied by minimal erythema.

Porphyria cutanea tarda. Bullae—especially on areas exposed to sun, friction, trauma, or heat—result from the characteristic photosensitivity that develops between the ages of 20 and 40. Papulovesicular lesions evolving to erosions or ulcers and scars may appear.

Tinea pedis. This fungal infection causes vesicles and scaling between the toes and, possibly, dry scaling over the entire sole. Severe infection causes in-

Drugs Causing Toxic Epidermal Necrolysis

A variety of drugs can trigger toxic epidermal necrolysis (TEN)—a rare but potentially fatal immune reaction characterized by a vesicular rash. TEN produces large, flaccid bullae that rupture easily, exposing extensive areas of denuded skin. The resulting loss of fluid and electrolytes—along with widespread systemic involvement—can lead to such life-threatening complications as pulmonary edema, shock, renal failure, sepsis, and disseminated intravascular coagulation. Here is a list of some drugs that can cause TEN:

- allopurinol
- aspirin
- chloramphenicol
- chlorpropamide
- gold salts
- nitrofurantoin
- penicillin
- phenolphtalein
- phenytoin
- primidone
- sulfonamides
- tetracycline

flammation, pruritus, and difficulty walking.

Toxic epidermal necrolysis. In this immune reaction to drugs or other toxins, vesicles and bullae are preceded by a diffuse, erythematous rash and followed by large-scale epidermal necrolysis and desquamation. Large, flaccid bullae develop after mucous membrane inflammation, a burning sensation in the conjunctivae, malaise, fever, and generalized skin tenderness. The bullae rupture easily, exposing extensive areas of denuded skin.

Infectious disease

Herpes simplex. This common viral infection produces vesicles on an erythematous base and usually affects the lips. About 25% of patients develop lesions on the genitalia. Vesicles are preceded by itching, tingling, burning or pain; develop singly or in groups; are 2 to 3 mm in size; and do not coalesce. They eventually rupture, forming a painful ulcer followed by a yellowish crust.

Environmental

Burns. Thermal burns that affect the epidermis and part of the dermis often cause vesicles and bullae, with erythema, swelling, pain, and moistness.

Insect bites. Vesicles appear on red hivelike papules and may become hemorrhagic.

Scabies. Small vesicles erupt on an erythematous base and may be located at the end of a curved, threadlike burrow. The lesions are 1 to 10 cm long, with a swollen nodule or red papule that contains the itch mite. Pustules and excoriations may also occur. Men may develop lesions on the glans, shaft, and scrotum; women may develop lesions on the nipples. Both sexes may develop lesions on the wrists, elbows, axillae, and waistline.

Clinical considerations

- A history should be obtained and an examination of the skin performed.
- Diagnostic tests include cultures of the lesions.
- A patient should be instructed not to touch the lesions and to wash his hands often.
- Antibiotics should be administered and topical corticosteroids applied, as ordered.
- The patient should be instructed to protect his skin from injury.

Rebound tenderness
(Blumberg's sign)

Description

A reliable indicator of peritonitis, rebound tenderness is intense, elicited abdominal pain caused by rebound of palpated tissue. The tenderness may be localized, as in an abscess, or generalized, as in perforation of an intraabdominal organ. Rebound tenderness usually occurs with abdominal pain, tenderness, and rigidity. When a patient has sudden, severe abdominal pain, this symptom is usually elicited to detect peritoneal inflammation.

Regression

Description

Regression is the return to a behavioral level appropriate to an earlier developmental age. This defense mechanism may occur in various psychiatric and organic disorders.

Repression

Description

Repression is the unconscious retreat from awareness of unacceptable ideas or impulses. This defense mechanism may occur normally or may accompany psychiatric disorders.

Retractions, costal and sternal

Description

A cardinal sign of respiratory distress in infants and children, retractions are visible indentations of the soft tissue covering the chest wall. They may be suprasternal (directly above the sternum and clavicles), intercostal (between the ribs), subcostal (below the lower costal margin of the rib cage), or substernal (just below the xiphoid process). Retractions may be mild or severe, producing barely visible to deep indentations.

Normally, infants and young children use abdominal muscles for breathing, unlike older children and adults who use the diaphragm. When breathing requires extra effort, accessory muscles assist respiration, especially inspiration. Retractions typically accompany accessory muscle use.

Eliciting Rebound Tenderness

To elicit rebound tenderness, the examiner places the patient in a supine position and pushes her fingers deeply and steadily into his abdomen, as shown above. Then she quickly releases the pressure. Pain that results from the rebound of palpated tissue—rebound tenderness—indicates peritoneal inflammation or peritonitis.

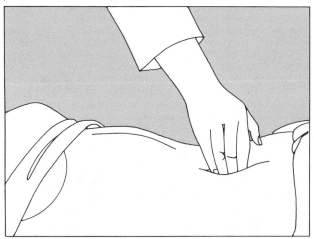

This symptom can also be elicited on a miniature scale by percussing the patient's abdomen lightly and indirectly (right). Better still, the examiner can simply ask the patient to cough. This allows her to elicit rebound tenderness without having to touch the patient's abdomen and may also increase his cooperation, since he won't associate exacerbation of his pain with her actions.

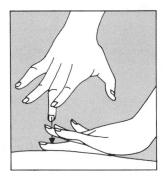

Possible causes

Eyes, ears, nose, throat

Epiglottitis. This life–threatening bacterial infection may precipitate severe respiratory distress with suprasternal, substernal, and intercostal retractions; stridor; nasal flaring; cyanosis; and tachycardia. Initially, it causes sudden onset of barking cough and high fever.

Laryngotracheobronchitis (acute). In this viral infection, substernal and intercostal retractions typically follow low to moderate fever, runny nose, poor appetite, barking cough, hoarseness, and inspiratory stridor.

Respiratory

Asthma attack. Intercostal and suprasternal retractions may accompany an attack. They are preceded by dyspnea, wheezing, a hacking cough, and pallor.

Bronchiolitis. Most common in children less than age 2, this acute lower respiratory tract infection may cause intercostal and subcostal retractions, nasal flaring, tachypnea, dyspnea, cough, restlessness, and possibly a slight fever. Periodic apnea may occur in infants less than 6 months old.

Pneumonia (bacterial). This disorder begins with signs of acute infection— such as high fever and lethargy—followed by subcostal and intercostal retractions, nasal flaring, dyspnea, tachypnea, grunting respirations, cyanosis, and productive cough.

Respiratory distress syndrome. Substernal and subcostal retractions are an early sign of this life–threatening syndrome, which affects premature infants shortly after birth.

Spasmodic croup. This disorder causes attacks of barking cough, hoarseness, dyspnea, and restlessness. As distress worsens, the child may display suprasternal, substernal, and intercostal retractions; nasal flaring; tachycardia;

Observing Retractions

When observing retractions in infants and children, care should be taken to note their exact location—an important clue to the cause and severity of respiratory distress. For example, subcostal and substernal retractions usually result from lower respiratory tract disorders, whereas suprasternal retractions usually result from upper respiratory tract disorders. Mild intercostal retractions alone may be normal. However, intercostal retractions accompanied by subcostal and substernal retractions may indicate moderate respiratory distress. Deep suprasternal retractions typically indicate severe distress.

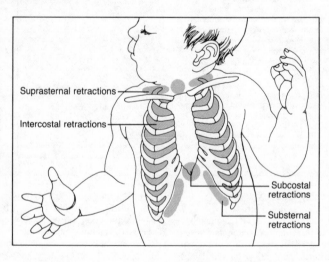

cyanosis; and an anxious, frantic expression. These attacks usually subside within a few hours but tend to recur.

Cardiovascular

Congestive heart failure. Usually linked to a congenital heart defect, this disorder may cause intercostal and substernal retractions along with nasal flaring, progressive tachypnea, and—in severe respiratory distress—grunting respirations, edema, and cyanosis.

Clinical considerations

• The patient should be assessed quickly for other signs of respiratory distress and the physician notified immediately.

• Emergency interventions should be anticipated to maintain a patent airway and adequate oxygenation.

• Diagnostic tests may include chest X-rays, sputum cultures, and arterial blood gas analysis.

• If the infant weighs less than 15 lb, he should be placed in an oxygen hood, as ordered. If he weighs more, he should be placed in a cool mist tent instead.

• As ordered, chest physical therapy with postural drainage should be performed to help mobilize and drain excess lung secretions.

Rhinorrhea
(Nasal discharge)

Description

Common but rarely serious, rhinorrhea is the free discharge of thin nasal mucus. It can be self-limiting or chronic, resulting from nasal, sinus, or systemic disorders or from basilar skull fractures. This sign can also result from sinus or cranial surgery, excessive use of vasoconstricting nose drops or sprays, or an irritant, such as tobacco smoke, dust, and fumes. Depending on the cause, the discharge may be clear, purulent, bloody, or serosanguineous.

Possible causes

Central nervous system

Basilar skull fracture. A tear in the dura can lead to cerebrospinal rhinorrhea, which increases when the patient lowers his head.

Cluster headache. In this disorder, rhinorrhea can accompany severe unilateral headache.

Eyes, ears, nose, throat

Ethmoiditis. In *acute bacterial ethmoiditis*, nasal discharge is yellow-gray or purulent; in *acute viral ethmoiditis*, it is mucoid. In *chronic ethmoiditis*, purulent discharge may be intermittent or persistent.

Mucormycosis. Rhinocerebral mucormycosis causes a thin, serosanguineous nasal discharge and ulceration or perforation of the nasal septum.

Nasal or sinus tumors. Nasal tumors can produce intermittent, unilateral bloody or serosanguineous discharge, possibly purulent and foul-smelling.

Rhinitis. Allergic rhinitis produces an episodic, profuse watery discharge. (Mucopurulent discharge indicates infection.) In *atrophic rhinitis*, nasal discharge is scanty, purulent, and foul-smelling. In *vasomotor rhinitis*, a profuse and watery nasal discharge accompanies chronic nasal obstruction, sneezing, recurrent postnasal drip, and pale, swollen turbinates.

Scleroma. This rare, progressive condition produces watery nasal discharge that later becomes foul-smelling and encrusted.

Sinusitis. Acute sphenoid sinusitis—a disorder affecting immunosuppressed, diabetic, elderly, and debilitated patients—produces purulent nasal discharge that leads to obstruction. In *chronic frontal sinusitis*, intermittent and purulent discharge may lead to nasal obstruction. In *chronic maxillary sinusitis*, mucopurulent discharge is intermittent and ipsilateral and may lead to unilateral nasal obstruction.

Infection

Common cold. An initial watery nasal discharge may become thicker and mucopurulent.

Drugs
Nasal sprays or drops containing vasoconstrictors may cause rebound rhinorrhea (rhinitis medicamentosa) if used longer than 3 weeks.
Treatments
Following sinus or cranial surgery, cerebrospinal rhinorrhea may occur.

Clinical considerations
• A history should be obtained and an examination of the nose performed.
• Diagnostic tests may include sinus X-rays, skull X-rays, computed tomography, and transillumination of the maxillary and frontal sinuses.
• Antihistamines, decongestants, analgesics, or antipyretics should be administered, as ordered.
• Fluids should be promoted to thin secretions.
• The patient should be warned to avoid using over-the-counter nasal sprays for more than 5 days, unless ordered.

Rhonchi

Description
Rhonchi are continuous adventitious breath sounds detected by auscultation. They are usually louder and lower-pitched than crackles—more like a hoarse moan or a deep snore, though they may be described as rattling or musical. However, sibilant rhonchi, or wheezes, are high-pitched.
  Rhonchi are heard over large airways, such as the trachea.

Mechanism
Rhonchi occur in pulmonary disorders when air flows through passages that have been narrowed by secretions, a tumor or foreign body, bronchospasm, or mucosal thickening. The resulting vibration of airway walls produces the rhonchi.

Possible causes
Respiratory
Adult respiratory distress syndrome. Fluid accumulation in this life-threatening disorder produces rhonchi and crackles.
Aspiration of a foreign body. A retained bronchial foreign body can cause inspiratory and expiratory rhonchi and wheezes due to increased secretions.
Asthma. An asthmatic attack can cause rhonchi, crackles, and commonly wheezes.
Bronchiectasis. This disorder causes lower-lobe rhonchi and crackles, which coughing may help relieve. Its classic sign is a cough that produces mucopurulent, foul-smelling, and possibly bloody sputum.
Bronchitis. Acute tracheobronchitis produces sonorous rhonchi and wheezes due to bronchospasm or increased mucus in the airways.
  In *chronic bronchitis*, auscultation may reveal scattered rhonchi, coarse crackles, wheezing, high-pitched piping sounds, and prolonged expirations.
Emphysema. This disorder may cause sonorous rhonchi, but faint, high-pitched wheezes are more typical, together with weight loss; a mild, chronic, productive cough with scant sputum; exertional dyspnea; accessory muscle use on inspiration; tachypnea; and grunting expirations.
Pneumonia. Bacterial pneumonias can cause rhonchi and a dry cough that later becomes productive.
Pulmonary coccidioidomycosis. This disorder causes rhonchi and wheezing.
Treatments
Respiratory therapy may produce rhonchi from loosened secretions and mucus.
Diagnostic tests
Pulmonary function tests or bronchoscopy can loosen secretions and mucus, causing rhonchi.

Clinical considerations
• A history should be obtained and a respiratory assessment performed.

• Diagnostic tests may include arterial blood gas analysis, pulmonary function studies, sputum analysis, and chest X-rays.

• To ease the patient's breathing, he may be placed in a semi–Fowler position, and repositioned every 2 hours. Or, if appropriate, increased activity should be encouraged to promote drainage of secretions.

• Deep breathing and coughing techniques and splinting should be taught, if necessary.

• Antibiotics, bronchodilators, and expectorants should be administered, as ordered.

• Humidification should be provided to thin secretions, to relieve inflammation, and to prevent drying.

• Pulmonary physiotherapy with postural drainage and percussion may also be provided to help loosen secretions.

• Fluids should be encouraged to help liquefy secretions and prevent dehydration.

Rockley's sign

Description

Rockley's sign is the difference in the angle created by two straight edges placed vertically against the orbits and zygomatic bones in a depressed fracture of the zygomatic arch. To detect this sign, two rulers or other straight-edged objects are rested on the outer edge of the ocular orbits and zygomatic arches. In a positive Rockley's sign, the angle on the affected side is smaller—the straight edge is more nearly parallel to the basic plane of the patient's face.

Romberg's sign

Description

Relatively uncommon, a positive Romberg's sign refers to a patient's inability to maintain balance when standing erect with his feet together and his eyes closed. It indicates a proprioceptive disorder or a disorder of the spinal tracts (the posterior columns) that carry proprioceptive information—the perception of one's position in space and joint movements and of pressure sensations—to the brain. Insufficient proprioceptive information causes an inability to execute precise movements or maintain balance without visual cues.

Possible causes

Central nervous system

Multiple sclerosis. A positive Romberg's sign is present in this disorder, along with other neurologic signs and symptoms.

Peripheral nerve disease. Besides a positive Romberg's sign, advanced disease may produce impotence, fatigue, and paresthesia, hyperesthesia, or anesthesia in the hands and feet.

Spinal cerebellar degeneration. In this disorder, a positive Romberg's sign accompanies decreased visual acuity, fatigue, paresthesias, loss of vibration sense, incoordination, ataxic gait, and muscle weakness and atrophy.

Spinal cord disease. A positive Romberg's sign may accompany fasciculations, muscle weakness and atrophy, and loss of proprioception, vibration, and other senses.

Tabes dorsalis. A positive Romberg's sign may occur, but burning extremity pain is this disorder's classic symptom.

Eyes, ears, nose, throat

Vestibular disorders. Besides a positive Romberg's sign, these disorders commonly cause vertigo.

Hematologic

Pernicious anemia. A positive Romberg's sign and loss of proprioception in the lower limbs reflect peripheral nerve and spinal cord damage.

Clinical considerations

• A history should be obtained and a neurologic examination performed.

• The patient should be assisted during ambulation and safety precautions taken, as necessary.

Rosenbach's sign

Description
Rosenbach's sign is the absence of the abdominal skin reflex, associated with intestinal inflammation and hemiplegia. This sign also refers to the fine, rapid tremor of gently closed eyelids in Graves' disease.

Rotch's sign

Description
Rotch's sign is dullness on percussion over the right lung at the fifth intercostal space. This sign occurs in pericardial effusion.

Rovsing's sign

Description
Rovsing's sign is pain in the right lower quadrant upon palpation and quick withdrawal of the fingers in the left lower quadrant. This referred rebound tenderness suggests appendicitis.

Rumpel–Leede sign

Description
Rumpel–Leede sign is extensive petechiae distal to a tourniquet placed around the upper arm, indicating capillary fragility in scarlet fever and in severe thrombocytopenia. To elicit this sign, the examiner places a tourniquet around the upper arm for 5 to 10 minutes and observes for distal petechiae.

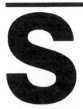

Salivation, decreased
(Dry mouth, xerostomia)

Description
Typically a common but minor complaint, diminished production or excretion of saliva most often results from mouth breathing. However, this symptom can also result from salivary duct obstruction, Sjögren's syndrome, the use of anticholinergics and other drugs, and the effects of radiation. It can even result from vigorous exercise or autonomic stimulation—for example, by fear.

Possible causes
Eyes, ears, nose, throat
Salivary duct obstruction. Usually associated with a salivary stone, this obstruction causes reduced salivation and local pain and swelling.
Musculoskeletal
Sjögren's syndrome. Diminished secretions from the lacrimal, parotid, and submaxillary glands produce the hallmarks of this disorder: decreased or absent salivation and dry eyes with a persistent burning, gritty sensation.
Drugs
Anticholinergics, antihistamines, tricyclic antidepressants, phenothiazines, clonidine hydrochloride, and narcotic analgesics may cause decreased salivation, which disappears after discontinuation of therapy.
Treatments
Excessive irradiation of the mouth or face from antineoplastic treatments or dental X–rays may cause transient decreased salivation due to salivary gland atrophy.

Clinical consideration
● A history should be obtained and salivary glands and ductal openings assessed (see *Assessing Salivary Glands and Ductal Openings*, p. 376).
● If markedly reduced salivation interferes with speaking, eating, or swallowing, the patient should be allowed extra time for these activities.
● Fluid intake should be increased and oral hygiene promoted.

Salivation, increased
(Polysialia, ptyalism)

Description
This uncommon symptom may result from gastrointestinal disorders, especially of the mouth. It also accompanies certain systemic disorders and may result from the effects of drugs and toxins. Saliva may also accumulate because of difficulty swallowing.

Possible causes
Eyes, ears, nose, throat
Stomatitis. Mucosal ulcers may be accompanied by moderately increased salivation, mouth pain, fever, and erythemia. Spontaneous healing usually occurs in 7 to 10 days, but scarring and recurrence are possible.
Infectious diseases
Syphilis. In secondary syphilis, mucosal ulcers cause increased salivation that may persist up to a year.

Assessing Salivary Glands and Ductal Openings

When a patient reports decreased salivation, the parotid and submaxillary glands should be assessed for enlargement and the ductal openings for salivary flow.

To detect an enlarged parotid gland, the examiner asks the patient to clench his teeth, thereby tensing the masseter muscle. Then she palpates the parotid duct (about 2″ [5 cm] long); she should be able to feel it against the tensed muscle, on the cheek below the zygomatic arch. Next, she checks the ductal orifice, opposite the second molar. Using a gloved finger, she palpates the orifice for enlargement and observes for drainage.

Next, she palpates the submaxillary gland. About the size of a walnut, it is located under the mandible, anterior to the angle of the jaw. Using a gloved finger, she palpates the floor of the mouth for enlargement of the submaxillary ductal orafice.

Finally, she tests both ductal openings for salivary flow. She places cotton under the patient's tongue, has him sip pure lemon juice, and then removes the cotton and observes salivary flow from each opening. She documents her findings.

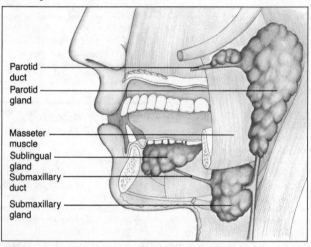

Parotid duct
Parotid gland
Masseter muscle
Sublingual gland
Submaxillary duct
Submaxillary gland

Tuberculosis. Certain forms of tuberculosis may produce solitary, irregularly shaped mouth or tongue ulcers, covered with exudate, that cause increased salivation.

Environmental

Mercury poisoning. Stomatitis—involving increased salivation and a metallic taste—commonly occurs in mercury poisoning.

Drugs

Increased salivation may occur in iodide toxicity, but the earliest symptoms are a brassy taste and a burning sensation in the mouth and throat. Associated findings include sneezing, irritated eyelids, and, commonly, pain in the frontal sinus.

Pilocarpine and other miotics used to treat glaucoma may be absorbed systemically, increasing salivation.

Cholinergics, such as bethanechol and neostigmine, may also cause this symptom.

Clinical considerations
• A history should be obtained and an oral examination performed.
• Though annoying to the patient, increased salivation does not require treatments beyond those needed to correct the underlying disorder.

Salt craving

Description
Craving salty foods is a compensatory response to the body's failure to adequately conserve sodium. Normally, the renal tubules reabsorb almost all sodium, allowing less than 1% of it to be excreted in the urine. This reabsorption is regulated by aldosterone, a hormone synthesized in the adrenal gland. However, primary adrenal insufficiency can reduce aldosterone levels, thereby impairing reabsorption and increasing excretion of sodium.

Scotoma

Description
A scotoma is an area of partial or complete blindness within an otherwise normal or slightly impaired visual field. Usually located within the central 30° area, the defect ranges from absolute blindness to a barely detectable loss of visual acuity. Typically, the patient can pinpoint the scotoma's location in the visual field.

A scotoma can result from retinal, choroid, or optic nerve disorders. It can be classified as absolute, relative, or scintillating. An *absolute scotoma* refers to the total inability to see all sizes of test objects used in mapping the visual field. A *relative scotoma*, in contrast, refers to the ability to see only large test objects. A *scintillating scotoma* refers to the flashes or bursts of light commonly seen during a migraine headache.

Possible causes
Central nervous system
Migraine headache. Transient scintillating scotomas, usually bilateral and often homonymous, can occur with a classic migraine aura.
Eyes, ears, nose, throat
Chorioretinitis. Inflammation of the choroid produces a paracentral scotoma.
Glaucoma. Prolonged elevation of intraocular pressure can cause an arcuate scotoma.
Macular degeneration. Any degenerative process or disorder affecting the fovea centralis results in a central scotoma.
Optic neuritis. Inflammation, degeneration, or demyelination of the optic nerve produces central, circular, or centrocecal scotoma. The scotoma may be unilateral with involvement of one nerve or bilateral with involvement of both nerves. It can vary in size, density, and symmetry. The patient may have severe visual loss or blurring, lasting up to 3 weeks, and pain—especially with eye movement.
Retinal pigmentary degenerations. These disorders cause premature retinal cell changes leading to cell death. One of these disorders, retinitis pigmentosa, initially involves loss of peripheral rods; the resulting annular scotoma progresses concentrically until only a central field of vision (tunnel vision) remains.

Clinical considerations
• A history should be obtained and an eye examination and visual field tests performed (see *Locating Scotomas*, p. 378).

Locating Scotomas

Scotomas, or blind spots, are classified according to the affected area of the visual field. The normal scotoma—shown in the temporal region of the right eye—appears in black in all the illustrations.

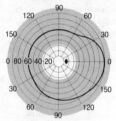

The *normally present scotoma* represents the position of the optic nerve head in the visual field. It appears between 10° and 20° on this chart of the normal visual field.

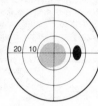

A *central scotoma* involves the point of central fixation. It is always associated with decreased visual acuity.

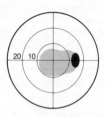

A *centrocecal scotoma* involves the point of central fixation and the area between the blind spot and the fixation point.

A *paracentral scotoma* affects an area of the visual field that is nasal or temporal to the point of central fixation.

An *arcuate scotoma* arches around the fixation point, usually ending on the nasal side of the visual field.

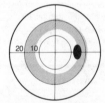

An *annular scotoma* forms a circular defect around the fixation point. It is common in retinal pigmentary degenerations.

Scrotal swelling

Description

Scrotal swelling occurs when a condition affecting the testicles, epididymis, or scrotal skin produces edema or a mass; the penis may or may not be involved. Scrotal swelling can be unilateral or bilateral and painful or painless. It can affect males of any age.

The sudden onset of painful scrotal swelling suggests torsion of a testicle or testicular appendages, especially in the prepubescent male. This emergency requires immediate surgery to untwist and stabilize the spermatic cord or to remove the appendage.

Possible causes
Genitourinary
Elephantiasis of the scrotum. In this disorder (common in some tropical countries), infection by a filaria worm obstructs lymphatic drainage, causing chronic gross scrotal edema and pain.

Epididymal cysts. Located in the head of the epididymis, these cysts produce painless scrotal swelling.

Epididymal tuberculosis. This disorder produces an enlarged scrotal mass separated from the testicle.

Epididymitis. Key features of inflammation are pain, extreme tenderness, and swelling in the groin and scrotum. The patient waddles to avoid pressure on the groin and scrotum during walking. He may have high fever, malaise, urethral discharge and cloudy urine, and lower abdominal pain on the affected side. His scrotal skin may be hot, red, dry, flaky, and thin.

Gumma. This rare, painless nodule can affect any bone or organ. If it affects the testicle, it causes edema.

Hernia. Herniation of bowel into the scrotum can cause swelling and a soft or unusually firm scrotum. Occasionally, bowel sounds can be auscultated in the scrotum.

Hydrocele. Fluid accumulation produces gradual scrotal swelling that is usually painless. The scrotum may be soft and cystic or firm and tense. Palpation reveals a round, nontender scrotal mass.

Idiopathic scrotal edema. Swelling occurs quickly in this disorder and usually disappears within 24 hours. The affected testicle is pink.

Orchitis (acute). Mumps may precipitate this disorder, which causes sudden painful swelling of one or, at times, both testicles.

Scrotal burns. Burns cause swelling within 24 hours of injury.

Scrotal trauma. Blunt trauma causes scrotal swelling with bruising and se-

vere pain. The scrotum may appear dark or bluish.

Spermatocele. This painless or painful cystic mass lies above and behind the testicle and contains opaque fluid and sperm. Its onset may be acute or gradual. Less than 1 cm in diameter, it is movable and may be transilluminated.

Testicular torsion. Most common before puberty, this urologic emergency causes scrotal swelling, sudden and severe pain, and possible elevation of the affected testicle within the scrotum.

Testicular tumor. Typically painless, smooth, and firm, a testicular tumor produces swelling and a sensation of excessive weight in the scrotum.

Torsion of a hydatid of Morgagni. Torsion of this small, pea–sized cyst severs its blood supply, causing a hard, painful swelling on the testicle's upper pole.

Treatments
An effusion of blood from *surgery* can produce a hematocele, leading to scrotal swelling.

Clinical considerations
• If testicular torsion is suspected, the patient should be prepared for surgery.
• If the patient is not in severe pain, a history should be obtained and a scrotal examination performed.
• A rolled towel should be placed between the patient's legs and under the scrotum to help reduce severe swelling. Or, if the patient has mild or moderate swelling, he should be advised to wear a loose–fitting athletic supporter lined with soft cotton dressings.
• Sitz baths should be given and heat or ice packs applied, as ordered, to decrease inflammation.
• Analgesics and antibiotics should be administered, as ordered.

Seeligmüller's sign

Description
Seeligmüller's sign is pupillary dilation on the affected side, in facial neuralgia.

Seizure, absence
(Petit mal seizure)

Description

Absence seizures are benign, generalized seizures thought to originate subcortically. These brief episodes of unconsciousness last 10 to 20 seconds and can occur 100 or more times a day, commonly causing periods of inattention. Absence seizures most often affect children between the ages of 4 and 12 and rarely persist beyond adolescence. Their first sign may be deteriorating school work and behavior. Their cause is not known.

Absence seizures occur without warning. The patient suddenly stops all purposeful activity and stares blankly ahead—unable to see, hear, or feel. Absence seizures may produce automatisms, such as repetitive lip smacking, or mild clonic or myoclonic movements, including mild jerking of muscles in the eyelids. The patient may drop objects he is holding, and muscle relaxation may cause him to drop his head or arms or to slump. After the attack, the patient resumes activity, typically unaware of the episode.

Absence status, a rare form of absence seizure, occurs as a prolonged absence seizure or as repeated episodes of these seizures. Usually not life–threatening, it occurs most commonly in patients with preexisting absence seizures.

Possible causes

Central nervous system
Idiopathic epilepsy. Frequently, absence seizures are accompanied by automatisms and learning disability.

Clinical considerations

• The occurrence and duration of the seizures should be assessed by reciting a series of numbers and then asking the patient to repeat them after the attack ends. He will be unable to do this. Or, if the seizures are occurring within minutes of each other, the patient should be asked to count for about 5 minutes. He will stop counting during a seizure, then resume when it is over. He should also be observed for accompanying automatisms.

• Diagnostic tests may include computed tomography scans and electroencephalography.

• The patient and his family should be taught about these seizures and how to recognize their onset, pattern, and duration. The child's teacher and school nurse should be included in the teaching process, if possible.

• If the seizures are being controlled with drug therapy, the importance of strict compliance should be emphasized.

Seizure, focal
(Simple partial seizure)

Description

Resulting from an irritable focus in the cerebral cortex, a focal seizure typically lasts about 30 seconds and does not alter the patient's level of consciousness. Its type and pattern reflect the location of the irritable focus. A focal seizure may be classified as motor or somatosensory. A focal motor seizure, in turn, includes a jacksonian seizure and epilepsia partialis continua. A somatosensory seizure includes visual, olfactory, and auditory seizures.

A *focal motor seizure* is a series of unilateral clonic (muscle jerking) and tonic (muscle stiffening) movements of one part of the body. The patient's head and eyes characteristically turn away from the hemispheric focus— most commonly the frontal lobe near the motor strip. A tonic–clonic contraction of the trunk or extremities may follow.

A *jacksonian motor seizure* typically begins with a tonic contraction of a finger, the corner of the mouth, or one foot. Clonic movements follow, spreading to other muscles on the same side of the body, moving up the arm or leg, and eventually involving the whole side. Or clonic movements may spread to the opposite side, becoming generalized and leading to loss of consciousness. In the postictal phase, the patient may display paralysis (Todd's paralysis) in the affected limbs that usually resolves within 24 hours.

Epilepsia partialis continua causes clonic twitching of one muscle group, usually in the face, arm, or leg. Twitching occurs every few seconds and persists for hours, days, or months without spreading. Spasms affect the distal arm and leg muscles more frequently than the proximal ones; in the face, they affect the corner of the mouth, one or both eyelids and, occasionally, the neck or trunk muscles unilaterally.

A *focal somatosensory seizure* affects a localized body area on one side. Usually, this seizure initially causes numbness, tingling, or crawling or "electric" sensations; rarely, it may cause pain or burning sensations in the lips, fingers, or toes. A *visual seizure* involves sensations of darkness or of stationary or moving lights or spots—usually red at first, then blue, green, and yellow. It can affect both visual fields or the visual field on the side opposite the lesion. The irritable focus is in the occipital lobe. In contrast, the irritable focus in an *auditory* or *olfactory seizure* is in the temporal lobe. In children more than in adults, focal seizures are likely to spread and become generalized. They typically cause the child's eyes, or his head and eyes, to turn to the side; in neonates, they cause mouth twitching, staring, or both.

Focal seizures in children can result from hemiplegic cerebral palsy, head trauma, child abuse, arteriovenous malformation, and Sturge–Weber syndrome. About 25% of febrile seizures may present as focal seizures.

Possible causes
Central nervous system
Brain abscess. Seizures can occur in the acute stage of abscess formation or after resolution of the abscess.

Brain tumor. Focal seizures are commonly the earliest indicators of a brain tumor.

Cerebrovascular accident (CVA). A major cause of seizures in patients over age 50, a CVA may induce focal seizures within 6 months after its onset.

Head trauma. Any head injury can cause seizures, but penetrating wounds are characteristically associated with focal seizures. These seizures most commonly arise 3 to 15 months after injury, decrease in frequency after several years, and eventually stop. The patient may have generalized seizures and a decreased level of consciousness that may progress to coma.

Multiple sclerosis. Rarely, this disorder begins with focal seizures; generalized seizures may also occur.

Neurofibromatosis. Multiple brain lesions cause focal seizures and, at times, generalized seizures.

Sarcoidosis. Multiple lesions from this disorder affect the brain, producing focal and generalized seizures.

Clinical considerations
• No emergency care is necessary during a focal seizure, unless it progresses to a generalized seizure. (See "Seizure, generalized tonic–clonic.")

• The patient should not be left unattended during the seizure.

• The physician should be notified immediately so he can witness the seizure, if possible.

• The patient's behavior should be recorded in detail, since it may be critical in locating the lesion in the brain.

• The patient may be requested to observe and record his seizures and to contact his physician if their character or frequency changes.

• The importance of complying with prescribed drug therapy should be emphasized to the patient.

• Diagnostic tests may include computed tomography scan and electroencephalography.

Seizure, generalized tonic–clonic
(Grand mal seizure)

Description
Like other types of seizure, a generalized tonic–clonic seizure reflects the paroxysmal, uncontrolled discharge of central nervous system (CNS) neurons, leading to neurologic dysfunction. Unlike most other types of seizure, this cerebral hyperactivity is not confined to the original focus or to a localized area but extends to the entire brain (see *What Happens in a Generalized Seizure*).

Generalized tonic–clonic seizures occur singly. The patient may be awake and active or sleeping. Possible complications include respiratory arrest due to airway obstruction from secretions, status epilepticus (occurring in 5% to 8% of patients), head or spinal injuries and bruises, Todd's paralysis, and, rarely, cardiac arrest. Life–threatening status epilepticus is marked by prolonged seizure activity or by rapidly recurring seizures with no intervening periods of recovery. It is commonly triggered by abrupt discontinuation of anticonvulsant drugs.

Generalized seizures may stem from brain tumors, vascular disorders, head trauma, infections, metabolic defects, drug and alcohol withdrawal syndromes, toxins, and genetic defects. These seizures may also stem from a focal seizure. In recurring seizures, or epilepsy, the cause may be unknown.

Between 75% and 90% of epileptic patients experience their first seizure before age 20. Many children between ages 3 months and 3 years experience generalized seizures associated with fever; some of these children later develop seizures without fever. Generalized seizures may also stem from inborn errors of metabolism, perinatal injury, brain infections, Reye's syndrome, Sturge–Weber syndrome, arteriovenous malformation, lead poisoning, hypoglycemia, and idiopathic causes. Rarely, the pertussis component of the DPT vaccine causes seizures.

Possible causes
Central nervous system
Alcohol withdrawal syndrome. Sudden withdrawal from chronic alcohol dependence may cause seizures 7 to 48 hours later and status epilepticus.

Barbiturate withdrawal. In chronically intoxicated patients, barbiturate withdrawal may produce generalized seizures 2 to 4 days after the last dose. Status epilepticus is possible.

Brain abscess. Generalized seizures may occur in the acute stage of abscess formation or after the abscess disappears.

Brain tumor. Generalized seizures may occur, depending on the tumor's location and type.

Cerebrovascular accident (CVA). Seizures (focal more often than generalized) occur within 6 months of an ischemic CVA.

Cerebral aneurysm. Occasionally, generalized seizures may occur with aneurysmal rupture.

Encephalitis. Seizures are an early sign of this disorder, indicating a poor prognosis; they may also occur after recovery as a result of residual damage.

Head trauma. In severe head trauma, generalized seizures occur at the time of injury. (Months later, focal seizures may occur.)

Hepatic encephalopathy. Late in this disorder, generalized seizures may occur.

Hypertensive encephalopathy. This life–threatening disorder may cause seizures.

Hypoxic encephalopathy. Besides generalized seizures, this disorder may produce myoclonic jerks and coma.

Idiopathic epilepsy. Frequently, the cause of recurrent seizures is unknown.

What Happens in a Generalized Seizure

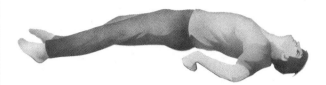

Before the Seizure

Prodromal signs and symptoms, such as myoclonic jerks, throbbing headache, and mood changes, may occur over several hours or days. Less common findings include abdominal pain or cramps, diarrhea or constipation, and facial pallor or redness. The patient may have premonitions of the seizure.

During the Seizure

If a generalized seizure begins with an *aura,* this indicates that irritability in a specific area of the brain quickly became widespread. Common auras include palpitations, epigastric distress rapidly rising to the throat, head or eye turning, and sensory hallucinations.

Next, *loss of consciousness* occurs as a sudden discharge of intense electrical activity overwhelms the brain's subcortical center. The patient falls and experiences brief, bilateral myoclonic contractures. Air forced through spasmodic vocal cords may produce a birdlike, piercing cry.

During the *tonic phase,* skeletal muscles contract for about 10 to 20 seconds. The patient's eyelids are drawn up, his arms are flexed, and his legs are extended. His mouth opens wide, then snaps shut; he may bite his tongue. His respirations cease because of respiratory muscle spasm, and initial pallor of the skin and mucous membranes (the result of impaired venous return) changes to cyanosis secondary to apnea. The patient arches his back and slowly lowers his arms. Other effects include dilated, nonreactive pupils; greatly increased heart rate and blood pressure; increased salivation and tracheobronchial secretions; and profuse diaphoresis.

During the *clonic phase,* lasting about 60 seconds, mild trembling progresses to violent contractures or jerks. Other motor activity includes facial grimaces (with possible tongue biting) and violent expiration of bloody, foamy saliva from clonic contractures of thoracic cage muscles. Clonic jerks slowly decrease in intensity and frequency. The patient is still apneic.

After the Seizure

The patient's movements gradually cease and he becomes unresponsive to external stimuli. Other postseizure features include stertorous respirations from increased tracheobronchial secretions, equal or unequal pupils (but becoming reactive), and urinary incontinence caused by brief muscle flaccidity. After about 5 minutes, the patient's level of consciousness increases, and he appears confused and disoriented. His muscle tone, heart rate, and blood pressure return to normal.

After several hours' sleep, the patient awakens exhausted and may experience headache, sore muscles, and amnesia from the seizure.

Multiple sclerosis. This disorder rarely produces generalized seizures.

Neurofibromatosis. Multiple brain lesions in this disorder cause focal and generalized seizures.

Endocrine

Hypoparathyroidism. Worsening tetany causes generalized seizures.

Genitourinary

Chronic renal failure. End–stage renal failure produces rapid onset of twitching, trembling, myoclonic jerks, and generalized seizures.

Musculoskeletal

Sarcoidosis. Lesions may affect the brain, causing generalized and focal seizures.

Metabolic

Hypoglycemia. Generalized seizures usually occur in late stages of severe hypoglycemia.

Hyponatremia. Seizures develop when serum sodium levels fall below 125 mEq/liter.

Intermittent acute porphyria. Generalized seizures are a late sign of this disorder, indicating severe CNS involvement.

Obstetrics–Gynecology

Eclampsia. Generalized seizures are a hallmark of this disorder.

Drugs

Toxic blood levels of aminophylline, theophylline, lidocaine, meperidine, penicillins, and cimetidine may cause generalized seizures. Phenothiazines, tricyclic antidepressants, alprostadil, amphetamines, isoniazid, and vincristine may cause seizures in patients with preexisting epilepsy.

Diagnostic tests

Contrast agents used in radiologic tests may cause generalized seizures.

Clinical considerations

• If the seizure is *witnessed* by a health care professional, someone should remain with the patient while someone else notifies the physician.

• If the seizure is *not witnessed* by a health care professional, a description of the seizure should be obtained from anyone who witnessed it.

• Care should focus on observing the seizure, protecting the patient from injury, and preventing airway obstruction.

• If the seizure lasts longer than 4 minutes or if a second seizure occurs before full recovery from the first, status epilepticus should be suspected. Measures should be taken to preserve airway patency and to start an I.V. Supplemental oxygen should be administered and cardiac monitoring initiated, as ordered.

• Observations and the intervals between seizures should be recorded.

• The patient should be monitored for recurring seizure activity; seizure precautions should be taken.

• When the patient's condition permits, a history of seizure activity should be obtained and a neurologic examination performed.

• Diagnostic tests may include computed tomography scan and electroencephalography.

• Strict compliance with drug therapy should be emphasized to the patient and his family.

• Family members should be asked to observe and record seizure activity to ensure proper treatment.

Seizure, psychomotor
(Complex partial seizure, temporal lobe seizure)

Description

A psychomotor seizure occurs when a focal seizure begins in the temporal lobe and causes an alteration in consciousness—usually confusion. A psychomotor seizure can occur at any age, but incidence usually increases during adolescence and adulthood. Two thirds of patients also have generalized seizures.

Typically, an aura—most often a complex hallucination or illusion—precedes a psychomotor seizure. The hallucination may be audiovisual (images with sounds), auditory (abnormal or normal sounds or voices from the patient's past), or olfactory (unpleasant smells, such as rotten eggs or burning materials). Other types of auras include feelings of déjà vu, unfamiliarity with surroundings, or depersonalization. Some patients become fearful or anxious or have an unpleasant feeling in the epigastric region that rises toward the chest and throat. The patient usually recognizes the aura and lies down before losing consciousness.

A period of unresponsiveness follows the aura. The patient may experience automatisms, appear dazed and wander aimlessly, perform inappropriate acts (such as undressing in public), be unresponsive, utter incoherent phrases, or, rarely, go into a rage or tantrum. After the seizure, he is confused, drowsy, and amnesic for the seizure. Behavioral automatisms rarely last longer than 5 minutes, but postseizure confusion and amnesia may persist.

Between attacks, the patient may exhibit slow and rigid thinking, outbursts of anger and aggressiveness, tedious conversation, a preoccupation with naive philosophical ideas, diminished libido, mood swings, and paranoid tendencies.

Psychomotor seizures in children may resemble absence seizures. They can result from birth injury, abuse, infections, or neoplasms. In about one third of patients, their cause is unknown.

Repeated psychomotor seizures commonly lead to generalized seizures. Typically, the child wanders aimlessly (an automatism) during a seizure and may develop frightening hallucinations.

Possible causes

Central nervous system

Brain abscess. If the brain abscess is in the temporal lobe, psychomotor seizures commonly occur in the acute phase or after the abscess disappears.
Head trauma. Severe trauma to the temporal lobe (especially from a penetrating injury) can produce psychomotor seizures months or years later. The seizures may decrease in frequency and eventually stop. Head trauma also causes generalized seizures and behavior and personality changes.

Herpes simplex encephalitis. If the herpes simplex virus attacks the temporal lobe, psychomotor seizures can occur.

Temporal lobe tumor. Psychomotor seizures may be the first sign of this disorder.

Clinical considerations

- One staff member should remain with the patient during the seizure while another notifies the physician.
- Unless the patient is angry or violent, he should be led gently to a safe area and calmly encouraged to sit down.
- A staff member should remain with the patient until he is fully alert, at which time he should be reoriented.
- When the patient's condition permits, a history of seizure activity should be obtained and a neurologic examination performed.
- Diagnostic tests may include electroencephalography and computed tomography scans.

Setting–sun sign
(Sunset eyes)

Description

Setting–sun sign describes the position of an infant's or young child's eyes as a result of pressure on cranial nerves III, IV, and VI. Both eyes are forced downward so that an area of sclera shows above the irises; in some patients, the irises appear to be forced outward.

Setting–sun sign reflects increased intracranial pressure (ICP). Typically, increased ICP results from space–occupying lesions—such as tumors—or from an accumulation of fluid in the brain's ventricular system, as occurs in hydrocephalus. It also results from intracranial bleeding or cerebral edema.

Setting–sun sign may be intermittent—for example, it may disappear when the infant is upright, because this position slightly reduces ICP. The sign may be elicited in a normal infant under 4 weeks old by suddenly changing his head position. It can also be elicited in a normal infant up to 9 months old by placing a bright light before his eyes and removing it quickly.

Shallow respirations

Description
Respirations are shallow when a diminished volume of air enters the lungs during inspiration. In an effort to obtain enough air, the patient with shallow respirations usually breathes at an accelerated rate. However, as he tires or as his muscles weaken, this compensatory increase in respirations diminishes, leading to inadequate gas exchange and such signs as dyspnea, cyanosis, confusion, agitation, loss of consciousness, and tachycardia.

Shallow respirations may develop suddenly or gradually and may last briefly or become chronic. They are a key sign of respiratory distress and neurologic deterioration. Causes include inadequate central respiratory control over breathing, neuromuscular disorders, increased resistance to airflow into the lungs, respiratory muscle fatigue or weakness, voluntary alterations in breathing, and decreased activity from prolonged bed rest.

In children, shallow respirations commonly indicate a life–threatening condition, such as idiopathic (infant) respiratory distress syndrome, acute epiglottitis, diphtheria, or aspiration of a foreign body.

Possible causes
Central nervous system
Amyotrophic lateral sclerosis. Respiratory muscle weakness in this disorder causes progressive shallow respirations.

Coma. Rapid, shallow respirations result from neurologic dysfunction or restricted chest movement.

Guillain–Barré syndrome. Progressive ascending paralysis causes rapid or progressive onset of shallow respirations.

Multiple sclerosis. Muscle weakness causes progressive shallow respirations.

Muscular dystrophy. With progressive thoracic deformity and muscle weakness, shallow respirations may occur along with waddling gait, contractures, scoliosis, lordosis, and muscle atrophy or hypertrophy.

Myasthenia gravis. Progression of this disorder causes respiratory muscle weakness marked by shallow respirations, dyspnea, and cyanosis.

Parkinson's disease. Fatigue and weakness lead to progressive shallow respirations.

Spinal cord injury. Diaphragmatic breathing and shallow respirations may occur in injury to the C5 to C8 area.

Respiratory
Adult respiratory distress syndrome. Initially, this life–threatening syndrome produces rapid, shallow respirations and dyspnea, at times after the patient appears stable.

Asthma. In this disorder, bronchospasm and hyperinflation of the lungs cause rapid, shallow respirations.

Atelectasis. Decreased lung expansion or pleuritic pain causes sudden onset of rapid, shallow respirations.

Bronchiectasis. Increased secretions obstruct air flow in the lungs, leading to shallow respirations and a productive cough with copious, foul–smelling, mucopurulent sputum (a classic finding).

Chronic bronchitis. Airway obstruction causes chronic shallow respirations.

Emphysema. Increased breathing effort causes muscle fatigue, leading to chronic shallow respirations.

Flail chest. In this disorder, decreased air movement results in rapid, shallow respirations, paradoxical chest wall motion from rib instability, tachycardia, hypotension, ecchymoses, cyanosis, and pain over the affected area.

Pleural effusion. In this disorder, restricted lung expansion causes shallow respirations, beginning suddenly or gradually.

Pneumonia. Pulmonary consolidation results in rapid, shallow respirations.

Pneumothorax. This disorder causes sudden onset of shallow respirations and dyspnea.

Pulmonary edema. Pulmonary vascular congestion causes rapid, shallow respirations.

Pulmonary embolism. This disorder causes sudden rapid, shallow respirations and severe dyspnea with anginal or pleuritic chest pain.

Upper airway obstruction. Partial airway obstruction causes acute shallow respirations with sudden gagging and dry, paroxysmal coughing; hoarseness; stridor; and tachycardia.

Musculoskeletal

Kyphoscoliosis. Skeletal cage distortion can eventually cause rapid, shallow respirations from reduced lung capacity.

Environmental

Botulism. In this disorder, progressive muscle weakness and paralysis initially cause shallow respirations. Within 4 days, the patient develops respiratory distress from respiratory muscle paralysis.

Tetanus. In this now rare disorder, spasm of the intercostal muscles and the diaphragm causes shallow respirations.

Drugs

Narcotics, sedatives and hypnotics, tranquilizers, neuromuscular blockers, magnesium sulfate, and anesthetics can produce slow, shallow respirations.

Treatments

After *abdominal* or *thoracic surgery*, pain associated with chest splinting and decreased chest wall motion may cause shallow respirations.

Clinical considerations

• The patient should be assessed for signs and symptoms of impending respiratory failure or arrest.

• If the patient is not in severe respiratory distress, a history should be obtained and a physical examination performed.

• Diagnostic tests may include complete blood count, arterial blood gas analysis, pulmonary function tests, chest X–rays, and bronchoscopy.

• The patient should be positioned in a semi– or high–Fowler position.

• Humidified oxygen, bronchodilators, mucolytics, expectorants, or antibiotics should be administered, as ordered.

• The patient should be instructed to cough and deep–breathe every hour to clear secretions and to counteract possible hypoventilation. If the patient is unable to reposition himself, he should be turned frequently according to a regular schedule.

• Chest physiotherapy, incentive spirometry, or intermittent positive–pressure breathing may be required.

Siegert's sign

Description

Siegert's sign is the presence of short, inwardly curved little fingers, typically appearing in Down's syndrome.

Signorelli's sign

Description

Signorelli's sign is extreme tenderness on palpation of the area anterior to the mastoid; associated with meningitis.

Simon's sign

Description

Simon's sign is incoordination of the movements of the diaphragm and thorax, occurring early in meningitis.

Skin, bronze

Description
Bronze skin tone tends to appear at pressure points—such as the knuckles, elbows, toes, and knees—and in creases on the palms and soles. Eventually, this hyperpigmentation may extend to the buccal mucosa and gums before covering the entire body. It may stem from endocrine disorders, malnutrition, biliary cirrhosis, and certain drugs.

Because bronzing develops gradually, it is sometimes mistaken for a suntan. However, the hyperpigmentation can affect the entire body, not just sun–exposed areas; sun exposure deepens the bronze color of exposed areas, but this effect gradually fades. In fair–skinned patients, the bronze tone can range from light to dark. It also varies with the disorder.

Mechanism
Bronze skin results from excess circulating melanin.

Possible causes
Endocrine
Adrenal hyperplasia. In this disorder, the entire skin assumes a dark bronze tone within a few months.
Adrenal insufficiency. In this disorder, bronze skin is a classic sign that may precede other features of hypoadrenalism by many years.
Gastrointestinal
Biliary cirrhosis. This disorder causes bronze skin from melanosis of exposed areas of jaundiced skin: eyelids, palms, neck, and chest or back.
Hematologic
Hemochromatosis. An early sign is progressive, generalized bronzing accented by metallic gray–bronze skin on sun–exposed areas, genitals, and scars. Mucous membranes are affected less often.
Metabolic
Malnutrition. As weight loss depletes body nutrients, bronzing develops along with apathy, lethargy, anorexia, weakness, and slow pulse and respirations.
Drugs
Prolonged therapy with high doses of phenothiazines may cause gradual bronzing of the skin.

Clinical considerations
• A history should be obtained and a physical examination performed.
• Diagnostic tests may include adrenocorticotropic hormone stimulation test, thyroid function studies, complete blood count, electrolyte analysis, electrocardiography, and a computed tomography scan of the pituitary.

Skin, clammy

Description
Clammy skin is moist, cool, and often pale. It typically accompanies shock, acute hypoglycemia, anxiety reactions, dysrhythmias, and heat exhaustion.

Mechanism
Clammy skin is a sympathetic response to stress, which triggers release of the hormones epinephrine and norepinephrine. These hormones cause cutaneous vasoconstriction and secretion of cold sweat from eccrine glands, particularly on the palms, forehead, and soles. It also occurs as a vasovagal reaction to severe pain.

Possible causes
Cardiovascular
Cardiogenic shock. Generalized cool, moist, pale skin accompanies confusion and restlessness, hypotension, tachycardia, tachypnea, narrowing pulse pressure, cyanosis, and oliguria.
Dysrhythmias. Cardiac dysrhythmias may produce generalized cool, clammy skin, mental status changes, dizziness, and hypotension.
Hypovolemic shock. In this common form of shock, generalized pale, cold, clammy skin accompanies subnormal body temperature, hypotension with

Clammy Skin: A Key Finding

Clammy skin commonly accompanies emergency conditions, such as shock, acute hypoglycemia, and dysrhythmias. The typical clinical situations described below show what to do when clammy skin is detected.

Clammy skin is detected in a patient who appears anxious and restless.

His vital signs should be taken quickly. If tachypnea, tachycardia, hypotension, or a weak, irregular pulse is present:

Shock should be suspected and the physician notified at once.

The patient should be placed in a supine position in bed and his legs elevated 20° to 30° to promote perfusion to vital organs.

An I.V. line should be inserted for administration of drugs, fluids, or blood, if ordered. Also, supplemental oxygen should be given, and cardiac monitoring initiated.

Clammy skin and possible tremors are detected in a patient who appears irritable and anxious and reports persistent hunger.

His vital signs should be quickly taken. If hypotension is present:

Acute hypoglycemia should be suspected and the physician notified at once.

Blood should be drawn immediately for glucose studies, and a drop of blood tested with a glucose reagent strip. An I.V. line should be inserted and administration of a 50-ml bolus of dextrose 50% anticipated. Also, cardiac monitoring should be initiated.

Clammy skin is detected in a patient with changes in mental status, such as confusion.

His vital signs should be taken quickly. If hypotension and changes in pulse rate and rhythm are present:

Dysrhythmias should be suspected and the physician notified at once.

An I.V. line should be inserted and administration of antiarrhythmic drugs anticipated. Also, supplemental oxygen should be given and cardiac monitoring initiated.

narrowing pulse pressure, tachycardia, tachypnea, and rapid, thready pulse.

Endocrine
Acute hypoglycemia. Generalized cool, clammy skin or diaphoresis may accompany irritability, tremors, palpitations, hunger, headache, tachycardia, and anxiety.

Psychiatric
Anxiety. An acute anxiety attack often produces cold, clammy skin on the forehead, palms, and soles.

Infection
Septic shock. The cold shock stage causes generalized cold, clammy skin.

Environmental
Heat exhaustion. In the acute stage, generalized cold, clammy skin accompanies an ashen-gray appearance, headache, confusion, syncope, giddiness, and a normal or subnormal temperature.

Clinical considerations

• Vital signs should be taken and a quick assessment performed to identify conditions that require emergency intervention (see *Clammy Skin: A Key Finding*, p. 389).

Skin, mottled

Description

Mottled skin is patchy discoloration indicating primary or secondary changes of the deep, middle, or superficial dermal blood vessels. It can result from hematologic, immune, or connective tissue disorders; chronic occlusive arterial disease; dysproteinemias; immobility; exposure to heat or cold; or shock. Or it can be a normal reaction, such as the diffuse mottling (cutis marmorata) that occurs when exposure to cold causes venous stasis in cutaneous blood vessels.

Mottling that occurs with other signs and symptoms most often affects the extremities, usually indicating restricted blood flow. For example, livedo reticularis, a characteristic network pattern of reddish blue discoloration, occurs when vasospasm of the mid-dermal blood vessels slows local blood flow in dilated superficial capillaries and small veins. Shock causes mottling from systemic vasoconstriction.

Possible causes

Cardiovascular
Acrocyanosis. In this rare disorder, anxiety or exposure to cold can cause vasospasm in small cutaneous arterioles. This results in persistent symmetrical blue and red mottling of the affected hands and feet.

Acute arterial occlusion. Initial signs include temperature and color changes. Pallor may change to blotchy cyanosis and livedo reticularis. Color and temperature demarcation develop at the level of obstruction.

Arteriosclerosis obliterans. Atherosclerotic buildup narrows intraarterial lumens, resulting in reduced blood flow through the affected artery. Obstructed blood flow to the extremities (most often the lower) produces such peripheral signs and symptoms as leg pallor, cyanosis, blotchy erythema, and livedo reticularis.

Buerger's disease. This form of vasculitis produces unilateral or asymmetrical color changes and mottling, particularly livedo networking in the lower extremities. It also typically causes intermittent claudication and erythema along extremity blood vessels. During exposure to cold, the feet are cold, cyanotic, and numb; later they're hot, red, and tingling.

Hypovolemic shock. Vasoconstriction from shock commonly produces skin mottling, initially in the knees and elbows. As shock worsens, mottling becomes generalized. Early signs: sudden onset of pallor, cool skin, restlessness, thirst, tachypnea, and slight tachycardia. As shock progresses, associated findings include cool, clammy skin; rapid, thready pulse; hypotension; narrowed pulse pressure; decreased urine output; subnormal temperature; confusion; and decreased level of consciousness.

Idiopathic or primary livedo reticularis. Symmetrical, diffuse, initially asymptomatic mottling can involve the hands, feet, arms, legs, buttocks, and trunk. Initially, networking is intermittent and most pronounced on exposure to cold or stress; eventually, mottling persists even with warming.

Periarteritis nodosa. Cutaneous findings may include asymmetrical, patchy livedo reticularis, palpable nodules along the distribution of medium-sized arteries, erythema, purpura, muscle wasting, ulcers, gangrene, and peripheral neuropathy.

Musculoskeletal
Rheumatoid arthritis. This disorder may cause skin mottling.

Systemic lupus erythematosus. This connective tissue disorder can cause livedo reticularis, most commonly on the outer arms.

Hematologic
Polycythemia vera. This hematologic disorder produces livedo reticularis, hemangiomas, purpura, rubor, ulcerative nodules, and scleroderma-like lesions.

Environmental
Thermal exposure. Prolonged thermal exposure, as from a heating pad or hot water bottle, may cause erythema abigne—a localized, reticulated brown-to-red mottling.

Treatments
Prolonged immobility may cause bluish, asymptomatic mottling, most noticeably in dependent extremities.

Clinical considerations
• Vital signs should be taken and a quick assessment performed to identify conditions that require emergency intervention (see *Mottled Skin: Know What to Do*).
• If the patient is not in distress, a history should be obtained and a physical examination performed.
• Typically, mottled skin results from chronic conditions. The patient should be instructed to avoid tight clothing

---

Mottled Skin: Know What to Do

If the patient's skin is mottled at the elbows and knees, or all over, and is pale, cool, and clammy, he may be developing *hypovolemic shock*. His vital signs should be taken quickly and tachycardia or a weak, thready pulse noted. He should be observed for flat neck veins and assessed for anxiety. If these signs and symptoms are present, he should be placed in a supine position in bed with his legs elevated 20° to 30°. The physician should be notified immediately. Oxygen should be administered by nasal cannula or face mask and cardiac monitoring begun. A large-bore I.V. line should be inserted for rapid fluid administration; and preparations made to assist with insertion of a central line or a Swan-Ganz catheter. Indwelling catheter insertion should be anticipated to monitor urine output.

Localized mottling in a pale, cool extremity that the patient says feels painful, numb, and tingling may signal *acute arterial occlusion*. His distal pulses should be checked immediately; if they are absent or diminished, the physician should be notified at once. An I.V. line should be inserted in an unaffected extremity, and the patient prepared for arteriography or immediate surgery, as ordered.

---

and overexposure to cold or to heating devices, such as hot water bottles and heating pads.

Skin, scaly

Description
Scaly skin varies in texture from fine and delicate to branny, coarse, or stratified. Scales are typically dry, brittle, and shiny, but they can be greasy and dull.

Their color ranges from whitish gray, yellow, or brown to a silvery sheen.

Usually benign, scaly skin occurs in fungal, bacterial, and viral infections (cutaneous or systemic), in lymphomas, and in lupus erythematosus; it is common in inflammatory skin diseases. A form of scaly skin—generalized fine desquamation—commonly follows prolonged febrile illness, sunburn, or thermal burn. Red patches of scaly skin that appear or worsen in the winter result from dry skin (or from actinic keratosis, common in the elderly). Drugs also cause scaly skin. Aggravating factors include cold, heat, immobility, and frequent bathing.

Mechanism

Scaly skin results when cells of the uppermost skin layer (stratum corneum) desiccate and shred, causing excessive accumulation of loosely adherent flakes of normal or abnormal keratin. Normally, skin cell loss is imperceptible; the appearance of scale indicates increased cell proliferation secondary to altered keratinization.

Possible causes
Musculoskeletal

Discoid lupus erythematosus. This cutaneous form of lupus may occur without systemic manifestations. Separate or coalescing lesions (macules, papules, or plaques), ranging from pink to purple, are covered with a yellow or brown crust. Enlarged hair follicles are filled with scale. Telangiectasia may be present. After this inflammatory stage, the lesions heal with hypopigmentation or hyperpigmentation and nontractile scarring and atrophy. The disorder commonly involves the face or sun-exposed areas of the neck, ears, scalp, lips, and oral mucosa. Alopecia may also occur.

Systemic lupus erythematosus. This disorder produces a bright red maculopapular eruption with fine scales. Patches are sharply defined and involve the nose and malar regions of the face in a butterfly pattern—a primary sign. Similar characteristic rashes appear on other body surfaces; scaling occurs along the lower lip or anterior hair line.

Skin

Bowen's disease. This common form of intraepidermal carcinoma causes painless, erythematous plaques that are widely distributed, raised, and indurated with a thick, hyperkeratotic scale and possibly ulcerated centers.

Dermatitis. Exfoliative dermatitis begins with rapidly developing generalized erythema. Desquamation with fine scales or thick sheets of all or most of the skin surface may cause life-threatening hypothermia.

In *nummular dermatitis*, round, pustular lesions often ooze purulent exudate, itch severely, and rapidly become encrusted and scaly. Lesions appear on the extensor surfaces of the limbs, posterior trunk, and buttocks.

Seborrheic dermatitis begins with erythematous, scaly papules that progress to larger scaly plaques, possibly involving the genitalia along with the scalp, chest, eyebrows, back axillae, and umbilicus. Pruritus accompanies the scaling.

Dermatophytosis. Tinea capitis produces lesions with reddened, slightly elevated borders and a central area of dense scaling; these lesions may become inflamed and pus-filled (kerions). Patchy alopecia and itching may also occur. *Tinea pedis* causes scaling and blisters between the toes. The squamous type produces diffuse, fine, branny scaling. Adherent and silvery white, it is most prominent in skin creases and may affect the entire dorsum of the foot. *Tinea corporis* produces crusty lesions. As they enlarge, their centers heal, causing the classic ringworm shape.

Lichen planus. In this disorder, flat, violent lesions with a fine scale most commonly affect the lumbar region, genitalia, ankles, and anterior lower legs.

Parpsoriasis (chronic). This disorder produces small or moderate-sized papules—with a thin, adherent scale—on the trunk, hands, and feet. Removal of the scale reveals a shiny brown surface.

Pityriasis. Pityriasis rosea—an acute, benign, and self-limiting disorder—produces widespread scales. It begins with an erythematous, raised, oval herald patch anywhere on the body. A few days or weeks later, yellow-tan or erythematous patches with scaly edges erupt on the trunk and limbs and sometimes on the face, hands, and feet. Pruritus also occurs.

Pityriasis rubra pilaris, an uncommon disorder, initially produces seborrheic scaling on the scalp, progressing to the face and ears. Later, scaly, red patches develop on the palms and soles, becoming diffuse, thick, fissured, hyperkeratotic, and painful. Lesions also appear on the hands, fingers, wrists, and forearms and then on wide areas of the trunk, neck, and limbs.

Psoriasis. Silvery white, micaceous scales in this disorder cover erythematous plaques that have sharply defined borders. Psoriasis most commonly appears on the scalp, chest, elbows, knees, back, buttocks, and genitals. Associated signs and symptoms include nail pitting, pruritus, arthritis, and sometimes pain from dry, cracked, encrusted lesions.

Tinea versicolor. This benign fungal skin infection typically produces macular hypopigmented, fawn-colored, or brown patches of varying sizes and shapes. All are slightly scaly. Lesions frequently affect the upper trunk, arms, and lower abdomen, sometimes the neck, and, rarely, the face.

Neoplastic

Lymphoma. Hodgkin's disease and non-Hodgkin's lymphoma commonly cause scaly rashes. *Hodgkin's disease* may cause scaling dermatitis with pruritus that begins in the legs and spreads to the entire body. Remission and recurrence are common.

Non-Hodgkin's lymphoma initially produces erythematous patches with some scaling that later become interspersed with nodules. Pruritus and discomfort are common; later, tumors and ulcers form.

Infectious disease

Syphilis (secondary). Papulosquamous, slightly scaly eruptions characterize this disorder. A ring-shaped pattern of copper-red papules usually forms on the face, arms, palms, soles, chest, back, and abdomen.

Drugs

Many drugs can produce scaling patches. Among them: penicillins, sulfonamides, barbiturates, quinidine, diazepam, phenytoin, and isoniazid.

Clinical considerations

- A history should be obtained and the entire skin surface examined.
- Diagnostic tests may include a Wood's light examination, skin scraping, and skin biopsy.
- The patient should be taught proper skin care depending on the causative disorder.

Skin turgor, decreased

Description

Skin turgor is the skin's elasticity. It is determined by observing the time required for the skin to return to its normal position after being stretched or pinched (see *Assessing Skin Turgor,* p. 394).

Decreased skin turgor results from dehydration, or volume depletion, which moves interstitial fluid into the vascular bed to maintain circulating blood volume, leading to slackness in the skin's dermal layer. It is a normal finding in the elderly and in people with rapid weight loss; it also occurs in disorders affecting the gastrointestinal, renal, endocrine, and other systems.

Assessing Skin Turgor

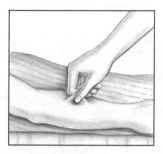 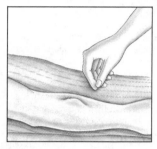

To assess skin turgor in an adult, the examiner picks up a fold of skin over the sternum or the arm, as shown at left. (In an infant, she rolls a fold of loosely adherent skin on the abdomen between her thumb and forefinger.) Then she releases it. Normal skin will immediately return to its previous contour. In decreased skin turgor, the fold of skin will "hold," as shown at right, for up to 30 seconds.

Soto-Hall sign

Description
The Soto-Hall sign is pain in the area of a lesion, occurring on passive flexion of the spine. To elicit this sign, the patient is placed supine, and his spine progressively flexed from the neck downward. The patient will complain of pain at the area of the lesion.

Spasmodic torticollis

Description
Spasmodic torticollis is intermittent or continuous spasms of the shoulder and neck muscles that turn the head to one side. Often transient and idiopathic, this sign can occur in extrapyramidal disorders. It can also occur in patients with shortened neck muscles (see "Dystonia").

Spider angioma
(Arterial spider, spider nervus, stellate angioma, vascular spider)

Description
A spider angioma is a fiery red vascular lesion with an elevated central body, branching spiderlike legs, and a surrounding flush (see *Spider Angioma*). A form of telangiectasia, this characteristic lesion ranges from a few millimeters to several centimeters in diameter and may be singular or multiple. Most commonly, it appears on the face and neck; less commonly, on the shoulders, thorax, arms, backs of the hands and fingers, and mucous membranes of the lips and nose. Rarely does it appear below the waist on the lips, ears, nail beds, or palms. On palpation, the angioma may be slightly warmer than the surrounding skin and may have a pulsating central body.

Spider Angioma

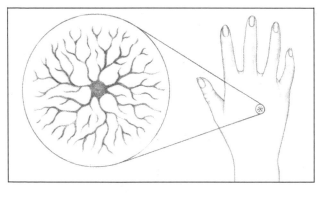

Spider angiomas are most commonly associated with cirrhosis. They may also erupt in the 2nd to 3rd months of pregnancy, enlarge and multiply, then disappear about 6 weeks after delivery. Occasionally, a few lesions may persist. These lesions may also appear in normal patients—especially the elderly—but are smaller and fewer in number (nine or less). They may persist indefinitely or spontaneously disappear.

Treatment is not indicated for spider angiomas during pregnancy. However, cautery, electrodesiccation, or freezing may be used to treat them in the patient with cirrhosis.

Spine sign

Description
Spine sign is resistance to anterior flexion of the spine, resulting from pain in poliomyelitis.

Splenomegaly

Descripion
Splenomegaly is an abnormal enlargement of the spleen. Because splenomegaly commonly occurs in many disorders, it is not a diagnostic sign by itself. In fact, an enlarged spleen may occur in as many as 5% of normal adults. Usually, though, this sign points to infection, trauma, or hepatic, autoimmune, neoplastic, or hematologic disorders.

Because the spleen functions as the body's largest lymph node, splenomegaly can result from any process that triggers lymphadenopathy. For example, it may reflect reactive hyperplasia (a response to infection or inflammation), proliferation or infiltration of neoplastic cells, extramedullary hemopoiesis, phagocytic cell proliferation, increased blood cell destruction, or vascular congestion associated with portal hypertension.

Possible causes
Respiratory
Sarcoidosis. This granulomatous disorder may produce splenomegaly and hepatomegaly, possibly accompanied by vague abdominal discomfort.
Cardiovascular
Infective endocarditis (subacute). This infection usually causes an enlarged, but nontender, spleen.
Gastrointestinal
Cirrhosis. About one third of patients with advanced cirrhosis develop moderate to marked splenomegaly.
Hepatitis. Splenomegaly may occur in this disorder. More characteristic findings include hepatomegaly, vomiting, jaundice, and fatigue.
Hypersplenism (primary). In this syndrome, splenomegaly accompanies signs of pancytopenia—anemia, neutropenia, or thrombocytopenia.
Pancreatic cancer. This cancer may cause moderate to severe splenomegaly if tumor growth compresses the splenic vein.
Splenic rupture. Splenomegaly may result from massive hemorrhage in this disorder.
Musculoskeletal
Felty's syndrome. Splenomegaly is characteristic in this syndrome that occurs in chronic rheumatoid arthritis.
Hematologic
Polycythemia vera. Late in this disorder, the spleen may become markedly enlarged, resulting in easy satiety, abdominal fullness, and left upper quadrant or pleuritic chest pain.
Thrombotic thrombocytopenic purpura. This disorder may produce splenomegaly and hepatomegaly accompanied by fever, generalized purpura, jaundice, pallor, vaginal bleeding, and hematuria.
Metabolic
Amyloidosis. Marked splenomegaly may occur here—the result of excessive protein deposits in the spleen.
Neoplastic
Leukemia. Moderate to severe splenomegaly is an early sign of both acute and chronic leukemia. In chronic granulocytic leukemia, splenomegaly is sometimes painful.
Lymphoma. Moderate to massive splenomegaly is a late sign here.
Infection
Brucellosis. In severe cases of this rare infection, splenomegaly is a major sign.
Histoplasmosis. Acute disseminated histoplasmosis commonly produces splenomegaly and hepatomegaly.
Malaria. Splenomegaly is common in malaria.
Infectious disease
Infectious mononucleosis. A common sign of this disorder, splenomegaly is most pronounced during the second and third weeks of illness.

Clinical considerations
• Splenomegaly may be detected by *light* palpation under the left costal margin (see *How to Palpate for Splenomegaly*). Unfortunately, this technique is not always advisable or effective.
• If the patient has a history of abdominal or thoracic trauma, the abdomen should *not* be palpated, because this may aggravate internal bleeding.
• If splenic rupture is suspected, the patient should be assessed for signs and symptoms of shock; the physician should be notified immediately if any signs or symptoms are present.
• Splenomegaly may need to be confirmed by a computed tomography or radionuclide scan.

Spoon nails

Description
Spoon nails refers to a malformation of the nails characterized by a concave instead of the normal convex outer surface. This commonly occurs in severe hypochromic anemia but occasionally may be hereditary.

How to Palpate for Splenomegaly

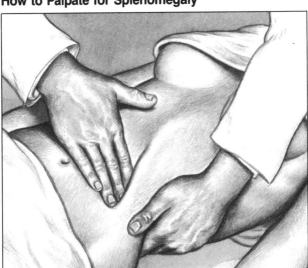

Detecting splenomegaly requires skillful and gentle palpation to avoid rupturing the enlarged organ. The steps below should be followed carefully:

• The examiner places the patient in a supine position and stands at her right side. He places his left hand under the left costovertebral angle and pushes lightly to move the spleen forward. Then he presses his right hand gently under the left front costal margin.

• The examiner tells the patient to take a deep breath and then exhale. As she exhales, he moves his right hand along the tissue contours under the ribs' border, feeling for the spleen's edge. The enlarged spleen should feel like a firm mass that bumps against the fingers. *Important:* Palpation must begin low enough in the abdomen to catch the edge of a massive spleen.

• The examiner grades the splenomegaly as slight (1 to 4 cm below the costal margin), moderate (4 to 8 cm below the costal margin), or great (8 cm or more below the costal margin).

• The examiner repositions the patient on her right side with her hips and knees flexed slightly to move the spleen forward. Then he repeats the palpation procedure.

Stellwag's sign

Description
Stellwag's sign is incomplete and infrequent blinking. It is usually related to exophthalmos in Graves' disease.

Stepping reflex

Description
The stepping reflex refers to spontaneous stepping movements in the neonate that simulate walking. This re-

ciprocal flexion and extension of the legs disappears at about age 4 weeks. To elicit this sign, the infant is held erect with the soles of his feet touching a hard surface. Scissoring movements with persistent extension and crossing of the legs or asymmetrical stepping is abnormal, possibly indicating central nervous system damage.

Strunsky's sign

Description

Strunsky's sign is pain on plantar flexion of the toes and forefoot, caused by inflammatory disorders of the anterior arch. To detect this sign, the examiner has the patient assume a relaxed position with his foot exposed. She then grasps the toes and quickly plantarflexes the toes and forefoot.

Stertorous respirations

Description

Stertorous respirations are characterized by a harsh, rattling, or snoring sound. This common sign occurs in about 10% of normal individuals, especially middle-aged, obese men. It may be aggravated by the use of alcohol or sedatives before bed, which increases oropharyngeal flaccidity, and by sleeping in the supine position, which allows the relaxed tongue to slip back into the airway.

The major pathologic causes of stertorous respirations are obstructive sleep apnea and life-threatening upper airway obstruction associated with an oropharyngeal tumor or with uvular or palatal edema. This obstruction may also occur during the postictal phase of a generalized seizure when mucous secretions or a relaxed tongue blocks the airway.

In children, the most common cause of stertorous respirations is nasal or pharyngeal obstruction secondary to tonsillar or adenoid hypertrophy or the presence of a foreign body.

Occasionally, stertorous respirations are mistaken for stridor, which is another sign of upper airway obstruction. However, stridor indicates laryngeal or tracheal obstruction, whereas stertorous respirations signal higher airway obstruction.

Mechanism

Stertorous respirations usually result from the vibration of relaxed oropharyngeal structures during sleep or coma, causing partial airway obstruction. Less often, these respirations result from retained mucus in the upper airway.

Possible causes
Respiratory

Airway obstruction. Regardless of its cause, partial airway obstruction may lead to stertorous respirations accompanied by wheezing, dyspnea, and tachypnea. It may lead to cardiopulmonary arrest.

Obstructive sleep apnea. Loud and disruptive snoring is a major characteristic of this syndrome, which commonly affects the obese. Typically, the snoring alternates with periods of sleep apnea, which usually end with loud, gasping sounds. Alternating tachycardia and bradycardia may occur. Episodes of snoring and apnea recur in a cyclic pattern throughout the night.

Treatments

Endotracheal surgery, intubation, or *suction* may cause significant palatal or uvular edema, resulting in stertorous respirations.

Clinical considerations

• A quick respiratory assessment should be performed and the physician notified of signs or symptoms of respiratory distress. Emergency equipment should be kept readily available.

• If stertorous respirations are detected while the patient is sleeping, his breathing pattern should be observed for 3 to 4 minutes and recorded.

• Corticosteroids or antibiotics and cool, humidified oxygen should be administered, as ordered, to reduce palatal or uvular inflammation and edema.

• Layngoscopy and bronchoscopy may be performed to rule out airway obstruction.

Stool, clay-colored

Description
Pale, putty-colored stools usually result from hepatic, gallbladder, or pancreatic disorders. Commonly, these stools are associated with jaundice.

Mechanism
Normally, bile pigments give the stool its characteristic brown color. However, hepatocellular degeneration or biliary obstruction may interfere with the formation or release of these pigments into the intestine, resulting in clay-colored stools.

Possible causes
Gastrointestinal
Bile duct cancer. Frequently a presenting sign of this cancer, clay-colored stools may be accompanied by jaundice, pruritus, and weight loss.
Biliary cirrhosis. Clay-colored stools typically follow unexplained pruritus that worsens at bedtime, weakness, fatigue, weight loss, and vague abdominal pain; these features may be present for years.
Cholangitis (sclerosing). Characterized by fibrosis of the bile ducts, this chronic inflammatory disorder may cause clay-colored stools, chronic or intermittent jaundice, pruritus, and right upper abdominal pain.
Cholelithiasis. Stones in the biliary tract may cause clay-colored stools, especially when they obstruct the common bile duct (choledocholithiasis). However, if the obstruction is intermittent, the stools may alternate between normal and clay color.

Hepatic carcinoma. Before clay-colored stools occur in this disorder, the patient usually has weight loss, weakness, and anorexia.
Hepatitis. In *viral hepatitis,* clay-colored stools signal the start of the icteric phase and are typically followed by jaundice within 1 to 5 days.

In cholestatic *nonviral hepatitis,* clay-colored stools occur with other signs of viral hepatitis.
Pancreatic cancer. Common bile duct obstruction associated with this insidious cancer may cause clay-colored stools.
Pancreatitis (acute). This disorder may cause clay-colored stools, dark urine, and jaundice.
Treatments
Biliary surgery may cause bile duct stricture, resulting in clay-colored stools.

Clinical considerations
• A history should be obtained and a physical examination performed.
• Diagnostic tests may include liver enzyme and serum bilirubin levels and stool analysis.

Stridor

Description
Stridor is a loud, harsh, musical respiratory sound. It results from obstruction in the trachea or larynx and is usually heard during inspiration. This sign may also occur during expiration in severe upper airway obstruction. It may begin as low-pitched "croaking" and progress to high-pitched "crowing" as respirations become more vigorous.

Life-threatening upper airway obstruction can stem from foreign body aspiration, increased secretions, intraluminal tumor, localized edema or muscle spasms, and external compression by a tumor or aneurysm.

Stridor is a major sign of airway obstruction in the pediatric patient.

Assisting with Emergency Endotracheal Intubation

For a patient with stridor, the doctor may order emergency endotracheal intubation to establish a patent airway and administer mechanical ventilation. The caregiver should be prepared to assist with tube insertion or to insert the tube herself, if hospital protocol allows. These essential steps should be followed:

• The necessary equipment should be gathered. If ordered, a respiratory technician or another nurse should be asked to set up the mechanical ventilator.

• The procedure should be explained to the patient.

• The patient should be placed flat on his back with a small blanket or pillow under his head. This position aligns the axis of the oropharynx, posterior pharynx, and trachea.

• The cuff on the endotracheal tube should be checked for leaks.

• After intubation, the cuff should be inflated, using the minimal leak technique.

• Tube placement should be checked by auscultating for bilateral breath sounds; the patient should be observed for chest expansion and the endotracheal tube's opening felt for warm exhalations.

• An oral airway or bite block should be inserted.

• The tube and airway should be secured with tape applied to skin treated with compound benzoin tincture.

• Secretions should be suctioned from the patient's mouth and endotracheal tube, as needed.

• Oxygen should be administered and/or mechanical ventilation initiated, as ordered.

After the patient has been intubated, secretions should be suctioned at least every 2 hours and cuff pressure checked once every shift (any air leaks should be corrected with the minimal leak technique). The patient should be prepared for chest X-rays to check tube placement. As needed, he should be restrained and reassured.

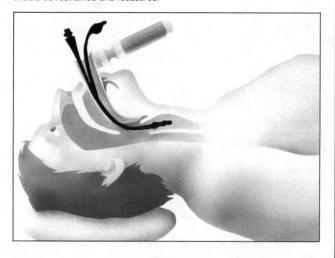

When you hear this sign, you must intervene quickly to prevent total airway obstruction. This emergency can happen more rapidly in a child because his airway is narrower than an adult's.

Possible causes
Respiratory
Airway trauma. Local trauma to the upper airway commonly causes acute obstruction, resulting in the sudden onset of stridor.

Anaphylaxis. In a severe allergic reaction, upper airway edema causes stridor and other signs of respiratory distress: nasal flaring, wheezing, accessory muscle use, intercostal retractions, and dyspnea.

Aspiration of a foreign body. Sudden stridor is characteristic in life-threatening aspiration of a foreign body.

Laryngeal tumor. Stridor is a late sign here and may be accompanied by dysphagia, dyspnea, enlarged cervical nodes, and pain that radiates to the ear.

Laryngitis (acute). This disorder may cause severe laryngeal edema, resulting in stridor and dyspnea. Its chief sign, though, is mild to severe hoarseness, perhaps with transient voice loss.

Mediastinal tumor. Often asymptomatic at first, this tumor may eventually compress the trachea and bronchi, resulting in stridor.

Cardiovascular
Thoracic aortic aneurysm. If this aneurysm compresses the trachea, it may cause stridor accompanied by dyspnea, wheezing, and a brassy cough.

Metabolic
Hypocalcemia. In this disorder, laryngospasm can cause stridor.

Endocrine
Retrosternal thyroid. This anatomic abnormality causes stridor, dysphagia, cough, hoarseness, and tracheal deviation.

Environmental
Inhalation injury. Within 48 hours after inhalation of smoke or noxious fumes, the patient may develop laryngeal edema and bronchospasms, resulting in stridor.

Treatments
After *prolonged intubation*, the patient may have laryngeal edema and stridor when the tube is removed. *Neck surgery,* such as thyroidectomy, may cause laryngeal paralysis and stridor.

Diagnostic tests
Bronchoscopy or *laryngoscopy* may precipitate laryngospasm and stridor.

Clinical considerations
• Vital signs should be taken and the airway assessed for partial obstruction.

• If airway obstruction is detected, one staff member should clear the airway with back blows or abdominal thrusts (Heimlich maneuver), while another notifies the physician. (Abrupt cessation of stridor signals complete obstruction in which the patient has inspiratory chest movement but absent breath sounds. Unable to talk, he quickly becomes lethargic and loses consciousness.)

• Emergency equipment should be kept readily available and preparations made for intubation or emergency tracheostomy and mechanical ventilation (see *Assisting with Emergency Endotracheal Intubation*).

• When the patient's condition permits, a history should be obtained and a physical examination performed.

• Diagnostic tests may include arterial blood gas analysis and chest X-rays.

Succussion splash

Description
A succussion splash is a splashing sound heard over a hollow organ or body cavity, such as the stomach or thorax, after rocking or shaking the patient's body. Indicating the presence of fluid or air and gas, this sound may be auscultated in pyloric or intestinal obstruction, a large hiatal hernia, or

hydropneumothorax. However, it may also be auscultated over a normal, empty stomach.

Sucking reflex

Description
The sucking reflex is an involuntary circumoral sucking movement in response to stimulation. Present at about 26 weeks gestational age, this reflex is initially weak and not synchronized with swallowing. It persists through infancy, becoming more discriminating during the first few months and disappearing by age 1. To elicit this response, a finger is placed in the infant's mouth. Rhythmic sucking movements are normal. Weakness or absence of these movements may indicate elevated intracranial pressure.

Syncope

Description
Syncope (or fainting) refers to transient loss of consciousness associated with impaired cerebral oxygenation. It usually occurs abruptly and lasts for seconds to minutes. Typically, the patient lies motionless with his skeletal muscles relaxed but sphincter muscles controlled. However, the depth of unconsciousness varies; some patients can hear voices or see blurred outlines, whereas others are unaware of their surroundings.

In many ways, syncope simulates death: the patient is strikingly pale with a slow, weak pulse, hypotension, and almost imperceptible breathing. If loss of consciousness lasts for 5 to 20 seconds, the patient may develop convulsive, tonic-clonic movements. However, the common sequelae of a convulsive seizure—confusion, headache, and drowsiness—do not follow syncope.

Syncope may result from cardiac and cerebrovascular disorders, hypoxemia, and postural changes in the presence of autonomic dysfunction. It may also follow vigorous coughing (tussive syncope) and emotional stress, injury, shock, or pain (vasovagal syncope, or the common faint). Hysterical syncope may also follow emotional stress but is not accompanied by other vasodepressor effects.

Possible causes
Central nervous system
Transient ischemic attack. Marked by transient neurologic deficits, these attacks may produce syncope and decreased level of consciousness.
Vagal glossopharyngeal neuralgia. In this disorder, localized pressure may trigger pain in the base of the tongue, pharynx, larynx, tonsils, and ear, resulting in syncope that lasts for several minutes.
Cardiovascular
Aortic arch syndrome. This syndrome produces syncope. The patient may have weak or abruptly absent carotid pulses and unequal or absent radial pulses.
Aortic stenosis. A cardinal late sign, syncope is accompanied by exertional dyspnea and anginal chest pain.
Cardiac dysrhythmias. Any dysrhythmia that decreases cardiac output and impairs cerebral circulation may cause syncope. Usually, other effects develop first, such as palpitations, pallor, confusion, diaphoresis, dyspnea, and hypotension. But in Adams-Stokes syndrome, syncope may occur several times daily without warning.
Carotid sinus hypersensitivity. Syncope is triggered here by compression of the carotid sinus, for example, or by wearing a tight collar. Usually, syncope lasts several minutes and is followed by mental clarity.
Orthostatic hypotension. Syncope occurs when the patient rises quickly from a recumbent position. It follows a drop of 10 to 20 mm Hg or more in systolic or diastolic blood pressure.

Hematologic
Hypoxemia. Regardless of its cause, hypoxemia may produce syncope.

Drugs
Quinidine commonly causes syncope—and possibly sudden death—associated with ventricular fibrillation. Prazosin may cause severe orthostatic hypotension and sycope, usually after the first dose. Occasionally, griseofulvin, levodopa, and indomethacin produce syncope, too.

Clinical considerations
If syncope is witnessed:
- The patient should be placed in a supine position, with his legs elevated and tight clothing loosened.
- Airway patency and vital signs should be assessed.
- If tachycardia, bradycardia, or an irregular pulse is detected, the physician should be notified and preparations made for cardiopulmonary resuscitation.

If syncope is *not witnessed:*
- A description of the episode should be obtained from the patient.
- Vital signs should be taken and the patient examined for injuries that may have occurred during a syncope-related fall.
- The physician should be notified.
- The patient should be advised to pace his activities, to rise slowly from a recumbent position, to avoid standing still for a prolonged time, and to sit or lie down as soon as he feels faint.

T

Tachycardia

Description
Tachycardia is a heart rate greater than 100 beats/minute. Usually, the patient also complains of palpitations or of his heart "racing." This common sign normally occurs in response to emotional or physical stress, such as excitement, exercise, pain, and fever. It may also result from use of stimulants, such as caffeine and tobacco. More importantly, though, tachycardia may be an early sign of a life-threatening disorder, such as cardiogenic or septic shock. When assessing for tachycardia, recognize that normal rates for children are higher than for adults (see *Normal Pediatric Vital Signs,* pp. 408 and 409.) In children, tachycardia may result from patent ductus arteriosus as well as from many of the adult causes.

Mechanism
Tachycardia represents the heart's effort to deliver more oxygen to body tissues by increasing the rate at which blood passes through the vessels. This sign can reflect overstimulation within the sinoatrial node, the atrium, the atrioventricular node, or the ventricles. Reduced cardiac output may lead to or result from tachycardia.

Possible causes
Central nervous system
Neurogenic shock. Tachycardia or bradycardia may occur.

Respiratory
Adult respiratory distress syndrome (ARDS). Besides tachycardia, ARDS causes crackles, rhonchi, dyspnea, tachypnea, nasal flaring, and grunting respirations.
Chronic obstructive pulmonary disease (COPD). Although the clinical picture varies widely in COPD, tachycardia is a common sign.
Pneumothorax. Life-threatening pneumothorax causes tachycardia and other signs of distress, such as severe dyspnea and chest pain, tachypnea, and cyanosis.
Pulmonary embolism. In this disorder, tachycardia is usually preceded by sudden dyspnea and anginal or pleuritic chest pain.

Cardiovascular
Aortic insufficiency. Accompanying tachycardia in this disorder are a "water-hammer" bounding pulse and a large, diffuse apical heave.
Aortic stenosis. Typically, this valvular disorder causes tachycardia, a weak, thready pulse, and an atrial or ventricular gallop.
Cardiac contusion. The result of blunt chest trauma, this contusion may cause tachycardia, substernal pain, dyspnea, and palpitations.
Cardiac dysrhythmias. Tachycardia may occur with a regular or irregular heart rhythm.
Cardiac tamponade. In life-threatening cardiac tamponade, tachycardia commonly occurs with pulsus paradoxus, dyspnea, and tachypnea.
Cardiogenic shock. Although many features of cardiogenic shock appear in

other types of shock, they are usually more profound here. Accompanying tachycardia are weak, thready pulse; narrowing pulse pressure; hypotension; tachypnea; cold, pale, clammy, and cyanotic skin; oliguria; restlessness; and altered level of consciousness.

Congestive heart failure. Especially common in left heart failure, tachycardia may be accompanied by ventricular gallop, fatigue, dyspnea (exertional and paroxysmal nocturnal), and orthopnea.

Hypertensive crisis. Life-threatening hypertensive crisis is characterized by tachycardia, tachypnea, diastolic blood pressure that exceeds 120 mm Hg, and systolic blood pressure that may exceed 200 mm Hg.

Hypovolemic shock. Slight tachycardia is an early sign of life-threatening hypovolemic shock.

Myocardial infarction. This life-threatening disorder may cause tachycardia or bradycardia. Its classic symptom, however, is crushing substernal chest pain that may radiate to the left arm, jaw, neck, or shoulder.

Orthostatic hypotension. Tachycardia accompanies the characteristic signs in this condition: dizziness, syncope, pallor, blurred vision, diaphoresis, and nausea.

Endocrine

Adrenocortical insufficiency. In this disorder, tachycardia commonly occurs with a weak, irregular pulse.

Pheochromocytoma. Characterized by sustained or paroxysmal hypertension, this rare tumor may also cause tachycardia and palpitations.

Thyrotoxicosis. Tachycardia is a classic feature of this thyroid disorder, as are an enlarged thyroid, nervousness, heat intolerance, weight loss despite increased appetite, diaphoresis, diarrhea, tremors, and palpitations.

Hematologic

Anemia. Tachycardia and bounding pulse are characteristic in anemia.

Hypoxemia. Tachycardia may accompany tachypnea, dyspnea, and cyanosis.

Metabolic

Diabetic ketoacidosis. This life-threatening disorder commonly produces tachycardia and a thready pulse. Its cardinal sign, though, is Kussmaul's respirations—abnormally rapid, deep breathing.

Hyperosmolar hyperglycemic nonketotic coma. Rapidly deteriorating level of consciousness is typically accompanied by tachycardia, hypotension, tachypnea, seizures, oliguria, and severe dehydration with poor skin turgor and dry mucous membranes.

Hypoglycemia. A common sign of hypoglycemia, tachycardia is accompanied by hypothermia, nervousness, trembling, fatigue, malaise, weakness, headache, hunger, nausea, diaphoresis, and moist, clammy skin.

Hyponatremia. Tachycardia is one effect of this electrolyte imbalance.

Immunologic

Anaphylactic shock. In life-threatening anaphylactic shock, tachycardia and sudden hypotension develop within minutes after exposure to an allergen, such as penicillin or an insect sting.

Psychiatric

Alcohol withdrawal syndrome. Tachycardia can occur with tachypnea, profuse diaphoresis, fever, insomnia, and anorexia.

Infection

Septic shock. Initially, septic shock produces chills, sudden fever, tachycardia, tachypnea, and possibly nausea, vomiting, and diarrhea.

Drugs

Various drugs affect the nervous system, circulatory system, or heart muscle, resulting in tachycardia. Examples of these include sympathomimetics; phenothiazines; anticholinergics, such as atropine; thyroid drugs; vasodilators, such as hydralazine and nifedipine; nitrates, such as nitroglycerin; and alpha-adrenergic blockers, such as phentolamine. Alcohol intoxication may also cause tachycardia.

Treatments
Cardiac surgery and *pacemaker malfunction* or *wire irritation* may cause tachycardia.

Diagnostic tests
Cardiac catheterization and *electrophysiologic studies* may induce transient tachycardia.

Clinical considerations
• Vital signs should be taken and the level of consciousness assessed.

• If the patient's blood pressure is increased or decreased beyond its normal range, the physician should be notified, oxygen administered, and cardiac monitoring begun. Emergency resuscitation equipment should be kept readily available.

• When the patient's condition permits, a history should be obtained and a physical examination performed.

• Diagnostic tests may include ambulatory and 12-lead EKGs, blood work, and pulmonary function studies.

Tachypnea

Description
Tachypnea is an abnormally fast respiratory rate—20 breaths or more per mintue. It is easily detected by unobtrusively counting the patient's respirations. Generally, tachypnea indicates the need to increase minute volume—the amount of air breathed each minute. It may be accompanied by an increase in tidal volume—the volume of air inhaled or exhaled per breath—resulting in hyperventilation. When assessing a child for tachypnea, the caregiver should recognize that the normal respiratory rate varies with the child's age (see *Normal Pediatric Vital Signs,* pp. 408 and 409).

Mechanism
Tachypnea may result from reduced arterial oxygen tension or arterial oxygen content, decreased perfusion, or increased oxygen demand. Heightened oxygen demand, for example, may result from exertion, anxiety, pain, and fever. Generally, respirations increase by 4 breaths/minute for every 1° F. rise in body temperature.

Tachypnea may also occur as a compensatory response to metabolic acidosis and may result from pulmonary irritation, stretch receptor stimulation, or neurologic disorders that upset medullary respiratory control.

Possible causes
Central nervous system
Head trauma. When trauma affects the brain stem, the patient may display central neurogenic hyperventilation, a form of tachypnea marked by rapid, even, and deep respirations.

Neurogenic shock. Tachypnea is characteristic in this life-threatening type of shock. It commonly occurs with apprehension, bradycardia or tachycardia, oliguria, fluctuating body temperature, and decreased level of consciousness that may progress to coma. The patient's skin is warm, dry, and perhaps flushed. He may experience nausea and vomiting.

Respiratory
Adult respiratory distress syndrome. In this life-threatening disorder, tachypnea and apprehension may be the earliest features. Tachypnea gradually worsens as fluid accumulates in the patient's lungs, causing them to stiffen.

Aspiration of a foreign body. Life-threatening upper airway obstruction may result from aspiration of a foreign body. In *partial obstruction,* the patient abruptly develops a dry, paroxysmal cough with rapid, shallow respirations.

Asthma. Tachypnea is common in life-threatening asthmatic attacks, which commonly occur at night.

Bronchiectasis. Although this disorder may produce tachypnea, its classic sign is a chronic productive cough with copious, mucopurulent, foul-smelling sputum and, occasionally, hemoptysis.

Bronchitis (chronic). Mild tachypnea may occur in this form of chronic obstructive pulmonary disease, but it is not typically a predominant sign.

Emphysema. This chronic pulmonary disorder commonly produces tachypnea accompanied by dyspnea on exertion.

Flail chest. Tachypnea usually appears early in this life-threatening disorder.

Interstitial fibrosis. In this disorder, tachypnea develops gradually and may become severe.

Lung abscess. In this abscess, tachypnea is usually paired with dyspnea and accentuated by fever. However, the chief sign is a productive cough with copious, purulent, foul-smelling, often bloody sputum.

Lung, pleural, or mediastinal tumor. This tumor may cause tachypnea along with dyspnea on exertion, cough, hemoptysis, and pleuritic chest pain.

Pneumonia (bacterial). A common sign in this infection, tachypnea is usually preceded by a painful, hacking, dry cough that rapidly becomes productive.

Pneumothorax. Tachypnea is a common sign of life-threatening pneumothorax. Typically it is accompanied by severe, sharp, and commonly unilateral chest pain.

Pulmonary edema. An early sign of this life-threatening disorder, tachypnea is accompanied by dyspnea on exertion, paroxysmal nocturnal dyspnea, and later, orthopnea.

Pulmonary embolism (acute). Tachypnea occurs suddenly in life-threatening pulmonary embolism and is usually accompanied by dyspnea. The patient may complain of anginal or pleuritic chest pain.

Pulmonary hypertension (primary). In this rare disorder, tachypnea is a late sign accompanied by dyspnea on exertion, general fatigue, weakness, and syncopal episodes. The patient may complain of anginal chest pain on exertion that may radiate to the neck.

Cardiovascular

Cardiac dysrhythmias. Depending on the patient's heart rate, tachypnea may occur along with hypotension, dizziness, palpitations, weakness, and fatigue.

Cardiac tamponade. In life-threatening tamponade, tachypnea may accompany tachycardia, dyspnea, and pulsus paradoxus.

Cardiogenic shock. Although signs of cardiogenic shock resemble signs of other types of shock, they are usually more severe. Besides tachypnea, the patient commonly has cold, pale, clammy, cyanotic skin; hypotension; tachycardia; narrowed pulse pressure; a ventricular gallop; oliguria; decreased level of consciousness; and neck vein distention.

Hypovolemic shock. An early sign of life-threatening hypovolemic shock, tachypnea is accompanied by cool, pale skin; restlessness; thirst; and mild tachycardia. As shock progresses, the patient's skin becomes clammy; his pulse, increasingly rapid and thready.

Hematologic

Anemia. Tachypnea may occur in this disorder, depending on the duration and severity of anemia.

Metabolic

Hyperosmolar hyperglycemic nonketotic coma. Rapidly deteriorating level of consciousness occurs with tachypnea, tachycardia, hypotension, seizures, oliguria, and signs of dehydration.

Immunologic

Anaphylactic shock. In this type of shock, tachypnea develops within minutes after exposure to an allergen, such as penicillin or insect venom.

Psychiatric

Alcohol withdrawal syndrome. A late sign in the acute phase of this syndrome, tachypnea typically is accompanied by anorexia, insomnia, tachycardia, fever, and diaphoresis.

Neoplastic

Mesothelioma (malignant). Often related to asbestos exposure, this pleural mass initially produces tachypnea and dyspnea on mild exertion.

Infection

Septic shock. Early in septic shock, the patient usually has tachypnea accompanied by sudden fever, chills, and possibly nausea, vomiting, and diarrhea.

Normal Pediatric Vital Signs

Vital signs	Newborn	2 years	4 years	6 years
Respiratory rate/minute				
Girls	28	26	25	24
Boys	30	28	25	24
Blood pressure (mm Hg)				
Girls	—	98/60	98/60	98/64
Boys	—	96/60	96/60	98/62
Pulse rate/minute				
Girls	130	110	100	100
Boys	130	110	100	100

Note: These values apply to children at rest.

Drugs
Tachypnea may result from an overdose of salicylates.

Clinical considerations
• A quick cardiopulmonary assessment should be performed. If cyanosis, chest pain, dyspnea, tachycardia, and hypotension are detected, the physician should be notified and emergency equipment kept readily available. The patient should be placed in a semi-Fowler position and given oxygen, as ordered.
• When the patient's condition permits, a history should be obtained and a physical examination performed.
• Diagnostic tests may include arterial blood gas analysis, chest X-rays, and an EKG.
• Vital signs should be closely monitored.

Tangentiality

Description
Tangentiality is speech characterized by tedious detail that prevents ever reaching the point of the statement. This occurs in schizophrenia and organic brain disorders.

Taste, abnormal

Description
This symptom refers to several types of taste impairment. *Ageusia*, for example, refers to complete loss of taste; *hypogeusia*, partial loss of taste; and *dysgeusia*, distorted sense of taste. In

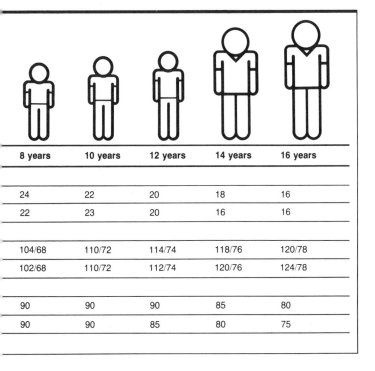

8 years	10 years	12 years	14 years	16 years
24	22	20	18	16
22	23	20	16	16
104/68	110/72	114/74	118/76	120/78
102/68	110/72	112/74	120/76	124/78
90	90	90	85	80
90	90	85	80	75

cacogeusia, food may taste unpleasant or even revolting. Taste abnormalities may result from trauma, infection, vitamin or mineral deficiency, neurologic or oral disorders, and the effects of drugs. Also, since tastes are most accurately perceived in a fluid medium, mouth dryness may interfere with taste.

Two major nonpathologic causes of impaired taste are aging, which normally reduces the number of taste buds, and heavy smoking (especially pipe smoking), which dries the tongue.

Mechanism
The sensory receptors for taste are the taste buds—concentrated over the tongue's surface and scattered over the palate, pharynx, and larynx. These buds can differentiate among sweet, salty, sour, and bitter stimuli. More complex flavors are perceived by taste and olfactory receptors together. In fact, much of what constitutes taste is actually smell; food odors typically stimulate the olfactory system more strongly than related food tastes stimulate the taste buds.

Any factor that interrupts transmission of taste stimuli to the brain may cause taste abnormalities (see *Tracing Taste Pathways to the Brain,* p. 410).

Possible causes
Central nervous system
Basilar skull fracture. When this fracture affects the cranial nerves, it may cause impaired taste. Usually, the patient is unable to taste aromatic flavors, although he can still correctly identify sweet, salty, sour, and bitter stimuli.

Tracing Taste Pathways to the Brain

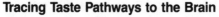

Normally, taste buds produce taste sensations by generating nerve impulses that are transmitted to the brain. When the pathway to the brain is interrupted by damage to the taste buds or the nerves that supply them, or by lesions of the temporal or parietal lobe, taste abnormalities may develop.

Third-order neurons carry the impulses from the thalamus to the sylvian fissure in the parietal cortex, where these impulses are interpreted as tastes.

Taste impulses from the front of the tongue pass to the lingual part of the trigeminal nerve, the chorda tympani, the facial nerve, and then to the brain stem.

Taste impulses from the back of the tongue and mouth move along the glossopharyngeal nerve to the lower brain stem.

Taste impulses from the base of the tongue and other pharyngeal areas travel through the vagus nerve to the brain stem.

Second-order neurons carry the impulses from the brain stem to the thalamus.

Taste impulses synapse in the brain stem at the tractus solitarius.

Bell's palsy. Taste loss involving the anterior two thirds of the tongue is common in this disorder.

Thalamic syndromes. Dejerine-Roussy syndrome, for example, may produce a distorted sense of taste.

Immunologic

Sjögren's syndrome. In this autosomal recessive disorder, impaired taste sense results from extreme mouth dryness associated with inadequate production of saliva.

Metabolic

Vitamin B_{12} deficiency. In this vitamin deficiency, hypogeusia is accompanied by an impaired sense of smell, anorexia, weight loss, abdominal discomfort, and glossitis.

Zinc deficiency. This mineral deficiency is common in patients with idiopathic hypogeusia, suggesting that zinc plays an important role in normal taste sensation.

Neoplastic

Oral cancer. Approximately half of all oral tumors involve the tongue, especially the posterior portion and the lateral borders. These tumors may destroy or damage test buds, resulting in impaired taste.

Infection

Common cold. Although impaired taste sense is a common complaint here, it is usually secondary to loss of smell.

Influenza. After this viral infection, the patient may have hypogeusia or dysgeusia.

Viral hepatitis (acute). Hypogeusia frequently precedes the jaundice of hepatitis by 1 to 2 weeks.

Drugs

Drugs that may distort taste include penicillamine, captopril, griseofulvin, lithium, rifampin, antithyroid preparations, procarbazine, vincristine, and vinblastine.

Treatments

Irradiation of the head or neck may cause excessive dryness of the mouth, resulting in impaired taste.

Clinical considerations

• A history should be obtained and the patient's taste and smell faculties evaluated.

• The patient should be instructed to modify his diet, if necessary, so that he can distinguish and enjoy as many tastes as possible.

Tearing, increased
(Epiphora)

Description

Tears normally bathe the eyes, keeping the epithelium moist and flushing away foreign bodies. Excessive production of this clear fluid—or lacrimation—results from stimulation of the lacrimal glands.

Lacrimation may be classified as psychic or neurogenic. *Psychic lacrimation* normally occurs in response to emotional or physical stress, such as pain; it is the most common cause of increased tearing. *Neurogenic lacrimation* is triggered by reflex stimulation associated with ocular trauma or inflammation or with exposure to environmental irritants, such as strong light, dry or hot wind, or airborne allergens. This type of lacrimation may also accompany eyestrain, yawning, vomiting, and laughing. (For information on decreased tearing, see *Causes of Decreased Tearing*, p. 412.)

Possible causes

Eyes, ears, nose, throat

Blepharophimosis. Increased tearing and exposure keratitis—corneal inflammation with incomplete lid closure—are common signs.

Conjunctival foreign bodies and abrasions. Increased tearing may accompany localized conjunctival injection, severe eye pain, and photophobia.

Conjunctivitis. Typically, increased tearing is accompanied by conjunctival injection and itching in this disorder.

Causes of Decreased Tearing

Decreased tearing, or hyposecretion, makes the patient's eyes uncomfortably dry. Usually, this sympton is associated with aging. However, it may also result from the following causes:

Anticholinergics. Decreased tearing commonly follows administration of anticholinergic (mydriatic) agents, such as atropine, scopolamine, cyclopentolate, and tropicamide.

Bonnevie-Ullrich syndrome. Characterized by congenital absence of the lacrimal gland, this syndrome also causes decreased tearing.

Keratoconjunctivitis sicca (dry eye syndrome). In this syndrome, atrophy of the lacrimal glands curtails tear production.

Ocular trauma. Decreased tearing may accompany healing and scar formation following acute ocular trauma.

Sarcoidosis. Decreased tearing results from inflammation of the lacrimal and salivary glands in this syndrome.

Stevens-Johnson syndrome. In this syndrome, decreased tearing is accompanied by purulent conjunctivitis and severe eye pain.

Vitamin A deficiency. Typically, this vitamin deficiency causes decreased tearing and poor night vision.

Treatment of nontraumatic decreased tearing usually involves a preparation of artificial tears in drops or ointment.

Corneal abrasion. Marked by severe corneal pain that is aggravated by blinking, this injury also causes increased tearing.

Corneal foreign body. When a foreign body lodges in the cornea, the patient will have increased tearing, blurred vision, a foreign body sensation, photophobia, eye pain, miosis, and conjunctival injection.

Corneal ulcers. In this vision-threatening disorder, increased tearing is accompanied by severe photophobia and eye pain.

Dacryocystitis. Increased tearing and purulent discharge are the chief complaints in this disorder, which is typically unilateral.

Episcleritis. Commonly unilateral, this disorder causes increased tearing, photophobia, and —if the sclera is inflamed —eye pain and tenderness on palpation.

Lid contractions. Here, increased tearing usually results from stricture of the canaliculi.

Punctum misplacement. Increased tearing is characteristic when ectropion involves the punctum, causing misplacement.

Raeder's syndrome. This syndrome is characterized by periodic symptomatic attacks for 5 minutes or longer. The patient may have increased tearing, ptosis, abnormal pupillary response, ipsilateral headache, and anhidrosis of the face and neck.

Scleritis. This rare, chronic disorder causes increased tearing, photophobia, and severe eye pain with tenderness on palpation.

Trachoma. An early sign of this disorder, increased tearing is accompanied by visible conjunctival follicles, red and edematous eyelids, pain, photophobia, and exudation.

Endocrine

Thyrotoxicosis. This disorder may cause increased tearing, usually in both eyes.

Skin

Psoriasis vulgaris. When these lesions affect the eyelids and extend into the conjunctiva, they may cause irritation with increased tearing and a foreign body sensation.

Infection

Herpes zoster. Increased tearing usually occurs when herpes zoster affects the trigeminal nerve.

Drugs

Miotics, such as pilocarpine, may increase tearing.

Clinical considerations

• A history should be obtained and an eye examination performed.

• Diagnostic tests may include culture and sensitivity testing of tear specimens and the Schirmer's test to measure production and secretion and to irrigate the lacrimal drainage system.

• The patient may be isolated until the results of tear specimen culture and sensitivity tests are obtained.

• The patient should be advised not to touch the unaffected eye to avoid possible cross-contamination.

Tenesmus, rectal

Description

Rectal tenesmus is the spasmodic contraction of the anal sphincter with a persistent urge to defecate and involuntary, ineffective straining. This occurs in inflammatory bowel disorders, such as ulcerative colitis and Crohn's disease, and in rectal tumors. Often painful, rectal tenesmus accompanies passage of small amounts of blood, pus, or mucus.

Tenesmus, urinary

Description

Urinary tenesmus is the persistent, ineffective, painful straining to empty the bladder, This results from irritation of nerve endings in the bladder mucosa, caused by infection or an indwelling catheter.

Terry's nails

Description

Terry's nails refers to nails with a white, opaque surface over more than 80% of the nail and a normal pink distal edge. This sign is often associated with cirrhosis.

Thornton's sign

Description

Thornton's sign is severe flank pain resulting from nephrolithiasis.

Thrill

Description

A thrill is a palpable sensation resulting from the vibration of a loud murmur or from turbulent blood flow in an aneurysm. Thrills are associated with heart murmurs of grades IV to VI and may be palpable over major arteries (see "Bruits" and "Murmurs").

Tibialis sign

Description

Tibialis sign is the involuntary dorsiflexion and inversion of the foot upon brisk, voluntary flexion of the patient's knee and hip, occurring in spastic paralysis of the lower limb.

To detect this sign, the patient is placed in a supine position with his leg flexed at the hip and knee so that the thigh touches the abdomen. Or he can be placed prone with his leg flexed at the knee so that the calf touches the thigh. If this sign is present, dorsiflexion of the great toe or of all toes and inversion of the foot may be observed. Normally, plantar flexion of the foot occurs with this action.

Tics

Description

A tic is an involuntary, repetitive movement of a specific group of muscles—usually those of the face, neck, shoulders, trunk, and hands. Typically, this sign occurs suddenly and intermittently. It may involve a single isolated movement, such as lip smacking, grimacing, blinking, sniffing, tongue thrusting, throat clearing, hitching up one shoulder, or protruding the chin. Or it may involve a complex set of movements. Mild tics, such as twitching of an eyelid, are especially common.

Usually, tics are psychogenic and may be aggravated by stress or anxiety. However, they are also associated with one rare affliction—Gilles de la Tourette's syndrome. Psychogenic tics, though, often begin between the ages of 5 and 10 as voluntary, coordinated, and purposeful actions that the child feels compelled to perform to decrease anxiety. Unless the tics are severe, the child may be unaware of them. The tics may subside as the child matures, or they may persist into adulthood.

To distinguish tics from minor seizures, the examiner must remember that tics are not associated with transient loss of consciousness or amnesia.

Psychotherapy and administration of tranquilizers may relieve the source of anxiety causing the tic. Many patients with Gilles de la Tourette's syndrome receive haloperidol or pimozide to control tics and reduce anxiety.

Tinel's sign

Description

Tinel's sign is the presence of distal paresthesias on percussion over an in-

jured nerve in an extremity, as in carpal tunnel syndrome. To elicit this sign in the patient's wrist, the area over the median nerve on the wrist's flexor surface is tapped. This sign indicates a partial lesion or the early regeneration of the nerve.

Tinnitus

Description

Tinnitus literally means ringing in the ears, although many other abnormal sounds fall under this term. For example, tinnitus may be described as the sound of escaping air, running water, or the inside of a seashell, or as a sizzling, buzzing, or humming noise. Occasionally, it is described as a roaring or musical sound. This common symptom may be unilateral or bilateral and constant or intermittent. Although the brain can adjust to or suppress constant tinnitus, intermittent tinnitus may be so disturbing that some patients contemplate suicide as their only source of relief.

Commonly resulting from ear disorders, tinnitus may also stem from cardiovascular and systemic disorders and from the effects of drugs. Nonpathologic causes of tinnitus include acute anxiety and presbycusis.

Tinnitus can be classified in several ways. *Subjective tinnitus* (nonvibratory or nonpulsatile tinnitus) is heard only by the patient, while *objective tinnitus* (vibratory or pulsatile tinnitus) is also heard by the observer who places a stethoscope near the patient's affected ear. *Tinnitus aurium* refers to noise that the patient hears in his ears; *tinnitus cerebri*, to noise that he hears in his head.

Mechanism

No matter how tinnitus is classified, its pathophysiology remains the same. This symptom reflects stimulation of sensory auditory neurons, resulting in transmission of a sound impulse.

Possible causes

Eyes, ears, nose, throat

Acoustic neuroma. An early symptom of this eighth cranial nerve tumor, tinnitus precedes unilateral sensorineural hearing loss and vertigo.

Ear canal obstruction. When cerumen or a foreign body blocks the ear canal, tinnitus may occur with conductive hearing loss, itching, and a feeling of fullness or pain in the ear.

Eustachian tube patency. Normally, the eustachian tube remains closed, except during swallowing. However, persistent patency of this tube can cause tinnitus, audible breath sounds, loud and distorted voice sounds, and a sense of fullness in the ear.

Glomus jugulare or tympanicum tumor. Usually, vibratory tinnitus is the first symptom of this tumor.

Labyrinthitis (suppurative). In this disorder, tinnitus may accompany sudden, severe attacks of vertigo, unilateral or bilateral sensorineural hearing loss, nystagmus, dizziness, nausea, and vomiting.

Ménière's disease. Most common in men between the ages of 55 and 65, this labyrinthine disease is characterized by attacks of low-pitched tinnitus, vertigo, and fluctuating sensorineural hearing loss. Usually, these attacks are unilateral and last from 10 minutes to several hours; they occur over a few days or weeks followed by a remission.

Ossicle dislocation. Acoustic trauma—such as a slap on the ear—may cause ossicle dislocation, resulting in tinnitus, sensorineural hearing loss, and bleeding from the middle ear.

Otitis externa (acute). Although not a major complaint, tinnitus may result if debris in the external ear canal impinges on the tympanic membrane.

Otitis media. This infection may cause tinnitus and conductive hearing loss. However, its more characteristic features include ear pain, a red and bulging tympanic membrane, high fever, chills, and dizziness.

Otosclerosis. In this disorder, the patient may describe ringing, roaring, or whistling tinnitus or a combination of these sounds.

Palatal myoclonus. In this disorder, muscles of the palate contract rhythmically—either intermittently or continuously—causing a clicking sound in the ear and vibratory tinnitus.

Tympanic membrane perforation. In this disorder, tinnitus and hearing loss go hand-in-hand. However, tinnitus is usually the chief complaint in a small perforation; hearing loss, in a larger one. Typically, these symptoms develop suddenly and may be accompanied by pain, vertigo, and a feeling of fullness in the ear.

Cardiovascular

Atherosclerosis of the carotid artery. In this disorder, the patient has constant tinnitus that can be stopped by applying pressure over the carotid artery.

Hypertension. Bilateral, high-pitched tinnitus may occur in severe hypertension.

Intracranial arteriovenous malformation. A large malformation may cause pulsating tinnitus accompanied by a bruit over the mastoid process.

Musculoskeletal

Cervical spondylosis. In this degenerative disorder, osteophytic growths may compress the vertebral arteries, resulting in tinnitus. Typically, a stiff neck and pain aggravated by activity produce tinnitus.

Hematologic

Anemia. Severe anemia may produce mild, reversible tinnitus accompanied by dim vision, syncope, and irritability.

Environmental

Noise. Chronic exposure to noise, especially high-pitched sounds, may damage the ear's hair cells, causing tinnitus and a bilateral hearing loss. These symptoms may be temporary or permanent.

Drugs

An overdose of salicylates frequently causes reversible tinnitus. Quinine, alcohol, and indomethacin may also cause reversible tinnitus. Common drugs that may cause irreversible tinnitus include the aminoglycoside antibiotics (especially kanamycin, streptomycin, and gentamicin) and vancomycin.

Clinical considerations
• A history should be obtained and an ear examination performed.
• Since tinnitus usually cannot be treated successfully, the patient must tolerate this symptom. Vasodilators, tranquilizers, and anticonvulsants may be ordered.
• If appropriate, the patient should be encouraged to consider biofeedback training or a tinnitus masker.
• A tinnitus masker produces a band of noise about 1800 Hz, which helps block out tinnitus without hampering hearing. Also, a hearing aid may be prescribed to amplify environmental sounds, thereby obscuring tinnitus. At times, a device that combines features of a masker and hearing aid may be used to block out tinnitus.

Tommasi's sign

Description
Tommasi's sign is the absence of hair on the posterolateral calf, occurring in males with gout.

Tongue, enlarged

Description
An enlarged tongue is an increase in the tongue's size, causing it to protrude from the mouth. Its causes include Down's syndrome, acromegaly, lymphangioma, Beckwith's syndrome, and congenital micrognathia. An enlarged tongue can also stem from cancer of the tongue, amyloidosis, and neurofibromatosis.

Tongue, fissured

Description
Tongue fissures are shallow or deep grooves of the dorsum of the tongue. Usually a congenital defect, tongue fissures occur normally in about 10% of the population. However, deep fissures may promote collection of food particles, leading to chronic inflammation and tenderness.

Tongue, hairy

Description
Hairy tongue is hypertrophy and elongation of the tongue's filiform papillae. Normally, white, the papillae may turn yellow, brown, or black from bacteria, food, tobacco, coffee, or dyes in drugs and food. Hairy tongue may also result from antibiotic therapy, irradiation of the head and neck, chronic debilitating disorders, and habitual use of mouthwashes containing oxidizing or astringent agents.

Tongue, magenta cobblestone

Description
Magenta cobblestone tongue is swelling and hyperemia of the tongue, forming rows of elevated fungiform and filiform papillae that give the tongue a magenta-colored, cobblestone appearance. It is most often a sign of vitamin B_2 (riboflavin) deficiency.

Tongue, red

Description
Red tongue is a patchy or uniform redness (ranging from pink to magenta)

of the tongue, which may be swollen and smooth, rough, or fissured. It usually indicates glossitis, resulting from emotional stress or nutritional disorders, such as pernicious anemia, Plummer-Vinson syndrome, pellagra, sprue, and folic acid and vitamin B deficiency.

Tongue, smooth

Description
A smooth tongue is the absence or atrophy of the filiform papillae, causing a smooth (patchy or uniform), glossy, red tongue. This primary sign of undernutrition results from anemia and vitamin B deficiency.

Tongue, swollen

Description
A swollen tongue results from edema of the tongue. It is most commonly associated with pernicious anemia, pellagra, hypothyroidism, and allergic angioneurotic edema.

Tongue ulcers

Description
Tongue ulcers are circumscribed necrotic lesions of the dorsum, margin, tip, and inferior surface of the tongue. Ulcers most commonly result from biting, chewing, or burning of the tongue. They may also stem from Type I herpes simplex virus, tuberculosis, histoplasmosis, and cancer of the tongue.

Tongue, white

Description
A white tongue refers to a uniform white coating or plaques on the tongue. Lesions associated with a white tongue may be premalignant or malignant and may require a biopsy. *Necrotic white lesions*—collections of cells, bacteria, and debris—are painful and can be scraped from the tongue. They often appear in children, commonly resulting from candidiasis and thermal burns. *Keratotic white lesions*—thickened, keratinized patches—are usually asymptomatic and cannot be scraped from the tongue. These lesions commonly result from alcohol use and local irritation from tobacco smoke or other substances.

Tonic neck reflex

Description
The tonic neck reflex is the extension of the limbs on the side to which the head is turned and flexion of the opposite limbs. In the neonate, this normal reflex appears between 28 and 32 weeks gestational age, diminishes as voluntary muscle control increases, and disappears by 4 months of age. The absence or persistence of this reflex may indicate central nervous system damage. To elicit this response, the infant is placed supine, then his head is turned to one side.

Tooth discoloration

Description
Tooth discoloration is a bluish yellow or gray cast to the teeth that may result from hypoplasia of the dentin and pulp, nerve damage, or caries. Yellow teeth may indicate caries. Mottling and staining suggest fluorine excess and may also be associated with the effects of certain drugs, such as tetracycline. Tooth discoloration (and small tooth size) may occur in osteogenesis imperfecta.

Tophi

Description
Tophi are deposits of sodium urate crystals in cartilage, soft tissue, synovial membranes, and tendon sheaths, producing painless nodular swellings, a classic symptom of gout. Tophi appear commonly on the ears, hands, and feet. They may erode the skin, producing open lesions, and cause gross deformity, limiting joint mobility. Inflammatory flare-ups may occur.

Tracheal deviation

Description
Normally, the trachea is located at the midline of the neck—except at the bifurcation, where it shifts slightly toward the right. Visible deviation from its normal position signals an underlying condition that can compromise pulmonary function and possibly cause respiratory distress (see *Detecting Slight Tracheal Deviation*). A hallmark of life-threatening tension pneumothorax, this sign occurs in disorders that produce mediastinal shift due to asymmetrical thoracic volume or pressure. In elderly persons, tracheal deviation to the right often stems from an elongated, atherosclerotic aortic arch, but this deviation is not considered abnormal.

Possible causes
Respiratory
Atelectasis. Extensive lung collapse can produce tracheal deviation toward the affected side.
Mediastinal tumor. Often asymptomatic in its early stages, this tumor, when large, can press against the trachea and nearby structures, causing tracheal deviation and dysphagia.
Pleural effusion. A large pleural effusion can shift the mediastinum to the contralateral side, producing tracheal deviation.
Pulmonary fibrosis. Asymmetrical fibrosis can cause tracheal deviation as the mediastinum shifts toward the affected side.
Pulmonary tuberculosis. With a large cavitation, tracheal deviation toward the affected side accompanies asymmetrical chest excursion, dullness on percussion, increased tactile fremitus, amphoric breath sounds, and inspiratory crackles.
Tension pneumothorax. This acute, life-threatening condition produces tracheal deviation toward the unaffected side.

Cardiovascular
Thoracic aortic aneurysm. This disorder usually causes the trachea to deviate to the right.

Endocrine
Retrosternal thyroid. This anatomic abnormality can displace the trachea. The gland is felt as a movable neck mass above the suprasternal notch.

Gastrointestinal
Hiatal hernia. Intrusion of abdominal viscera into the pleural space causes tracheal deviation toward the unaffected side.

Musculoskeletal
Kyphoscoliosis. This disorder can cause rib cage distortion and mediastinal shift, producing tracheal deviation toward the compressed lung.

Clinical considerations
If the patient exhibits signs of respiratory distress:
• The physician should be notified immediately and emergency equipment kept readily available.
• The patient should be placed in a semi-Fowler position and given oxygen, as ordered.
• Preparations should be made for possible intubation or chest tube insertion.

If no signs of respiratory distress are present:
• A history should be obtained and a physical examination performed.

Detecting Slight Tracheal Deviation

Although gross tracheal deviation will be visible, detection of slight deviation requires palpation and perhaps even an X-ray. Palpation is attempted first.

With the tip of the index finger, the examiner locates the patient's trachea by palpating between the sternocleidomastoid muscles. Then she compares the trachea's position to an imaginary line drawn vertically through the suprasternal notch. Any deviation from midline is usually considered abnormal.

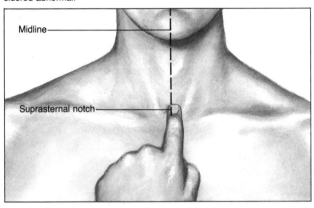

Midline

Suprasternal notch

• Diagnostic tests may include chest X-ray, EKG, and arterial blood gas analysis.

• Because tracheal deviation usually signals a severe underlying disorder that can cause respiratory distress at any time, the patient's respiratory and cardiac status should be monitored and emergency equipment kept readily available.

Tracheal tugging
(Cardarelli's sign, Castellino's sign, Oliver's sign)

Description

Tracheal tugging is a visible recession of the larynx and trachea that occurs in synchrony with cardiac systole. It commonly results from an aneusysm or a tumor near the aortic arch and may signal dangerous compression or obstruction of major airways. The tugging movement, best observed with the patient's neck hyperextended, reflects abnormal transmission of aortic pulsations because of compression and distortion of the heart, esophagus, great vessels, airways, and nerves.

Possible causes

Cardiovascular

Aortic arch aneurysm. A large aneurysm can distort and compress surrounding tissues and structures, producing tracheal tugging.

Endocrine

Thymoma. This rare tumor can cause tracheal tugging if it develops in the anterior mediastinum.

Neoplastic

Hodgkin's lymphoma. Development of a tumor adjacent to the aortic arch can cause tracheal tugging.

Non-Hodgkin's lymphoma. Tracheal tugging may reflect anterior mediastinal lymphadenopathy or tumor development next to the aortic arch.

Clinical considerations

If the patient exhibits signs of respiratory distress:

• The physician should be notified immediately and emergency equipment kept readily available.

• The patient should be placed in a semi-Fowler position and given oxygen, as ordered.

• Preparations should be made for possible intubation.

If no signs of respiratory distress are present:

• A history should be obtained and a physical examination performed.

• Diagnostic tests may include chest X-ray, computed tomography scan, lymphangiography, aortography, bone marrow biopsy, liver biopsy, echocardiography, and a complete blood count.

• The patient should be observed for signs and symptoms of respiratory depression.

Transference

Description

Transference is an unconscious process of transferring feelings and attitudes originally associated with important figures, such as parents, to another. Used therapeutically in psychoanalysis, transference can also occur in other settings and relationships.

Tremors

Description

Tremors are rhythmic, purposeless, quivering movements resulting from the involuntary, alternating contraction and relaxation of opposing groups of skeletal muscles. They are typical of extrapyramidal or cerebellar disorders and can also result from certain drugs.

Tremors can be characterized by their location, amplitude, and frequency. They are classified as resting, intention, or postural. *Resting tremors* occur only when an extremity is at rest and subside with movement. They include the classic pill–rolling tremor of Parkinson's disease. Conversely, *intention tremors* occur only with movement and subside with rest. *Postural (or action) tremors* appear when an extremity or the trunk is actively held in a particular posture or position. A slow postural tremor is known as an *essential tremor*. Tremors may also be elicited, such as asterixis—the characteristic flapping tremor in hepatic failure (see "Asterixis").

Stress or emotional upset tends to aggravate a tremor; alcohol use often diminishes it.

Possible causes

Central nervous system

Benign familial essential tremor. This disorder of early adulthood produces a bilateral essential tremor that typically begins in the fingers and hands and may spread to the head, jaw, lips, and tongue. Laryngeal involvement may result in a quavering voice.

Cerebellar tumor. Intention tremor may be an early sign of this disorder.

General paresis. This effect of neurosyphilis may cause an intention tremor accompanied by clonus, a positive Babinski's reflex, ataxia, Argyll Robertson pupils, and a diffuse, dull headache.

Multiple sclerosis (MS). Intention tremor may be an early sign of MS. Like the disorder's other effects, it tends to wax and wane.

Thalamic syndrome. Central midbrain syndromes are heralded by contralateral ataxic tremors and other abnormal movements. *Anteromedial–inferior thalamic syndrome* produces varying combinations of tremor, deep sensory loss, and hemiataxia.

Parkinson's disease. Tremors, a classic early sign of this degenerative disease, begin in the fingers and may eventually affect the foot, eyelids, jaw, lips, and tongue. The slow, regular, rhythmic resting (or occasionally intention) tremor takes the form of flexion–extension or abduction–adduction of the fingers or hand, or pronation–supination of the hand. Flexion–extension of the fingers combined with abduction–adduction of the thumb yields the characteristic pill–rolling tremor.

Leg involvement produces flexion–extension foot movement. Lightly closing the eyelids causes them to flutter. The jaw may move up and down, and the lips may purse. The tongue, when protruded, may move in and out of the mouth in tempo with tremors elsewhere in the body. The rate of the tremor holds constant over time, but amplitude varies.

Endocrine

Thyrotoxicosis. Neuromuscular effects of this disorder include a rapid, fine intention tremor of the hands and tongue, along with clonus, hyperreflexia, and Babinski's reflex.

Hematologic

Porphyria. Involvement of the basal ganglia in porphyria can produce resting tremor with rigidity, accompanied by chorea and athetosis.

Metabolic

Alkalosis. Severe alkalosis may produce a severe intention tremor, along with twitching, carpopedal spasms, agitation, diaphoresis, and hyperventilation.

Hypercapnia. Elevated PCO_2 levels may result in a rapid, fine intention tremor.

Hypoglycemia. Acute hypoglycemia may produce a rapid, fine intention tremor accompanied by confusion, weakness, tachycardia, diaphoresis, and cold, clammy skin.

Kwashiorkor. Coarse intention and resting tremors may occur in the advanced stages of this rare disease.

Wernicke's disease. Intention tremor is an early sign of this thiamine deficiency.

Wilson's disease. This disorder of abnormal copper metabolism produces slow "wing–flapping" tremors in the arms and pill–rolling tremors in the hands; these appear early in the disease and progressively worsen.

Psychiatric

Alcohol withdrawal syndrome. Acute alcohol withdrawal following long–term dependence may first be manifested by resting and intention tremors that appear as soon as 7 hours after the last drink and progressively worsen.

Environmental

Manganese toxicity. Early signs of manganese poisoning include resting tremor, chorea, propulsive gait, cogwheel rigidity, personality changes, amnesia, and masklike facies.

Drugs

Phenothiazines (particularly piperazine derivatives, such as fluphenazine) and other antipsychotics may cause resting and pill–rolling tremors. Infrequently, metoclopramide and metyrosine also cause these tremors. Lithium toxicity, sympathomimetics (such as terbutaline and pseudoephedrine), amphetamines, and phenytoin can all cause essential tremors that disappear with dose reduction.

Clinical considerations

• A history should be obtained and a physical examination performed.

• Severe intention tremors may interfere with the patient's ability to perform activities of daily living. The patient should be assisted with these activities as necessary, and precautions taken against possible injury during such activities as walking or eating.

Trendelenburg's test

Description

Trendelenburg's test is a demonstration of valvular incompetence of the saphenous vein and inefficiency of the communicating veins at different levels. To perform this test, the examiner raises the patient's legs above the heart level until the veins empty; then she rapidly lowers them. If the valves are incompetent, the veins immediately distend.

Performing the Jaw Jerk Test

If the patient reports difficulty in opening his mouth, the jaw jerk test should be performed, because even slight trismus may indicate an otherwise asymptomatic, mild localized tetanus. To elicit this important reflex, the examiner asks the patient to relax his jaw and slightly open his mouth. Then the examiner places her index finger over the middle of the patient's chin and firmly taps it with a reflex hammer.

Normally, this tap produces sudden jaw closing. Then an inhibitory mechanism abruptly halts motor nerve activity, and the mouth remains closed. In trismus, however, this inhibitor mechanism fails and motor nerve activity increases, causing immediate spasm of jaw muscles.

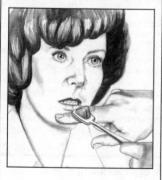

Trismus
(Lockjaw)

Description

Trismus is a prolonged and painful tonic spasm of the masticatory jaw muscles. It is a characteristic early symptom of tetanus, but can also result from drug therapy. Occasionally, a milder form may be associated with neuromuscular involvement in other disorders, or with infection or disease of the jaw, teeth, parotid glands, or tonsils. A jaw jerk test is performed to determine the presence of trismus (see *Performing the Jaw Jerk Test*).

Mechanisn

Trismus is produced by the neuromuscular effects of tetanospasmin, a potentially lethal exotoxin.

Possible causes

Central nervous system
Seizure disorders. Trismus, along with spasms of other facial muscles, a limb, and the trunk, commonly occurs during a generalized tonic–clonic seizure.

Eyes, ears, nose, throat
Temporomandibular joint syndrome. This syndrome causes trismus, facial pain, and mandibular dysfunction.

Metabolic
Hypocalcemia. Severe hypocalcemia can produce trismus and cramping spasms in virtually all muscle groups, except those of the eye.

Environmental
Tetanus. This acute, life–threatening infection is heralded by trismus, typically appearing within 14 days of initial infection. The painful spasms increase in frequency and intensity during the initial disease stage, then gradually subside.

Strychnine poisoning. In this potentially fatal condition, tonic seizures characterized by trismus, leg muscle rigidity, and respiratory muscle spasm follow early symptoms of irritability and twitching.

Rabies. Trismus often develops after a prodromal period of fever, headache, photophobia, hyperesthesia, and increasing restlessness and agitation.

Drugs

Phenothiazines (particularly the piperazine derivatives, such as fluphenazine) and other antipsychotics may produce an acute dystonic reaction marked by trismus, involuntary facial movements, and tonic spasms in the limbs. These complications usually occur early in drug therapy, sometimes after the initial dose.

Clinical considerations

• A history should be obtained and a neurologic examination performed.

• A quiet environment should be maintained, the patient's room darkened, and all stimulation kept to a minimum.

• Sedatives should be administered, as ordered.

• If the patient has tetanus, ryngeal or respiratory muscle spasm is a constant threat during the acute phase. Vital signs should be monitored frequently and oxygen and emergency airway equipment kept readily available.

• As ordered, human tetanus immune globulin, which neutralizes unbound toxins, should be administered. The patient should be told about the importance of annual booster injections to ensure immunization.

Troisier's sign

Description

Troisier's sign is the enlargement of a single lymph node, usually in the left supraclavicular group. It indicates metastasis from a primary carcinoma in the upper abdomen, often the stomach. To detect this sign, the examiner has the patient sit erect facing her. She palpates the region behind the sternocleidomastoid muscle as the patient performs Valsalva's maneuver. Although the enlarged node often lies so deep that it escapes detection, it may rise and become palpable with this maneuver.

Trousseau's sign

Description

Trousseau's sign is a test for latent tetany in which carpal spasm is induced by inflating a sphygmomanometer cuff on the upper arm for four minutes to a pressure between the patient's diastolic and systolic readings. The patient's head and fingers assume the "obstetrical hand" position, with wrist and metacarpophalangeal joints flexed, interphalangeal joints extended, and fingers and thumb adducted (see also "Carpopedal Spasm").

Tunnel vision
(Gunbarrel vision, tubular vision)

Description

Tunnel vision is typically described as the sensation of looking through a tunnel or gun barrel (see *Comparing Tunnel Vision and Normal Vision*, p. 424). It may be unilateral or bilateral and usually develops gradually. This abnormality occurs in chronic open–angle glaucoma, advanced retinal degeneration, and laser photocoagulation therapy. The sensation results from severe constriction of the visual field that leaves only a small central area of sight.

Tunnel vision is also a common complaint of malingerers and can be verified or discounted by visual field examination performed by an ophthalmologist.

Possible causes

Eyes, ears, nose, throat

Chronic open–angle glaucoma. In this insidious disorder, bilateral tunnel vi-

Comparing Tunnel Vision and Normal Vision

The patient with tunnel vision experiences drastic constriction of his peripheral visual field. The diagrams here convey the extent of this constriction, comparing test findings for normal and tunnel vision.

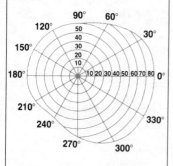

Normal field of vision in the right eye, as shown on a perimetry chart.

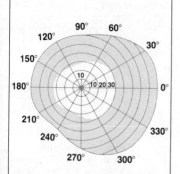

Tunnel vision in the right eye, as shown on a perimetry chart.

sion occurs late and slowly progresses to complete blindness.

Retinal pigmentary degeneration. This group of hereditary disorders, such as retinitis pigmentosa, produces an annular scotoma that progresses concentrically, causing tunnel vision and eventually resulting in complete blindness, usually by age 50.

Treatments

Tunnel vision can result from *laser photocoagulation therapy*, which aims to correct retinal detachment.

Clinical considerations

• A history should be obtained to determine the progression of vision loss and an ophthalmologic examination performed.
• Diagnostic tests include tonometry, perimeter cuts, and visual field tests.
• To protect the patient from injury, all potentially dangerous objects should be removed and the patient oriented to his surroundings.
• The patient should be taught to move his eyes from side to side when he walks to avoid bumping into objects.

Twitching

Description

Twitching is a nonspecific, intermittent contraction of muscles or muscle bundles (see "Fasciculations" and "Tics").

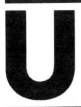

Uremic frost

Description
Uremic frost is a fine white powder, believed to be urate crystals, that covers the skin. It is a characteristic sign of end-stage renal failure, or uremia. Urea compounds and other waste substances that cannot be excreted by the kidneys in urine are excreted in sweat, and remain as powdery deposits on the skin when the sweat evaporates. The frost typically appears on the face, neck, axillae, groin, and genitalia.

Because of advances in managing renal failure, uremic frost is now relatively rare. However, it does occur in patients with chronic renal failure who, because of their advanced age or the severity of their accompanying illnesses (such as extensive neurologic deterioration), do not undergo dialysis.

Urinary frequency

Description
Urinary frequency refers to increased incidence of the urge to void. Usually resulting from decreased bladder capacity, frequency is a cardinal sign of urinary tract infection. However, it can also stem from other urologic disorders, neurologic dysfunction, and pressure on the bladder from a nearby tumor or from organ enlargement (as with pregnancy).

Urinary frequency may be reported by the patient with polyuria—an increase in total daily urine output (see "Polyuria").

Possible causes
Central nervous system
Multiple sclerosis (MS). Urinary frequency, urgency, and incontinence are common urologic findings in MS.

Spinal cord lesion. Incomplete cord transection results in urinary frequency and urgency when voluntary control of sphincter function weakens. Added urologic effects may include hesitancy and bladder distention.

Gastrointestinal
Rectal tumor. The pressure exerted by this tumor on the bladder may cause urinary frequency.

Genitourinary
Benign prostatic hypertrophy. Prostatic enlargement causes urinary frequency, along with nocturia and possibly incontinence and hematuria.

Bladder calculus. Bladder irritation may lead to urinary frequency and urgency, dysuria, hematuria, and suprapubic pain from bladder spasms.

Bladder cancer. Urinary frequency, dribbling, and nocturia may develop from bladder irritation.

Prostatic cancer. In advanced stages, urinary frequency may occur.

Prostatitis. Acute prostatitis commonly produces urinary frequency, along with urgency, dysuria, nocturia, and purulent urethral discharge.

Urethral stricture. Bladder decompensation produces urinary frequency, along with urgency and nocturia.

Urinary tract infection. Affecting the urethra (urethritis), the bladder (cystitis), or the kidneys (pyelonephritis), this common cause of urinary frequency also may produce urgency, dysuria, hematuria, cloudy urine, and, in males, urethral discharge.

Musculoskeletal

Reiter's syndrome. In this self-limiting syndrome, urinary frequency occurs with other symptoms of acute urethritis 1 to 2 weeks after sexual contact.

Psychiatric

Anxiety neurosis. Morbid anxiety produces urinary frequency and other types of genitourinary dysfunction, such as dysuria, impotence, and frigidity.

Obstetrics-Gynecology

Reproductive tract tumor. A tumor in the female reproductive tract may compress the bladder, causing urinary frequency.

Treatments

Radiation therapy may cause bladder inflammation, leading to urinary frequency.

Clinical considerations

• A history should be obtained and a physical examination performed.

• Diagnostic tests may include urinalysis, culture and sensitivity tests, imaging tests, ultrasonography, cystoscopy, and cystometry.

Urinary hesitancy

Description

Hesitancy is difficulty starting a urinary stream. It can result from a urinary tract infection, a partial lower urinary tract obstruction, a neuromuscular disorder, or use of certain drugs. Occurring at all ages and in both sexes, it is most common in older men with prostatic enlargement. Hesitancy usually arises gradually, often going unnoticed until urinary retention causes bladder distention and discomfort.

Possible causes

Central nervous system

Spinal cord lesion. A lesion below the micturition center that has destroyed the sacral nerve roots causes urinary hesitancy, tenesmus, and constant dribbling from retention and overflow incontinence.

Genitourinary

Benign prostatic hypertrophy. Clinical features of this disorder depend on the extent of prostatic enlargement and the lobes affected. Urinary hesitancy is an early characteristic finding in this disorder.

Prostatic cancer. In advanced stages of this disorder, urinary hesitancy may occur.

Urethral stricture. Partial obstruction of the lower urinary tract secondary to trauma or infection produces urinary hesitancy, tenesmus, and decreased force and caliber of the urinary stream.

Urinary tract infection. Urinary hesitancy may be associated with this infection.

Drugs

Anticholinergics and drugs with anticholinergic properties (such as tricyclic antidepressants and some nasal decongestant preparations and cold remedies) may cause urinary hesitancy.

Clinical considerations

• A history should be obtained and a physical examination performed.

• Diagnostic tests may include cystometrography or observation cystourethroscopy.

• The patient's voiding pattern should be monitored and the bladder palpated frequently to assess for distention.

• Heat treatments should be applied to the perineum or the abdomen to enhance muscle relaxation and aid urination.

• Credé's maneuver may be used to start urinary flow.

Urinary urgency

Description

Urinary urgency is a sudden compelling urge to urinate, accompanied by bladder pain. It is a classic symptom of urinary tract infection. As inflammation decreases bladder capacity, discomfort results from the accumulation of even small amounts of urine. Repeated, frequent voiding in an effort to alleviate this discomfort produces urine output of only a few milliliters at each voiding.

Urgency without bladder pain may point to an upper motor neuron lesion that has disrupted bladder control.

Possible causes

Central nervous system

Amyotrophic lateral sclerosis (ALS). ALS occasionally produces urinary urgency.

Multiple sclerosis (MS). Urinary urgency can occur with or without the frequent urinary tract infections that often accompany MS. Like the other variable effects of MS, urinary urgency may wax and wane.

Spinal cord lesion. Urinary urgency can result from incomplete cord transection when voluntary control of sphincter function weakens.

Genitourinary

Bladder calculus. Bladder irritation can lead to urinary urgency and frequency, dysuria, hematuria, and suprapubic pain from bladder spasms.

Urethral stricture. Bladder decompensation produces urinary urgency, frequency, and nocturia.

Urinary tract infection. Urinary urgency is commonly associated with this infection.

Musculoskeletal

Reiter's syndrome. In this self-limiting syndrome that primarily affects males, urgency occurs with other symptoms of acute urethritis 1 to 2 weeks after sexual contact.

Treatments

Radiation therapy may irritate and inflame the bladder, causing urinary urgency.

Clinical considerations

• A history should be obtained and a physical examination performed.

• Diagnostic tests may include urinalysis, culture and sensitivity studies, and possibly neurologic tests.

• Unless contraindicated, the patient's fluid intake should be increased to dilute the urine and diminish the feeling of urgency.

• Antibiotics and urinary anesthetics (such as phenazopyridine) should be administered, as ordered.

Urine cloudiness

Description

Cloudy, murky, or turbid urine reflects the presence of bacteria, mucus, leukocytes or erythrocytes, epithelial cells, fat, or phosphates (in alkaline urine). It is characteristic of urinary tract infection but can also result from prolonged storage of a urine specimen at room temperature.

Urticaria
(Hives)

Description

Urticaria is a vascular skin reaction characterized by the eruption of pruritic wheals—smooth, slightly elevated patches with well-defined erythematous margins and pale centers. It is produced by the local release of histamine or other vasoactive substances as part of a hypersensitivity reaction. (See *Recognizing Common Skin Lesions,* pp. 362 and 363.)

Acute urticaria evolves rapidly and usually has a detectable cause, commonly hypersensitivity to certain drugs, foods, insect bites, inhalants or contactants, or emotional stress. (See *Common Drugs that Cause Urticaria,* p. 428.) Although individual lesions usually subside within 12 to 24 hours, new crops of lesions may erupt continuously, thus prolonging the attack.

Urticaria lasting longer than 6 weeks is classified as chronic. The lesions

Common Drugs That Cause Urticaria

Many drugs can produce urticaria. Among the most common are:

aspirin	morphine
atropine	penicillin
codeine	quinine
dextrans	sulfonamides
immune serums	vaccines
insulin	

Also, radiographic contrast medium commonly produces urticaria, especially when administered intravenously.

may recur for months or years, and the underlying cause is usually unknown. Occasionally, a diagnosis of psychogenic urticaria is made.

Angioedema, or giant urticaria, is characterized by the acute eruption of wheals involving the mucous membranes and, occasionally, the arms, legs, or genitals.

Urticaria is usually treated with a bland skin emollient or one containing menthol and phenol, antihistamines, systemic corticosteroids, or, if stress is a suspected contributing factor, tranquilizers. Tepid baths and cool compresses may also enhance vasoconstriction and decrease pruritus. The patient should be taught to avoid the causative agent, if identified.

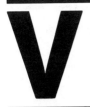

Vaginal bleeding, abnormal

Description

Abnormal vaginal bleeding is the passage of blood from the vagina at times other than menses. It may indicate abnormalities of the uterus, cervix, ovaries, fallopian tubes, or vagina. It may also indicate an abnormal pregnancy (see also "Menorrhagia," "Metrorrhagia," and "Vaginal bleeding, postmenopausal").

Vaginal bleeding, postmenopausal

Description

Postmenopausal vaginal bleeding is bleeding that occurs 6 or more months after menopause. It is an important indicator of gynecologic cancer. However, it can also result from infection, local pelvic disorders, estrogenic stimulation, and physiologic thinning and drying of the vaginal mucous membranes. It usually occurs as slight, brown or red spotting either spontaneously or following coitus or douching, but it may also occur as oozing of fresh blood or as bright red hemorrhage. Many patients—especially those with a history of heavy menstrual flow—minimize the importance of this bleeding, seriously delaying diagnosis.

Possible causes

Obstetrics-Gynecology

Atrophic vaginitis. When bloody staining occurs, it usually follows coitus or douching.

Cervical cancer. Early invasive cervical cancer causes vaginal spotting or heavier bleeding, usually after coitus or douching but occasionally spontaneously.

Cervical or endometrial polyps. These small, pedunculated growths may cause spotting (possibly as a mucopurulent, pink discharge) after coitus, douching, or straining at stool. Endometrial polyps are often asymptomatic, however.

Endometrial cancer. Bleeding occurs early and can be brownish and scant or bright red and profuse. It often follows coitus or douching. Bleeding later becomes heavier, more frequent, and of longer duration, and may be accompanied by pelvic, rectal, lower back, and leg pain.

Ovarian tumors (feminizing). Estrogen-producing ovarian tumors can stimulate endometrial shedding and cause heavy bleeding unassociated with coitus or douching.

Vaginal cancer. Characteristic spotting or bleeding may be preceded by a thin, watery vaginal discharge. Bleeding may be spontaneous but usually follows coitus or douching.

Drugs

Excessive or prolonged estrogen administration is the most common drug cause of postmenopausal vaginal bleeding.

Clinical considerations

• An obstetric and gynecologic history should be obtained and a gynecologic examination performed.

• Diagnostic tests may include ultrasonography to outline a cervical or uterine tumor; endometrial biopsy and dilation and fractional curettage to obtain tissue for histologic examination; testing for occult blood in the stool; and vaginal and cervical cultures to detect infection.

• If ordered, estrogen drug therapy should be discontinued until a diagnosis is made.

Vein sign

Description

Vein sign is a palpable, bluish cordlike swelling along the line formed in the axilla by the junction of the thoracic and superficial epigastric veins. This sign appears in tuberculosis and obstruction of the superior vena cava.

Venous hum

Description

A venous hum is a functional or innocent murmur heard above the clavicles throughout the cardiac cycle. Loudest during diastole, it is low-pitched, rough, or noisy. The hum often accompanies a thrill or, possibly, a high-pitched whine. It is best heard by applying the bell of the stethoscope to the medial aspect of the right supraclavicular area, with the patient seated upright (see *Detecting a Venous Hum*).

A venous hum is a common and normal finding in children and pregnant women. However, it also occurs in hyperdynamic states, such as anemia and thyrotoxicosis. The hum results from increased blood flow through the internal jugular veins, especially on the

Detecting a Venous Hum

To detect a venous hum, the examiner has the patient sit upright, then places the bell of the stethoscope over his right supraclavicular area. She gently lifts his chin and turns his head toward the left, which increases the loudness of the hum (top). If she still cannot hear the hum, she presses his jugular vein with her thumb (bottom). The hum will disappear with pressure but will suddenly return, temporarily louder than before, when she releases her thumb—a result of the turbulence created by pressure changes.

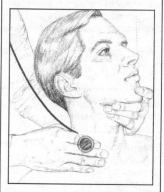

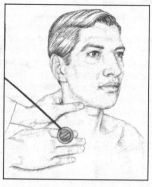

right side, which causes audible vibrations in the tissues.

Occasionally, a venous hum may be mistaken for an intracardiac murmur or a thyroid bruit. However, a venous hum disappears with jugular vein compression and waxes and wanes with head-turning. In contrast, both an intracardiac murmur and a thyroid bruit persist despite jugular compression and head-turning.

Possible causes
Endocrine
Thyrotoxicosis. This disorder may cause a loud venous hum, audible whether the patient is sitting or supine.
Hematologic
Anemia. A venous hum is common with severe anemia (hemoglobin level below 7 g/dl).

Clinical considerations
• A history should be obtained to determine if the patient has had anemia or thyroid disorders and a physical examination performed.
• Diagnostic tests may include an EKG, complete blood count, and thyroid hormone (T_3 and T_4) assays.

Vertigo

Description
Vertigo is an illusion of movement in which the patient feels that he is revolving in space (subjective vertigo) or that his surroundings are revolving around him (objective vertigo). He may complain of feeling pulled sideways, as though drawn by a magnet.

A common symptom, vertigo usually begins abruptly and may be temporary or permanent, mild or severe. It worsens when the patient moves and often subsides when he lies down. Frequently, it is confused with dizziness—a sensation of imbalance and lightheadedness that does not include a whirling sensation. However, unlike dizziness, vertigo is often accompanied by nausea, vomiting, nystagmus, and tinnitus or hearing loss. Although limb coordination is unaffected, vertiginous gait may occur.

Vertigo may result from neurologic or otologic disorders that affect the equilibratory apparatus (the vestibule, semicircular canals, eighth cranial nerve, vestibular nuclei in the brain stem and their temporal lobe connections, and eyes). However, this symptom may also result from alcohol intoxication, hyperventilation, postural changes (benign postural vertigo), and the effects of certain drugs, tests, and procedures.

Possible causes
Central nervous system
Brain stem ischemia. This condition produces sudden, severe vertigo that becomes episodic and later persistent.
Head trauma. Persistent vertigo, occurring soon after injury, accompanies spontaneous or positional nystagmus and, if the temporal bone is fractured, hearing loss.
Multiple sclerosis (MS). Episodic vertigo may occur early and become persistent.
Posterior fossa tumor. In this disorder, positional vertigo lasts for a few seconds.
Eyes, ears, nose, throat
Acoustic neuroma. This tumor of the eighth cranial nerve causes mild, intermittent vertigo several months after onset of unilateral sensorineural hearing loss.
Labyrinthitis. Severe vertigo begins abruptly with this inner ear infection. Vertigo may occur in a single episode or may recur over months or years.
Ménière's disease. In this disease, labyrinthine dysfunction causes abrupt onset of vertigo, lasting minutes, hours, or days. Unpredictable episodes of severe vertigo and unsteady gait may cause the patient to fall. During an attack, any sudden motion of the head or eyes can precipitate nausea and vomiting.

Vestibular neuritis. In this disorder, severe vertigo usually begins abruptly and lasts several days, without tinnitus or hearing loss.

Infection
Herpes zoster. Infection of the eighth cranial nerve produces sudden onset of vertigo accompanied by facial paralysis, hearing loss in the affected ear, and herpetic vesicular lesions in the auditory canal.

Drugs
High doses and toxic levels of certain drugs may produce vertigo. These include salicylates, aminoglycosides (such as streptomycin and gentamicin), antibiotics (such as minocycline, capreomycin, and polymyxin), quinine, and oral contraceptives. Alcohol intoxication may also produce vertigo.

Treatments
Middle ear surgery may cause vertigo that lasts for several days. In addition, administration of *overly warm* or *cold ear drops* or *irrigating solutions* may cause vertigo.

Diagnostic tests
Caloric testing (irrigating the ears with warm or cold water) can induce vertigo.

Clinical considerations

• A history should be obtained and a neurologic examination performed.
• Diagnostic tests may include electronystagmography and X-rays of the middle and inner ears.
• Precautions should be taken to ensure the patient's safety, such as keeping the side rails up if he is in bed or assisting him to a chair if he is standing when vertigo occurs. The patient should always be assisted while ambulating.
• The patient's room should be darkened and his environment kept quiet.
• Drugs to control nausea and vomiting and meclizine or dimenhydrinate to decrease labyrinthine irritability should be administered, as ordered.

Violent behavior

Description
Violent behavior refers to the use of physical force to violate, injure, or abuse an object or person. It is marked by sudden loss of self-control. This behavior may also be self-directed. It may result from organic and psychiatric disorders and the effects of drugs.

Possible causes
Psychiatric disorders
Violent behavior occurs as a protective mechanism in response to a perceived threat in psychotic disorders, such as schizophrenia. A similar response may occur in personality disorders, such as antisocial or borderline personality.

Organic disorders
Many disorders may cause violent behavior due to metabolic and neurologic dysfunction. Common causes include epilepsy, brain tumor, encephalitis, head injury, endocrine disorders, metabolic disorders (such as uremia and calcium imbalance), and severe physical trauma.

Drugs
Various drugs, such as lidocaine and procaine penicillin, may cause violent behavior as an adverse effect. Alcohol abuse or withdrawal, hallucinogens, amphetamines, and barbiturate withdrawal may also cause violent behavior.

Clinical considerations
• Other persons should stay calm and remain at a distance from the patient until help is obtained.
• The patient should be encouraged to move to a quiet location—free of noise, activity, and people—to avoid being frightened or stimulated further.
• The patient should be reassured and told that he is safe.
• Any violent threats the patient makes should be taken seriously and those at whom the threats are directed should be informed.

• Enough personnel should be obtained for a show of force or, if necessary, for subduing the patient.
• Drugs to combat psychotic symptoms should be given, as ordered.
• When the patient's behavior is under control, the onset of violent behavior should be determined. If onset is recent, a medical history should be obtained and a physical examination performed.

Vision, blurred

Description

Blurred vision is the loss of visual acuity with indistinct visual details. It may result from eye injury, neurologic and eye disorders, or disorders with vascular complications, such as diabetes mellitus. Visual blurring may also result from mucus passing over the cornea, refractive errors, improperly fitted contact lenses, or the effects of drugs.

Possible causes

Central nervous system

Brain tumor. Visual blurring may occur with a brain tumor.

Cerebrovascular accident (CVA). Brief attacks of bilateral visual blurring may precede or accompany a CVA.

Concussion. Immediately or shortly after blunt head trauma, vision may be blurred, double, or temporarily lost.

Migraine headache. This disorder may cause visual blurring and paroxysmal attacks of severe, throbbing, unilateral or bilateral headache.

Multiple sclerosis. Blurred vision, diplopia, and paresthesias may occur early in this disorder.

Eyes, ears, nose, throat

Cataract. This painless disorder causes gradual visual blurring. Other effects include halo vision (an early sign), visual glare in bright light, progressive vision loss, and a gray pupil that later turns milky white.

Conjunctivitis. Visual blurring may be accompanied by photophobia, pain, burning, tearing, itching, and a feeling of fullness around the eyes.

Corneal abrasions. Visual blurring may occur with severe eye pain, photophobia, redness, and excessive tearing.

Corneal foreign bodies. Visual blurring may accompany a foreign body sensation, excessive tearing, photophobia, intense eye pain, miosis, conjunctival injection, and a dark corneal speck.

Diabetic retinopathy. Retinal edema and hemorrhage produce gradual blurring, which may progress to blindness.

Dislocated lens. Dislocation of the lens, especially beyond the line of vision, causes visual blurring and (with trauma) redness.

Eye tumor. If the tumor involves the macula, visual blurring may be the presenting symptom.

Glaucoma. In *acute closed-angle glaucoma,* an ocular emergency, unilateral visual blurring and severe pain begin suddenly.

In *chronic closed-angle glaucoma,* transient visual blurring and halo vision may precede pain and blindness.

Hereditary corneal dystrophies. Visual blurring may remain stable or may progressively worsen throughout life.

Hyphema. Blunt eye trauma with hemorrhage into the anterior chamber causes visual blurring.

Iritis. Acute iritis causes sudden visual blurring.

Optic neuritis. Inflammation, degeneration, or demyelinization of the optic nerve usually causes an acute attack of visual blurring and vision loss.

Retinal detachment. Sudden visual blurring may be the initial symptom of this disorder. Blurring worsens, accompanied by visual floaters and recurring flashes of light. Progressive detachment increases vision loss.

Retinal vein occlusion (central). This disorder causes gradual unilateral visual blurring and varying degrees of vision loss.

Senile macular degeneration. This retinal disorder may cause visual blurring (initially worse at night) and slowly or rapidly progressive vision loss.

Serous retinopathy (central). Visual blurring may accompany darkened vision in the affected eye.

Temporal arteritis. Most common in women over age 60, this disorder causes sudden blurred vision accompanied by vision loss and a throbbing unilateral headache in the temporal or frontotemporal region.

Uveitis (posterior). This disorder may produce insidious onset of blurred vision.

Vitreous hemorrhage. Sudden unilateral visual blurring and varying vision loss occur with this condition.

Cardiovascular

Hypertension. This disorder may cause visual blurring and a constant morning headache that decreases in severity during the day.

Drugs

Visual blurring may stem from the effects of cycloplegics, guanethidine, reserpine, clomiphene, phenylbutazone, thiazide diuretics, antihistamines, anticholinergics, and phenothiazines.

Clinical considerations

• If the patient reports visual blurring accompanied by sudden, severe eye pain, a history of trauma, or sudden vision loss, the physician should be notified immediately (see *Managing Sudden Vision Loss*, p. 434).

• If the patient is not in distress, a history should be obtained and an eye examination and visual acuity test performed

• Diagnostic tests may include tonometry, slit-lamp examination, X-rays of the skull and orbit, and, if a neurologic lesion is suspected, a computed tomography scan.

• If necessary, the patient should be oriented to his surroundings and his safety ensured.

Vision loss

Description

Vision loss is the inability to perceive visual stimuli. It can be sudden or gradual and temporary or permanent. The deficit can range from a slight impairment of vision to total blindness. It results from ocular, neurologic, and systemic disorders, as well as from trauma and reactions to certain drugs.

Possible causes

Central nervous system

Concussion. Immediately or shortly after blunt head trauma, vision may be blurred, double, or lost. Generally, vision loss is temporary.

Eyes, ears, nose, throat

Amaurosis fugax. In this disorder, recurrent attacks of unilateral vision loss may last from a few seconds to a few minutes. Vision is normal at other times.

Cataract. Typically, painless and gradual visual blurring precedes vision loss. As the cataract progresses, the pupil turns milky white.

Diabetic retinopathy. Retinal edema and hemorrhage lead to visual blurring, whch may progress to blindness.

Endophthalmitis. Typically, this intraocular infection follows penetrating trauma, intravenous drug use, or intraocular surgery, causing possibly permanent unilateral vision loss; a sympathetic inflammation may affect the other eye.

Glaucoma. This disorder produces visual blurring that may progress to total blindness. *Acute closed-angle glaucoma* is an ocular emergency that may produce blindness within 3 to 5 days.

Chronic closed-angle glaucoma has a gradual onset and usually produces no symptoms, although blurred or halo vision may occur. If untreated, it progresses to blindness and extreme pain.

Chronic open-angle glaucoma is usually bilateral, with an insidious onset and a slowly progressive course. It causes peripheral vision loss, aching eyes, halo vision, and reduced visual acuity (especially at night).

Hereditary corneal dystrophies. Some dystrophies cause vision loss with associated pain, photophobia, tearing, and corneal opacities.

Keratitis. This inflammation of the cornea may lead to complete unilateral vision loss.

Ocular trauma. Following eye injury, sudden unilateral or bilateral vision loss may occur. Vision loss may be total or partial, and permanent or temporary.

Optic neuritis. An umbrella term for inflammation, degeneration, or demyelinization of the optic nerve, optic neuritis usually produces temporary but severe unilateral vision loss.

Retinal artery occlusion (central). This painless ocular emergency causes sudden, unilateral vision loss, which may be partial or complete.

Retinal detachment. Depending on the degree and location of detachment, painless vision loss may be gradual or sudden and total or partial. Macular involvement will cause total blindness. With partial vision loss, the patient may describe visual field defects or a shadow or curtain over the visual field, as well as visual floaters.

Retinal vein occlusion (central). Most common in geriatric patients, this painless disorder causes a unilateral decrease in visual acuity with variable vision loss.

Senile macular degeneration. Occurring in elderly patients, this disorder causes painless blurring or loss of central vision. Vision loss may proceed slowly or rapidly, eventually affecting both eyes. Visual acuity may be worse at night.

Stevens-Johnson syndrome. Corneal scarring from associated conjunctival lesions produces marked vision loss.

Temporal arteritis. Vision loss and visual blurring with a throbbing, unilateral headache characterize this disorder.

Managing Sudden Vision Loss

Sudden vision loss can signal central retinal artery occlusion or acute closed-angle glaucoma—ocular emergencies that require immediate intervention. If a patient reports sudden vision loss, an ophthalmologist should be notified immediately for an emergency examination, and the following interventions may be performed.

For a patient with suspected central retinal artery occlusion, the examiner performs light massage over his closed eyelid. She increases his carbon dioxide level, as ordered, by administering a set flow of oxygen and carbon dioxide through a Venturi mask. Or she has the patient rebreathe in a paper bag to retain exhaled carbon dioxide. These steps will dilate the artery and, possibly, restore blood flow to the retina.

For a patient with suspected acute closed-angle glaucoma, the examiner helps the physician measure intraocular pressure with a tonometer, as ordered. (She can also estimate intraocular pressure without a tonometer by placing her fingers over the patient's closed eyelid. A rock-hard eyeball usually indicates increased intraocular pressure.) She should expect to administer timolol drops and I.V. acetazolamide to help decrease intraocular pressure.

Trachoma. This rare disorder may initially produce varying vision loss and a mild infection resembling bacterial conjunctivitis.

Uveitis. Inflammation of the uveal tract may result in unilateral vision loss. *Anterior uveitis* produces moderate to severe eye pain, severe conjunctival injection, photophobia, and a small, nonreactive pupil. *Posterior uveitis* may produce insidious onset of blurred vision, conjunctival injection, visual floaters, pain, and photophobia.

Vitreous hemorrhage. In this condition, sudden unilateral vision loss may result from intraocular trauma, ocular tumors, or systemic disease (especially diabetes, hypertension, sickle cell anemia, or leukemia). Visual floaters and partial vision with a reddish haze may occur. The patient's vision loss may be permanent.

Endocrine
Pituitary tumor. As a pituitary adenoma grows, blurred vision progresses to hemianopia and, possibly, unilateral blindness.

Musculoskeletal
Paget's disease. Bilateral vision loss may develop as a result of bony impingements on the cranial nerves.

Infection
Herpes zoster. When this disorder affects the nasociliary nerve, bilateral vision loss occurs.

Drugs
Chloroquine therapy may cause gradual vision loss that is not arrested by discontinuing the drug; prolonged use causes irreversible vision loss. Phenylbutazone may cause vision loss and increased susceptibility to retinal detachment. Digitalis derivatives, indomethacin, ethambutol, quinine sulfate, and methanol toxicity may also cause vision loss.

Clinical considerations
• If the patient reports sudden vision loss, the physician should be notified immediately, since such loss can signal an ocular emergency (see *Managing Sudden Vision Loss,* p. 435).
• If the patient's vision loss occurred gradually, a history should be obtained and an eye examination and visual acuity performed.
• The patient should be oriented to his environment and all persons should announce themselves before approaching the patient.
• Steps should be taken to provide for the patient's safety.

Visual floaters

Description
Visual floaters are particles of blood or cellular debris that move about in the vitreous. As these enter the visual field, they appear as spots or dots. Chronic floaters may occur normally in elderly or myopic patients. However, the sudden onset of visual floaters often signals retinal detachment, an ocular emergency.

Possible causes
Eyes, ears, nose, throat
Retinal detachment. Floaters and light flashes appear suddenly in the portion of the visual field where the retina is detached. As the retina detaches further (a painless process), gradual vision loss occurs, likened to a cloud or curtain falling in front of the eyes.

Uveitis (posterior). This disorder may cause visual floaters accompanied by gradual eye pain, photophobia, blurred vision, and conjunctival injection.

Vitreous hemorrhage. Rupture of retinal vessels produces a shower of red or black dots or a red haze across the visual field.

Clinical considerations
• If the patient reports sudden onset of visual floaters, retinal detachment should be suspected and the physician notified. Eye movements should be restricted until a diagnosis is made.

• If the patient's condition permits, a history should be obtained and an eye examination and visual acuity test performed.

• Bed rest and a calm environment should be provided.

• The patient should be told not to touch or rub his eyes and to avoid straining or sudden movements.

• If bilateral eye patches are necessary—as with retinal detachment—the patient's safety must be ensured.

• All persons should identify themselves when approaching the patient, and the patient should be kept oriented to time.

• Treatment may involve eye patches, surgery, corticosteroids, or other drug therapy.

Vomiting

Description

Vomiting is the forceful expulsion of gastric contents through the mouth. Characteristically preceded by nausea, vomiting results from a coordinated sequence of abdominal muscle contractions and reverse esophageal peristalsis.

A common sign of GI disorders, vomiting also occurs with fluid and electrolyte imbalances; infections; and metabolic, endocrine, labyrinthine, central nervous system, and cardiac disorders. It can also result from drug therapy, surgery, and radiation.

Vomiting occurs normally during the first trimester of pregnancy, but its subsequent development may signal complications. It can also result from stress, anxiety, pain, alcohol intoxication, overeating, or ingestion of distasteful foods or liquids.

Possible causes

Central nervous system

Increased intracranial pressure. Projectile vomiting that is *not* preceded by nausea is a sign of increased intracranial pressure.

Vomitus: Characteristics and Causes

When a sample of the patient's vomitus is collected, it should be observed carefully for clues to the underlying disorder. Vomitus may indicate the following:

Bile-stained (greenish) vomitus
Obstruction below the pylorus, as from a duodenal lesion

Bloody vomitus
Upper GI bleeding, as from gastritis or peptic ulcer if bright red; if dark red, as from esophageal or gastric varices

Brown vomitus with a fecal odor
Intestinal obstruction or infarction

Burning, bitter-tasting vomitus
Excessive hydrochloric acid in gastric contents

Coffee-ground vomitus
Digested blood from slowly bleeding gastric or duodenal lesion

Undigested food
Gastric outlet obstruction, as from gastric tumor or ulcer

Migraine headache. Nausea and vomiting are prodromal symptoms.

Eyes, ears, nose, throat

Labyrinthitis. Nausea and vomiting commonly occur with this acute inner ear inflammation.

Ménière's disease. This disorder causes sudden, brief, recurrent attacks of nausea and vomiting.

Cardiovascular

Congestive heart failure. Nausea and vomiting may occur, especially in right-heart failure.

Myocardial infarction. Nausea and vomiting may occur here, but the cardinal symptom is severe substernal chest pain that may radiate to the left arm, jaw, or neck.

Endocrine

Adrenal insufficiency. Common GI findings in the disorder include vomiting, nausea, anorexia, and diarrhea.

Thyrotoxicosis. Nausea and vomiting may accompany the classic findings.

Gastrointestinal

Appendicitis. Vomiting and nausea may follow or accompany abdominal pain.

Cholecystitis (acute). In this disorder, nausea and mild vomiting often follow severe upper quadrant pain that may radiate to the back or shoulders.

Cholelithiasis. Nausea and vomiting accompany severe right upper quadrant or epigastric pain following ingestion of fatty foods.

Cirrhosis. Insidious early symptoms of cirrhosis typically include nausea and vomiting, anorexia, aching abdominal pain, and constipation or diarrhea.

Gastric cancer. This rare cancer may produce mild nausea, vomiting (possibly of mucus or blood), anorexia, upper abdominal discomfort, and chronic dyspepsia.

Gastritis. Nausea and vomiting of mucus or blood are common here, especially after ingestion of alcohol, aspirin, spicy foods, or caffeine.

Gastroenteritis. This disorder causes nausea, vomiting (often of undigested food), diarrhea, and abdominal cramping.

Hepatitis. Vomiting often follows nausea as an early sign of viral hepatitis.

Intestinal obstruction. Nausea and vomiting (bilious or fecal) frequently occur with obstruction, especially of the upper small intestine.

Mesenteric artery ischemia. This life-threatening disorder may cause nausea and vomiting and severe cramping abdominal pain, especially after meals.

Mesenteric venous thrombosis. Insidious or acute onset of nausea, vomiting, and abdominal pain occur here.

Pancreatitis (acute). Vomiting, usually preceded by nausea, is an early symptom of pancreatitis.

Peptic ulcer. Nausea and vomiting may follow sharp or burning epigastric pain, especially when the stomach is empty or after ingestion of alcohol, caffeine, or aspirin.

Peritonitis. Nausea and vomiting usually accompany acute abdominal pain in the area of inflammation.

Ulcerative colitis. Vomiting, nausea, and anorexia may occur here, but the most common sign is recurrent diarrhea with blood, pus, and mucus.

Genitourinary

Renal and urologic disorders. Cystitis, pyelonephritis, calculi, and other disorders of this system can cause vomiting.

Metabolic

Electrolyte imbalances. Such disturbances as hyponatremia, hypernatremia, hypokalemia, and hypercalcemia frequently cause nausea and vomiting.

Metabolic acidosis. This imbalance may produce nausea and vomiting.

Obstetrics-Gynecology

Ectopic pregnancy. Vomiting, nausea, vaginal bleeding, and lower abdominal pain occur in this potentially life-threatening disorder.

Hyperemesis gravidarum. Unremitting nausea and vomiting that last beyond the first trimester characterize this disorder of pregnancy. Vomitus contains undigested food, mucus, and small amounts of bile early in the disorder; later, it has a "coffee-grounds" appearance.

Preeclampsia. Nausea and vomiting are common in this disorder of pregnancy.

Environmental

Food poisoning. Certain toxins, such as *Salmonella,* cause vomiting, nausea, and diarrhea.

Motion sickness. Nausea and vomiting may be accompanied by headache, dizziness, fatigue, diaphoresis, and dyspnea.

Drugs

Drugs that commonly cause vomiting include antineoplastic agents, opiates, ferrous sulfate, levodopa, oral potassium, chloride replacements, estrogens, sulfasalazine, antibiotics, quinidine, anesthetic agents, and overdoses of digitalis and theophylline.

Treatments

Radiation therapy may cause nausea and vomiting if it disrupts the gastric mucosa. Nausea and vomiting are common after *surgery*, especially abdominal surgery.

Clinical considerations

• A history and description of the vomitus should be obtained and a physical examination performed (see *Vomitus: Characteristics and Causes,* p. 437).

• Because projectile vomiting *unaccompanied* by nausea may indicate increased intracranial pressure—a life-threatening emergency—the physician should be notified immediately.

• Antiemetics should be administered, as ordered.

• Vital signs and fluid intake and output should be monitored.

• Because pain can precipitate or intensify nausea and vomiting, ordered pain medications should be administered promptly.

• Since prolonged vomiting can cause dehydration, electrolyte imbalances, and metabolic alkalosis, the patient's fluid, electrolyte, and acid-base status should be monitored.

• The patient should be encouraged to breathe deeply to ease his nausea and help prevent further vomiting.

• The patient's room should be kept fresh and clean-smelling by removing bedpans and emesis basins promptly after use.

W

Weight gain, excessive

Description
Weight gain occurs when ingested calories exceed body requirements for energy, causing increased adipose tissue storage. It can also occur when fluid retention causes edema. When weight gain results from overeating, emotional factors—most commonly anxiety, guilt, and depression—and social factors may be the primary causes.

Among the elderly, weight gain often reflects a sustained food intake in the presence of the normal, progressive fall in basal metabolic rate. Among women, a progressive weight gain occurs with pregnancy, whereas a periodic weight gain usually occurs with menstruation.

Weight gain, a primary symptom of many endocrine disorders, also occurs with conditions that limit activity, especially cardiovascular and pulmonary disorders. It can also result from drug therapy that increases appetite or causes fluid retention and from cardiovascular, hepatic, and renal disorders that cause edema.

Possible causes
Cardiovascular
Congestive heart failure. Despite anorexia, weight gain may result from edema.

Endocrine
Acromegaly. This disorder causes moderate weight gain.
Diabetes mellitus. The increased appetite associated with this disorder may lead to weight gain, although weight loss sometimes occurs instead.
Hypercortisolism. Excessive weight gain, usually over the trunk and the back of the neck (buffalo hump), characteristically occurs in this disorder.
Hyperinsulinism. This disorder increases appetite, leading to weight gain.
Hypogonadism. Weight gain is common in prepubertal and postpubertal hypogonadism.
Hypothalamic dysfunction. Such conditions as Laurence-Moon-Biedl and Morgagni-Stewart-Morel syndromes cause a voracious appetite with subsequent weight gain.
Hypothyroidism. In this disorder, weight gain occurs despite anorexia.

Gastrointestinal
Pancreatic islet cell tumor. This disorder causes excessive hunger, which leads to weight gain.

Genitourinary
Nephrotic syndrome. In this syndrome, weight gain results from edema. In severe cases, anasarca develops—increasing body weight up to 50%.

Obstetrics-Gynecology
Preeclampsia. In this disorder, rapid weight gain (exceeding the normal weight gain of pregnancy) may accompany nausea and vomiting, epigastric pain, elevated blood pressure, and blurred or double vision.
Sheehan's syndrome. Most common in women who experience severe obstetric hemorrhage, this syndrome may cause weight gain.

Drugs
Corticosteroids, phenothiazines, and tricyclic antidepressants cause weight gain from fluid retention and increased

appetite. Other drugs that can lead to weight gain include oral contraceptives, which cause fluid retention; cyproheptadine, which increases appetite; and lithium, which can induce hypothyroidism.

Clinical considerations
• A history should be obtained and a physical examination and nutritional assessment performed (see *Assessing Nutritional Status*).
• Psychological counseling may be necessary for patients with weight

gain, particularly when it results from emotional problems or when uneven weight distribution alters body image.
• The patient should be told to consult a physician before beginning an exercise program.

Weight loss, excessive

Description
Weight loss can reflect decreased food intake, increased metabolic require-

---

Assessing Nutritional Status

To help assess the nutritional status of a patient with excessive weight loss or gain, the examiner measures his skin-fold thickness and midarm circumference and calculates his midarm muscle circumference. Skin-fold measurements reflect adipose tissue mass (subcutaneous fat accounts for about 50% of the body's adipose tissue). Midarm measurements reflect skeletal muscle and adipose tissue mass.

The examiner uses the steps described on the next page to gather these measurements. Then she expresses them as a percentage of standard by using this formula:

$$\frac{\text{actual measurement}}{\text{standard measurement}} \times 100 = \underline{\quad}\%$$

Standard anthropometric measurements vary according to the patient's age and sex, and can be found in a chart of normal anthropometric values. The abridged chart below lists standard arm measurements for adult men and women.

Test	Standard	
Triceps skin fold	Men	12.5 mm
	Women	16.5 mm
Midarm circumference	Men	29.3 cm
	Women	28.5 cm
Midarm muscle circumference	Men	25.3 cm
	Women	23.2 cm

A triceps or subscapular skin-fold measurement below 60% of the standard value indicates severe depletion of fat reserves; a measurement between 60% and 90% indicates moderate to mild depletion; and above 90% indicates significant fat reserves. A midarm circumference of less than 90% of the standard value indicates caloric deprivation; greater than 90% indicates adequate or ample muscle and fat. A midarm muscle circumference of less than 90% indicates protein depletion; over 90% indicates adequate or ample protein reserves.

(continued)

Assessing Nutritional Status *(continued)*

To measure the triceps skinfold, the examiner locates the midpoint of the patient's upper arm, using a nonstretch tape measure. She marks the midpoint with a felt-tip pen. Then she grasps the skin with her thumb and forefinger about 1 cm above the midpoint, places the calipers at the midpoint, and squeezes them for about 3 seconds. She records the measurement registered on the handle gauge to the nearest 0.5 mm. She takes two more readings and averages all three to compensate for any measurement error.

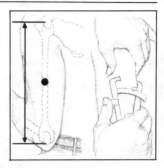

To measure the subscapular skinfold, the examiner uses her thumb and forefinger to grasp the skin just below the angle of the scapula, in line with the natural cleavage of the skin. She applies the calipers and proceeds as she would when measuring the triceps skinfold. Subscapular and triceps skinfold measurements are reliable measurements of fat loss or gain during hospitalization.

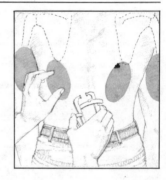

To measure midarm circumference, the examiner returns to the midpoint she marked on the patient's upper arm. Then she uses a tape measure to determine arm circumference at this point. This measurement reflects skeletal muscle and adipose tissue mass and helps evaluate protein and calorie reserves. *To calculate midarm muscle circumference,* she multiplies the triceps skin-fold thickness (in centimeters) by 3.143, and subtracts this figure from the midarm circumference. Midarm muscle circumference reflects muscle mass alone, providing a more sensitive index of protein reserves.

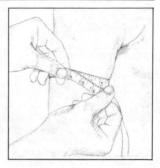

ments, or a combination of the two. Its causes include endocrine, neoplastic, GI, and psychiatric disorders; nutritional deficiencies; infections; and neurologic lesions that cause paralysis and dysphagia. However, weight loss may accompany conditions that prevent sufficient food intake, such as painful oral lesions, ill-fitting dentures, and loss of teeth. It may be the metabolic sequela of poverty, fad diets, excessive exercise, and certain drugs.

Weight loss may occur as a late sign in such chronic diseases as congestive heart failure and renal disease. In these diseases, however, it is the result of anorexia (see "Anorexia").

Possible causes
Eyes, ears, nose, throat
Stomatitis. Inflammation of the oral mucosa (usually red, swollen, and ulcerated) in this disorder causes weight loss due to decreased eating.
Respiratory
Pulmonary tuberculosis. This disorder causes gradual weight loss, along with fatigue, weakness, anorexia, night sweats, and low-grade fever.
Endocrine
Adrenal insufficiency. Weight loss occurs in this disorder, along with anorexia, weakness, fatigue, irritability, syncope, nausea, vomiting, abdominal pain, and diarrhea or constipation.

Diabetes mellitus. Weight loss may occur with this disorder, despite increased appetite (polyphagia).

Thyrotoxicosis. In this disorder, increased metabolism causes weight loss.
Gastrointestinal
Crohn's disease. Weight loss occurs with chronic cramping, abdominal pain, and anorexia.

Esophagitis. Painful inflammation of the esophagus leads to temporary avoidance of eating and subsequent weight loss.

Gastroenteritis. Malabsorption and dehydration cause weight loss in this disorder. The loss may be sudden in acute viral infections or reactions, or gradual in parasitic infection.

Ulcerative colitis. Weight loss is a late sign of this disorder, which is initially characterized by bloody diarrhea with pus or mucus.

Whipple's disease. This rare disease causes progressive weight loss along with abdominal pain, diarrhea, steatorrhea, arthralgia, fever, hyperpigmentation, lymphadenopathy, and splenomegaly.
Hematologic
Leukemia. Acute and *chronic leukemia* cause progressive weight loss.
Psychiatric
Anorexia nervosa. This psychogenic disorder, most common in young women, is characterized by a severe, self-imposed weight loss ranging from 10% to 50% of premorbid weight, which typically was normal or not more than 5 lb (2.3 kg) over ideal weight.

Depression. Weight loss may occur with severe depression.
Neoplastic
Lymphoma. Hodgkin's disease and *non-Hodgkin's lymphoma* cause gradual weight loss.
Drugs
Amphetamines and inappropriate dosage of thyroid preparations commonly lead to weight loss. Laxative abuse may cause a malabsorptive state that leads to weight loss. Chemotherapeutic agents cause stomatitis, which, when severe, causes weight loss.

Clinical considerations
• A history should be obtained and a physical examination and nutritional assessment performed (see *Assessing Nutritional Status,* pp. 441 and 442).
• If weight loss stems from anorexia nervosa or depression, the patient should be referred for psychological counseling.
• If weight loss is due to chronic disease, hyperalimentation or tube feedings should be administered, as ordered, to maintain nutrition and to prevent edema, poor healing, and muscle wasting.
• A dietitian should be consulted if the patient needs dietary instruction.

Weill's sign

Description
Weill's sign is the absence of expansion in the subclavicular area of the affected side on inspiration, occurring in infantile pneumonia.

Westphal's sign

Description
Westphal's sign is the absence of the knee jerk reflex, occurring in tabes dorsalis.

Wheezing
(Sibilant rhonchi)

Description
Wheezes are adventitious breath sounds with a high-pitched, musical, squealing, creaking, or groaning quality. When they originate in the large airways, they can be heard by placing an unaided ear over the chest wall or at the mouth. When they originate in smaller airways, they can be heard by placing a stethoscope over the anterior or posterior chest. Unlike crackles and rhonchi, wheezes cannot be cleared by coughing.

Assessing Abnormal Breath Sounds

To assess airflow through the patient's respiratory system and to detect abnormal breath sounds, the examiner follows the auscultation sequences shown here.
She has the patient take full, deep breaths, and compares sound variations from one side to the other. She notes the location and timing of any abnormal breath sounds, and characterizes them as follows:
• *Wheezes* sound like high-pitched, musical squeaks. They may be detected anywhere in the chest and are usually more prominent on expiration.
• *Rhonchi* are loud, low, coarse, rattling sounds that may be sonorous, bubbling, or rumbling. They are generally detected in larger airways during expiration.
• *Crackles* are popping, nonmusical sounds that may be high- or low-pitched. They may be detected anywhere in the chest and are usually heard best during inspiration.

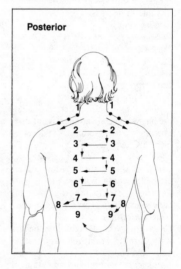

Posterior

Usually, prolonged wheezing occurs during expiration when bronchi are shortened and narrowed. Causes include bronchospasm; mucosal edema; partial obstruction from a tumor, a foreign body, or secretions; and extrinsic pressure, as in tension pneumothorax or goiter. With airway obstruction, wheezing occurs during inspiration.

Possible causes
Respiratory

Aspiration of a foreign body. Partial obstruction by a foreign body produces sudden onset of wheezing.

Aspiration pneumonitis. Wheezing may accompany tachypnea and marked dyspnea.

Asthma. Wheezing is an initial and cardinal sign of asthma. It is heard at the mouth during expiration.

Bronchial adenoma. This insidious disorder produces unilateral, possibly severe, wheezing.

Bronchiectasis. Excessive mucus commonly causes intermittent and localized or diffuse wheezing.

Bronchitis (chronic). This disorder causes wheezing that varies in severity, location, and intensity.

Bronchogenic carcinoma. Obstruction may cause localized wheezing.

Chemical pneumonitis (acute). Mucosal injury causes increased secretions and edema, leading to wheezing and dyspnea.

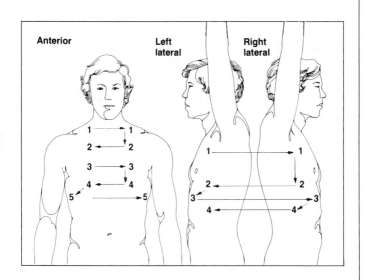

Emphysema. Mild to moderate wheezing may occur in this form of COPD.

Pneumothorax (tension). This life-threatening disorder causes respiratory distress with possible wheezing, dyspnea, tachycardia, tachypnea, and sudden, severe, sharp chest pain (often unilateral).

Pulmonary coccidioidomycosis. This disorder may cause wheezing and rhonchi along with a cough.

Pulmonary edema. Wheezing may occur with this life-threatening disorder.

Pulmonary embolus. Rarely, diffuse, mild wheezing occurs in this disorder.

Pulmonary tuberculosis. In late stages, fibrosis causes wheezing.

Tracheobronchitis. Auscultation may detect wheezing, rhonchi, and crackles.

Wegener's granulomatosis. This disorder may cause mild to moderate wheezing if it compresses major airways.

Endocrine

Thyroid goiter. This disorder may be asymptomatic, or it may cause wheezing, dysphagia, and respiratory difficulty related to a compressed airway.

Immunologic

Anaphylaxis. This allergic reaction can cause tracheal edema or bronchospasm, resulting in severe wheezing and stridor.

Clinical considerations

If the patient is in *acute* respiratory distress:

• A quick respiratory assessment should be performed and the physician notified of the findings.

• The patient should be assisted to a semi-Fowler position and given oxygen.

• Preparations should be made for intubation and emergency resuscitation.

• The patient should be suctioned, as needed, and encouraged to cough and breathe slowly and deeply.

If the patient is *not* in acute respiratory distress:

• A history should be obtained and a respiratory assessment performed, with abnormal breath sounds noted (see *Assessing Abnormal Breath Sounds*, pp. 444 and 445).

• Diagnostic tests may include chest X-rays, arterial blood gas analysis, and sputum culture.

• The patient may be placed in a semi-Fowler position to facilitate breathing.

• Unless contraindicated, the patient should be encouraged to increase his activity level to promote drainage and prevent pooling of secretions.

• The patient should be instructed to perform regular deep breathing and coughing exercises.

• The patient should be encouraged to drink plenty of fluids to liquefy secretions and prevent dehydration.

• Respiratory therapy treatments and air humidification may be necessary to relieve mucous membrane inflammation and to thin secretions.

• Antibiotics, bronchodilators, mucolytics, and expectorants should be administered, as ordered.

Wilder's sign

Description

Wilder's sign is a subtle twitching of the eyeball on medial or lateral gaze. This early sign of Graves' disease is discernible as a slight jerk of the eyeball when the patient changes the direction of his gaze.

Wristdrop

Description

In wristdrop, the hand remains flexed due to paresis of the extensor muscles of the hand and fingers. This weakness may be slight or severe and temporary or permanent. Wristdrop may occur unilaterally and suddenly with a radial nerve injury, or bilaterally and gradually with neurologic disorders, such as myasthenia gravis, Guillain-Barré syndrome, and multiple sclerosis.

Possible causes

Central nervous system
Guillain-Barré syndrome. Wristdrop may occur in this syndrome, but the primary neurologic sign is muscle weakness that typically begins in the legs and ascends to the arms and facial nerves within 24 to 72 hours.

Multiple sclerosis. This disorder may cause wristdrop, but the earliest symptoms are usually diplopia, blurred vision, and paresthesia.

Myasthenia gravis. In this disorder, wristdrop may occur if the extensor muscles are affected.

Radial nerve injury. Compression, severance, or inflammation of the radial nerve causes a loss of motor and sensory function in the involved area. Wristdrop may occur; it may be temporary if injury is incomplete.

Clinical considerations

• A history should be obtained and a neurologic examination performed.
• The patient should be given assistance with activities of daily living.
• Physical therapy is indicated to strengthen weak muscles.
• Occupational therapy may be indicated to provide assistive devices, such as a swivel spoon with a cuff that enables the patient to feed himself.
• Splints may be used to prevent contractures.

Yawning, excessive

Description

Excessive yawning is a persistent involuntary opening of the mouth, accompanied by attempted deep inspiration. In the absence of sleepiness, excessive yawning may indicate cerebral hypoxia.

DISEASES AND DISORDERS PROFILE

Diseases and disorders are rarely diagnosed by an individual sign or symptom. Accurate diagnosis requires familiarity with the patterns in which signs and symptoms occur in disease. This chart outlines classic patterns or profiles of 100 major diseases and disorders. Here is a list of those appearing in the chart.

1. Acquired immune deficiency syndrome (AIDS)
2. Addison's disease
3. Adult respiratory distress syndrome (ARDS)
4. Alzheimer's disease
5. Amyotrophic lateral sclerosis (ALS)
6. Angina pectoris
7. Ankylosing spondylitis
8. Aortic aneurysm, abdominal
9. Appendicitis
10. Asthma
11. Benign prostatic hypertrophy (BPH)
12. Breast cancer
13. Bronchitis, acute
14. Bronchitis, chronic
15. Carbon monoxide poisoning
16. Cardiac tamponade
17. Carpal tunnel syndrome
18. Cerebrovascular accident (CVA)
19. Cholecystitis, acute
20. Cirrhosis
21. Colorectal cancer
22. Congestive heart failure, left
23. Congestive heart failure, right
24. Crohn's disease
25. Croup (laryngotracheobronchitis)
26. Cushing's syndrome
27. Cystitis
28. Deep-vein thrombophlebitis (DVT)
29. Diabetes mellitus
30. Diabetic ketoacidosis (DKA)
31. Disseminated intravascular coagulation (DIC)
32. Diverticulitis
33. Ectopic pregnancy
34. Emphysema
35. Encephalitis
36. Endometriosis
37. Epiglottitis
38. Fibrocystic breast disease
39. Gastritis
40. Gastrointestinal bleeding
41. Glomerulonephritis, acute
42. Gout
43. Guillain-Barré syndrome
44. Hemothorax
45. Hepatic encephalopathy (hepatic coma)
46. Hepatitis, viral
47. Herniated disk, lumbar
48. Herpes genitalis
49. Hiatal hernia
50. Hodgkin's disease
51. Hyperthyroidism (Graves' disease)
52. Hypothyroidism (myxedema)
53. Increased intracranial pressure
54. Insulin shock
55. Intestinal obstruction
56. Irritable bowel syndrome
57. Lead poisoning
58. Leukemia, acute
59. Leukemia, chronic
60. Lung cancer
61. Meningitis
62. Mitral stenosis
63. Multiple myeloma
64. Multiple sclerosis (MS)
65. Myasthenia gravis
66. Myocardial infarction (MI)
67. Osteoarthritis
68. Pancreatitis, acute
69. Parkinson's disease
70. Pelvic inflammatory disease (PID)
71. Peptic ulcer
72. Pericarditis
73. Peritonitis
74. Pleural effusion
75. Pneumonia, bacterial
76. Pneumonia, viral
77. Pneumothorax
78. Premenstrual syndrome (PMS)
79. Pulmonary edema
80. Pulmonary embolism (PE)
81. Pulmonary hypertension
82. Pyelonephritis, acute
83. Raynaud's disease
84. Renal calculi
85. Reye's syndrome
86. Rheumatoid arthritis
87. Shock, anaphylactic
88. Shock, cardiogenic

Diseases and Disorders Profile (continued)

89. Shock, hypovolemic
90. Shock, neurogenic
91. Shock, septic
92. Sickle-cell crisis
93. Sinusitis, acute bacterial
94. Subacute bacterial endocarditis (SBE)

95. Subarachnoid hemorrhage
96. Systemic lupus erythematosus (SLE)
97. Toxic shock syndrome (TSS)
98. Transient ischemic attack (TIA)
99. Ulcerative colitis
100. Urethritis

Disease or Disorder	Signs and Symptoms
Acquired immune deficiency syndrome (AIDS)	Signs and symptoms vary greatly, but may include: • Fever • Anorexia • Weight loss • Diarrhea • Fatigue • Lymphadenopathy • Nonproductive cough • Manifestations of opportunistic diseases, such as reddish purple lesions of Kaposi's sarcoma; whitish mucoid exudate of candidiasis; tachypnea, possibly crackles (rales), rhonchi, and cyanosis associated with *Pneumocystis carinii* pneumonia
Addison's disease	• Progressive weakness and fatigue • Weight loss • Loss of secondary sex characteristics and libido in females • Mental status changes (depression, irritability, and restlessness) • Blue-gray hyperpigmentation on exposed areas of body and on mucous membranes • Salt craving • Hypotension and syncope • Poor coordination • Abdominal pain
Adult respiratory distress syndrome (ARDS)	• Dyspnea • Tachypnea • Tachycardia • Diaphoresis • Cyanosis • Cough productive of pink, frothy sputum • Diffuse crackles (rales), wheezes, and rhonchi • *With worsening hypoxemia*—restlessness, agitation, anxiety, altered level of consciousness
Alzheimer's disease	• Progressive mental deterioration (personality changes, progressive dementia, amnesia, decreased attention span, faulty concentration, loss of abstract thinking, hyperactivity, irritability, difficulty comprehending written and verbal speech)

(continued)

Diseases and Disorders Profile *(continued)*

Disease or Disorder	Signs and Symptoms
Alzheimer's disease *(continued)*	• Motor disturbances (expressive and receptive aphasia, echolalia, apraxia, spatial disorientation, repetitive movements, slow reflexes, shuffling gait, incontinence)
Amyotrophic lateral sclerosis (ALS)	• Motor disturbances (fasciculations accompanied by muscle weakness and atrophy, especially in forearms and hands; impaired speech; difficulty chewing, swallowing, and breathing; choking; excessive drooling; urinary frequency and urgency, and difficulty initiating a stream) • Paresthesias • Depression • Inappropriate laughter and crying spells (caused by bulbar palsy)
Angina pectoris	• Chest pain (may be dull or burning or described as pressure, tightness, or heaviness; increases and fades gradually; may be felt in abdomen; may radiate to jaw, teeth, face, left arm, neck, shoulders, upper abdomen, or back) • Anxiety and diaphoresis • Dyspnea • Tachycardia • Palpitations (possible)
Ankylosing spondylitis	Signs and symptoms progress unpredictably; sudden disease remission, exacerbation, or arrest may occur at any stage. Signs and symptoms may include: • Intermittent low back pain that is most severe in the morning or after a period of inactivity, is unrelieved by rest, and may radiate down the thighs • Stiffness and limited mobility of lumbar spinal region • Pain and limited chest expansion (due to thoracic spine involvement) • Peripheral arthritis involving shoulders, hips, and knees • Kyphosis (with advanced disease) • Tenderness over the site of inflammation • Mild fatigue, fever, anorexia, weight loss • Iritis (occasional)
Aortic aneurysm, abdominal	An abdominal aortic aneurysm usually produces no signs or symptoms, but physical assessment will reveal: • Pulsating mass in the periumbilical area • Systolic bruit over the aorta

Diseases and Disorders Profile *(continued)*

Disease or Disorder	Signs and Symptoms
Aortic aneurysm, abdominal *(continued)*	• Tenderness on deep palpation • Intermittent abdominal or lower back pain that radiates to the flank and groin (with a large aneurysm) Signs and symptoms of aneurysmal rupture include: • Severe, persistent abdominal and back pain • Subcutaneous ecchymosis in the flank or groin • Signs and symptoms of hemorrhage and shock (weakness, diaphoresis, tachycardia, hypotension)
Appendicitis	• Epigastric or periumbilical pain that later localizes in right lower quadrant at McBurney's point • Anorexia • Nausea • Vomiting • Abdominal rigidity • Rebound tenderness • Mild fever • Constipation (occurs late) • Sudden cessation of abdominal pain (with perforation or infarction of the appendix)
Asthma	• Mild wheezing, audible wheezing progressing to severe dyspnea • Chest tightness • Cough productive of thick mucus • Tachypnea • Nasal flaring • Diaphoresis • Flushed skin • Intercostal and supraclavicular retraction • Accessory chest muscle use • Possible signs and symptoms of eczema or allergic rhinitis
Benign prostatic hypertrophy (BPH)	• Changes in voiding patterns (urinary hesitancy, dribbling, reduced urinary stream force, straining, possible retention) • Nocturia • Burning on urination (in presence of urinary tract infection)
Breast cancer	• Nontender, irregularly shaped, fixed breast nodule • Bloody nipple discharge • Breast dimpling • Nipple deviation or retraction • Peau d'orange • Axillary lymphadenopathy • Breast pain (rare)

(continued)

Diseases and Disorders Profile *(continued)*

Disease or Disorder	Signs and Symptoms
Bronchitis, acute	• Cough (may or may not be productive) • Coarse rhonchi or wheezes • Nasal discharge • Fever • Malaise
Bronchitis, chronic	• Dyspnea on exertion • Abundant sputum production; sputum may be white, gray, or yellow • Tachypnea • Cyanosis • Edema • Digital clubbing (in late stages) • Wheezing
Carbon monoxide poisoning	Acute poisoning may cause: • Altered level of consciousness (amnesia, fatigue, confusion, seizures, coma) • Headache and dizziness • Motor disturbances (muscle twitching; transient hemiplegia, aphasia, and athetoid movements; parkinsonism in later years) • Sensory deviations (visual disturbances, multiple neuritis) • Nausea and vomiting • Cherry-red skin and mucous membranes • Hypertension and bounding pulse Gradual poisoning may cause: • Fever • Excessive sweating • Decreased exercise tolerance • Dyspnea on exertion • Signs and symptoms of increasing intracranial pressure
Cardiac tamponade	• Beck's triad (diminished or muffled heart sounds, jugular vein distention, hypotension) • Pulsus paradoxus • Narrowed pulse pressure • Tachycardia • Dyspnea • Diaphoresis • Pallor or cyanosis • Anxiety • Restlessness
Carpal tunnel syndrome	Signs and symptoms may affect one or both hands and may include: • Weakness, pain, burning, numbness, or tingling in the thumb, forefinger, and middle finger but not in the fourth or fifth finger

Diseases and Disorders Profile *(continued)*

Disease or Disorder	Signs and Symptoms
Carpal tunnel syndrome *(continued)*	• Pain possibly radiating up the arm; may be constant or intermittent • Pain that worsens at night or in the morning • Inability to make a fist with the affected hand • Atrophic nails • Dry, shiny skin
Cerebrovascular accident (CVA)	Signs and symptoms vary depending on the location of the lesion, but may include: When CVA affects the middle cerebral artery— • Motor disturbances (aphasia, dysphasia, contralateral hemiparesis or hemiplegia) • Sensory deviations (pain and tenderness in the affected arm or leg, numbness, tingling) • Altered level of consciousness (LOC) (decreased LOC, progressing to coma) When CVA affects the carotid artery— • Headache • Motor disturbances (weakness, contralateral paralysis or paresis) • Sensory deviations (contralateral numbness and sensory changes, ipsilateral visual disturbances, transient blindness) • Altered LOC (confusion, memory deficit) When CVA affects the vertebral and basilar arteries— • Motor disturbances (contralateral weakness, diplopia, poor coordination, dysphagia, ataxia) • Sensory deviations (visual field defects, numbness around the lips and mouth, dizziness, blindness, deafness) • Altered LOC (amnesia, confusion, loss of consciousness) When CVA affects the anterior cerebral artery— • Motor disturbances (impaired motor function, including weakness, loss of coordination, and incontinence) • Sensory deviations (numbness in the lower leg or foot, impaired vision) • Altered LOC (confusion, personality changes) When CVA affects the posterior cerebral artery— • Motor disturbances (contralateral hemiplegia) • Sensory deviations (visual field defects, impaired pain and temperature sensation, cortical blindness) • Altered LOC (coma)
Cholecystitis, acute	• Sudden onset of severe, cramping pain in epigastrium or right upper quadrant; may be referred to back or right scapula; often follows ingestion of fatty foods; usually subsides after about 1 hour and is followed by a dull ache *(continued)*

Diseases and Disorders Profile (continued)

Disease or Disorder	Signs and Symptoms
Cholecystitis, acute (continued)	• Nausea and vomiting • Low-grade fever • Chills • Indigestion, belching, and flatulence • Jaundice (may occur with obstruction of common bile duct)
Cirrhosis	Early signs and symptoms are vague, and may include: • Mild right upper quadrant pain (worsens as disease progresses) • Nausea • Vomiting • Anorexia • Constipation or diarrhea Late signs and symptoms result from hepatic insufficiency and portal hypertension, and may include: • Hepatic encephalopathy (decreased level of consciousness progressing to coma, slurred speech, asterixis, peripheral neuritis, paranoia, and hallucinations) • Bleeding tendencies (epistaxis, easy bruising, bleeding gums) • Skin changes (severe pruritus, extreme dryness, poor tissue turgor, abnormal pigmentation, spider angiomas, palmar erythema) • Jaundice • Hepatomegaly • Ascites and peripheral edema • Fetor hepaticus (musty breath odor) • Pain in right upper quadrant that worsens when patient sits upright or leans forward • Fever • Upper GI bleeding (from esophageal varices) • Testicular atrophy and gynecomastia (in men) • Menstrual irregularities • Loss of chest and axillary hair
Colorectal cancer	Early signs and symptoms are typically vague and depend on the location and function of the bowel segment containing the tumor. They may include: With right colon tumor— • Black, tarry stools • Abdominal aching, pressure, or cramps With left colon tumor— • Rectal bleeding • Intermittent abdominal fullness or cramping • Rectal pressure • Obstipation, diarrhea, or ribbon- or pencil-shaped stools • Pain that is relieved by passage of stool or flatus

Diseases and Disorders Profile (continued)

Disease or Disorder	Signs and Symptoms
Colorectal cancer (continued)	• Dark or bright red blood and mucus in stool With rectal tumor— • Change in bowel habits (morning diarrhea or obstipation alternating with diarrhea) • Blood or mucus in stool • Sensation of incomplete evacuation • Rectal pain (occurs late)
Congestive heart failure (left ventricular)	• Dyspnea on exertion • Orthopnea • Paroxysmal nocturnal dyspnea • Cough productive of frothy, pink sputum • Crackles and wheezes • Fatigue and weakness • Palpitations and tachycardia • Cyanosis or pallor • Pulsus alternans • Oliguria
Congestive heart failure (right ventricular)	• Fatigue and weakness • Dizziness and syncope • Hepatomegaly • Ascites • Dependent peripheral edema • Jugular vein distention • Nausea, vomiting, anorexia, abdominal distention • Tachycardia • Weight gain • Oliguria
Crohn's disease	• Cramping pain in lower right quadrant • Nausea • Mild, urgent diarrhea • Low-grade fever • Abdominal tenderness • Flatulence • Weight loss • Weakness and malaise
Croup (laryngotracheobronchitis)	• Inspiratory stridor • Sharp, barking cough • Hoarse or muffled breath sounds • Fever • Scattered crackles
Cushing's syndrome	• Weakness and fatigue • Weight gain • Moon face • Acne • Thoracic kyphosis

(continued)

Diseases and Disorders Profile *(continued)*

Disease or Disorder	Signs and Symptoms
Cushing's syndrome *(continued)*	• Supraclavicular fat pad development • Purple striae on arms, abdomen, and thighs • Easy bruising, petechiae • Peripheral edema • Loss of muscle mass • Mental status changes (irritability, emotional lability, depression, psychosis) • Amenorrhea • Gynecomastia • Hirsutism
Cystitis	• Dysuria, urinary frequency, and urgency • Cloudy urine or hematuria • Lower back or flank pain • Fever • Nausea and vomiting (possible) • Inflamed genital area (possible)
Deep-vein thrombophlebitis (DVT)	Signs and symptoms may vary with the site and length of the affected vein. They may include: • Pain and swelling of the affected extremity • Cyanotic skin in the affected area (with severe venous obstruction) • Positive Homans' sign (spasm and pain in calf muscles with dorsiflexion of the foot) • Fever and chills (possible)
Diabetes mellitus	• Polyuria • Polydipsia • Polyphagia • Weight loss • Fatigue • Dry skin and mucous membranes
Diabetic ketoacidosis (DKA)	• Anorexia • Nausea and vomiting • Polyuria • Weakness • Malaise • Kussmaul's respirations • Fruity breath odor • Abdominal pain • Decreased level of consciousness (if untreated)
Disseminated intravascular coagulation (DIC)	• Bleeding problems (abnormal or prolonged bleeding from venipuncture sites, drainage tubes, suture lines, or body orifices; hemoptysis; hematuria; occult blood in stool; vital sign changes [possibly indicating internal bleeding]; increasing abdominal girth [with GI bleeding]; petechiae or

Diseases and Disorders Profile *(continued)*

Disease or Disorder	Signs and Symptoms
Disseminated intravascular coagulation (DIC) *(continued)*	ecchymoses; visual disturbances; excessive menstrual bleeding; altered level of consciousness [with CVA]) • Clotting problems (cool, mottled skin; absent peripheral pulses; cyanosis of fingers, toes, earlobes, or tip of the nose; calf swelling and pain on dorsiflexion; altered level of consciousness [with CVA])
Diverticulitis	• Lower left quadrant pain • Nausea • Constipation occurring with onset of pain • Low-grade fever • Abdominal tenderness (with severe disease)
Ectopic pregnancy	• Lower abdominal pain (may be stabbing, sharp, or dull; unilateral or bilateral; constant or intermittent) • Nausea • Vomiting • Amenorrhea (in 75% of patients) • Vaginal spotting or bleeding (with tubal pregnancy) • Tachycardia and hypotension (possible)
Emphysema	• Dyspnea • Chronic cough • Anorexia and weight loss • Malaise • Barrel chest • Accessory chest muscle use • Prolonged expiration with grunting • Tachypnea • Peripheral cyanosis • Digital clubbing
Encephalitis	All viral forms of encephalitis have similar clinical features, including: • Fever • Headache • Vomiting • Evidence of meningeal irritation (nuchal rigidity, back pain) • Motor disturbances (paralysis, ataxia) • Altered level of consciousness (seizures; lethargy or restlessness progressing to stupor and coma; coma may persist for days, weeks, or longer after acute phase subsides) • Personality changes • Mental deterioration

(continued)

Diseases and Disorders Profile *(continued)*

Disease or Disorder	Signs and Symptoms
Endometriosis	• Constant menstrual pain referred to the rectum and lower sacral or coccygeal regions • Dyspareunia (with uterosacral involvement or vaginal extension) • Pain on defecation (with rectovaginal segment and colon involvement) • Dysuria (bladder involvement) • Nausea and vomiting (with small bowel and appendix involvement) • Excessive, prolonged, or frequent uterine bleeding with no specific pattern
Epiglottitis	• Dyspnea (in severe cases, apnea) • High fever • Inspiratory stridor (rare in adults) • Severe sore throat, with cherry-red, enlarged epiglottis • Cough • Hoarseness • Substernal retractions on inspiration (possible)
Fibrocystic breast disease	• Thickened, nodular areas in breast(s) • Nodule-related pain and tenderness, especially in the premenstrual phase of the menstrual cycle • Slight serous nipple discharge
Gastritis	• Epigastric pain slightly left of midline • Indigestion • Nausea • Vomiting (possible hematemesis) • Diarrhea • Melena
Gastrointestinal (GI) bleeding	From upper GI structures: • Abdominal pain • Vomiting (bright red vomitus indicates acute bleeding; dark red vomitus suggests less recent bleeding) • Bloody diarrhea (with acute bleeding) • Melena (with chronic bleeding) • Weakness • Tachycardia • Diaphoresis • Fainting From lower GI structures: • Pain and abdominal cramping • Rectal bleeding • Bloody diarrhea (possible pus or mucus in stool)

Diseases and Disorders Profile *(continued)*

Disease or Disorder	Signs and Symptoms
Glomerulonephritis, acute	Signs and symptoms, which usually appear within 1 to 3 weeks after streptococcal infection of the throat or skin, may include: • Mild to moderate edema • Oliguria (possible anuria) • Hematuria • Proteinuria • Fatigue • Mild to severe hypertension • Costovertebral angle tenderness
Gout	• Severe joint pain of sudden onset • Immobility, swelling, tenderness, inflammation, and warmth of affected joints • Dusky-red or cyanotic appearance of affected joints • Thickened, wrinkled, desquamated skin over affected joints • Low-grade fever (occasionally) • Painless tophi
Guillain-Barré syndrome	Signs and symptoms usually appear after an upper respiratory infection, and may include: • Motor disturbances (muscle weakness in legs, extending to arms and face within 24 to 72 hours and progressing to total paralysis and respiratory failure; possible flaccid quadriplegia; cranial nerve paralysis; ocular paralysis) • Sensory deviations (paresthesias that disappear before muscle weakness occurs)
Hemothorax	• Chest pain • Tachypnea • Mild to severe dyspnea • Tachycardia • Diaphoresis • Dusky skin color • Hemoptysis • Bloody, frothy sputum • Mild to severe hypotension • Altered level of consciousness (possible)
Hepatic encephalopathy (hepatic coma)	This disorder progresses through four stages, with the signs and symptoms described below: • Prodromal stage—mild confusion, euphoria, or depression, vacant stare, inappropriate laughter, forgetfulness; inability to concentrate, slow mentation, slurred speech, untidiness, lethargy, belligerence, minimal asterixis • Impending stage—obvious obtundation, aberrant behavior, definite asterixis, constructional apraxia *(continued)*

Diseases and Disorders Profile *(continued)*

Disease or Disorder	Signs and Symptoms
Hepatic encephalopathy (hepatic coma) *(continued)*	• Stuporous stage (patient can still be aroused)—marked confusion, incoherent speech; asterixis, noisiness, abusiveness, violent behavior • Comatose stage (patient cannot be aroused, responds only to painful stimuli)—positive Babinski's sign, hepatic fetor (musty breath odor)
Hepatitis, viral	Signs and symptoms of Types A, B, and non-A non-B hepatitis are similar but most severe with Type B, possibly leading to massive liver necrosis and death. Hepatitis typically occurs in two phases, with the signs and symptoms described below: • Prodromal phase—mental and physical fatigue; nausea and vomiting; mild right upper quadrant pain; anorexia; diarrhea; headache; hives or skin rash; angioneurotic edema; flulike symptoms (sore throat, cough, irritated nasal mucosa, fever between 100° and 104° F. [37.8° C. to 40° C.]); low-grade fever (with Type B); joint pain (possible) • Icteric phase—dark yellow urine, clay-colored stool, jaundice (except with non-A non-B hepatitis), lymphadenopathy, weight loss, hepatomegaly
Herniated disk, lumbar	• Low back pain, which may radiate to the buttocks, legs, and feet • Muscle spasms • Sensory deviations (decreased sensation, paresthesias, absent reflexes over dermatomes, voiding or defecating difficulties) • Muscle weakness and atrophy in affected extremities
Herpes genitalis	In males, signs and symptoms may include: • Oval or round penile ulcers (may also occur in anal or rectal areas or on the oropharynx) • Fever • Malaise • Dysuria In females, signs and symptoms may include: • Blisters and ulcers covering extensive areas of the vulva and perianal skin • Pruritus, burning, and tingling in genital area preceding eruption of lesions • Severe vulvar pain after appearance of lesions • Fever • Malaise • Watery vaginal discharge with appearance of lesions • Dysuria and urinary retention (possible)

Diseases and Disorders Profile *(continued)*

Disease or Disorder	Signs and Symptoms
Hiatal hernia	• Dysphagia • Heartburn • Nocturnal regurgitation (aggravated by lying down, relieved by standing)
Hodgkin's disease	• Painless lymph node enlargement, beginning in the cervical area and advancing to the axillary, inguinal, mediastinal, and mesenteric regions • Possible fever • Generalized pruritus, which may be mild to severe • Anorexia and weight loss (with advanced disease)
Hyperthyroidism (Graves' disease)	Because hyperthyroidism profoundly affects every body system, a wide range of signs and symptoms may occur. Classic findings include: • Enlarged thyroid gland • Nervousness • Heat intolerance • Weight loss despite increased appetite • Increased sweating • Diarrhea • Tremor • Palpitations and tachycardia • Exophthalmos • Smooth, warm, flushed skin • Fine, thin hair and friable nails
Hypothyroidism (myxedema)	• Fatigue • Memory lapses • Cold intolerance • Unexplained weight gain • Constipation • Cold, dry skin, hair loss, and brittle nails • Puffy face, hands, and feet • Periorbital edema • Slow speech and hoarseness • Bradycardia and signs of poor peripheral circulation • Menorrhagia, decreased libido, and infertility
Increased intracranial pressure	• Headache • Vomiting • Unequal pupils • Slow, dysrhythmic respirations • Confusion progressing to coma • Muscle weakness, progressing to paralysis, hyperreflexia, and, finally, decerebrate rigidity • Bradycardia • Increased blood pressure • Papilledema (possible)

(continued)

Diseases and Disorders Profile *(continued)*

Disease or Disorder	Signs and Symptoms
Insulin shock	• Diaphoresis • Tremors • Increased blood pressure, pulse rate, and respirations • Headache and confusion • Incoordination • Seizures, possibly followed by coma and death
Intestinal obstruction	Small-bowel obstruction: • Severe, colicky abdominal pain in the epigastric or periumbilical area • Nausea and vomiting (occurs early) • Constipation (occurs late) • Abdominal distention (diffuse or only in the epigastric area; occurs late) • Signs and symptoms of hypovolemic shock if obstruction is not treated promptly Large-bowel obstruction: • Colicky abdominal pain; may be referred to the lumbar spinal area; less severe than with small-bowel obstrution • Possible nausea • Vomiting (may contain fecal material; occurs late) • Constipation • Abdominal distention
Irritable bowel syndrome	• Lower abdominal pain, usually relieved by defecation or passage of gas • Diarrhea alternating with constipation or normal bowel function • Small stools containing visible mucus • Possible dyspepsia and abdominal distention
Lead poisoning	• Extreme irritability • Anorexia • Burning sensation in the mouth and esophagus • Abdominal pain • Diarrhea or constipation • Nausea and vomiting • Focal or generalized seizures • Paralysis following seizures • Polyneuritis • Lethargy, delirium, progressing to coma
Leukemia, acute	• Abnormal bleeding (bleeding from the nose and gums, prolonged menses, easy bruising) • Lymphadenopathy (generalized or involving only the cervical nodes) • Splenomegaly • Fatigue

Diseases and Disorders Profile *(continued)*

Disease or Disorder	Signs and Symptoms
Leukemia, acute *(continued)*	• Low-grade or high-grade fever • Chills • Headache • Shortness of breath • Tinnitus • Abdominal or bone pain
Leukemia, chronic	• Fatigue • Anorexia and weight loss • Bone tenderness • Possible lymphadenopathy • Hepatomegaly and splenomegaly • Low-grade fever • Edema • Pruritus
Lung cancer	• Absent or mild cough, or chronic cough pattern that changes in some way • Dyspnea on exertion • Anorexia and weight loss • Weakness • Possible fever • Possible hemoptysis • Possible chest pain
Meningitis	• Fever and chills • Malaise • Headache • Nausea and vomiting • Nuchal rigidity • Positive Brudzinski's sign • Positive Kernig's sign • Exaggerated and symmetrical deep-tendon reflexes • Opisthotonos
Mitral stenosis	• Dyspnea on exertion, paroxysmal nocturnal dyspnea, and orthopnea • Hemoptysis • Cough • Fatigue • Facial flushing • Atrial fibrillation • Localized, delayed, rumbling, low-pitched diastolic murmur at or near apex; possible loud S_2 with elevated pulmonary pressure • Peripheral edema • Abdominal and extremity pain

(continued)

Diseases and Disorders Profile (continued)

Disease or Disorder	Signs and Symptoms
Multiple myeloma	• Pain in bones and muscles, which may become severe • Fever • Malaise • Weight loss • Peripheral neuropathy • Pathologic fractures and bone deformities (with disease progression)
Multiple sclerosis (MS)	Signs and symptoms vary widely but may include: • Sensory deviations (paresthesia and vision impairment) • Motor disturbances (slurred speech, intention tremor, nystagmus, spastic paralysis, poor coordination, loss of proprioception, ataxia, transient muscle weakness, incontinence, or urinary retention) • Emotional disturbances (mood swings, irritability, euphoria, or depression)
Myasthenia gravis	• Motor disturbances (progressive muscle weakness during activity, respiratory muscle impairment during myasthenic crisis, difficulty supporting head due to neck muscle weakness, dysarthria, dysphagia) • Diplopia • Ptosis • Lack of facial expression • Nasal vocal tone
Myocardial infarction (MI)	• Chest pain (persistent, crushing substernal pain that may radiate to the left arm, jaw, neck, or shoulder blades; may be described as "heavy," "squeezing," or "crushing"; may last 12 hours or more; is not relieved by nitroglycerin; may build rapidly or in waves to maximum intensity within a few minutes) • Nausa and vomiting (may accompany chest pain) • Dyspnea and, possibly, orthopnea, cough, and wheezing • Fatigue • Apprehension, sense of impending doom • Possible irregular heart beat • Tachycardia or bradycardia and weak pulses • Normal or decreased blood pressure • Fever 24 hours after onset of infarction • Significant murmurs, diminished gallop rhythm, pericardial friction rub and rales (heard on auscul-

Diseases and Disorders Profile (continued)

Disease or Disorder	Signs and Symptoms
Myocardial infarction (MI) (continued)	tation); murmurs may precede or accompany rupture of septum or papillary muscle • Possible distended neck veins, diaphoresis, pallor, cyanosis, and shock
Osteoarthritis	• Joint pain (particularly after exercise or weight bearing), relieved by rest; aching pain during weather changes • Joint stiffness in the morning and after exercise, relieved by rest • Joint swelling and tenderness without redness or warmth • Heberden's nodes in distal joints, Bouchard's nodes in proximal joints (with interphalangeal joint involvement)
Pancreatitis, acute	• Nausea and vomiting • Severe radiating pain on the left side • Abdominal rigidity
Parkinson's disease	• Motor disturbances (tremor; characteristic rhythmic, unilateral pill-rolling movement of thumb and forefinger; muscle rigidity; resistance to passive movement; akinesia or bradykinesia; inability to initiate and perform volitional motor activities; slow, shuffling Parkinson's gait [may be retropulsive or propulsive]; arm rigidity when walking; hand tremor at rest) • Sensory deviations (thermal paresthesia, hyperhydrosis, pain in one or both arms) • Minor intellectual deficits • Fatigue • Postural deformities of arms, legs, and trunk • Eczema • Micrographia • Low-pitched, monotonic speech pattern
Pelvic inflammatory disease (PID)	• Profuse, purulent vaginal discharge • Possible temperature elevation and malaise • Lower abdominal pain
Peptic ulcer	• Dyspepsia • Gnawing, burning epigastric pain 1 to 3 hours after eating, relieved by food or antacids
Pericarditis	• Chest pain of sudden onset (precordial or substernal; pleuritic; radiating to left neck, shoulder, back, or epigastrium; exacerbated by lying down or swallowing)

(continued)

Diseases and Disorders Profile (continued)

Disease or Disorder	Signs and Symptoms
Pericarditis (continued)	• Fever • Tachycardia • Pericardial friction rub
Peritonitis	• Sudden, severe abdominal pain • Nausea and vomiting • Fever • Pallor • Increased sweating • Hypotension • Tachycardia • Abdominal rigidity, rebound tenderness • Decreased bowel sounds
Pleural effusion	• Chest pain (pleuritic; may radiate to neck, shoulders, or abdomen) • Dyspnea • Tachycardia • Displaced heart sounds • Gallop heart rhythms • Decreased breath sounds • Dullness over affected area • Absent or diminished voice sounds
Pneumonia, bacterial	• Productive cough • Pleuritic chest pain • Fever and chills
Pneumonia, viral	• Fever • Malaise • Myalgia • Headache • Sore throat • Chills of sudden onset • Nonproductive cough that becomes productive
Pneumothorax	• Sudden, sharp, pleuritic pain exacerbated by chest movement, breathing, and coughing • Asymmetrical chest-wall movement • Shortness of breath, which may become severe • Cough
Premenstrual syndrome (PMS)	Signs and symptoms vary greatly and may include any combination of the following: • Behavioral changes (mild to severe personality changes, nervousness, irritability, agitation, sleep disturbances, fatigue, lethargy, depression) • Neurologic changes (headache, vertigo, syncope, paresthesia of the arms and legs, exacerbation of epilepsy)

Diseases and Disorders Profile *(continued)*

Disease or Disorder	Signs and Symptoms
Premenstrual syndrome (PMS) *(continued)*	• Respiratory disturbances (increased susceptibility to colds, exacerbation of allergic rhinitis and asthma) • Gastrointestinal disturbances (abdominal bloating [most common], diarrhea or constipation, appetite changes, exacerbation of spastic colitis) • Edema • Temporary weight gain • Palpitations • Backache • Exacerbation of skin problems • Breast enlargement and tenderness • Oliguria • Easy bruising
Pulmonary edema	• Dyspnea, orthopnea • Cough productive of pink, frothy sputum • Tachypnea • Tachycardia and possible dysrhythmias • Crackles • Hypotension (if cardiac output drops)
Pulmonary embolism (PE)	• Sudden onset of dyspnea • Possible pleuritic chest pain • Hemoptysis • Tachycardia • Cyanosis • Diaphoresis • Low-grade fever
Pulmonary hypertension	• Dyspnea on exertion • Fatigue • Syncope • Possible evidence of right ventricular heart failure (peripheral edema, ascites, neck vein distention, hepatomegaly)
Pyelonephritis, acute	• Sudden fever and chills • Nausea and vomiting • Flank pain • Costovertebral angle tenderness • Kidney tenderness • Dysuria, hematuria
Raynaud's disease	• Pain in hands after exposure to cold or stress • Cold fingers and hands without change in radial or ulnar pulses • Blanching, cyanosis, and redness of the fingers • Numbness, tingling, and swelling of fingers or hands

(continued)

Diseases and Disorders Profile *(continued)*

Disease or Disorder	Signs and Symptoms
Renal calculi	• Pain that typically travels from the costovertebral angle to the flank, suprapubic region, and external genitalia; may become severe • Fever and chills • Hematuria, pyuria, and, rarely, anuria • Possible back and abdominal pain
Reye's syndrome	The following signs and symptoms occur in five stages, following a brief recovery period from a viral infection: • Vomiting • Lethargy and rapidly changing mental status • Increase in blood pressure, pulse, and respirations • Motor disturbances (Stage I—none; Stage II—hyperactive reflexes; Stage III—decorticate rigidity; Stage IV—decerebrate rigidity and large, fixed pupils; Stage V—loss of deep-tendon reflexes, flaccidity) • Seizures (Stage V) • Altered level of consciousness (Stage I—lethargy; Stage II—coma; Stage III—deepening coma; Stages IV and V—deep coma)
Rheumatoid arthritis	• Joint stiffness, warmth, swelling, and, with active disease progression, deformities • Vague arthralgias and myalgias • Limited range of motion • Fatigue • Malaise • Anorexia • Persistent low-grade fever • Lymphadenopathy (generalized or proximal to the involved joints) • Possible rheumatoid nodules • Muscle atrophy
Shock, anaphylactic	• Respiratory distress (dyspnea, wheezing, choking, airway obstruction, cyanosis) • Vascular collapse (rapidly falling blood pressure, tachycardia, weak pulse, diaphoresis) • Dermatologic changes (urticaria, erythema, angioedema, pruritus) • Gastrointestinal complaints (nausea, vomiting, abdominal cramps, diarrhea)
Shock, cardiogenic	Although many of the following signs and symptoms occur in other shock syndromes, they are usually more profound in cardiogenic shock: • Cold, pale clammy skin • Hypotension, with narrowing pulse pressure

Diseases and Disorders Profile *(continued)*

Disease or Disorder	Signs and Symptoms
Shock, cardiogenic *(continued)*	• Tachycarida • Rapid, shallow respirations • Restlessness • Decreased level of consciousness • Cyanosis • Oliguria
Shock, hypovolemic	• Cold, pale, clammy skin • Hypotension, with narrowing pulse pressure • Tachycardia • Rapid, shallow respirations • Decreased level of consciousness • Oliguria
Shock, neurogenic	• Warm, dry, possibly flushed skin • Apprehension or restlessness, possibly progressing to drowsiness, stupor, or coma • Bradycardia • Full, regular pulses • Tachypnea • Hypotension • Fluctuating body temperature • Oliguria • Nausea and vomiting
Shock, septic	Signs and symptoms of septic shock vary according to the stage of shock, the causative organism, and the patient's age. They may include: Early stage— • Oliguria • Sudden fever (over 101° F. [38.3° C.]) • Chills • Nausea, vomiting, diarrhea • Prostration Late stage— • Restlessness, apprehension, irritability, altered level of consciousness • Tachycardia • Hypotension • Tachypnea, hyperventilation • Hypothermia • Thirst
Sickle cell crisis	• Fatigue • Dyspnea • Joint swelling and pain • Pallor • Tachycardia, systolic murmurs • Headache • Pain in legs, abdomen, and chest • Fever

(continued)

Diseases and Disorders Profile *(continued)*

Disease or Disorder	Signs and Symptoms
Sinusitis, acute bacterial	• Nasal congestion • Difficulty breathing through the nose • Possible purulent nasal discharge • Low-grade fever • Sore throat • Malaise • Nausea and anorexia • Pain and swelling over the affected sinus • Periorbital edema
Subacute bacterial endocarditis (SBE)	• Persistent fever • Weakness, fatigue • Anorexia, weight loss • Arthralgia • Night sweats • Dyspnea (in approximately 50% of cases) • Sudden change in preexisting heart murmur or development of new murmur • Petechiae of the skin and buccal, pharyngeal, and/or conjunctival mucosa • Splinter hemorrhages beneath the nails • Finger and toe clubbing (with longstanding disease) • Osler's nodes and Janeway lesions (rare)
Subarachnoid hemorrhage	• Sudden, severe headache • Nausea and vomiting • Focal or generalized seizures • Motor disturbances (depending on area of brain affected and degree of bleeding or ischemia, these may include hemiparesis, aphasia, ataxia, vertigo, syncope, and facial weakness) • Sensory deviations (visual impairment, with pressure on optic nerve or chiasm; double vision, with third, fourth, and fifth cranial nerve compression) • Altered level of consciousness (irritability, stupor progressing to coma) • Fever • Irregular respirations • Dilated and fixed pupils • Papilledema, retinal hemorrhage • Bilateral Babinski's reflex, positive Brudzinski's and Kernig's signs • Nuchal rigidity • Signs of increased intracranial pressure

Diseases and Disorders Profile (continued)

Disease or Disorder	Signs and Symptoms
Systemic lupus erythematosus (SLE)	• Arthralgia (most common in fingers, hands, wrists, ankles, and knees) • Facial erythema (butterfly rash) • Photosensitivity • Weakness, fatigue • Fever • Anorexia, weight loss • Alopecia
Toxic shock syndrome (TSS)	• Sudden high fever • Nausea, vomiting • Hypotension • Photophobia • Abdominal pain • Myalgia, arthralgia • Headache
Transient ischemic attack (TIA)	Signs and symptoms of TIA depend on the location of the affected artery, and may include: • Double vision, unilateral blindness • Speech deficits (slurring or thickness) • Ataxia • Unilateral weakness and numbness • Falling (due to weakness in the legs and dizziness) • Decreased level of consciousness
Ulcerative colitis	• Cramping abdominal pain • Anorexia, nausea, and vomiting • Profuse, episodic, bloody diarrhea, possibly containing mucus • Weight loss • Low-grade fever
Urethritis	• Urinary frequency and urgency, hematuria, dysuria • Fever • Edema and erythema of urinary meatus and vulva • Urethral and/or vaginal discharge

REFERENCES AND ACKNOWLEDGMENTS

REFERENCES

Adams, Raymond, and Victor, Maurice. *Principles of Neurology,* 3rd ed. New York: McGraw-Hill Book Co., 1985.

American Hospital Formulary Service: Drug Information '87. Bethesda, Md.: American Society of Hospital Pharmacists.

Assessment. Nurse's Reference Library. Springhouse, Pa.: Springhouse Corp., 1982.

Avery, Mary E., and Taeusch, H. William, Jr. *Shaffer's Diseases of the Newborn,* 5th ed. Philadelphia: W.B. Saunders Co., 1984.

Bates, Barbara. *A Guide to Physical Examination,* 4th ed. Philadelphia: J.B. Lippincott Co., 1987.

Baum, Gerald L., ed. *Textbook of Pulmonary Diseases,* 3rd ed. Boston: Little, Brown & Co., 1983.

Behrman, Richard E., and Vaughan, Victor C., III. *Nelson Textbook of Pediatrics,* 12th ed. Philadelphia: W.B. Saunders Co., 1983.

Blacklow, Robert S., ed. *MacBryde's Signs and Symptoms: Applied Pathologic Physiology and Clinical Interpretation,* 6th ed. Philadelphia: J.B. Lippincott Co., 1983.

Braunwald, Eugene, ed. *Heart Disease: A Textbook of Cardiovascular Medicine,* 2 vols. Philadelphia: W.B. Saunders Co., 1984.

Bricker, Neal S., and Kirschenbaum, Michael A. *The Kidney: Diagnosis and Management.* New York: John Wiley & Sons, 1984.

Brunner, Lillian, and Suddarth, Doris. *Textbook of Medical-Surgical Nursing,* 5th ed. Philadelphia: J.B. Lippincott Co., 1984.

Bullock, Barbara, et al., eds. *Pathophysiology: Adaptations and Alterations in Function.* Boston: Little, Brown & Co., 1984.

Cardiovascular Disorders. Nurse's Clinical Library. Springhouse, Pa.: Springhouse Corp., 1984.

Danforth, David N., ed. *Obstetrics and Gynecology,* 4th ed. Philadelphia: J.B. Lippincott Co., 1982.

Diseases, 2nd ed. Nurse's Reference Library. Springhouse, Pa.: Springhouse Corp., 1986.

Duane, Thomas D., and Jaeger, Edward A., eds. *Clinical Ophthalmology.* Philadelphia: Harper & Row Publishers, 1983.

Endocrine Disorders. Nurse's Clinical Library. Springhouse, Pa.: Springhouse Corp., 1984.

Glauser, Frederick L., ed. *Signs and Symptoms in Pulmonary Medicine.* Philadelphia: J.B. Lippincott Co., 1983.

Greenspan, Francis S., and Forsham, Peter H., eds. *Basic and Clinical Endocrinology.* Los Altos, Calif.: Lange Medical Pubns., 1983.

Horwitz, L., and Groves, B. *Signs and Symptoms in Cardiology.* Philadelphia: J.B. Lippincott Co., 1985.

Hurst, J.W., et al. *The Heart,* 6th ed. New York: McGraw-Hill Book Co., 1985.

Jacobs, Margaret, and Geels, Wilma. *Signs and Symptoms in Nursing Interpretation and Management.* Philadelphia: J.B. Lippincott Co., 1985.

Kempe, C. Henry, et al., eds. *Current Pediatric Diagnosis and Treatment,* 8th ed. Los Altos, Calif.: Lange Medical Pubns., 1984.

Krause, Marie V., and Mahan, Kathleen. *Food, Nutrition and Diet Therapy: A Textbook of Nutritional Care,* 7th ed. Philadelphia: W.B. Saunders Co., 1984.

Krupp, Marcus A., et al., eds. *Current Medical Diagnosis and Treatment.* Los Altos, Calif.: Lange Medical Pubns., 1985.

Loustau, A., and Lee, K. "Dealing With the Dangers of Dysphagia," *Nursing85* 15(2):47-50, February 1985.

Lucente, Frank E., and Sobol, Stephen M. *Essentials of Otolaryngology.* New York: Raven Press Pubs., 1983.

Malasanos, Lois, et al. *Health Assessment,* 3rd ed. St. Louis: C.V. Mosby Co., 1985.

Metz, Robert, and Larson, Eric B. *Blue Book of Endocrinology.* Philadelphia: W.B. Saunders Co., 1984.

Moschella, Samuel L., and Hurley, Harry J. *Dermatology,* 2nd ed. Philadelphia: W.B. Saunders Co., 1985.

Nursing88 Drug Handbook. Springhouse, Pa.: Springhouse Corp., 1988.

Peckham, Ben M., and Shapiro, Sander S. *Signs and Symptoms in Gynecology.* Philadelphia: J.B. Lippincott Co., 1983.

Petersdorf, Robert G., and Adams, Raymond D., eds. *Harrison's Principles of Internal Medicine,* 10th ed. New York: McGraw-Hill Book Co., 1983.

Phipps, Wilma J., et al. *Medical-Surgical Nursing: Concepts and Clinical Practice,* 3rd ed. St. Louis: C.V. Mosby Co., 1986.

Respiratory Disorders. Nurse's Clinical Library. Springhouse, Pa.: Springhouse Corp., 1984.

Rudy, Ellen B. *Advanced Neurological and Neurosurgical Nursing.* St. Louis: C.V. Mosby Co., 1984.

Shafer, William G., et al. *Textbook of Oral Pathology,* 4th ed. Philadelphia: W.B. Saunders Co., 1983.

Sleisenger, Marvin H., and Fordtran, John S. *Gastrointestinal Disease: Pathophysiology, Diagnosis, Management,* 3rd ed. Philadelphia: W.B. Saunders Co., 1983.

Smith, Donald R. *General Urology,* 11th ed. Los Altos, Calif.: Lange Medical Pubns., 1984.

Spiro, Howard M. *Clinical Gastroenterology,* 3rd ed. New York: Macmillan Publishing Co., 1983.

Suitor, Carol J., and Crowley, Merrily F. *Nutrition: Principles and Application in Health Promotion,* 2nd ed. Philadelphia: J.B. Lippincott Co., 1984.

Swanson, Phillip D. *Signs and Symptoms in Neurology.* Philadelphia: J.B. Lippincott Co., 1984.

Thomas, D.O. "Are You Sure It's Only Croup?" *RN* 47(12):40-43, December 1984.

Vaughan, Daniel, and Asbury, Taylor. *General Ophthalmology,* 10th ed. Los Altos, Calif.: Lange Medical Pubns., 1983.

Whaley, Lucille F., and Wong, Donna L. *Nursing Care of Infants and Children,* 3rd ed. St. Louis: C.V. Mosby Co., 1986.

Wyngaarden, James B., and Smith, Lloyd H. *Cecil Textbook of Medicine,* 16th ed. Philadelphia: W.B. Saunders Co., 1982.

ACKNOWLEDGMENTS

pp. 236-37: Scale adapted from M.H. Klaus and A.A. Fanaroff, *Care of the High Risk Neonate,* 2nd ed. (St. Louis: C.V. Mosby Co., 1979, p. 79). Used with permission of the publisher.

INDEX

C

D

E

F

G

H

I

J

K

O

P